For the ninth edition of *Dossey & Keegan's Holistic Nursing: A Handbook for Practice*, the cover design (photo credit given to Devante Heyward/Getty Images) pays tribute to the enduring legacy of this transformative text, first published in 1988 and cherished across generations of nurses. The image is inspired by the natural meeting place of great elemental forces, perhaps "where the Pacific Ocean laps at the mountain's base," or other sacred landscapes of such immense power and awe. The artwork evokes the serenity and resilience of holistic nursing practice, guided by nature's supreme flow and limitless depth.

You are invited to contemplate how the image's grand motion and vibrant, yet sublime, colors of the natural world might reawaken ancient knowing and inspire contemporary understandings of health, healing, and well-being. These sensations stir the "passions of ancient and contemporary concepts of presence, healing, harmony, and human consciousness embedded in holistic nursing."

We hope that this text ignites all the senses, invites inner reflection, and deepens awareness of the sacred connections between self, others, the living world, and all that is. Infused with the expansive visions of Barbara Dossey and Lynn Keegan, this edition stands as both a scholarly guide and a sensorial experience of holistic wisdom.

Ninth Edition

American Holistic Nurses Association SEAL OF DISTINCTION

Dossey & Keegan's

Holistic Nursing

A Handbook for Practice

Deborah A. Shields, PhD, RN, CCRN, QTTT, AHN-BC, SGAHN
Professor Emerita, Capital University School of Nursing, Columbus, Ohio
Staff Nurse, Perioperative Care and System Education (retired)
OhioHealth, Columbus, Ohio
President, Ohio Heart of Healing, Bremen, Ohio

Karen M. Avino, EdD, MSN, RN, AHN-BC, HWNC-BC, SGAHN
Chief Executive Officer, Integrative Nurse Coach Academy, Miami, Florida
President, International Nurse Coaching Association, Miami, Florida

Tracy L. Hoag, DHSc, MSN, RN, AHN-BC
Assistant Professor of Nursing, Capital University, Columbus, Ohio

Caroline E. Ortiz, PhD, MPH, RN, NC-BC
Associate Professor, Pacific College of Health and Science
New York, New York
Director at Large, American Holistic Nurses Credentialing Corporation, Cedar Park, Texas

JONES & BARTLETT
LEARNING

World Headquarters
Jones & Bartlett Learning
25 Mall Road
Burlington, MA 01803
978-443-5000
info@jblearning.com
www.jblearning.com

Jones & Bartlett Learning books and products are available through most bookstores and online booksellers. To contact Jones & Bartlett Learning directly, call 800-832-0034, fax 978-443-8000, or visit our website, www.jblearning.com.

Substantial discounts on bulk quantities of Jones & Bartlett Learning publications are available to corporations, professional associations, and other qualified organizations. For details and specific discount information, contact the special sales department at Jones & Bartlett Learning via the above contact information or send an email to specialsales@jblearning.com.

31036-8

Production Credits
Vice President, Innovative Learning and Assessment Solutions: Ada Woo
Senior Director, Content Production and Delivery: Christine Emerton
Director, Product: Melissa Kleeman-Moy
Manager, Content Development: Carol Brewer Guerrero
Senior Outsourcing Specialist: Elisabeth Williams
Content Coordinator: Rachelle Soden
Content Management: MPS Limited
Manager, Intellectual Properties and Content Production: Kristen Rogers
Content Production Manager: John Fuller
Senior Intellectual Property Specialist (eBook): Angela Dooley
Senior Product Marketing Manager: Lindsay White
Director, Product Fulfillment: Aaron McKinzie
Purchasing Manager: Wendy Kilborn
Composition: S4Carlisle Publishing Services
Project Management: S4Carlisle Publishing Services
Cover Design: MPS Limited
Text Design: S4Carlisle Publishing Services
Media Developer: Faith Brosnan
Intellectual Property Specialist: Robin Silverman
Cover Image (Title Page, Part Opener, Chapter Opener):
© Devante Heyward/ iStock/Getty Images Plus/Getty Images
Printing and Binding: Sheridan Michigan

Library of Congress Cataloging-in-Publication Data
Library of Congress Cataloging-in-Publication Data unavailable at time of printing.
LCCN: 2025041444

6048

Printed in the United States of America
31 30 29 28 27 26 10 9 8 7 6 5 4 3 2 1

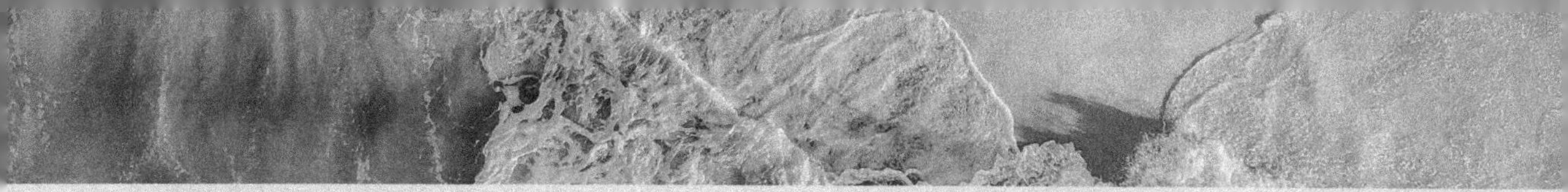

The Pedagogy

Dossey & Keegan's Holistic Nursing: A Handbook for Practice, Ninth Edition enhances understanding through various strategies that address students' learning needs while also fostering excitement about the topic. This interactive approach addresses different learning styles, making it the perfect book to ensure mastery of essential concepts for both undergraduate and graduate students, as well as professional nurses. The types of pedagogical aids found in most chapters are outlined below.

Nurse Healer Objectives

These objectives give faculty and students a quick overview of the key information in each chapter and act as a checklist to help guide and focus their study.

Definitions

Keywords and terms are outlined and defined at the start of each chapter.

Nursing Situations

These narratives illuminate the chapter content, offering real-life situations to explore and reflect on—to experience the art and science of holistic nursing.

Integration/Implications

Consider how the chapter content informs:

- *Clinical Practice*
- *Education*
- *Research*
- *Policy*
- *Global Health*

Experiential Activities

Pause and reflect on what you are learning about yourself and the art and science of holistic nursing.

References

Continue your exploration by reading from the comprehensive list of text and electronic references and resources.

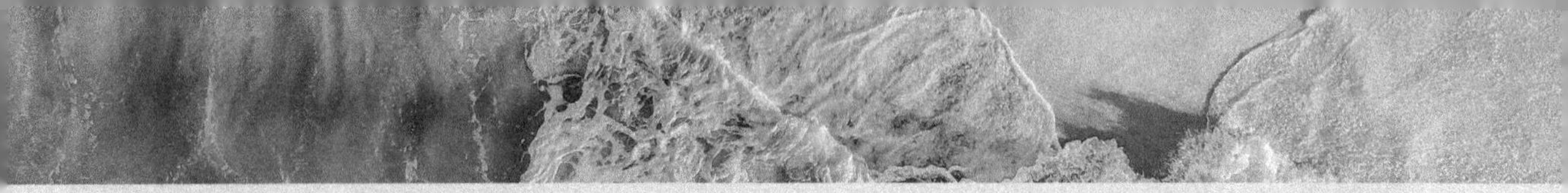

Editors

Deborah A. Shields, PhD, RN, CCRN, QTTT, AHN-BC, SGAHN
Professor Emerita
Capital University School of Nursing, Columbus, Ohio
Staff Nurse, Perioperative Care and System Education (retired)
OhioHealth, Columbus, Ohio
President, Ohio Heart of Healing, Bremen, Ohio

Karen M. Avino, EdD, MSN, RN, AHN-BC, HWNC-BC, SGAHN
Chief Executive Officer
Integrative Nurse Coach Academy
Miami, Florida
President
International Nurse Coaching Association
Miami, Florida

Tracy L. Hoag, DHSc, MSN, RN, AHN-BC
Assistant Professor of Nursing
Capital University
Columbus, Ohio

Caroline E. Ortiz, PhD, MPH, RN, NC-BC
Associate Professor
Pacific College of Health and Science
New York, New York
Director at Large
American Holistic Nurses Credentialing Corporation
Cedar Park, Texas

With Special Gratitude to the Original Authors

Barbara Montgomery Dossey, PhD, RN, AHN-BC, FAAN, HSGAHN
International Co-Director
Nightingale Initiative for Global Health
Santa Fe, New Mexico; Washington, District of Columbia; Ottawa, Canada; Geneva, Switzerland

Lynn Keegan, PhD, RN, AHN-BC, FAAN, HSGAHN
Holistic Nursing Consultants
Carmel, Indiana
Past President, American Holistic Nurses Association, Topeka, Kansas

The Flame of Florence Nightingale's Legacy

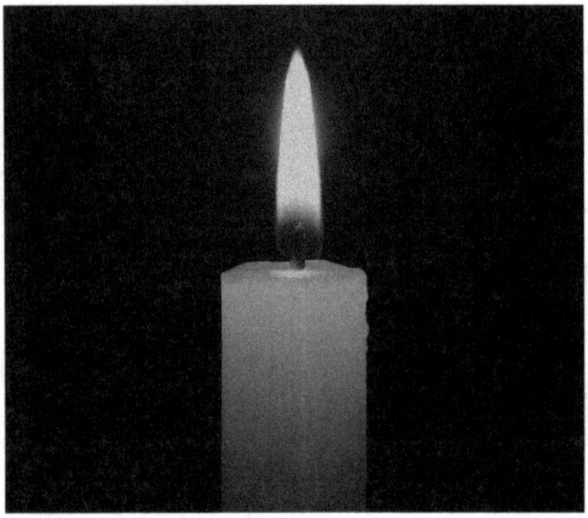

© irin-k/ShutterStock

Today, our world needs healing and to be rekindled with Love.
Once, Florence Nightingale lit her beacon of lamplight to comfort the wounded
And her Light has blazed a path of service across a Century to us,
Through her example and through the countless Nurses and Healers who have followed in her footsteps.

Today, we celebrate the flame of Florence Nightingale's Legacy.
Let that same Light be rekindled to burn brightly in our hearts.
Let us take up our own Lanterns of Caring, each in our own ways.
To more brightly walk our own paths of service to the World.
To more clearly share our own Noble Purpose with each other.

May Human Caring become the Lantern for the 21st Century.
May we better learn to care for ourselves, for each other and for all Creation.
Through our Caring, may we be the Keepers of that Flame.
That Our Spirits may burn brightly
To kindle the hearts of our children and great-grandchildren
As they too follow in these footsteps.

Deva-Marie Beck, PhD, RN, DTM
International Co-Director, Nightingale Initiative for Global Health
Washington, District of Columbia, and Santa Fe, New Mexico

To Our Colleagues In Nursing

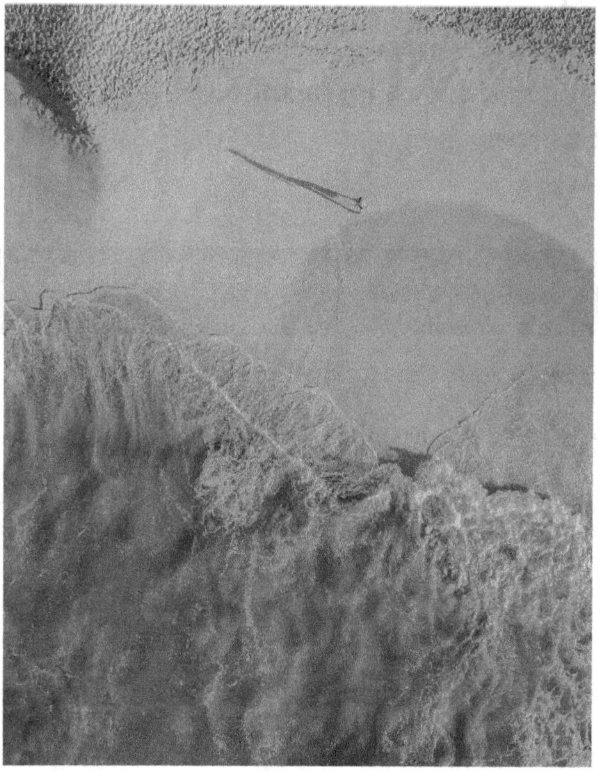

When a nurse
Encounters another
Something happens
What occurs
Is never a neutral event
A pulse taken
Words exchanged
A touch
A healing moment
Two persons
Are never
The same

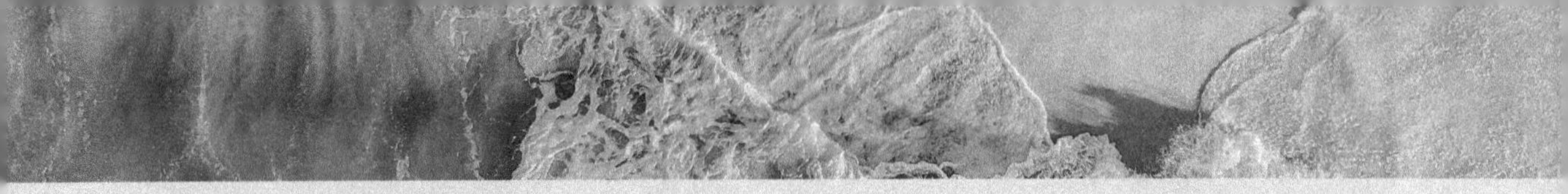

Brief Contents

Contents

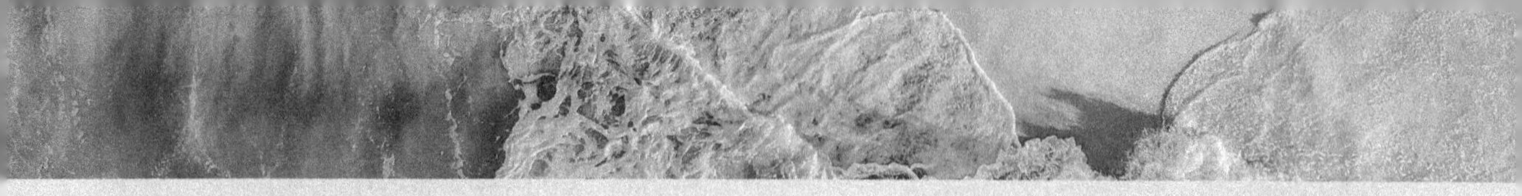

Foreword

Holistic nurses have the potential to be a powerful force, bringing our trusted caring and compassion for suffering into advocacy for a better world (Beck & Dossey, 2024). In an ever-changing world, disease, illness, and suffering continue to be prevalent. As such, holistic nurses must continue to engage in seeking, applying, and expanding the best knowledge, skills, art, and science of care to their patients, their culture, and themselves. By fostering excellence in holistic care within their chosen health field domain, nurses can contribute to a more compassionate and effective healthcare system.

Holistic nurses are poised to step forward as visionary leaders, empowered by Florence Nightingale (1820–1910), the philosophical founder of modern secular nursing and the first nursing theorist, who stands among the most accomplished reformers and activists in healthcare and social equity history (Dossey, 2010).

In the inaugural edition of *Holistic Nursing: A Handbook for Practice* (1988), questions were explored related to universal ethical commitment to holism, caring, and healing, as well as the exploration of body-mind-spirit-cultural-environmental dimensions. The first edition featured four core authors, followed by subsequent editions with just two authors and two/three editors. Over the decades, the text evolved into a well-known work edited by four master-mentored nursing editors and a collection of skilled and knowledgeable contributors.

In this *Ninth Edition*, we persist in advocating for a "both/and" approach rather than an "either/or" approach when integrating contemporary medical and surgical therapies with healing rituals and complementary modalities. From the very beginning, we have delved into three fundamental questions:

1. What do we understand about the essence of healing?
2. What practical steps can we take daily to facilitate healing?
3. How can we serve as catalysts in the healing process?

Holistic Nursing: A Handbook for Practice, Ninth Edition now incorporates new topics that effectively address healthcare advancements in practice, education, research, and health policy decisions at local to global levels. In light of the current moment, we now include these three critical questions:

1. Do our holistic nursing core values align with the integration of emerging arts and sciences of holism that address individual, population, environmental, and planetary health gaps and disparities?
2. How can we enhance our healing, caring, compassion, and overall well-being with innovative approaches?
3. What are our responsibilities and commitments as global citizens?

Holistic nurses face the challenge of actively participating in the 17 UN Sustainable Development Goals (SDGs) of the 2030 Agenda. These goals are divided into five themes: People, Planet, Peace, Prosperity, and Partnership (Dossey et al., 2019; United Nations, n.d.). Each theme provides practical ideas related to practice, education, research, and health policies that aim for the harmonious coexistence of humans and the planet. By reflecting on the ongoing dynamic between the AHNA Core Values and these themes, holistic nurses can effectively integrate them into their practice. This integration underscores the urgent need for a shift in consciousness and advocacy for the SDGs, which prioritize the survival of both humans and the planet (Rosa et al., 2019).

In the 21st century, holistic nursing advocacy demands nurses who comprehend relationship-centered care and human flourishing. These nurses possess integral and integrative nursing and nurse coaching skills that guide behavioral change strategies, promote health, maintain it, and prevent diseases (Dossey et al., 2015).

One of the key themes we introduced in the first edition of this text, published 38 years ago, was self-care. Since then, nurses have come to recognize the significance of self-assessment and self-care, understanding that these principles are the foundation of caring for others. Self-care conferences are now led by holistic nurses and are widely attended across the country. This text presents diverse perspectives and strategies that empower individuals to make efficient, effective, and cost-effective choices for self-care. These choices are pivotal in transforming health care from a disease-centric model to one that prioritizes health and wellness.

Nursing's primary focus is on human health, encompassing individuals, communities, and the world. Nurses are educated and prepared, physically, emotionally, mentally, and spiritually, to effectively accomplish the tasks required on the ground with their care teams, promoting people's health.

If today's nurses, midwives, and allied health professionals are nurtured and supported in innovative ways, they can become like Florence Nightingale—effective advocates for and exemplars of healing, leadership, and global action leading to a healthier world (Nightingale Initiative for Global Health, n.d.). This empowerment can bolster nursing's ranks and help the world recognize and appreciate its vital contributions.

Holistic Nursing: A Handbook for Practice, Ninth Edition challenges nurses to embark on a transformative journey of self-discovery and identify their growing capacity for change and healing. It encourages us to recognize ourselves as global citizens committed to saving the planet through engaged actions. This exploration fosters a compassionate power to heal ourselves and others. This inner healing allows us to return to the roots of nursing, where healer and healing have always been understood. By carrying Florence Nightingale's vision for healing, leadership, and global action forward into the 21st century and beyond, we can embody her famous quote, "My work is my must." Nightingale's shining example invites us to discover and embrace our own "must" and explore our own meaning, purpose, and spirituality (Dossey, 2010).

Barbara Montgomery Dossey
Lynn Keegan

References

Beck, D. M., & Dossey, B. M. (2024). Remembering Nightingale in her turbulent times: Introducing the Theory of Integral Nursing in our turbulent times. *International Nursing Review*. 72(3), e13064. https://doi.org/10.1111/inr.13064

Dossey, B. M. (2010). *Florence Nightingale: Mystic, Visionary, Healer*. Commemorative Edition. F. A. Davis.

Dossey, B. M., Luck, S., & Schaub, B. G. (2015). *Nursing Coaching: Integrative Approaches for Health and Healing*. International Nurse Coach Association.

Dossey, B. M., Rosa, W. E., & Beck, D. M. (2019). Nursing and the Sustainable Development Goals: From Nightingale to now. *American Journal of Nursing*, 119(5), 44–49.

Nightingale Initiative for Global Health. (n.d.). http://www.nightingaledeclaration.net

Rosa, W. E., Dossey, B. M., Watson, J., Beck, D. M., & Upvall, M. J. (2019). The United Nations Sustainable Development Goals: The ethic and ethos of holistic nursing. *Journal of Holistic Nursing*, 37(4), 381–393.

United Nations (UN). *Transforming our World: The 2030 Agenda for Sustainable Development*. https://sustainabledevelopment.un.org/content/documents/21252030%20Agenda%20for%20Sustainable%20Development%20web.pdf

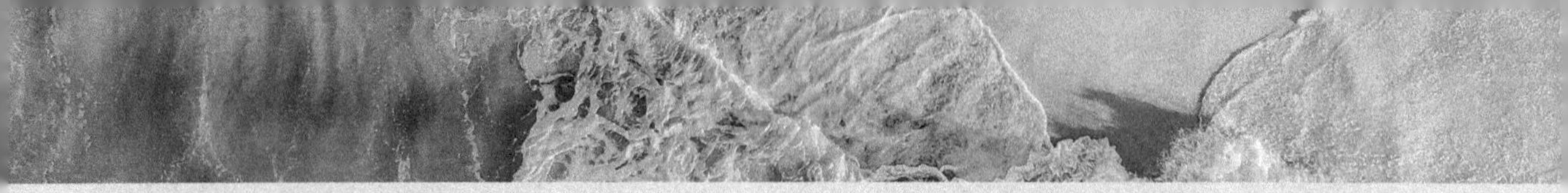

Preface

At a time when our world feels increasingly divided by politics and policies, disaster and war, skin color, classifications, attitudes, and competing interests, this text celebrates what brings us together. As holistic nurses, we value life's intricate and delicate interconnections. We know that nursing is not art OR science; it is the essence of those gorgeous things combined. We know the ultimate goal is not health or wellness; it is the promotion of becoming and being.

Holistic nurses honor the profound connection we share with the individuals, communities, and populations we serve, while affirming that nurses must first offer loving care to themselves.

Don't let the idealism of this holistic philosophy feel out of reach.

You are here because you recognize your value as a healer, and you understand that caring for yourself is a foundational first step. You are also here because you want to learn, grow, and contribute to a vision of nursing that is innovative, imaginative, and rooted in holism.

To do this sacred work, we need support, and we need each other. The ninth edition of *Dossey and Keegan's Holistic Nursing: A Handbook for Practice* is both a resource and a place of connection.

For those who have owned every edition of this handbook since 1988, this version will feel fresh yet familiar. The updated content is organized around the five core values that guide holistic nursing:

- holistic philosophies, theories, and ethics
- self-reflection, self-development, and self-care
- the holistic caring process
- holistic communication, therapeutic relationships, healing environments, and cultural care
- holistic education and research.

The text culminates with a section on advanced concepts and meaningful reflections. The original authors and the editors of this edition have collaborated with nursing experts to bring you knowledge, skills, and attitudes that are responsive to today's healthcare realities, yet firmly rooted in the timeless ideals of holism. These chapters reflect evolving approaches in holistic nursing and offer the insight of seasoned voices in the field.

And for those of you who are new to this *Handbook*, we welcome you. Our hope is to share that holistic nursing is not just about *doing*, it is about *being*. The light you bring to nursing is both needed and deeply appreciated.

In a wounded world, holistic nurses remain resolute as instruments of healing. Shine on.

Deborah A. Shields
Karen M. Avino
Tracy L. Hoag
Caroline E. Ortiz

Acknowledgments

Nothing would be published were it not for a team dedicated to the work and willing to collaborate; communicate; be patient, honest, and respectful; and put ego aside for the sake of the work. This is the team that, together, created *Dossey and Keegan's Holistic Nursing: A Handbook for Practice, Ninth Edition.*

To the members of our publishing team at Jones & Bartlett Learning, a huge thank you for sharing your knowledge of the publishing world and keeping this on track.

To our contributing chapter authors, who selflessly share their wisdom, we are deeply grateful. Your heartfelt contributions to the *Ninth Edition* are the threads of art and science in this tapestry of hope. Some of you have been part of earlier editions, and others are new to the *Handbook*. Each one of you is a treasured part of the team.

And to our beloved mentors, Dr. Barbara Dossey and Dr. Lynn Keegan, we give our heartfelt thanks and feel blessed in your presence. You have stood by us, believed in us, trusted, guided, nudged and, importantly, loved us. No matter the need or question, you responded; not always giving us the answer, but rather illuminating the way. You have taught us the true meaning of mentorship by living it, and we have each grown as holistic nurses.

Deborah A. Shields
Karen M. Avino
Tracy L. Hoag
Caroline E. Ortiz

Learning and Teaching Resources

Student Resources

Each new purchase of the print textbook includes:

- A Navigate eBook with eBook Quizzes

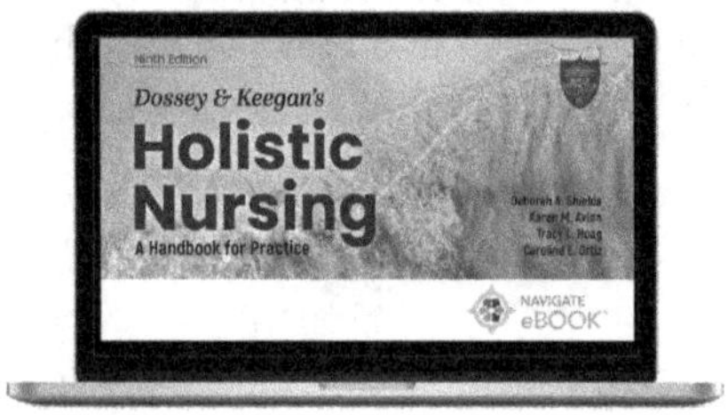

Instructor Resources

Qualified instructors can receive the full suite of Instructor Resources, including the following:

- Slides in PowerPoint format
- Test Bank in LMS-compatible formats (Chapter Quizzes, Midterm, Final Exam)
- Instructor Manual
- Syllabus

We Value Your Feedback

Do you love this text? Spot an error you'd like to report? Follow this QR code to give us your observations and suggestions for improvement.

Contributors

Hyochol Ahn, PhD, APRN, ANP-BC, FAAN
Dean and Professor
The University of Arizona College of Nursing
Tucson, Arizona

Marjorie S. Anderson, MS, RN, PMHCNS-BC (retired), QTTT, SGAHN
Global Academy of Holistic Nursing
Topeka, Kansas
American Holistic Nurses Association
Topeka, Kansas
Therapeutic Touch International Association
Delmar, New York
Ohio Heart of Healing
Bremen, Ohio

Veda L. Andrus, EdD, MSN, RN, HN-BC, HSGAHN
Vice President, Education and Program Development
The Birch Tree Center for Healthcare Transformation
Tucson, Arizona

Karen M. Avino, EdD, MSN, RN, AHN-BC, HWNC-BC, SGAHN
Chief Executive Officer
Integrative Nurse Coach Academy
Miami, Florida
President
International Nurse Coaching Association
Miami, Florida

Charlotte D. Barry, PhD, RN, FAAN
Professor Emerita
Florida Atlantic University
Christine E. Lynn College of Nursing
Boca Raton, Florida

Deva-Marie Beck, PhD, RN, DTM, HSGAHN
International Co-Director
Nightingale Initiative for Global Health
Washington, D.C, & Santa Fe, New Mexico

Janet Booth, MA, RN, NC-BC
End-of-Life Nurse Coach & Educator
Self-employed
Boulder, Colorado

Margaret McGrath Brown, MSN, RN, AHN-BC, HWNC-BC
Director of Compassion and Caring for Colleagues
Lehigh Valley Health Network-Jefferson Health
Allentown, Pennsylvania

Jennifer S. Browning, DNP, MS, APRN-CNP, ACHPN
Advanced Practice Lead for APP Quality and Professional Development
Palliative Medicine Nurse Practitioner
The James at The Ohio State University Wexner Medical Center
Columbus, Ohio

Margaret A. Burkhardt, PhD, RN, AHN, SGAHN
Associate Professor Emerita
Robert C. Byrd Health Sciences Center, West Virginia University School of Nursing
Morgantown, West Virginia
Past President, American Holistic Nurses Association
Topeka, Kansas

Carey S. Cadieux, PhD, RN, AHN-BC, RYT, FAAN
Associate Professor of Nursing
Decker College of Nursing, Binghamton University
Binghamton, New York

Barbara Montgomery Dossey, PhD, RN, AHN-BC, FAAN, HSGAHN
International Co-Director
Nightingale Initiative for Global Health
Santa Fe, New Mexico; Washington, District of Columbia; Ottawa, Canada; Geneva, Switzerland

Joan C. Engebretson, DrPH, AHN-BC, RN, FAAN
Professor Emerita
Cizik School of Nursing
The University of Texas Health Science Center at Houston
Houston, Texas

Helen L. Erickson, PhD, RN, AHN-BC, FAAN, SGAHN
Global Academy of Holistic Nursing
Co-Founder & Executive Director
Society for the Advancement of Modeling – Role Modeling (SAM-RM)
Theory Expert & Elder
University of Texas - Professor Emeritus
University of Texas - Endowed Lectureship in Holistic Nursing
Austin, Texas

Margaret E. Erickson, PhD, RN, MSN, CNS, APRN, APHN-BC, SGAHN
CEO
American Holistic Nurses Credentialing Corporation
Topeka, Kansas

Wyona M. Freysteinson, PhD, MN, RN, FAAN, SGAHN
Professor
Nelda C. Stark School of Nursing
Texas Woman's University
Houston, Texas

Heather Janiszewski Goodin, PhD, RN, AHN-BC, CPN
Dean and Professor
Capital University School of Nursing
Columbus, Ohio

Shirley C. Gordon, PhD, RN, ANH-BC, HWNC-BC, NCSN-E, SGAHN
Professor (retired)
Tequesta, Florida

Diane L. Gullett, PhD, RN, MPH
Faculty, Nursing Program
FVI School of Nursing & Technology
Miramar, Florida

Lorrine Hall, MSN, RN, AMB-BC, AHN-BC
Registered Nurse
Department of Veterans Affairs
Atlanta, Virginia
Trauma Recovery Program
Atlanta, Georgia

Mary Anne Hanley, RN, PhD, QTTT, SGAHN
Treasurer, Global Academy of Holistic Nursing
Secretary, Therapeutic Touch Dialogues, Inc.
Topeka, Kansas

Mary A. Blaszko Helming, PhD, APRN, FNP-BC, AHN-BC
Professor Emerita
Quinnipiac University School of Nursing
Associate Professor
Hamden, Connecticut
Goodwin University School of Nursing
Family Nurse Practitioner
East Hartford, Connecticut

Mary Enzman Hines, PhD, APRN, CNS, CPNP-PC, APHN-BC, SGAHN
Professor Emeritus
University of Colorado
Colorado Springs, Colorado
Co-Owner and Certified Pediatric Nurse Practitioner and Advanced Practice Holistic Nurse
Integrative Pediatric Health Care, LLC
Denver, Colorado

Denise J. Joswiak, BSN, RN, HNB-BC, RA™, CCA
Educator, Consultant
Essential Health
Mendota Heights, Minnesota

Lynn Keegan, PhD, RN, AHN-BC, FAAN, HSGAHN
Holistic Nursing Consultants
Carmel, Indiana
Past President, American Holistic Nurses Association

Chiyoung Lee, PhD, RN
Assistant Professor
The University of Arizona College of Nursing
Tucson, Arizona

Marian Bianco Long, RN, MSN, AHN-BC, retired
Educational Retreat Contractor; American Holistic Nurses Association
Long Holistic Services, LLC
Grayling, Michigan

Carla Mariano, EdD, RN, AHN-BC, FAAIM, SGAHN
Professor
Pacific College of Health and Science
New York, New York
Adjunct Associate Professor, New York University
New York, New York
Past President, American Holistic Nurses Association

Deborah McElligott, DNP, ANP-BC, AHN-BC, HWNC-BC
Nurse Practitioner
Center for Wellness and Integrative Medicine
Katz Institute for Women's Health, Northwell Health
Lake Success, New York
Clinical Assistant Professor
Donald and Barbara Zucker School of Medicine Hofstra/Northwell
Uniondale, New York

Mitzie Rains Meyers, PhD, RN, CNE, AHN-BC
Adjunct Nursing Faculty
University of Northern Colorado
Greeley, Colorado

Mary Gail Nagai-Jacobson, RN, BSN, MSN
Community Health Resource Nurse
San Marcos and Wimberley, Texas

Caroline E. Ortiz, PhD, MPH, RN, NC-BC
Associate Professor
Pacific College of Health and Science
New York, New York
Director at Large
American Holistic Nurses Credentialing Corporation
Topeka, Kansas

Janet F. Quinn, PhD
Director, HaelanWorks
Lafayette, Colorado

Jennifer Rasmussen, RN, MPH
Education Fellow
Planetary Health Alliance
Johns Hopkins Bloomberg School of Public Health
Washington, District of Columbia

Jennifer L. Reich, PhD, MA, RN, NC-BC, GHAN
Nurse Coach, Author, Poet
Faculty: American Holistic Nurses' Association (AHNA) Integrative Healing Arts Program
Phoenix, Arizona

Marci Resnicoff, MSN, RN, AHN-BC, HWNC-BC
Holistic Nurse and Health & Wellness Nurse Coach
Brooklyn, New York
President, American Holistic Nurses Credentialing Corporation
Topeka, Kansas

Heidi Honegger Rogers, DNP, FNP-C, APHN-BC, FNAP
Associate Professor
University of New Mexico College of Nursing
Albuquerque, New Mexico

William E. Rosa, PhD, MBE, APRN, FAANP, FPCN, FAAN
Assistant Attending Behavioral Scientist
Department of Psychiatry and Behavioral Sciences
Memorial Sloan Kettering Cancer Center
New York, New York

Bonney Gulino Schaub, RN, MS, PMHCNS, NC-BC
Co-Director, Huntington Meditation and Imagery Center
Founder and Director, Transpersonal Nurse Coaching
Huntington, New York

Marie M. Shanahan, MA, BSN, RN, HN-BC, HSGAHN
President and CEO
The Birch Tree Center for Healthcare Transformation
Tucson, Arizona

Deborah A. Shields, PhD, RN, CCRN, QTTT, AHN-BC, SGAHN
Professor Emerita
Capital University School of Nursing
Columbus, Ohio
Staff Nurse Perioperative Care and System Education (retired)
OhioHealth
Columbus, Ohio
President, Ohio Heart of Healing

Sharon Stout-Shaffer, PhD, RN, SGAHN
Professor Emeritus
Capital University
Columbus, Ohio
Adjunct Professor
Heritage University
Nursing Education Specialist
S4Netquest

Lucia M. Thornton, ThD, MSN, RN
Consultant and Educator
Developer of the Model of Whole-Person Caring
Past President American Holistic Nurses Association
Past President Academy of Integrative Health and Medicine

Stephanie Van Hope, DNP, RN, NC-BC
Founder
Holistic Psychedelic Nurses Collective
Woodbourne, New York

Mary Beth White, MS, RN, NP Emeritus, NC-BC
Faculty Huntington Meditation and Imagery Center
Huntington, New York

Shu-Fen Wung, PhD, MS, RN, ACNP-BC, FAAN
Professor
University of California, Davis, Betty Irene Moore School of Nursing
Sacramento, California

Debra Rose Wilson PhD, MSN, RN, AHN-BC, CHT, SGAHN
Professor and Lenora C. Reuther Chair of Excellence
Austin Peay State University School of Nursing
Clarksville, Tennessee

Toyoko Yasui, DNP, MSN, RN, AHN-BC, OCN, HWNC-BC, CCAP, CHTP
Holistic Nurse Coordinator
White Plains Hospital
White Plains, New York
Private Practice/Consultant in Holistic Nursing

Katherine E. Zychowski, PhD
Assistant Professor
University of New Mexico – Health Sciences
Albuquerque, New Mexico

With heartfelt gratitude, we acknowledge our dear colleague, Dr. Carolyn "Carla" Mariano (July 10, 1945–March 21, 2025), for her lifelong dedication to nurses and her immense contributions to the "being" and "doing" of holistic nursing. Because of her deep commitment and perseverance, holistic nursing is recognized by the American Nurses Association (ANA) as a nursing specialty with national board certification granted by the American Holistic Nurses Credentialing Corporation (AHNCC).

"Remember, you're doing the best you can under the circumstances." C.M.

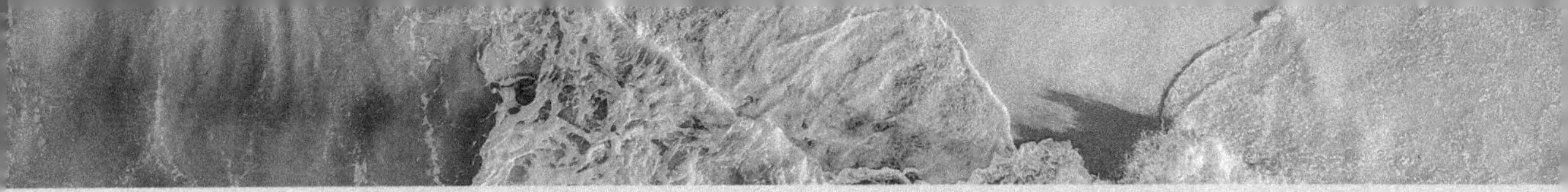

Reviewers

The editors and publisher also wish to thank the reviewers, whose valuable feedback contributed greatly to the preparation of this new edition.

Gloria Browning, PhD, MSN, RN, HN-BC
University of Tennessee—Martin
Martin, Tennessee

Joyce Burr, PhD, RN, AHN-BC
University of Central Florida
Orlando, Florida

John D. Chovan, PhD, DNP, APRN, CNP, CNS, PMHNP-BC, PMHCNS-BC
Professor & Chair, Department of Nursing
Otterbein University
Westerville, Ohio

Doris Clark, PhD, RN, CNE
Bowie State University
Bowie, Maryland

Faith L. Johnson, RN, BSN, MA, EdD
Adjunct Professor
Ottawa University
Surprise, Arizona

Lauren A. Loyd, MSN, RN-BC, CNE
MidAmerica Nazarene University
Bennington, Nebraska

Kristin M. McHale, DNP, RN, AHN-BC
Augsburg University
Minneapolis, Minnesota

Carol Persoon Reid, BAN, MS, PhD
Professor of Nursing
Metropolitan State University
St. Paul, Minnesota

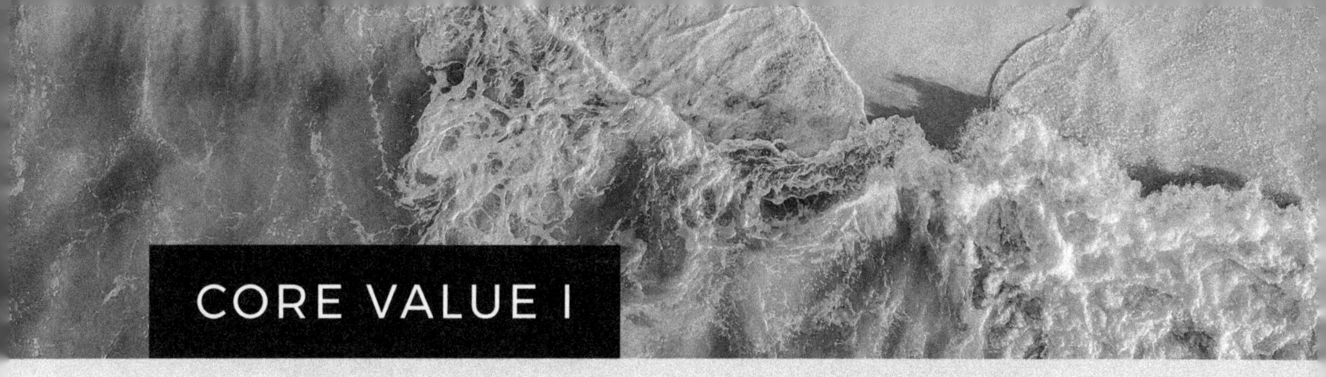

CORE VALUE I

Holistic Philosophies, Theories, and Ethics

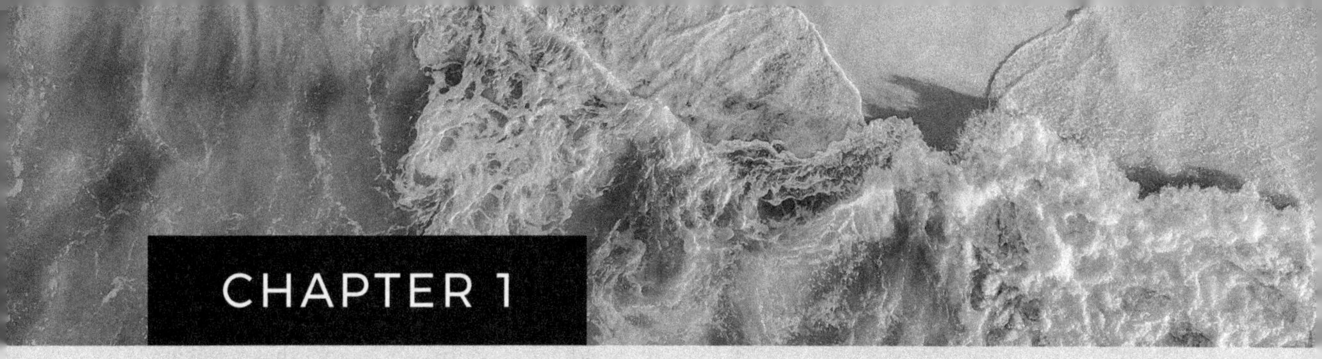

CHAPTER 1

Global Holistic Nursing

Deva-Marie Beck, Barbara Montgomery Dossey, and William E. Rosa

NURSE HEALER OBJECTIVES

- Define global health.
- Define global citizenship.
- Define global citizen nurse.
- Examine the 17 United Nations Sustainable Development Goals (SDGs) and their relevance to you as a global citizen nurse.
- Examine how a Pledge to Planetary Citizenship empowers you as a global nurse.

DEFINITIONS

Global citizenship: Holding a worldview of inclusiveness with all humanity and identifying as belonging to a world community and expressing shared values within this community (United Nations, 2024b).

Global citizen nurse: A nurse who is engaged with people from across nations and beyond borders; they do not necessarily travel from their country of origin, but rather participates in a shift in consciousness to see nursing as globally inclusive (Rosa & Shaw, 2017).

Global health: Refers to practice, research, and study that is focused on the advancement of health and equity for all persons and populations through interdisciplinary and multisector partnerships, recognition of global interdependence, and inclusion of planetary health (Wilson et al., 2016).

Planetary citizenship: A way to invite healing into the fractured aspects of the human-animal-Earth experience and to identify global nurses as planetary leaders, planetary advocates, and planetary change agents (Rosa, 2017).

Introduction: A New Holistic Nursing Philosophical Understanding Becomes Our "North Star"

Challenging health needs are not isolated problems in far-off places. They exist in every community and country around the world, from grassroots to global health. With globalization as our ongoing reality, today's health concerns also demonstrate humanity's interconnectedness as a crucial component of everyone's health and well-being. In addition, global citizenship is emerging to explore and discover new levels of solutions—innovative tools and tasks for us as global citizens. Our tools are related to the communication of interconnected and holistic information. Our tasks include the sharing of information as public advocacy (Servaes, 2003). As we make our own shifts to encompass global citizenship in our own personal and professional lives, we can carry a global holistic nursing vision as an expanded awareness—and the sharing of this awareness—that everything we do impacts holistic health and healing everywhere, grassroots to global. This new holistic nursing philosophical understanding is our "North Star."

The Global Health Mirrors Holistic Health

The original definition of *global health* was established in the preamble of the *Constitution of the World Health Organization*. The first World Health Organization (WHO) director, General Dr. Brock Chisholm, a Canadian veteran of both World War I and World War II, proposed the name "World Health Organization" as serving all peoples in all nations. In keeping with Dr. Chisholm's vision, the WHO Constitution also established health as "a state of complete physical, mental and social well-being and not merely the absence of disease or infirmity" (WHO, 2024a).

The WHO Constitution also declares health to be a fundamental right of every human being and recognizes that "the health of all peoples is fundamental to the attainment of peace and security" (WHO, 2024a). Chisholm also believed that the well-being of humanity is dependent on the world's emotional and mental health (Kolappa et al., 2013).

These global health definitions mirror holistic health. Just as holistic health is based on attention to all aspects of an individual—physical, mental, emotional, spiritual, existential, sexual, cultural, and social at the personal microlevel (American Nurses Association and American Holistic Nurses Association, 2019)—the previously provided global definitions of *health* are *holistic* at the macrolevel. Individual holistic health is a significant component of global holistic health.

Globalization and Nurses as Global Citizens

The word *globalization* describes the growing interdependence occurring in all components of life. While this certainly applies to the world's economies, it equally applies to many cultures and most professions (Peterson Institute for International Economics, 2019). Influenced by cross-border trade in goods and services and through technology, globalization also includes significant flows of people and information sharing—across these cultures and professions—within groups, as well as from individuals.

Nurses are a globalized workforce of 29 million, providing the vast majority of primary healthcare services worldwide (WHO, 2024b). As major participants in the achievement of health on a global scale, they have recently been acknowledged in an unprecedented way with the 2020 bicentennial of Florence Nightingale's birth—as WHO's International Year of the Nurse and the Midwife (WHO, 2023). This recognition heralds the impact and influence that nurses already have and can further strengthen, within groups and from individuals, on both the policy and the practice required for healthy people, worldwide.

With a timeless relevance to globalization and recognition of the need for individual participation to achieve a better world, Florence Nightingale wrote a remarkably visionary article, published in the then-popular *Fraser's Magazine* in 1873:

> What will the world be on August 11, 1999? What we have made of it.... What 1999 will be, whether all these things are the same then as now, or worse, or better, depends, of course, in its proportion upon what we are doing now, or upon what we are not [italics hers] doing now.... In 1999, shall we not wish to have worked out what life, family life, social life, political life should [italics hers] be? And not to have taken for granted that family life, social life, political life are to be as they are. (Nightingale, 1873, p. 25)

As in Nightingale's query, nurses are challenged to rediscover the essence of our profession and become an even more genuinely healing profession, as authentic, committed healers, and leaders around the world (Beck & Dossey, 2025). With the continuing reality of globalization and the recognition of nursing's value to leverage globalization toward better health for all peoples, nurses are being seen—and increasingly see themselves—as never before, as global citizens, as major stakeholders and influencers to envision and achieve what it takes to have a healthy humanity.

Global citizenship can be defined as holding a worldview of inclusiveness with all humanity—identifying as belonging to a world community and expressing shared values within this community (United Nations, 2024b). A global citizen nurse does not necessarily travel from their country of origin but rather participates in a shift in consciousness to see nursing as globally inclusive. While caring for patients, families, and communities from this perspective, global citizen nurses are engaged with people from across nations and beyond borders (Rosa & Shaw, 2017).

With this shift in consciousness—to see ourselves in global citizen roles—nurses are emerging with an updated awareness of nursing's caring, compassionate, and committed contract with society.

Living in Fragile and Uncertain Times

We live in globally fragile and uncertain times (Rosa et al., 2019a). The United Nations notes that humanity is now in an age of "polycrisis" where the world's peoples are still faltering from COVID-19 impacts, while also enduring more severe climate changes. Intensifying wildfires, heatwaves, droughts, flooding, and increasing sea level rise are frequently catastrophic, with recent increases in war, conflict, and resulting human rights violations (United Nations, 2023a). As of 2023, 110 million people, including 35 million refugees, have been displaced—the highest number recorded. As well, migration deaths reached nearly 7,000 in 2022, surpassing pre-pandemic levels (United Nations, 2023a).

Another United Nations report further established that one million of Earth's species face extinction (UN News, 2019). This report reviewed about 15,000 scientific and government sources and was compiled by 145 expert authors from 50 countries. This report included, for the first time, Indigenous and local knowledge as well as scientific studies—the first comprehensive overview of its kind in 15 years. This report also established overwhelming evidence that human activities are the cause of nature's decline, including overfishing, bush meat hunting and poaching, deforestation, climate change, pollution, and invasive alien species (UN News, 2019).

Determinants of Health and Calls for Sustainable Development

Still keenly relevant to today, Florence Nightingale called for better conditions for women, children, the poor, and the hungry and for better education programs for marginalized people (Dossey et al., 2019). She identified environmental health determinants, including clean air, water, food, and housing, and social health determinants, including poverty, education, family relationships, and employment (Dossey et al., 2017).

In our times, and for nearly six decades, the aforementioned social and environmental issues are and have been understood as key factors in achieving global development (Beck, 2017). Starting with the United Nations' First and Second Development Decades in the 1960s and 1970s, the United Nations convened a series of conferences and summits focused on development issues, notably for environmental concerns during the 1972 Human Environment Conference in Stockholm and the 1992 Earth Summit in Rio de Janiero (Beck, 2017).

Arising directly from these global gatherings and discussions, eight United Nations Millennium Development Goals (MDGs)—focused on poverty, hunger, illiteracy, gender inequalities, premature death of children, maternal mortality, disease, and environmental degradation—were identified to be achieved between 2000 and 2015 (United Nations, 2024a). Based on what was learned from this 2000–2015 effort, all 193 member states adopted 17 United Nations SDGs (**Figure 1-1**) in 2015, covering an all-encompassing series of development issues—defined as the UN 2030 Agenda for Sustainable Development (the 2030 Agenda)—aimed to be achieved by 2030 (Rosa et al., 2019b).

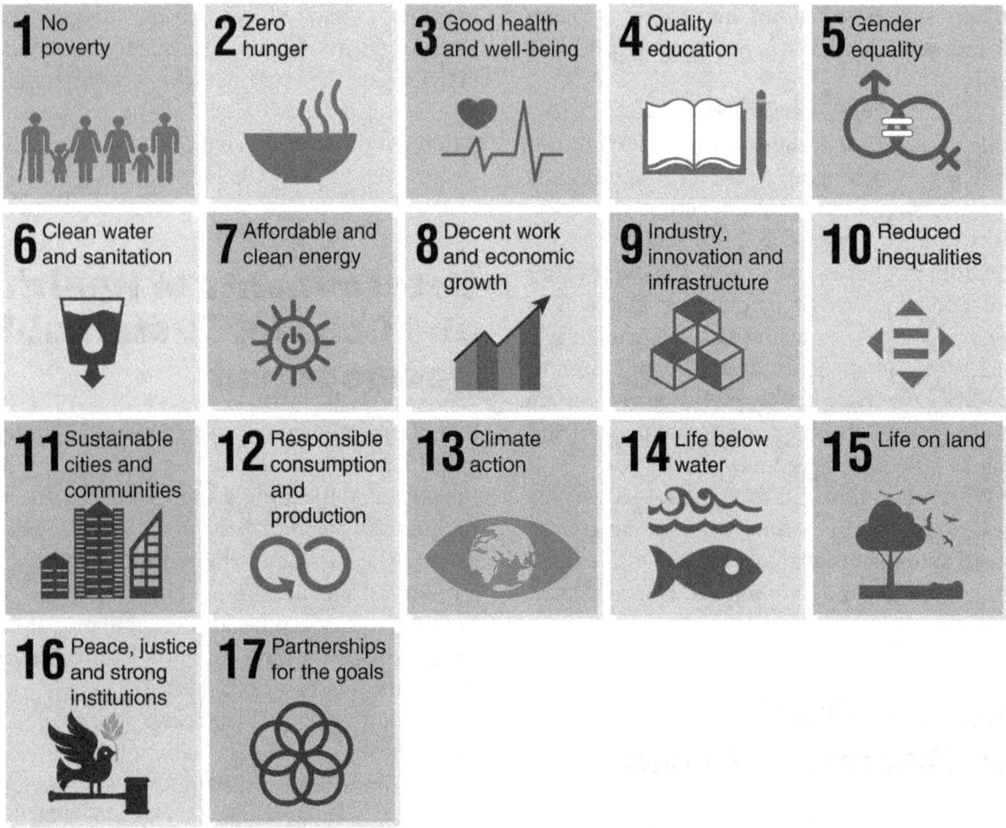
1 No poverty
2 Zero hunger
3 Good health and well-being
4 Quality education
5 Gender equality
6 Clean water and sanitation
7 Affordable and clean energy
8 Decent work and economic growth
9 Industry, innovation and infrastructure
10 Reduced inequalities
11 Sustainable cities and communities
12 Responsible consumption and production
13 Climate action
14 Life below water
15 Life on land
16 Peace, justice and strong institutions
17 Partnerships for the goals

Figure 1-1 United Nations SDGs.

"The content of this publication has not been approved by the United Nations and does not reflect the views of the United Nations or its officials or Member States." https://www.un.org/sustainabledevelopment/sustainable-development-goals/

Holistic Nursing Core Values and the Sustainable Development Goals[1]

The ANA and AHNA's *Holistic Nursing: Scope and Standards of Practice* (WHO, 2024a) have established five Core Values to provide an important framework for holistic nurses' mission. In review, these are the five Core Values:

- Core Value 1: Holistic Philosophies, Theories, and Ethics
- Core Value 2: Holistic Nurse Self-Reflection, Self-Development, and Self-Care
- Core Value 3: Holistic Nursing Process
- Core Value 4: Holistic Communication, Therapeutic Relationships, Healing Environments, and Cultural Care
- Core Value 5: Holistic Education and Research

These Core Values connect the dots between holistic nursing clinical practice and the United Nations 2030 Agenda and 17 SDGs—local to global (Beck, 2017), as described in **Table 1-1**.

1 This section has been adapted from Rosa, W. E., Dossey, B. M., Watson, J., Beck, D. M., & Upvall, M. J. (2019). The United Nations sustainable development goals: The ethic and ethos of holistic nursing. *Journal of Holistic Nursing, 37*(4), 381–393.

Table 1-1 The 17 SDGs Accompanied by Holistic Statements of Commitment

UN SDGs	Statements of Commitment
1. No poverty	■ We recognize the predictors and sequelae of poverty are multidimensional and complex; they include institutionalized marginalization, greed, and power imbalances; they are historically rooted and politically sustained. We are committed to eradicating poverty and the divisive implications of its pathology.
2. Zero hunger	■ We acknowledge the importance of food security and the consequences of hunger on the overall wellness of individuals, families, and communities. We are committed to wiping out hunger, improving sustainable access to food, and advocating systems to redistribute nutritional resources equitably.
3. Good health and well-being	■ We honor the role of nursing to promote, procure, and protect the health and well-being of all peoples everywhere and expand our scope to include the vitality of animal species and the planet at large. We are committed to elevating the health and well-being of all life to invite a future of wholeness and thriving.
4. Quality education	■ We understand the crucial nature of a quality education for all human beings and its role in attaining sociopolitical and economic equity. We are committed to individualizing education to clients across the spectrum of care to ensure ease, quality, and the advancement of health literacy for all.
5. Gender equality	■ We walk beside all women who continue on the path toward true equity in respect, salary, and opportunity; we include all those underrepresented and disenfranchised individuals from across the gender identity spectrum to be a part of the equality movement. We are committed to creating safe spaces and environments that role model true inclusivity and equality for all people of all genders.
6. Clean water and sanitation	■ We note the repeated threats to health and survival imposed by a lack of clean water and sanitation throughout history, often disproportionately witnessed in low-resource settings across continents. We are committed to ensuring clean water and sanitation for all communities and regarding it as an unresolved social justice issue.
7. Affordable and clean energy	■ We have witnessed the threats to environmental welfare due to unsustainable sourcing of energy, threats that continue to endanger the future of communities worldwide. We are committed to partnering with organizations and systems that seek affordable and clean energy to build a long-term path to environmental well-being.
8. Decent work and economic growth	■ We have experienced the debilitating outcomes of unemployment and imbalanced economic opportunity, making health and happiness both difficult and impossible. We are committed to addressing these imbalances and advocating systems that promote opportunity and growth for all.
9. Industry, innovation, and infrastructure	■ We in high-resource countries often overlook the lifesaving graces of progressive industry, openly competitive innovation, and reliable infrastructure; we in low-resource countries seek the security and safety that are elusive without it. We are committed to seeking new ways of promoting industry, sparking innovation, and collaborating to lay systemic infrastructure to serve all.
10. Reduced inequalities	■ We admit the impact of inequalities inherent to the hierarchies that determine welfare in society, within nations, between nations, among peoples, and within systems and professions. We are committed to confront inequality and identify solutions to heal the wounds at the systems level.

(*continues*)

Table 1-1 The 17 SDGs Accompanied by Holistic Statements of Commitment *(continued)*

UN SDGs	Statements of Commitment
11. Sustainable cities and communities	■ We see that the whole must be sustained if the world is to make it; the unity of the global and planetary village is of utmost importance at this time of uncertainty. We are committed to advancing the needs of our cities and communities to ensure our collective sustainability.
12. Responsible consumption and production	■ We call for the responsible use and production of material goods across systems, particularly throughout hospitals, notorious contributors to waste. We are committed to working with systems at all levels and finding opportunities to increase accountability for consumption and production practices.
13. Climate action	■ We continue to learn of how devolving climate stability is becoming a volatile predictor of planetary survival; ultimately, the climate will determine the welfare of life on the planet. We are committed to promote climate awareness and knowledge and to taking informed action for positive change.
14. Life below water	■ We are deeply affected by the well-being of our rivers, lakes, and oceans and are dependent upon these waters for survival. We are committed to environmental activism and conservation efforts that protect our waters and the life below them.
15. Life on land	■ We seek healing for all life on land, within the human species but also between species and in concert with our forests, deserts, and land ecosystems. We are committed to defending the welfare of all life on land in order to sustain nature for the healing and wholeness of all those yet to come and all suns yet to rise.
16. Peace, justice, and strong institutions	■ We bear witness to a world that is deeply wounded from a lack of peace and glaring injustice; we seek the strength of institutions that are founded on compassion and the recognition of an interdependent humanity. We are committed to being peacemakers, calling for justice, and supporting institutions whose strength is born from the well-being of its people.
17. Partnerships for the goals	■ We know we cannot do this alone; the path is long, the stakeholders diverse, and the needs great; the partnerships that advance equity must reflect mutual respect and benefit at all levels. We are committed to seeking, creating, and role modeling such partnerships for the sake of self, other, system, and planet.

Reproduced from Rosa, W. E., Dossey, B. M., Watson, J., Beck, D.-M., & Upvall, M. J. (2019). The United Nations sustainable development goals: The ethic and ethos of holistic nursing. *Journal of Holistic Nursing, 37*(4), 381–393. doi:10.1177/0898010119841723

People, Planet, Peace, Prosperity, and Partnership

The United Nations 2030 Agenda is a global framework of action for five themes (United Nations, 2023b): People, Planet, Peace, Prosperity, and Partnership (**Figure 1-2**). These themes provide an ideal way to learn and teach about the UN 2030 Agenda and can become an education process, toward human-planet thriving, to reflect upon an ongoing dynamic flow between the AHNA Core Values (**Figure 1-3**) and these five themes (**Figure 1-4**). Global holistic nurses can integrate these Core Values with these five themes, understanding, further, the necessity to shift consciousness and advocate for the SDGs that are about human and planetary survival (Dossey et al., 2019).

A Global Panel for Global Challenges

In 2017, a Global Advisory Panel on the Future of Nursing and Midwifery (GAPFON) was convened to review relevant research and release a related

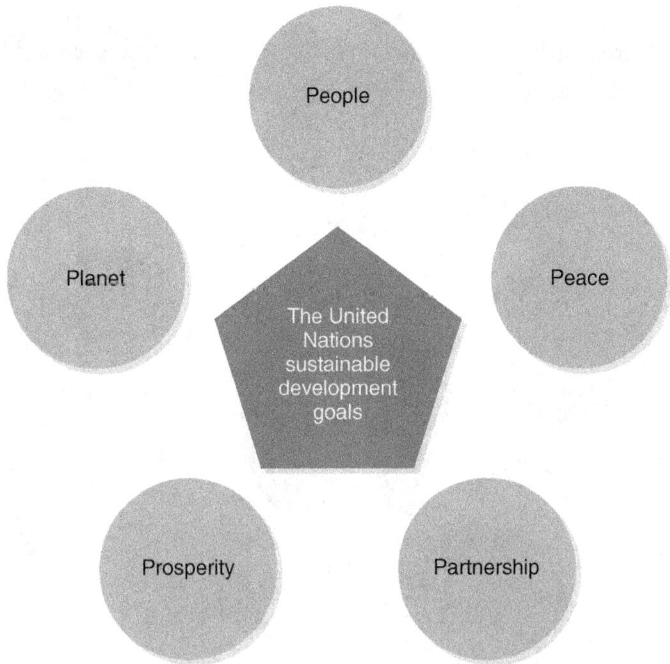

Figure 1-2 UN Sustainable Development Goals and five themes.

Reproduced from Rosa, W. E., Dossey, B. M., Watson, J., Beck, D. M., & Upvall, M. J. (2019). The United Nations sustainable development goals: The ethic and ethos of holistic nursing. *Journal of Holistic Nursing, 37*(4), 381–393. doi:10.1177/0898010119841723

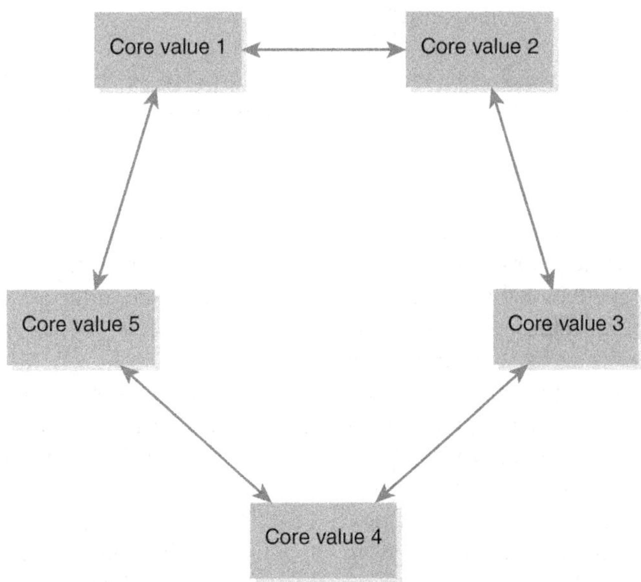

Figure 1-3 American Holistic Nurses Association Core Values.

Reproduced from Rosa, W. E., Dossey, B. M., Watson, J., Beck, D.-M., & Upvall, M. J. (2019). The United Nations sustainable development goals: The ethic and ethos of holistic nursing. *Journal of Holistic Nursing, 37*(4), 381–393. doi:10.1177/0898010119841723

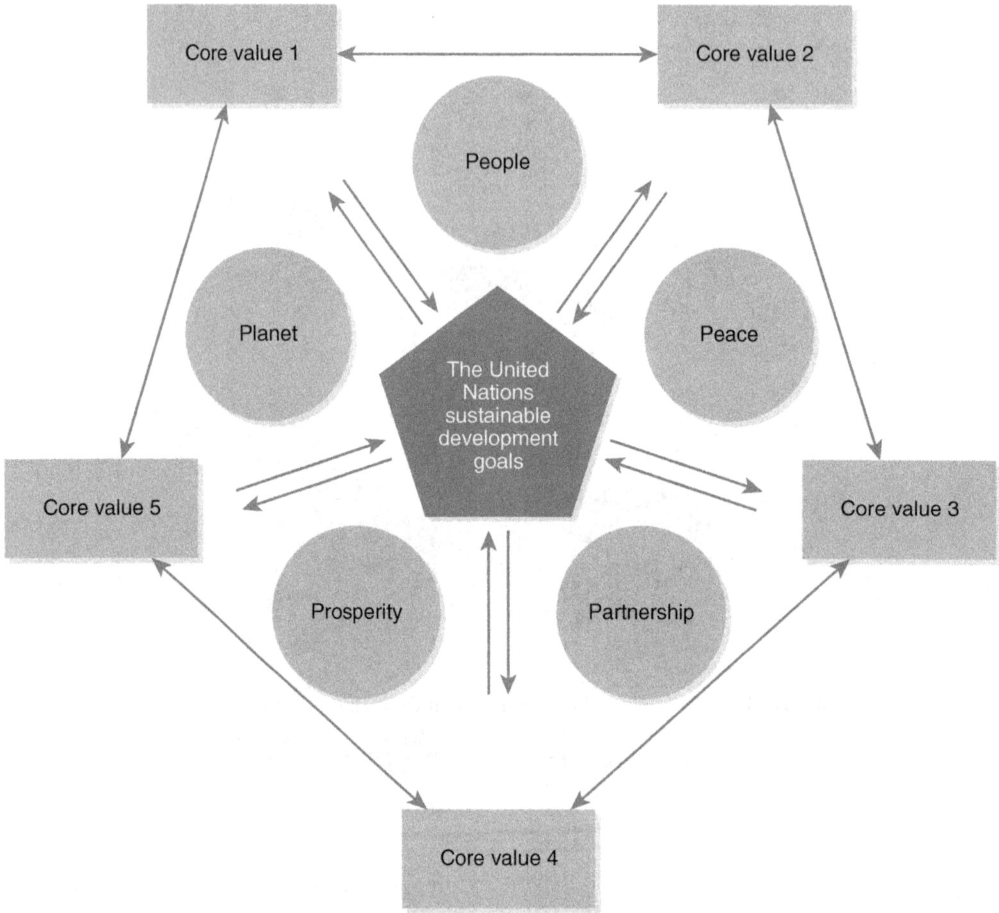

Figure 1-4 Sustainable Development Goals and Core Values: A framework for health and healing.

Reproduced from Rosa, W. E., Dossey, B. M., Watson, J., Beck, D.-M., & Upvall, M. J. (2019). The United Nations sustainable development goals: The ethic and ethos of holistic nursing. *Journal of Holistic Nursing, 37*(4), 381–393. doi:10.1177/0898010119841723

summary report (Wilson et al., 2016). Representing the culmination of three years of efforts led by the Sigma Theta Tau International Nursing Honorary Society, this report synthesized data on the challenges of global health care and the priority of nursing's professional issues gathered at high-level meetings in each of seven global regions. A related task force searched for and reviewed articles published in English, Spanish, and Portuguese between 2005 and 2015, developed summaries, listed key elements, identified prevalent themes, and developed consensus definitions.

Two of these definitions developed through consensus by the GAPFON (Wilson et al., 2016)—for global health and for global nursing—are both lengthy but are worthwhile to quote, along with their original references, in entirety here (Wilson et al., 2016, pp. 1536–1537):

> Global health refers to an area for practice, study, and research that places a priority on improving health, achieving equity in health for all people (Smeeth & Kyobutungi, 2023) and ensuring health-promoting and sustainable sociocultural, political and economic systems (Kumar, 2012). Global health implies planetary health which equals human, animal,

> environmental and ecosystem health (Aliouche, 2022). It emphasizes transnational health issues, determinants, and solutions; involves many disciplines within and beyond the health sciences, and promotes interdependence and interdisciplinary collaboration. It a synthesis of population-based prevention with individual holistic care. (Wilson et al., 2016)
>
> Global nursing is the use of evidence-based nursing process to promote sustainable planetary health and equity for all people (Kumar, 2012). Global nursing considers social determinants of health, includes individual and population-level care, research, education, leadership, advocacy, and policy initiatives (Yatsu & Saeki, 2022). Global nurses engage in ethical practice and demonstrate respect for human dignity, human rights, and cultural diversity (Upvall et al., 2014). Global nurses engage in a spirit of deliberation and reflection in interdependent partnership with communities and other health care providers. (Cho & Kim, 2022)

Recognizing that increased globalization has led to expanded awareness of the importance of global health and global nursing among students and faculty in the health professions and among policy makers and practitioners everywhere, the GAPFON will use the research gained to guide the promotion, voice, and vision for nursing that will contribute to the advancement of the profession's contribution to global health (Wilson et al., 2016).

Our Planetary Citizen "North Star"

Upon consideration of global conditions, including the previously discussed global health issues and the related struggles nurses face, our outlook may appear bleak. But there is hope. The rapidly evolving field of global health calls for nursing's wisdom and advocacy that demonstrate a leading edge in response to our global challenges, yet continues firmly rooted in a nursing perspective and lens (NIGH, 2024b).

To these ends, a new Pledge to Planetary Citizenship (**Figure 1-5**) has been crafted to inspire our generation and the generations to come (Rosa, 2017).

Planetary citizenship is thus proposed to invite healing to the fractured aspects of human-animal-Earth experience. This *Pledge to Planetary Citizenship* encourages and supports us to identify as planetary leaders, planetary advocates, and planetary change agents (Rosa, 2017).

This pledge reflects a "North Star" that we can aim toward as global holistic nurses as we continue our practices, education, research, advocacy, and, most of all, our reflections, our meditations, and our prayers.

Implications

Clinical Practice

While nursing's clinical practice has traditionally centered on one-on-one interventions that have, over recent decades, included holistic approaches to acknowledge health as encompassing physical, emotional, and spiritual components, an emerging global citizen clinical practice participates in a shift in consciousness to see nursing as globally inclusive; that is, engaged with people from across nations and beyond borders (Rosa & Shaw, 2017).

Education

Recognizing the imperative to embed nursing education with global holistic nursing perspectives—at all levels, including continuing education across nurses' careers—teaching and learning about the United Nations 2030 Agenda and the related five themes of People, Planet, Peace, Prosperity, and Partnership, in the context of the AHNA Core Values, can become a strong foundation for integrating global citizenship into nursing's culture and through a nursing lens (American Nurses Association and American Holistic Nurses Association, 2019; Dossey et al., 2019; Rosa et al., 2019a).

I pledge to be a Planetary Citizen,
To strive continuously toward a universal experience of dignity,
To embrace cultural differences and confront human inequalities and disparities in an effort to know and promote peace,
And to lovingly, but directly, address all threats to planetary well-being, be they be human or environmental.

I pledge to be a Planetary Citizen,
To be a global nurse in the highest sense of the word,
Embracing nursing as the finest of arts and the most rooted of sciences,
To wield safety, inclusiveness, and social justice as tools to elevate consciousness and role-model compassion,
To be an advocate for healing and global activism,
A conduit for transformation and unity,
And a leader in the journey toward One Mind-One Health-One Planet.
I pledge to role-model kindness and respect as integral aspects of my Planetary Citizenship,
To carry the intention of unity in my words and actions,
To remain present to the global consequences of my choices,
To commit to creating healing environments at all levels, in all spaces, for all beings everywhere,
And to build relationships based on trust and awareness of a shared humanity.

I pledge to nurture a safe and inclusive world as a Planetary Citizen,
To release prejudices, divisive judgments, and aggression,
To forgive what is needed and return myself to wholeness,
To "Be the Change," live the virtues, and practice the values inherent to ethical engagement,
To accept people as they are and the world as it is in order to more fully embrace myself as I am.

I pledge to devote my energies to self-care, self-knowledge, and self-love as a Planetary Citizen,
Caring for myself as a sacred vessel,
Caring for my family as myself,
Caring for Others as my family,
And for the Planet as I do all Others,
And, in this way, caring for the Planet as myself, and the sacred mystery that It is.

I pledge partnership with all beings in an effort to realize Planetary Citizenship and a Planetary World,
To remain open, available and flexible,
To teach what I know and learn what I don't know,
To honor the light in all life,
And to leave the Planet better than I found it.

This is my solemn pledge and commitment.
William Rosa (2017)

Figure 1-5 A Pledge to Planetary Citizenship.

Nursing Situation

The Nightingale Initiative for Global Health (NIGH) is an international nongovernmental organization (INGO) that exemplifies nurses as global citizens who are developing global holistic nursing. Co-founded by Nightingale scholar nurses and aligned citizen activists, NIGH illustrates how Florence Nightingale remains a pillar of holistic nursing, still keenly relevant today (Beck, 2021). NIGH is guided by the *Theory of Integral Nursing* (TIN) arising from an in-depth study of Nightingale's life—and her value to today's nurses. This *Theory* builds an inclusive paradigm aiming to engage nursing's culture toward "deeper levels of meaning and understanding about our knowing, doing, and being" (see Chapter 4, Theory of Integral Nursing).

NIGH has become a catalytic movement assembled to promote global health concerns through education and worldwide public dissemination. While remembering Nightingale, NIGH also honors other nurses, midwives, healthcare workers, and concerned citizens, past and present, who have shown by their example how personal actions can make a significant difference (Beck, 2021). NIGH seeks to engage the common values and wisdom of millions and to act as a catalyst for the transformation of individuals, communities, and society toward the achievement of a healthy world (Beck, 2021).

In 2018, NIGH World was awarded "Special Consultative Status" with the United Nations Economic and Social Council (UN ECOSOC). This "Status" is the principal means by which the UN ECOSOC receives input from NGO voices into its deliberations at official public meetings, as well as in and through UN international conferences and related gatherings (NIGH, 2024b).

Through NIGH's growing grassroots-to-global outreach, its teams are reflecting the voices of nurses, midwives, teachers, and interdisciplinary groups of concerned citizens. Most recently, NIGH co-hosted the "Nurses' Voices Speaker Series," which are virtual sessions broadcasted in collaboration with the United Nations Institute for Training and Research (UNITAR) and UNITAR's CIFAL York Centre at York University in Toronto. Through this Series, more than 50 nursing leaders have shared their public voices from 30 nations and across all six regions of the WHO (NIGH, 2024c).

In earlier examples, NIGH teams were catalysts to celebrate the 2010 International Year of the Nurse and to promote this year with advocacy for achieving the UN MDGs (Cho & Kim, 2022). From 2012 to 2014, NIGH advocated for MDG # 5—Maternal Health—with its *Daring, Caring & Sharing to Save Mothers' Lives* awareness campaign, launched in New York City and, then, online. Over 24 months, NIGH's website achieved 3.5 million hits with 90,000 unique online visitors from 146 nations (NIGH, 2024b).

In 2004, the co-founders of the NIGH met, for the first time, during an international nursing conference convened in Toronto, while the SARS epidemic was raging in hospitals—with nurses and patients dying less than a mile from their meeting (NIGH, 2024). Aware of this tragedy, while remembering the seemingly impossible challenges that Nightingale faced and knowing that many nurses still see themselves as inheritors of Nightingale's legacy, NIGH's co-founders crafted the *Nightingale Declaration for a Healthy World* (NIGH, 2024a) (the Nightingale Declaration; **Figure 1-6**) to establish NIGH's credo, to renew our individual commitments to Nightingale's vision, and to see the possibility of what we each can achieve, in our time.

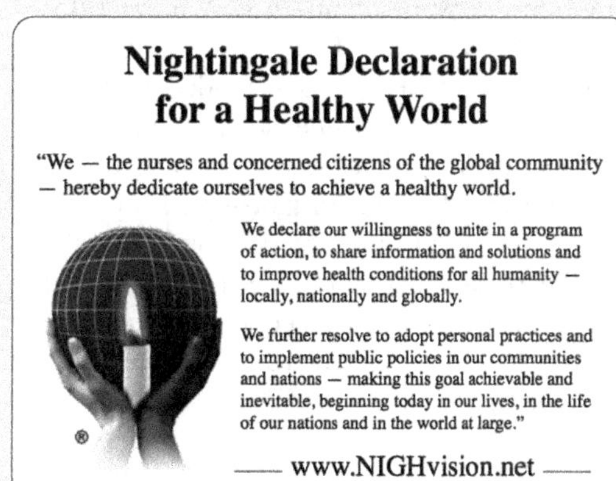
Nightingale Declaration for a Healthy World
"We — the nurses and concerned citizens of the global community — hereby dedicate ourselves to achieve a healthy world.
We declare our willingness to unite in a program of action, to share information and solutions and to improve health conditions for all humanity — locally, nationally and globally.
We further resolve to adopt personal practices and to implement public policies in our communities and nations — making this goal achievable and inevitable, beginning today in our lives, in the life of our nations and in the world at large."
www.NIGHvision.net

Figure 1-6 The Nightingale Declaration for a Healthy World.

The *Nightingale Declaration* was purposefully modeled after the *Preamble* (United Nations, 1945) to the founding *Charter of the United Nations* with the words, "We the peoples of the United Nations..." and became the foundational credo for all NIGH's activities. It clarifies and commits to our shared goals and purposes—to work together to build a better world for everyone.

During NIGH's initial launch, from 2006 to 2010, the *Nightingale Declaration* was signed by more than 25,000 nurses and concerned citizens, some who officially represented millions of organizational members worldwide (NIGH, 2024b). As of July 2024, this *Declaration* is available in 14 language versions, including all six official United Nations languages and the first Indigenous version in Kiswahili, also the official language of the African Union. Many more versions will be added to encourage and engage nurses and concerned citizens from across the world to bring their voices—through NIGH's UN ECOSOC "Special Consultative Status"—to the United Nations and into the decades ahead (NIGH, 2024b).

Research

With nursing research extending to encompass globalization issues through initiatives exemplified by the GAPFON, current and future qualitative and quantitative data can be gained to guide the promotion, voice, and vision for nursing that will contribute to the advancement of our profession's contribution to global health (Wilson et al., 2016).

Policy

Remembering the significant impact that Florence Nightingale had on the global health policy of her time, global holistic nurses can be inspired by her timeless challenge to consider whether "things are the same then as now, or worse, or better, [which] depends, of course, in its proportion upon what we are doing now, or upon what we are *not* doing now" (Nightingale, 1873). Beyond the one-on-one roles that nurses have tended to focus upon since Nightingale's time, she encouraged us to extend nursing's arena of effectiveness to the deeper and broader scale of global health policy. "Shall we not wish to have worked out what life, family life, social life, political life should be? And not to have taken for granted that family life, social life, political life are to be as they are" (Nightingale, 1873).

Conclusion

At this significant time in planetary existence, there has never been a more pressing need for the intersection of nursing philosophy with a staunch commitment to social justice, through proactive participation in the achievement of the United Nations 2030 Agenda. This challenge is no longer an optional extra in nurses' personal or professional lives. This has become imperative to procure health and well-being for the whole of the global village and to restore ecological integrity across the natural systems that govern all of life (Dossey et al., 2019).

Nurses have long been leaders in linking physiologic, social, environmental, and economic health determinants with an understanding of humanity as interconnected and interdependent and health as holistic. Now, global citizen nurses are developing person-centered interventions, while also expanding the envelope of nursing's arena to include population-centered interventions (Wilson et al., 2016). As well, instead of assuming unrealistic and unsustainable responsibilities for achieving the large tasks required to address the global health challenges that we—as a humanity—face, nurses are learning to foster sustainable transdisciplinary partnerships built on mutual benefit and respect (Dossey, 2025).

The many problems of global health will not be solved in a day, or a year, or even a generation. But, in our generation, we are encouraged, as holistic global citizen nurses, to use our wisdom and our advocacy to continually plant the seeds of our caring, compassion, and commitment—aimed to the "North Star" of planetary citizenship that can and will grow toward a healthy humanity, over time, in the decades and generations to come.

References

Aliouche, H. (2022). *What is planetary health*. News Medical Life Sciences. https://www.news-medical.net/health/What-is-Planetary-Health.aspx

American Nurses Association and American Holistic Nurses Association. (2019). *Holistic nursing: Scope and standards of practice* (3rd ed.). Nursesbooks.org.

Beck, D. M. (2017). A brief history of the United Nations and nursing: A healthy world is our common future. In W. Rosa (Ed.), *A new era in global health: Nursing and the United Nations 2030 Agenda for Sustainable Development* (pp. 57–83). Springer Publishing Company.

Beck, D. M. (2021). Creating the Nightingale Initiative for Global Health: Theoretical reflections to follow in Florence Nightingale's footsteps. *Revista Americana-Latino de Emfermagem, 30*(29), 1–11. https://doi.org/10.1590/1518-8345.4720.3430

Beck, D. M., & Dossey, B. M. (2025). Remembering Florence Nightingale in her turbulent times: Activating the Theory of Integral Nursing in our turbulent times. *International Nursing Review, 72*(3). https://doi.org/10.1111/inr.13064

Cho, M. K., & Kim, M. Y. (2022). Factors affecting the global health and competencies of nursing students. *International Journal of Environmental Research and Public Health, 19*(7), 4109. https://doi.org/10.3390/ijerph19074109

Dossey, B. M., & Keegan, L. (2016). *Holistic nursing: A handbook for practice*. Jones & Bartlett Learning.

Dossey, B. M., Beck, D. M., Oerther, S., & Manjrekar, P. (2017). Florence Nightingale's legacy: The rationale for an integral worldview in achieving the sustainable development goals. In W. Rosa (Ed.), *A new era in global health: Nursing and the United Nations 2030 Agenda for Sustainable Development* (pp. 149–178). Springer Publishing Company.

Dossey, B. M., Rosa, W. E., & Beck, D. M. (2019). Nursing and the sustainable development goals: From Nightingale to now. *American Journal of Nursing, 119*(5), 44–49.

Kolappa, K., Henderson, D. C., & Kishore, S. P. (2013). No physical health without mental health: Lessons unlearned. *Bulletin of the World Health Organization, 91*(1). https://doi.org/10.2471/BLT.12.115063

Kumar, S. (2012). Health promotion: An effective tool for global health. *Indian Journal of Community Medicine, 37*(1), 5–12. https://doi.org/10.4103/0970-0218.94009

NIGH. (2024a). *Nightingale declaration for a healthy world*. http://www.nighvision.net/nightingale-declaration.html

NIGH. (2024b). *The Nightingale Initiative for Global Health*. http://www.NIGHvision.net

NIGH. (2024c). *Nurses' voices speaker series*. https://www.nighvision.net/nurses-voices-speaker-series.html

Nightingale, F. (1873, July 8). A subnote of interrogation; What will our religion be in 1999? *Fraser's Magazine* (New Series), pp. 25–36.

Peterson Institute for International Economics. (2019). *What is globalization?* https://piie.com/microsites/globalization/what-is-globalization.html

Rosa, W. (2017). One mind, one health, one planet—A pledge to planetary citizenship. In W. Rosa (Ed.), *A new era in global health: Nursing and the United Nations 2030 Agenda for Sustainable Development* (pp. 517–527). Springer Publishing Company.

Rosa, W. E., Dossey, B. M., Watson, J., Beck, D. M., & Upvall, M. J. (2019a). The United Nations sustainable development goals: Ethics and ethos of holistic nursing. *Journal of Holistic Nursing, 37*(4), 381–393. https://doi.org/10.1177/0898010119841723

Rosa, W. E., & Shaw, H. K. (2017). Global nurse citizenship: Toward a safe and inclusive civil society. In W. Rosa (Ed.), *A new era in global health: Nursing and the United Nations 2030 Agenda for Sustainable Development* (pp. 85–107). Springer Publishing Company.

Rosa, W. E., Upvall, M. J., Beck, D. M., & Dossey, B. M. (2019b, May 21). Nursing and sustainable development: Furthering the global agenda in uncertain times. *OJIN, 24*(2), manuscript 1. https://doi.org/10.3912/OJIN.Vol24No02Man01

Servaes, J. (2003). By way of introduction. In J. Servaes (Ed.), *Approaches to development: Studies on communication for development*. UNESCO/UNESDOC Digital Library. https://unesdoc.unesco.org/ark:/48223/pf0000134647

Smeeth, L., & Kyobutungi, C. (2023). Reclaiming global health. *The Lancet, 401*(10377). https://doi.org/10.1016/S0140-6736(23)00327-6

United Nations. (1945). *Preamble to the United Nations charter*. https://www.un.org/en/sections/un-charter/preamble/index.html

United Nations. (2023a). *The Sustainable Development Goals Report 2023: Special edition*. https://unstats.un.org/sdgs/report/2023/

United Nations. (2023b). *Transforming our world: The 2030 Agenda for Sustainable Development*. https://sdgs.un.org/2030agenda

United Nations. (2024a). *End poverty: Millennium development goals and beyond 2015*. https://www.un.org/millenniumgoals/

United Nations. (2024b). *Global citizenship*. https://www.un.org/en/academic-impact/global-citizenship

UN News. (2019). *World is "on notice" as a major UN report shows one million species face extinction*. https://news.un.org/en/story/2019/05/1037941

Upvall, M. J., Leffers, J. M., & Mitchell, E. M. (2014). Introduction and perspectives of global health. In M. J. Upvall & J. M. Jeffers (Eds.), *Global health nursing: Building and sustaining partnerships* (pp. 1–17). Springer Publishing Company.

Wilson, L., Mendes, I. A., Klopper, H., Catrambone, C., Al-Maaitah, R., Norton, M. E., & Hill, M. (2016). "Global health" and "global nursing": Proposed definitions from the Global Advisory Panel on the Future of Nursing. *Journal of Advanced Nursing, 72*(7), 1529–1540. https://doi.org/10.1111/jan.12973

World Health Organization. (2023). *The International Year of the Nurse and the Midwife: Taking stock of outcomes and commitments*. https://www.who.int/publications/i/item/9789240081925

World Health Organization. (2024a). *Constitution*. https://www.who.int/about/governance/constitution

World Health Organization. (2024b). *Nursing and midwifery*. https://www.who.int/news-room/fact-sheets/detail/nursing-and-midwifery

Yatsu, H., & Saeki, A. (2022). Current trends in global nursing: A scoping review. *Nursing Open*, 9(3), 1575–1588. https://doi.org/10.1002/nop2.938

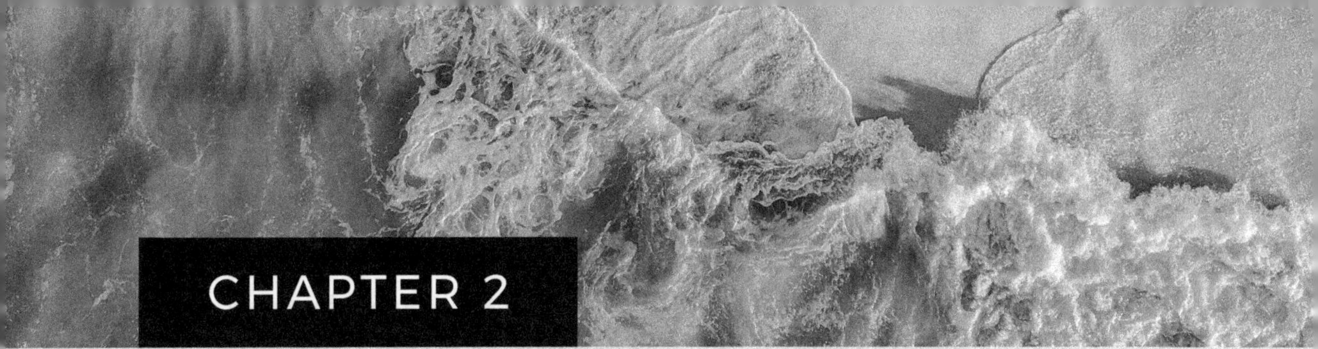

CHAPTER 2

The Integral Relations of Holistic Nursing and Society: Past, Present, and Future

Helen L. Erickson

NURSE HEALER OBJECTIVES

- Identify one change in society affected by nursing.
- Describe relations among nursing education, military needs, and changes in society.
- Describe the relations between the evolution of holistic nursing and U.S. society.
- Discuss the significance of nurses' ability to articulate the essence of their practice.
- Envision the potential of holistic nursing in the 21st century.

Holistic Nursing's Moral Commitment to Society

Holistic Nursing's Core Value One embodies the philosophy and theories that provide a framework for understanding the knowledge needed for practice and the ethics that guide the sacred actions of practice (American Holistic Nurses Association [AHNA], 2019). The close connection between knowledge and ethics gives rise to the professional discipline of nursing. Holistic nursing stresses the vital, inseparable relations between human beings' biophysical and spiritual needs, thus defining its role as a nursing specialty and clarifying its relations with society. The responsibility of holistic nurses is to use intentionality, presence, voice (Barrett, 2010), and enact ways of *knowing* and being (Rosch, 2009), all of which are integral to the discipline. Based on the belief that nursing is not medicine and medicine is not nursing (Nightingale, 1969), this reflects a holistic nurse's moral commitment—our covenant with society (Fowler, 2015).

This chapter expands on Cordeau's (2020) review of nursing history, focusing on its relations with society and explaining how holistic nursing emerged as a solution to societal needs. It examines the social factions that influenced the development of nursing, unresolved social issues, their impact on contemporary culture, and the implications for holistic nursing. The narrative highlights how modern culture evolved from early mercantilist values, Manifest Destiny, and the founders' vision of a democratic republic.

The assumptions are threefold: there are visible links that create indivisible relations between society and nursing; unresolved issues from the past will continue to reemerge during times of stress or change until they are resolved; and holistic nursing has an opportunity to act as a catalyst for healing that can transform society in the 21st century.

The chapter is organized by century, beginning with a brief discussion about 18th-century nursing, the impact of society's values on human care, and relations between nursing and society. It continues with the 19th and 20th centuries, exploring how nursing has been shaped by societal needs and emphasizing the emergence of holistic nursing as a significant aspect of the 21st century.

Nursing and Society in the 18th Century

1700: Emerging from the Dark Age of Nursing

Before the early 19th century, nursing in the U.S. colonies consisted of midwifery, wet nursing, and home-based care. These practices were cultural traditions that did not require formal education. Care was given by family members, the impoverished, uneducated individuals, or those with a religious calling in almshouses. Most nurses were women, while men occasionally helped the sick or injured, mainly transporting them. The first permanent hospital was founded in Pennsylvania in 1751 (University of Pennsylvania School of Nursing, n.d.).

When the American Revolutionary War started in 1775, the usual norms in the colonies were challenged. Most men went to battle, leaving few to help the injured or sick. Many were left on the battlefield. While prewar norms stressed different roles for men and women, the Revolutionary War changed them. Some women disguised themselves as men to fight with their relatives. Others, like Martha Washington and Abigail Adams, supported the troops by bringing supplies, providing food, washing clothes, and caring for the slightly wounded. Many helped as needed. Hundreds died from wounds or sickness within the first few weeks of the war.

1775: Relations Between Nursing and the Military

Three months into the war, the outlook was discouraging. There were no replacements, insufficient supplies, limited food, and no one to care for the sick and wounded. General Horatio Gates visited George Washington at Mount Vernon to discuss their options. He noted that the Continental Army was well established, but the "… sick (and wounded) suffered much for want of good female nurses" (Miller, 2018). Washington contacted the Continental Government to request funding to hire female nurses. Congress approved one nurse for every 10 sick or injured soldiers (Miller, 2018). Nurses were taking on a new role to meet society's needs.

1775: Medicine's Response to Nursing

Initially, many physicians opposed female nurses on the battlefield, limiting their roles to emptying chamber pots and changing and washing bedding. However, as the war progressed, perspectives shifted. Help was scarce; physicians began to request nurses to assist with anesthesia, hold injured limbs, and support other surgical needs. It became natural for nurses to care for soldiers after surgery and during recovery. They fed and bathed them, tidied and refreshed their beds, combed their hair, cleaned and treated wounds, and provided comfort that eased their suffering. Their compassion and care enhanced their innate ability to heal. While physicians and soldiers acknowledged that nurses' efforts saved lives, the specific activities and attitudes tied to these roles were not discussed or shared with the public. As a result, most members of society believed that physicians held full authority over soldier care and that nurses assisted simply by following physicians' orders. Nevertheless, nurses' unique contributions left a lasting effect on how the military viewed the need for nurses, laying the groundwork for future requests for them. Meanwhile, society resumed its view of women's roles in the community.

1787: The Formation of a New Society

In 1787, leaders of the new colonies gathered to discuss how they would unite the colonies and create a nation supported by mercantilism—an economy based on trade. They believed the new nation was destined to expand westward, from coast to coast. With access to coal and iron in the northern colonies, many felt that trade should focus on manufacturing goods. They believed the emigrant population could handle the labor, supplemented by indentured servants.

The Southern colonies protested: based on the principles of slavocracy; they had established the trade of tobacco and cotton grown in Virginia. Now, they sought to expand further into the South and cultivate rice. Without their established slave labor practices, they could not financially benefit from trade or grow as the United States expanded. After considerable debate, the newly formed colonial government reached a compromise that would support an economy rooted in the principles of slavocracy. The nation would consist of 13 states: 9 would be free of slavery, and 4 would remain slave states. The Constitution was drafted and ratified in 1788, setting the stage for social discourse that would shape their future.

Nursing and Society in the 19th Century

1820: The Missouri Compromise

By 1803, the size of the United States had doubled, and the population had grown to nearly 10 million people, including almost 1.6 million enslaved individuals. It was time to decide how to divide the remaining territory into states. Issues of States' Rights reemerged, rekindling old resentments from the signing of the Constitution and bringing slavocracy to the forefront of debate among the states. The Missouri Compromise of 1820 temporarily settled the issue: Maine would be a free state, Missouri a slave state, and the rest of the territory would be free.

1821: Most Nurses Are Women

During this period, nursing was seen as a woman's vocation—a fact rarely acknowledged in society. William Lloyd Garrison and Angelina and Sarah Grimké were among many who protested the oppression of women's rights as human beings, including their right to vote and participate in society. William Lloyd Garrison, owner of the newspaper *The Liberator*, advocated for the rights of all individuals, emphasizing the importance of freedom and education for both enslaved people and women (National Park Service, n.d.). The efforts of Garrison and the Grimké sisters laid the foundation for Florence Nightingale, Mary Seacole, Clara Barton, Mary Mahoney, and other female nurses who would soon become societal leaders, helping to foster a cultural shift that would take nearly another century to fully develop.

1831: Creating a Culture for the New Society

The new U.S. government focused on fulfilling its destiny—acquiring land from coast to coast. France and Spain had claimed the land where Native Americans had lived for at least 20,000 years (National Park Service; Archeology this Month, 2025). The U.S. government purchased it from them with plans to relocate and restrict the Native Americans to land often less suitable and unfamiliar. When many were unwilling to move, the military initiated skirmishes that often escalated to more serious battles across the territory. Thousands were killed, and others were forced to migrate. Sixty thousand were compelled to leave their homeland in the southeastern colonial territories, walking over 1,200 miles of tough terrain to Oklahoma. As many as 4,000 died during the journey (Klein, 2025). Meanwhile, other military forces helped facilitate the migration of new European immigrants coming to settle the land vacated by Native Americans. The government's dream of manifest destiny unfolded, further shaping a culture that valued human worth differently.

1835: The Liberator

Those who wanted to expand the cotton, tobacco, and rice industries in the United States were unhappy. They needed cheap labor but faced restrictions on dealing with slavery issues. Others were upset that slavery still existed but compromised for the sake of the new country. By the early 1830s, abolitionists supporting a slave-free stance backed the Missouri Compromise. This agreement limited slavery's expansion, making it more likely that the country could eventually free all slaves, both in the South and North. It was just a matter of time. William Lloyd Garrison formed the Anti-American Slavery Society, boldly asserting he would not stop until slavery ended. Garrison also actively focused on other social causes, including women's rights and education.

1850: Florence Nightingale: Mother of Nursing

Florence Nightingale was born in 1820 into an aristocratic British family that valued gender equality and Unitarian beliefs. Her father championed the education of both men and women, teaching her five languages, world history, and mathematics with the goal that she would use her education to serve society. At age 15, she had a spiritual experience that intensified her interest in humanitarian needs. Soon after, she combined her spiritual insights with her education, focusing on the humanistic needs of the sick and poor. She applied her mathematical skills to monitor her work and quickly gained recognition as a social reformer who used statistics to support her recommendations.

In 1850, Nightingale visited the Lutheran religious community at Kaiserswerth am Rhein in Germany, where the poor and sick received care from the Deaconess. Observing the Deaconess provide compassionate care to the sick and destitute, she decided to become a nurse. After completing her training in 1853, she returned to London and was soon appointed superintendent of the Hospital for the Care of Gentlewomen (Harley Street, n.d.).

The Crimean War started that year, and reports of injuries and deaths among British and French soldiers reached London. Nightingale contacted Sidney Herbert, the British Secretary of War, and volunteered to help. He agreed and assigned her the task of recruiting, organizing, and leading nurses to the battlefront in Scutari, Turkey. She successfully recruited 55 women, including 39 nurses and 15 nuns, arranged their travel, and departed unescorted for Scutari. They arrived in November 1854 to find sick and injured men starving and lying in filthy, unsanitary conditions. Nightingale ordered clean towels, bedding, soap, boilers to heat water, and other supplies to help them clean themselves and their environment, while directing the nurses on humane care for the wounded. Throughout the war, Nightingale organized and wrote notes to her nurses (Nightingale, 1915). She guided them in their work, emphasizing that nursing was a unique service, distinct from medicine, and highlighting the importance of each part of their role. She taught them how to provide compassionate care, and observe and record signs and symptoms of complications, health, and recovery. She insisted that they create and keep records to ensure continuity of care and assess their effectiveness (Nightingale, 1969).

1853: Mary Seacole

Mary Seacole was a Jamaican-born British citizen because of the island's colonization (National Library of Jamaica, 2025). She also kept track of reports about the war. Known as Mother Seacole, she believed that proper nutrition was essential for recovery when someone was sick or injured and declared her intention to go to Crimea to work with Florence Nightingale. Soon after her arrival, she offered her services but was turned down. Discouraged but still determined to provide nutritious food for the troops, she reached out to Alexis Soyer, a well-known chef in the area. He helped her set up a restaurant and bar where she prepared food and delivered it to the troops with little help. When she arrived with the food and supplies, she often changed dressings, comforted tired or injured soldiers, and listened to their stories (National Library of Jamaica, n.d.). After the war, Nightingale recognized Seacole for her efforts in providing nutritious food, kindness, and other caring actions that helped the soldiers survive and heal.

1859: Nursing's Shift from Providing Care to Healing

After the war, Nightingale compiled letters describing how to provide care and explaining why attending to the individual's human needs was nursing. She added comments and published *Notes on Nursing* in 1859. It provided a framework for nursing practice and offered evidence to establish nursing as a unique profession. She explained that medicine addresses the injury or illness of the soldier, while nurses focus on the care that "...puts the patient in the best condition for nature to act upon him" (Nightingale, 1969, p. 133). This was the first publication to clarify the core of nursing and its distinction from medicine. Nightingale also clearly stated that nursing must move from an informal activity in society to a role recognized by the community. Furthermore, nurses needed formal education based on scientific principles, emphasizing developing humanity's natural healing ability (Buhler-Wilkerson & D'Antonio, 2025).

Nightingale established the first nurse training program in 1860, at a time when most women could not attend school. Those who did typically focused on domestic skills and manners expected of a lady rather than the sciences needed for nursing. Her work paved the way for nurses and women to emerge and expand their societal roles, influencing the future of the United States.

In 1873, three schools influenced by Nightingale opened: Bellevue Training School for Nurses in New York, the Connecticut Training School for Nurses in New Haven, and the Boston Training School for Nurses at Massachusetts General Hospital.

1860: American Civil War and Nursing

As European society recovered from the Crimean War, social unrest grew in the United States. By 1861, living under Slavocratic principles contributed to the outbreak of the American Civil War. Thousands of men and women volunteered on both sides. Dorothea Dix, a champion of nondiscriminatory care, was appointed Superintendent of Union Army Nurses and tasked with organizing nursing services (Parry, 2006). Not well-prepared for administrative duties, Dix consulted Nightingale and relied on her expertise to meet the challenge. Her work laid the groundwork for the Union Sanitary Commission, which initially aimed to improve health care for sick and injured soldiers and later for civilians. Dix inspired over 3,000 women to volunteer in 400 hospitals with 400,000 beds.

1860: Civil War Nurses

Many women, including Harriet Tubman, volunteered during the Civil War (Bradford, 1886). Tubman escaped slavery early in the war, moved North, and served as a nurse for Black soldiers. She returned 13 times to the plantation where she had been enslaved to rescue her family and others still enslaved. Several other remarkable nurses of the American Civil War provided nondiscriminatory care to sick and wounded soldiers. Some included Clarissa Harlow Barton (Clara Barton), Susie King Taylor, Mary Ann Bickerdyke of the North, Sally Tomkins, and Phoebe Pember from the South (National Women's History Museum, n.d.). Each was recognized by Congress in 1892 for their outstanding contributions to society.

1861: Clara Barton and the Red Cross

Clarissa Barton, also known as Clara, organized groups of civilian men and women to provide impartial aid to wounded or sick soldiers. They carried water, prepared food, helped feed those in need, and assisted families in locating their loved ones—dead or alive—who had been separated by war. In 1881, Barton's efforts led to the formation of the International Federation of Red Cross and Red Crescent Societies (ICRC), a coalition of national Red Cross and Red Crescent organizations. Barton, who served as president of the Red Cross for 23 years, played a key role in passing the First Geneva Convention in the United States in 1864.

Today, the ICRC, with over 13,000 nurses, coordinates the world's largest humanitarian relief efforts during wars or natural disasters.

1865: Post-Civil War Society

Peace was declared on April 13, 1865, followed by a turbulent and uncertain period known as the Postwar Reconstruction Era (1865–1877). The government worked to reunite the seceded states while addressing the war's political, social, and economic legacies and managing the transition from an agricultural to an industrial economy. On December 11, 1865, the 13th Constitutional Amendment abolished slavery. In 1867, the United States purchased Alaska, furthering the dream of manifest destiny.

The 14th Amendment, ratified in 1868, granted citizenship to all people born or naturalized in the United States and prohibited depriving anyone of life, liberty, or property without due process. This amendment included Black men but not women. This difference was justified because the word "woman" was not in the Constitution. Many women disagreed, and Mary Mahoney was one of them. Spellman College for Black Women opened in 1870.

In 1870, Mary Eliza Mahoney, the daughter of two freed slaves, understood what inequality was like and vowed to secure the vote for women. She had worked as a janitor, cook, washerwoman, and nurse's aide, was able to attend nursing school at age 33 and was the first Black woman to complete a formal nursing program. She graduated Magna Cum Laude from Brown University in 1879, just as the country was entering the Jim Crow era when a series of laws aimed at preventing integration were passed. Mahoney never married or had children. Instead, she dedicated her life to society, focusing on educating Black nurses and advocating for women's suffrage. It was years of confronting segregation and Jim Crow laws before she realized her dream of voting (National Women's History Museum, n.d.). In the interim, the U.S. Government passed the 16th, 17th, and 18th amendments. The 16th and 17th amendments, ratified in 1913, prohibited the sale of liquor and gave the government the right to levy taxes and the states the right to elect Senators. The 18th Amendment prohibited the sale of liquor. The 19th amendment, ratified in 1920, gave women the right to vote. Mary Mahoney was one of the first to register to vote in Boston after the ratification of the 19th Amendment. Unfortunately, many Black women of the South could not register to vote until almost 50 years later (Spring, 2017). Spellman University opened the first nursing program for Black nurses in 1870.

When the five-month Spanish–American War broke out in April 1889, 15,000 nurses were called to serve; not all were trained. More than 280,000 soldiers participated; 3,000 died, with 2,000 deaths caused by disease. A postwar investigation indicated that nurses should be prepared for war, including care for those who contracted a disease as well as those who were injured. The Army Nurse Corps was established in 1901 to prepare nurses for many facets of the military. The United States acquired Puerto Rico and Guam as territories and the Philippines as protectorates. The founders' vision of manifest destiny was coming true.

1890: A Migration of Millions

After the war, millions migrated to the United States from Europe and other countries. Many more moved from the Southern states to the North. Many arrived in New York with little to no resources. Housing, food, clothing, and health services were urgently needed. Lillian Wald, a nurse, worked with hundreds of nurses who responded to society's humanitarian needs and helped establish the Henry Street Settlement and public health nursing. Some nurses worked for the government; others worked without pay. Wald's public housing project laid the foundation for President Johnson's Department of Housing and Urban Development (HUD), part of his Great Society program in the 1960s (Roterg, 2025).

By 2023, more than nine million people lived in public housing, and 467,211 public health nurses worked for state and federal agencies (AACN, 2024). Twenty-three public health nurses played various roles in the community, including serving as school nurses and case managers for families and individuals. Others collaborated with healthcare teams to develop and implement health promotion programs. Many acted as referral agents when needed, connecting people to social services.

1896: Nursing Organizes and Adapts

By the end of the century, nursing had defined its unique role and strengthened its ties with the community. Nurse educators founded the National League of Nursing (NLN) to standardize education (NLN, 2025); nurses from Canada and the United States formed the Associated Alumni of Trained Nurses of Canada and the United States (AATNCUS) to set ethical standards for nursing and support the NLN. Another cohort of nurses who were intent on supporting and promoting the international nursing profession, created the International Council of Nursing (American Association of Colleges of Nursing, 2024). Nursing was taking control of its role in society.

Nursing and Society in the 20th Century

1900: Nursing Evolves with a Growing U.S. Society

During the early years of the 20th century, the young society expanded and prospered. Newly discovered innovations such as electricity, improved transportation, telephones, typewriters, airplanes, cameras, new anesthesia, and vaccines contributed to better health and increased life expectancy. Society needed more educated nurses to meet the demands of a thriving population.

AATNCUS published the first edition of the *American Journal of Nursing* in 1900, and in 1901, the Colored Home and Training School graduated its first class of six students. Soon after, several State Nurse Associations were established, each aiming to prepare well-educated nurses needed in a growing society. Empowered by society's call and the support of nursing associations, nurses took on new roles. Lina Lavanceh Rogers was appointed the first public-school nurse in New York City.

As society evolved, nurses adapted. Sometimes, educational programs were secondary. Rather than hiring a nurse trained for a specific role, many roles were developed because society needed nurses to perform them. Educators recognized society's need and nursing adaptability and created educational programs to ensure that nurses acquired a core of knowledge that distinguished nursing from other professions.

New Zealand launched the first licensure and registration program for nurses in 1901. Meanwhile, in North Carolina, the first U.S. Nurse Practice Act was being developed. It became law and was adopted in 1903. The New Zealand Practice Act emphasized the importance of caring for the patient, the room, and the doctor. The U.S. Nurse Practice Act outlined the education and examination requirements for licensure. The integral relations between nursing and society continued to evolve. Nurses adapted to new roles as society changed, while simultaneously clarifying the essence of nursing.

1907: Formalizing Roles in Society

The School of Nurse-Midwives was established in 1907, and at the same time, Lillian Wald negotiated insurance payments for nursing care at home. In 1908, the NLN partnered with Columbia University to create an educational role for nurse faculty, and the Naval Nurse Corps was launched. Each of these developments formalized roles nurses performed for society's well-being.

Roles and educational opportunities expanded for educated white nurses, but not for Black nurses. Many were restricted from fully participating in society during the 20th century (Chamberlain University, n.d.). Most were still barred from enrolling in educational programs, and even after graduation, they faced restrictions from becoming registered nurses. In 1907, Ludie Andrews, a nurse who graduated from Spellman College, sued the Georgia State Board of Nursing for the right to take a nursing license exam. She won her lawsuit in 1919, years after serving society in multiple ways. Many other outstanding Black nurses worked tirelessly to ensure that Black nurses could become an integral part of society during the 20th century (Chamberlain University, n.d.).

1912: NLN Evolves and AATUCNS Splits

Nursing was progressing, but it still struggled to regulate itself and clearly define its role. The U.S. Bureau of Education published the first nursing status report in 1912. Adelaide Nutting, the author of the pre-report, stated that nursing could do more, but its education was limited by hospital administrators who controlled it (Nutting, 1912). The NLN took notice, changed its purpose and name, and became the National League of Nursing Education (NLNE). Building on Nightingale's work, NLNE challenged the standing premises that the care of the sick was overseen and directed by physicians. It declared nursing an independent profession that could operate with or without physicians, with or without collaboration, and that physicians should not order them.

AATUCNS recognized the importance of supporting organizations like the NLNE. The members created AATUCUS to support NLNE as an integral part of society. This legal move required them to remove references to Canada from their name. In 1912, AATUCUS became the American Nurses Association and the Canadian Nurses Association. Nursing was starting to build a power base and give voice to its unique societal role (Chamberlain University, n.d.).

1912: Rights of Sovereignty

Without restrictions, more hospital administrators, concerned about the quality and cost of nurses, launched programs tailored to their specific needs. This streamlined education model soon replaced the NLN's proposed model for professional practice and nursing's right to self-regulation. However, most nurses were women. Interconnected premises that affected their life were that physicians provided orders for nurses to follow, and the women's right to vote and nursing's right to define its core were questionable. The male-dominated government ignored the women's movement and focused on sovereignty issues; the 16th and 17th Amendments were passed in 1913, enabling federal taxation and states' direct election of Senators. The battles for women's suffrage and nurses' professional control remained ongoing.

Nursing education programs continued to evolve but not based on Nightingale's model of nursing. Both civilian and military nursing curricula were grounded in the Nurse Practice Acts but adapted to their respective systems' needs. Most continued to see the doctor's orders as the plan for care of the patient provided by all providers, including nursing . They ignored the 1912 Nutting Report on the Status of Nursing but recognized the NLNE. In 1915, the NLN published the first *Standard Curriculum Guide for Schools of Nursing* to promote standardization in education.

1914: WWI

Meanwhile, tensions in Europe increased as leaders argued over trade and land deals, held onto past resentments, and built up their military forces for defense. The assassination of Austria's Archduke in June 1914 triggered WWI. It then spread across the continent.

The United States adopted an isolationist stance but agreed to provide essential food and ammunition needed for Britain's war effort. In 1917, attacks on U.S. ships carrying supplies led to the United States joining the Allies. The American Red Cross mobilized 20,000 registered nurses for military service. They provided nondiscriminatory care to the wounded on the frontlines, risking their lives. One of them, Edith Cavell, lost her life to a German firing squad (Red Cross, 2025). Another, Olga Bing, documented her experiences through drawings. Her artwork is recognized for depicting the nondiscriminatory care that nurses provided to save lives on the battlefield during the war. When analyzed, her drawings reveal an ironic juxtaposition of the roles of nurses and soldiers. While nurses focused on saving lives, soldiers were engaged in combat and killing one another (Kenny & Kelley, 2019). Then, nature took its course, impacting the future of society.

1918: The Flu

The 1918 influenza pandemic affected one-fifth of the population and spread worldwide. The only known treatments focused on slowing the illness and managing complications like pneumonia. Common remedies included Vick's® VapoRub, aspirin, bed rest, sponge baths, whiskey, cough medicines, clean bedding, and hot soup, all best administered by nurses skilled in providing comforting care and monitoring for complications (Keeling, 2010). As the pandemic intensified, the U.S. military needed nurses in Europe to care for the sick and wounded, and in the United States to treat those sent home, as well as injured and sick German prisoners in the country (Clark, 2018).

Three strategies were launched to address the issue of protecting the home front. First, the U.S. Government assigned disabled, married, older, or non-white nurses to "home-defense" roles through the Red Cross. Non-white nurses not allowed to serve in Europe were tasked with caring for Germany's wounded soldiers, many of whom sympathized with the Nazis. Despite this, 1,800 Black nurses joined the Red Cross, and 18 other Black women became secretarial assistants for military administration in the Nurse Corps. Second, civilian hospitals established funded training programs that offered education, room, and board in exchange for students working as nurse aides and committing to a two-year work contract after graduation. Third, the Army School of Nursing adopted a similar model, with military personnel training students to serve as officers. These students worked as nursing aides during their training and vowed to serve two years after graduation. Although many students did not complete the military program, many continued working in military hospitals as aides or assistants after the WWI armistice in November 1918.

The Impact of the Unspoken Doctrine on Nursing

The perception that physicians were in charge of all care for hospitalized patients remained influential in many medical and certain nursing schools. Some institutions considered it an official policy until the early 21st century. With advances in medicine and technology, the nurturing, comforting care that General Gates saw as essential for saving lives in the 1700s was often viewed as unnecessary. Nursing care as Nightingale had defined it was considered a skill that women excelled in rather than a professional duty. As a result, many hospital programs focused on teaching students the necessary skills to facilitate the physician's plan of care rather than reinforcing the care of human needs. Nursing became increasingly vital to society, but the reasons for this remained unclear. It probably had little to do with General Gates' attitude; more likely, it was because nurses could be trusted to follow physicians' orders and were caring and kind.

1920: A Growing Society and Hope for the Future

After the 1918–1919 pandemic, the United States focused on rebuilding for the future. Many European immigrants and rural residents moved to cities for better opportunities. Technological advancements from WWI, such as mobile X-ray machines and blood banks, promised longer lifespans. Hospitals evolved into places for acute care and recovery with expert nursing care. Nurses continued to expand their roles in society. Nurse anesthetists, who had provided anesthesia since the Civil War, founded the American Association of Nurse Anesthetists.

1929: The Boom and the Crash

Society and nursing were thriving. Economic growth created jobs and improved lifestyles. Nurses were establishing independent roles in society, gaining professional autonomy. People saved money and deposited it; others invested in the stock market; and banks provided loans to farmers and stock investors, believing growth would continue. Interest rates rose from 12 to 20 percent over 10 years, signaling trouble ahead. By early 1928, signs of an economic slowdown appeared. The market was flooded with unnecessary products, and sales declined, especially in cars, radios, refrigerators, and agricultural goods, which affected the stock market, causing a sharp drop. People started losing jobs. Farmers could not repay their loans; investors lost money in the stock market and could not pay off their margin loans. Within a year, many farmers went bankrupt and lost their farms, and investors also went bankrupt. Banks shut down across the United States.

A recession hit, causing the Great Depression of 1929–1939, which affected every part of global society. Many people, including nurses, lost their jobs. People became malnourished, homeless, sick, and hopeless. Soup kitchens and other services opened to help low-income individuals. Many unemployed nurses volunteered their humanitarian services at these makeshift places for the respite of those in need, often serving soup and caring for the sick or injured for long hours each day.

1933: The Great New Deal

Roosevelt, elected U.S. President in 1933, immediately began supporting those in need through the Great New Deal programs. Three of his planned initiatives focused on the relations between nursing and society. First, the Federal Relief Fund paid nurses $25 a month to care for the sick and the depleted in rural areas. Second, the Civilian Conservation Corps created jobs for thousands of Americans, including roles for nurses to care for the workers. Third, the Social Security Act (SSA) provided relief for mothers, children, the disabled, and the uninsured, with nurses playing a key role in designing and delivering some of these services. Nurses did what they do best: they adapted, problem-solved, and provided services where needed (Pollitt & Reese, 1997).

The Black community continued to face limitations in the social services they received. In 1932, Aliene Carrington Ewell and 11 registered nurses (known collectively as the "12 Jewels") founded the Chi Eta Phi Sorority, promoting health programs for their community with the motto "Service for Humanity." Chi Eta Phi became a major provider of health promotion and disease prevention programs for Black communities. In 2025, they reported over 9,000 members with chapters across the United States and the Virgin Islands (Chi Eta Phi, n.d.).

1941: International Turmoil Escalates into World War II

As the United States recovered from the Great Depression of 1929, unrest grew in Europe and Southeast Asia. Japan attacked China in 1937, and Germany conquered Poland in 1939, followed by France and other European countries. Although the United States declared neutrality, nurses anticipated war and formed the Nursing Council on National Defense. Japan attacked Oahu on December 7, 1941. The United States, caught in the Southeast Asia conflict, joined the Allies in the European war that same day.

The following month, 26 allied nations gathered in New York City and signed an agreement to collaborate in winning the war. During World War II, 60,000 Army nurses and 14,000 Navy and Air Force nurses participated in military operations, providing anesthesia, assisting in surgeries, and caring for soldiers (ANC, n.d.). Over 200 nurses were captured as prisoners. A total of 201 lost their lives carrying out duties (The WWII Medical Research Center, n.d.). The relations between the military as protectors of the United States and nurses as caregivers for injured soldiers serving to defend was strengthened. This bond continued to shape the core of nursing and how the public viewed it.

1945: WWII and the Right to Health

The allied nations regrouped after the war, pledged to maintain international peace and security, and drafted the United Nations Charter. They agreed that human rights are essential for freedom, and health is a fundamental human right. The World Health Organization (WHO) was established in 1948 to develop programs that promote health and prevent the spread of disease globally. The preamble of the first WHO Charter defined *health* as complete physical, mental, and social well-being, not just the absence of disease or infirmity. Their Charter also stated that everyone has the right to health, and a healthy population is vital for peace and security (Schramme, 2023). Although it took several years and more wars for it to emerge, the stage was set for Deva-Marie Beck and Barbara Dossey to emphasize the integral relations between society and nursing as they created the Nightingale Initiative for Global Health, launched in 2006 (Beck, 2021).

1945: Society's Need for Nursing Role Expands

World War II led to new discoveries that benefited humanity during peacetime. Medicine determined that many wartime deaths were caused by limb infections or gangrene resulting from loss of circulation. Battlefield care involved applying tourniquets to stop blood loss, but transfer delays caused tissue necrosis and infections. Medical scientists focused on the best ways to treat arterial wounds, while biological scientists worked on disease prevention. Their work helped society manage epidemics during peace and war and saved lives in future conflicts.

1950: From Home Care to the Hospital

A polio epidemic emerged in the early 1950s. Polio had been a minor issue in the United States for years, with only a few scattered cases. The only known treatments were warm soaks and massages to ease painful muscle spasms. Most people received care at home; many died. When the epidemic appeared in the 1950s, healthcare professionals understood that polio was contagious, attacked the muscular system, and often caused paralysis that affected the respiratory system. The cause and transmission method were still unknown, but now, they had the iron lung to help people breathe during the acute phase and trained nurses to care for them (Dunphy, 2001).

Specialized isolated units, called intensive care units (ICUs), were created to group patients with similar medical conditions. The healthcare team, now led by nurses, customized care to each patient's needs. The nurses observed what helped patients breathe more easily, motivated their recovery, and shared their insights with the team. Many recovered enough to live full lives because of their specialized care during their illness.

Nurses developed keen observation skills, as described by Nightingale, and were able to teach these to their colleagues. They had not yet realized that their ability to combine the art and science of care was a scholarly activity or that they were emerging scholars. They did not understand that articulating the essence of nursing practice is vital for societal benefit and for overcoming the belief that physician's orders directed all care of the sick , a practice that was common in the hospitals of the time.

1950: Global Unrest Leading to War

During the polio epidemic in the United States, social unrest was increasing worldwide. Russia occupied East Berlin, was heavily involved in North Korea (Wilson Center, n.d.), and aimed to spread communism in Europe. When North Korea invaded South Korea, the United Nations authorized a police action led by the U.S. military in 1950. An armistice was signed in 1953, leaving North Korea under a communist regime and South Korea under the protection of the United States. Vietnam was also divided after WWII. In 1946, the North was influenced and supported by China. The French tried to recolonize the South to stop the spread of communism. By the mid-1950s, the French military was exhausted and making little progress in recolonization. WWII Allies worried that if South Vietnam fell to North Vietnam, communism might take over the entire Southeast Asia. The United States joined the conflict in 1955.

1955: Collaboration Saved Lives

With vaccines available, contagious diseases were no longer the primary concern during wartime. Medical efforts shifted toward addressing arterial damage, a recurring problem identified during World War II and the Korean War. Mobile Army Surgical Hospitals (MASH units) were strategically positioned near the battlefront throughout South Vietnam to reduce delays in medical care. Corpsmen, surgeons, and nurses worked together as a unified team. The team focused on saving limbs and lives using advanced resuscitation and surgical techniques. On the battlefield, corpsmen resuscitated soldiers, controlled bleeding with modern tourniquets, administered pain relief medication, and ensured rapid transport to nearby MASH units. Surgeons, assisted by nurses and corpsmen, diagnosed and treated injuries, while nurses provided critical bedside care and monitored for secondary complications from Agent Orange and other toxic herbicides. The fatality rate for severe wounds decreased from 4.5 percent in World War II to 2.5 percent during the Korean War and further declined to 2 percent in Vietnam (Army Medical Department, n.d.). The war required that society produce a steady stream of educated nurses.

1960s: Nurses Problem-Solve

Nurse educators aimed to find more cost-effective ways to produce a steady flow of trained nurses, while nurse theorists continued to explore the core of nursing. The educators emphasized the importance of speeding up the process of training nurses to meet society's diverse needs. Recognizing that many aspiring nurses lacked access to or funds for diploma or four-year college programs, they proposed that a two-year associate degree (ADN) focusing on basic nursing skills could help students progress faster than traditional diploma or BSN programs. This approach would enable students to start working sooner and gradually advance through higher levels of education.

Two-year ADN programs emerged in community colleges, allowing students to take the RN exam and then continue their degrees through RN-BSN programs at the same colleges. Many institutions developed RN-BSN programs to provide a clear pathway for these students, as well as for those graduating from diploma programs. Nursing was temporarily addressing a staffing shortage but was still working on clarifying role definitions. Nurse theorists contributed to the discussion.

In 1960, Virginia Henderson, building on Nightingale's work, published *Basic Principles of Nursing Care,* emphasizing that nurses should help patients meet their needs as if they could. She promoted nursing education in colleges instead of hospitals (Cordeau, 2020). Lydia Hall advocated for a nursing process she defined as the Three C Theory: care (nursing), cure (medicine), and core (patient needs). She also stated that those injured recover faster if professional nurses advocate for them during rehabilitation.

Ida Jean Orlando promoted a systematic approach emphasizing critical thinking, patient-centered care with goal-oriented tasks, evidence-based practice, and nursing intuition. She argued that nursing is a dynamic process rooted in interpersonal relationships and can be guided by Maslow's hierarchy of needs. Faye Abdellah, who published *Patient Centered Approaches in Nursing*, reminded nurses that doctors cure and nurses care. In 1965, she became the first nurse to serve as Deputy Surgeon General, continuing to advocate for the idea that doctors cure, nurses care (Cordeau, 2020). Nurses were moving closer to clarifying their unique roles but still working harmoniously with societal changes.

1964: Conundrum and the Nurse Training Act (NTA)

The government faced a dilemma: society needed more nurses for civilian hospitals, and the military required well-educated nurses for MASH units in Vietnam, but nursing education in colleges was costly. Congress proposed the Nurse Training Act to provide funds for new educational facilities, refurbishing existing ones, and offering loans to those aspiring to become nurses.

Three Black nurses, Mabel Staupers, Mary Elizabeth Carnegie, and Esteele Riddle Osborne, saw their opportunity. They presented research data showing that the main cause of a nursing shortage was the prohibition of people of color from enrolling in most nursing programs. Title VI of the Civil Rights Act, passed in 1965, outlawed such discrimination. The NTA was enacted on September 4, 1964, with a clause requiring compliance with the law as a condition for receiving funds. For the first time, individuals of color who wanted to become nurses were allowed to enroll in educational programs that had previously been limited to white students (Anchrum, 2025).

1965: A War-Weary Nation

Ten years into the Vietnam War, society was growing exhausted from the conflict. Daily protests erupted across the country. Thousands of soldiers had been killed, and many more were permanently maimed. Numerous people returned home with physical disabilities that limited their ability to work. Others suffered from PTSD and found it hard to reintegrate into society. Some developed chronic health problems caused by the toxic effects of Agent Orange, fumes from burning oil, and other herbicides. Some faced ostracism because of their participation in the war; most veterans felt alienated and struggled to reconnect with their communities. VA Veteran Centers opened, along with other services, but more support was still needed. It took time for the government to recognize the long-term effects of combat trauma and their societal impact. Many families became disenfranchised members of their communities (Ngô & Nguyễn, 2024).

1965: A Need for Social Services

By the mid-1960s, 70 percent of employed Americans had hospital insurance, but less than 50 percent of older adults were covered, and many others struggled to obtain insurance. Congress amended the Social Security Act, adding Medicare and Medicaid (National Association of Social Insurance, 2025). This allowed more people to access hospital and clinic care, which the WHO Charter considered a basic human right. It also shifted the cost of care from local hospitals to the U.S. government, reducing hospitals' income and causing a domino effect.

Most hospitals used to be non-profit and had limits on what they could charge. Their profit margins decreased since they received less money for a hospital stay. However, they needed more nurses to care for patients who previously could not access the hospital. Many non-profit hospitals were sold or turned into for-profit or different not-for-profit organizations, which operate under different rules. This change has led to higher hospital costs for everyone.

While the U.S. government addressed the humanitarian needs of older adults and those unable to care for themselves with the introduction of Medicare and Medicaid, it was a temporary solution (Berkowitz, 2005). The international community took a different approach. The United Kingdom, Sweden, Iceland, Norway, Denmark, and Finland adopted the WHO's stance and transitioned to a national healthcare system that offers equal access for all citizens. By 2025, 80 countries had adopted this model.

1970 and Beyond: "Shifting Paradigm" and Its Effect

As models of medical care evolved, Lawrence Weed proposed that medical students focus on identifying problems and objectively determining the best treatment approaches. This record-keeping method became known as the Problem-Oriented Medical Recording (POMR) system. The POMR system included four types of information in medical records: subjective notes, objective notes, assessment notes, and planning notes. This approach is known as SOAP charting.

Weed's proposal for integrating POMR and SOAP charting gained widespread acceptance across the continent, leading to significant changes in healthcare practices. Electronic records were created around medical diagnoses and adopted accordingly. Instead of using Orlando's nursing process based on Maslow's hierarchy of needs, nurses documented patients' responses to medical treatments aimed at addressing biomedical issues. As a result, traditional nursing skills like bed baths and nightly care were largely discontinued.

Many nurses aimed to address the humanistic aspects of nursing but were not instructed on how to incorporate these into their practice, nor were they recognized for attending to humanistic needs. Additionally, new graduates often focused primarily on tasks related to medical issues. Although some were interested in discussing patients' human needs, it was difficult to record this on standardized or electronic charts, which prioritized medical problems. Over time, the emphasis on individualized, holistic care gradually faded from their conscious practice. Nonetheless, many continued to provide compassionate care and engage with patients as individuals.

By the mid-1980s, there was a significant shift toward biomedical sciences in nursing, leading to the closure of hospital-based programs and an increase in community college–based programs. At the same time, medical advancements were rapidly progressing. Medical conditions once considered untreatable could now be managed, resulting in greater specialization in the medical field. Nursing also expanded with more graduate programs focused on roles related to these medical conditions.

1980s: Nursing's Voice in the Mid-Late 20th Century

During the later part of the 20th century, more nurse theorists published their views on nursing, including Martha Rogers, Margaret Newman, and Jean Watson (Cordeau, 2020). Other nurse theorists joined the discussion in the early 1980s. Each offered nurses alternative ways to think about their professional roles.

While the core of nursing was becoming clearer for some, it remained unclear for those in clinical practice. Many continued to struggle with adapting their roles to meet the specific needs of different societal groups. To make matters worse, graduate programs were often designed to prepare nurses for emerging societal roles without emphasizing the fundamental principles of holistic nursing.

1982: Holistic Nurses Gather

Inspired by Nightingale's holistic view, a group of nurses formed the American Holistic Nurses Association (AHNA) to promote compassionate, whole-person care in modern nursing. They emphasized holistic nursing as essential to humanistic caring and healing (Hanley et al., 2017). The AHNA outlined its values, principles, and standards of care, hosted conferences, and validated holistic practices. Membership grew, and publications clarified their stance. In 1995, they published the first edition of *Scope and Standards: Holistic Nursing* and started holistic nursing certification programs. A practice analysis study led to the creation of the American Holistic Nurses Credentialing Corporation (AHNCC), which held its first certification exam in 1998.

1983: The Prospective Payment System

Recognizing the high costs of Medicare and Medicaid, the government introduced the Prospective Payment System (PPS) in 1983. The PPS model used statistics to classify patients by their medical diagnosis and expected recovery time. Upon admission, patients were categorized based on a DRG (Diagnosis-Related Group) and assigned a fixed number of hospital days for which Medicare would reimburse (National Association of Social Insurance, 2025). The goal was to deliver quality care within those days, allowing patients to recover and go home. There was a limited period for receiving additional care. The hospital would assume responsibility for all expenses if patients were readmitted for the same condition within that period. Hospitals accepting Medicare or Medicaid patients had to agree to these terms to qualify for reimbursement.

With the PPS in place, federal funds supported research to identify best practices for reducing hospital stays while improving health outcomes. Studies found that early mobilization and walking after surgery led to faster recovery and fewer complications (Abeles et al., 2017). Others showed that patients could recover at home, avoiding extended hospital stays. As a result, surgeries were followed by discharge within a day or two, emphasizing rapid patient mobilization and discharge. Hospital stay durations decreased, and nursing education focused on a biomedical care model.

1983: Nursing's Relation to Society

That same year, the ANA drafted the first Social Policy Statement, defining society's expectations and nursing obligations. The document clearly stated that nursing had a contractual relationship with society but was not specific about how to define that relationship. It suggested that nursing identifies and treats symptoms related to medical diagnoses while also advocating for the health and well-being of society. Three more versions of Nursing's Social Policy Statement were published before it was proposed that nursing has a covenant with society that differs from a contract. This covenant is based on shared ethics and should guide nursing education and practice (Fowler, 2008a). Meanwhile, nursing continued to define its boundaries and Fowler continued to discuss the ethics of nursing's boundaries (2008b).

1984: The Metaparadigm

Hardy proposed that nursing adopt a paradigm to distinguish it from medicine in 1978. Fawcett (1984) analyzed the literature and identified four major constructs defining a metaparadigm: health, environment, person, and nursing. Nursing's metaparadigm gained widespread acceptance by 1986. The NLN used the metaparadigm to evaluate programs submitted for accreditation. It was expected that faculty would use the metaparadigm to shape their programs and develop courses necessary for its implementation. Faculty were challenged to demonstrate consistency and alignment among the school's mission and purpose, values and beliefs, and educational programs. They also needed to show how their programs related to society.

1990: About Nursing and Society

By the mid-1990s, the American Nurses Association recognized that many nurses struggled to clearly define their roles; some even confused them with those of medicine. Workgroups were formed to address this issue and offer recommendations. Marsha Fowler (2015) and colleagues released a new version of Nursing's Ethics, clarifying its principles and providing guidance for their application. Despite these efforts, educational models continued to focus on the biomedical model of care, which was supported by societal funding sources.

Although demonstration projects received sporadic funding from the NIH that supported nurses' work, few follow-up studies focused on individuals' humanistic needs. Society had come to trust nurses as genuine, trustworthy people, but it had not yet understood what nurses did to foster that trust. Nursing needed to clearly define its unique role in society so its members could be fully supported and empowered to uphold society's core values.

Society, Shifting Paradigms, and Holistic Nursing in the 21st Century

2001: Compassionate Care to the Maximum Possible

Early in the new century, studies were undertaken by The Institute of Medicine (IOM) to identify the needs for the 21st century, and it was recommended that consumers be included as active members of the healthcare team. Nursing practice should consist of compassionate, holistic care, and nurses should practice to their fullest abilities based on their education (IOM, 2011). The ANA updated its Scope and Standards for Practice, Code of Ethics, and Social Policy Statements. Nursing created new graduate nurse practitioner programs, while both nursing and medicine developed integrated healthcare and wellness coaching programs.

Holistic nursing recognized the movement, revised its documents, and established new certification programs. AHNA and AHNCC collaborated to develop standards and competencies for both basic and graduate holistic nurses. The first exams took place in 1999 and 2004, respectively. AHNA sought recognition of holistic nursing as a specialty and received it in 2006.

2004: Nursing, Society, War, and the 21st Century

Nursing and society were in transition at the turn of the century, with intersecting civil and military events affecting the well-being of society. Graduate enrollments increased, global rural-to-urban migration was underway, and new technology created an internet superhighway connecting communities worldwide. The world sought balance while adapting to these changes. However, it was distracted when an attack on New York City, Washington, D.C., and Shanksville, Pennsylvania, occurred on September 11, 2001, shocking the world. Suddenly, backed by the United Nations, the United States was at war with Afghanistan, which lasted until 2021, and by extension with Iraq from 2003 to 2011. About 2.5 million men and women from the United States were deployed to support these wars. Once again, more nurses were needed to support the war efforts and meet society's growing needs. Over 6,300 nurses, along with 3,000 women who fought as soldiers, served in the military during this period. Over 20,700 US soldiers were wounded and an additional 917 US soldiers died, including 139 women, 1,144 allied soldiers plus nearly 500 humanitarian workers, 72 journalists, more than 66,000 Afghan military and more than 47,000 Afgahn civilians died in this war (A-Mark Foundation, 2021). Strategies learned during Vietnam, combined with new science driven by the PPS model of civilian care, saved lives but left many with postwar sequelae requiring new and additional services. Nurses' demand grew as societies worldwide faced new challenges. The 19th century was ending, taking with it the comfort of societal familiarity. Time was fostering an international society, with all that this meant for countries organized around competition and otherness.

Technology has made the world smaller with the rise of the superhighway. Many barriers, such as distance, languages, and transportation, are being eliminated. People can now communicate and collaborate with others on the other side of the globe and translate languages through their computers or phones. Research findings are now shared widely through open-access publishing. Countries are working together to produce parts where resources are plentiful and transport them overnight to other nations to finish the production of cars, bicycles, kitchenware, and many other products used in society today. Artificial intelligence also promises to be a significant force in the 21st century. It is with these ways of knowing that holistic nurses can be change agents (National Academies of Sciences, Engineering, and Medicine, 2009).

Three nurses, Deva-Marie Beck, Barbara Dossey, and Louise Selanders, met at the ICN Centennial Conference in 1999 to share their views on nursing in the next century. They discussed the relevance of Nightingale's work in modern nursing and explored ways to "follow her footsteps into the 21st century" (NIGH, 2025). They envisioned a world where nurses, students, and concerned citizens are empowered to act as global advocates for health. As they invited nurses from around the world, their conversations led to the creation of the "Nightingale Initiative for Global Health" (NIGH), launched in 2006. They have spoken at the United Nations several times, worked with the World Health Organization and Nations Civil Society Development Forums, and in 2009, they received United Nations DPI-NGO Status. They have also sponsored several global group presentations, each recorded and available for others to learn from. NIGH has strengthened the international relations between nursing and society for those willing to "carry the lamp." To quote Beck,

> As nurses create our own shifts—to deepen our caring consciousness and reconnect with a renewed sense of "calling" in nursing—we can rekindle our own lamps and carry Nightingale's vision of caring, healing, and leading—with a broader awareness that everything we do affects health and healing everywhere. This is a fitting development because the word "nurse" comes from the Latin nutrire, meaning "nourish." Nurses—with exemplary empathy, compassion, caring, and wisdom—nourish countless people on their journeys from birth to death. (Beck, 2021)

2006: The APRN Movement

As graduate programs expanded to meet emerging roles proposed by the IOM studies, State Boards of Nursing faced pressure to approve them. A group of nurses representing the National Council of State Boards of Nursing (NCSBN) created a new designation that reflected these emerging advanced practice roles, called the Advanced Practice Registered Nurse (APRN). Recognized roles such as nurse midwives, nurse anesthetists, clinical nurse specialists, and newly established nurse practitioners were identified as APRNs. Future educational programs required standardized coursework aligned with each state's practice act, including three core courses applicable to all APRN programs. Licensure was granted to individuals who completed a recognized program based on the state's practice act and passed the role-specific certification exam. The Board of Nursing would also grant prescriptive authority within the state where the APRN practiced.

AHNCC and other organizations protested the limited scope of the APRN designation in 2004. In 2006, the role was approved as part of the Consensus Model. The announcement stated that others could apply for APRN status and be considered by the LACE committee (Licensure, Accreditation, Certification, Education, and Nursing Advocacy). AHNCC applied for the Advanced Practice Holistic Nursing (APHN) (American Holistic Nurses Credentialing Corporation, 2016) role to be recognized, but their application was denied.

2010: Society, Congress, the APHN, and a Covenant

Data had been circulating since the beginning of the century, indicating that 26 million U.S. citizens lacked healthcare insurance. People aged 18–24 were twice as likely to be uninsured compared to the overall population under 65. The percentage of Native American, Alaska Native, and Hispanic individuals without insurance was higher than that of white people, and the percentage of low-income, uninsured workers' families was higher than that of those with higher incomes. Despite this, the United States spends more per person on health care than any other country (The Commonwealth Fund, 2014).

Congress passed the Patient Protection and Affordable Care Act (ACA) in 2010. This law, aligned with the WHO's definition of health, reaffirming health as a human right. National recognition of health as a human right encouraged AHNCC to further pursue APRN status for the APHN-BC role. AHNCC drafted a position statement (AHNCC, 2013) and submitted another application explaining how the Advanced Holistic Nursing Certification program, standards, competencies, and courses met criteria for APRN status.

While waiting for a reply, the AHNCC Board and the CMTF collaborated to further clarify the role and create a corresponding examination for the APHN-BC nurse. Four courses were drafted to prepare students for prescriptive authority, paralleling the required courses for APRNs. The first examination was administered in 2013 (Erickson et al., 2013). The AHNCC application was denied because the role was unclear and lacked specification of the advanced practice role.

AHNCC created the Consensus Model Task Force (CMTF) of Holistic Nurses in 2014 with the charge to further clarify and define the APHN role and continue the appeal for a 5th role in the Consensus Model. The CMTF drafted a third application stating that all AHNCC certifications at the graduate level are based on graduate education while clarifying the APHN educational program that prepares the graduate nurse to practice to the fullest of their education.

The APHN worked to meet the charges, built on the AHN-BC role, and further clarified courses that prepared nurses to apply for APRN status. The *Foundations, Competencies, and Curricular Guidelines for Basic to Doctoral Holistic Nursing Education, First Edition* was published (AHNCC, 2017). It specified the curricular program needed for graduate-level holistic nurses and clarified how the three required courses included in the Consensus Model were addressed with comparable outcomes but based on the perspective of eudemonistic health rather than a biomedical model (American Holistic Nurses Credentialing Corporation, 2017). Another appeal was submitted to LACE and was rejected.

A follow-up discussion with members of LACE was requested. During the follow-up meeting they did not explain their reason for rejection. However, they mentioned that disseminating the

Compact Agreement for APRN Ratification was in progress and that adding another role could be confusing. Their final comments were that the APHN-BC appeared to meet the criteria, and AHNCC should try again with more specific details about the four required courses.

Webinars were created to explain the APHN-BC role and the required courses, and several sessions were presented at the AHNA conferences. The webinars were offered, and positive feedback was received. A third request was submitted to LACE, including tables and narratives comparing the APRN and the APHN, and details about the webinars.

However, it was also rejected. The rejection this time was twofold: the distribution of the Compact Agreement phase for the Consensus Model to the state Boards for ratification, and the perception that the role was redundant because all nurses are holistic. Both reasons confused the AHNCC leadership. The first issue arose because LACE members continued to state that new roles could be added, yet the APHN-BC was rejected because it was too late.

The second reason was confusing because ANA had designated holistic nursing as a specialty in 2006, while representatives of the NCSBN had recently claimed that all nurses are holistic. AHNCC sought advice from a colleague familiar with LACE's work. The colleague commented that the problem was threefold: members of LACE did not understand the value or essence of holistic nursing; did not understand the difference between clinical health, based on a biomedical model of health and holistic nursing, based on a eudemonistic model of health; and AHNCC was targeting the wrong group if they wanted recognition. The colleague proposed that, instead, AHNCC needed to partner with society.

The CMTF took time to reflect and read the current literature and concluded that holistic nursing is a specialty, and when the members share a common purpose, values, and/or beliefs, they create a cohort who has the potential to create a society where there are mutual relations between the members and their society. Thus, the society's well-being depends on how well the individual supports the beliefs and values of the society, and vice versa (Thomas, 2025).

The CMTF reflected on these perspectives, analyzed the paradigms of Nursing, and determined that ANA's recognition of holistic nursing as a specialty presents a dilemma—and that the dilemma could, in fact, be the solution to their problem with LACE. The question for holistic nursing to consider was the differing perspectives on what health means, and how the philosophies and dimensions of health should be taught and practiced.

Society, the Individual, and Nursing

Some may argue that nurses are members of healthcare teams serving society, and health is health—all nurses have a contract outlining each party's responsibilities. Marsha Fowler's 2015 version of Nursing's Social Policy Statement was revisited to better understand this issue.

Fowler, known for her work on nursing ethics, took a different approach to discuss the relations between nursing and society. She challenged the idea that nurses have a contract with society and suggested that, instead, the profession's ethics call for nursing to have a covenant with society (Fowler, 2015). She clarified that a contract is a business agreement between two entities that facilitates transactional communication. A covenant is a commitment aligned with the values and beliefs of oneness and the desire for the "common good" that is enacted using the ethics of the profession. She stated that it transforms the nature of oneself through the covenant relationship, which brings the nurse into solidarity with the other person. She stated, "I come to experience the covenant relationship, the solidarity of being with another, to know… intimately, ontologically, the shared human condition" (Fowler, 2015, p. 113).

She added that it is through these processes that nurses gain wisdom and an understanding of the common good, where social networks aim to create conditions that enable human individuals and groups to flourish and live an entirely genuine life.

Fowler's words reflected the values and beliefs of the CMTF. They concluded that a covenant exceeds a contract with society; it is a moral commitment that arises from a heartfelt understanding that this is one's purpose. The reward for the nurse is being with others, facilitating their healing, and sharing in their life journey. The holistic nurse's covenant is to become one with the individual or group within a society and to help them flourish.

Recognizing these self-truths, the CMTF affirmed that strengthening its covenant with society was more important than being recognized by LACE as APRNs. They committed to launching a new organization that would give voice to and disseminate the wisdom of holistic nurses. The goal was to provide a platform for affirming members as scholar and to create a community where dialogues could expand and clarify the wisdom of the scholars and their relations with society.

2020: New Relations

The Global Academy of Holistic Nursing (GAHN) was conceived by the CMTF and launched in March 2020 to promote holistic nursing globally. The first group of scholars was inducted in June 2020, and committees were formed to advance scholarship. Dialogues began to clarify holistic nursing scholarship, with recent discussions focusing on holistic nursing wisdom. An annual Congress provides opportunities to learn more about the organization, and proposals for curriculum development are underway, suggesting an integrated model for 21st-century nursing education. In 2023, GAHN and NIGH established a formal partnership, with NIGH hosting sessions where nursing students from around the world discuss nursing in the 21st century, the unique needs of their societies, uncertainties they face, and how they respond.

Validation in 2021 and 2025

In 2021, the IOM published *The Future of Nursing 2020 to 2030*, highlighting nursing's role in society and emphasizing health and well-being as a human right (National Academies of Sciences, Engineering, and Medicine, 2021). Nurses were given the go-ahead to step forward, take their role in society, and practice from a humanitarian perspective, remembering that humans are holistic beings. It confirmed society's need for holistic nurses.

Concurrently, faculty from Harvard University partnered with faculty from Baylor University who were interested in what affects a flourishing society. Together, they partnered with Gallup, Inc., and the Center for Open Science (COS) and created the Human Flourishing Program (2025), assuming that a flourishing society was integral with members who shared values and beliefs and perceived that they were flourishing (Thomas, 2025).

They clarified six factors of human life previously identified by VanderWheele (2017) thought to contribute to one's well-being: happiness, health, purpose, character, relations, and housing and financial stability. Each factor was assessed with two questions each. Data were collected over five years from 207,000 individuals representing 22 diverse countries.

The data indicated that the number one factor contributing to a flourishing life was to have purpose and meaning in life; perceiving stability in life—have financial security and a roof over one's head—was the least important factor. Indonesia had the highest overall flourishing score with all six factors considered, while the United States ranked 12th among the 22 countries. Factors influencing flourishing varied across countries (Harvard University's Human Flourishing Program, 2025). The Flourishing Program provides additional support for holistic nursing's covenant with society and provides direction for further collaboration with society. It is time for holistic nursing to step forth, to give voice to their beliefs, prepare nursing students accordingly, and proactively provide services to society as needed.

The Implications for Holistic Nursing

The first 25 years of the 21st century have been disruptive, sometimes chaotic, and often challenging for the global population. Political division among people and wars between nations have resulted in damage to many and the cost of life to others. Floods, tornadoes, and other natural disasters have added to the burden. Countries have pulled out of international treaties and agreements that provided support and resources needed, ultimately isolating and blaming others without considering the harm caused by such attitudes.

Relations within communities and across societies, marked by division among individuals, have created a culture of insecurity, mistrust, fear, anger, and hostility, which impacts the ability of groups and communities to compromise and work together. Societies worldwide face the risk of disintegration and collapse. The future lies ahead. The world is on the brink of a new time, what it will be like depends on what happens now. Holistic nurses are needed more than ever before.

It is time for holistic nurses to work together, to perceive their work as a service to individuals within a local society while envisioning its impact on the global society. To do this, holistic nurses must give voice to their covenant with society and their abilities to facilitate healing through compassionate, caring-healing processes and to articulate the significance of this way of knowing and being as foundational to the role of holistic nursing.

It is not the work of holistic nurses to promise to cure or solve every problem, but to commit to loving and accepting others unconditionally, to be a light in dark places, to provide the safe space where others can find the beauty within themselves, to learn, grow, heal and transition with grace wherever and whenever indicated.

To be change agents, holistic nurses must learn to trust themselves as facilitators who nurture others, know that small acts of kindness have power that takes on a sequence of changes, give meaning to life, and have the potential to affect the culture within a society. They can create healing spaces that will provide room and resources needed for the humans' natural propensity to take over, and in doing this they can initiate a healing process that has the potential to heal a nation and create global transformation. They can be a light during dark times and find meaning in their work through these acts.

It is with these ways of knowing and being that holistic nurses can be change agents. It is with voice coupled with small acts of kindness, respect, and compassion that holistic nurses can once again partner with society, to help it move through a time of distress to a new beginning or not. Each holistic nurse is challenged to reflect on their choice as an individual and as a member of a cohort of colleagues and determine what role they will perform in the remainder of the 21st century and beyond.

There is no possibility of not having an effect; we all affect the culture and well-being of those we interact with. In turn, this ripples out and affects the global society. The question for the reader to ponder is this: *What ripple-out effect do you want to impact the future of humanity*?

As Nightingale once commented, it will be what we make it (Nightingale, 1873).

Summary

This chapter explores the important link between holistic nursing and society, tracing its development from the 18th century to the present. It emphasizes the moral commitment of holistic nurses to their communities and highlights the importance of compassionate, patient-centered care. The discussion covers how historical events, such as wars and social movements, have influenced nursing practices and societal perceptions. It also examines the challenges that nurses face in communicating their unique role and the significance of their work. The chapter concludes with reflections on the future of holistic nursing and its potential to drive societal change and improve well-being, concluding with an invitation to holistic nursing to proactively participate in the future of society by doing what they do best.

References

Abeles, A., Kwasnicki, R., Pettengell, C., & Murphy, J. (2017). The relationship between physical activity and post-operative length of hospital stay: A systematic review. *International Journal of Surgery, 44*, 295–302.

A-Mark Foundation. (2023, September 18). Afghanistan war: U.S deaths and costs. *A-Mark Foundation*. https://amarkfoundation.org/reports/afghanistan-war-costs/.

American Association of Colleges of Nursing. (2024). *Nursing workforce fact sheet*. https://www.aacnnursing.org/news-data/fact-sheets/nursing-workforce-fact-sheet

American Holistic Nurses Credentialing Corporation. (2017). *Foundations, competencies, and curricular guidelines*. https://www.ahncc.org/wp-content/uploads/2018/10/ Foundations-Competencies-Curricular-Guidelines.pdf

American Holistic Nurses Credentialing Corporation. (2013). *APRN position statement for NCSBN*. https://www.ahncc.org/wp-content/uploads/2016/06/APRN_Position_Statement_for_NCSBN.pdf

Army Nurse Corps Association. (n.d.). *1940–1950*. https://e-anca.org/History/ANC-Eras/1940-1950

Anchrum, H. (2025). Through the eyes of Black nurses: The impact of the Nurse Training Act of 1964. *Policy, Politics & Nursing Practice, 26*(1), 56–64. https://doi.org/10.1177/15271544241296825

Army Medical Department. (n.d.). *Vietnam medical support*. https://achh.army mil/history/book-vietnam-medical support-chapter3

Barrett, E. (2010). Power as knowing participation in change: What's new and what's next. *Nursing Science Quarterly*, 23(1), 47–54. https://doi.org/10.1177/0894318409353797

Beck, D.-M. (2021). Creating the Nightingale Initiative for Global Health: Theoretical reflections to follow in Florence Nightingale's footsteps. *Revista Latino-Americana de Enfermagem, 29*, e3430. https://doi.org/10.1590/1518-8345.4720.3430

Berkowitz, E. (2005). Medicare and Medicaid: The past as prologue. *Health Care Financing Review, 27*(2), 11–23.

Bradford, S. (2017). *The historic biography of America's Joan of Arc: Harriet Tubman—the Moses of her people*. https://books.google.com/books/about/Harriet_Tubman.html?id=7GJ6FON5IlQC

Buhler-Wilkerson, K., & D'Antonio, P. (2025). Nursing. In *Encyclopedia Britannica*. https://www.britannica.com/science/nursing

Chamberlain University. (n.d.). *A celebration of 10 famous Black nurses in history*. https://www.chamberlain.edu/blog/a-celebration-of-10-famous-black-nurses-in-history

Chi Eta Phi. (n.d.) *Chi Eta Phi*. https://chietaphi.org

Clark, A. (2018). The army's first Black nurses were relegated to caring for Nazi prisoners of war. *Smithsonian Magazine*. https://www.smithsonianmag.com/history/armys-first-black-nurses-had-tend-to-german-prisoners-war-180969069/

Cordeau, M. (2020). Nursing history and the evolution of holistic nursing. In M. Helming, D. Shields, K. Avino, & W. Rosa (Eds.), *Dossey & Keegan's holistic nursing: A handbook for practice* (pp. 211-230). Jones & Bartlett Learning.

Dunphy, L. (2001). The steel cocoon: Tales of the nurses and patients of the iron lung, 1929–1955. *Nursing History Review, 9*(1), 3–20. https://doi.org/10.189/1062-8061.9.1.3

Erickson, H. L., Erickson, M. E., Campbell, J. A., Brekke, M. E., & Sandor, M. K. (2013). Validation of holistic nursing competencies: Role-delineation study, 2012. *Journal of Holistic Nursing, 31*(4), 291-302. https://doi.org/10.1177/0898010113491144

Fawcett, J. (1984). The metaparadigm of nursing: Present status and future refinements. Image. *The Journal of Nursing Scholarship, 16*(3), 84–87. https://doi.org/10.1111/j.1547-5069.1984.tb01393.x

Fowler, M. (Ed.). (2008a). *Guide to nursing's social policy statement: Understanding the profession from social contract to social covenant*. American Nurses Association.

Fowler, M. (Ed.). (2008b). *Guide to the Code of Ethics for Nurses: Interpretation and appreciation*. American Nurses Association.

Fowler, M. (2015). *Guide to nursing's social policy statement: Understanding the profession from social contract to social covenant* (2nd ed.). American Nurses Association.

Hanley, M. A., Coppa, D., & Shields, D. (2017). A practice-based theory of healing through therapeutic touch: Advancing holistic nursing practice. *Journal of Holistic Nursing, 35*(4), 369–381. https://doi.org/10.1177/0898010117721827

Harley Street. (n.d.). *Florence Nightingale*. https://www.harleystreet.com/why-harley-street/pioneers-past/florence-nightingale/

Harvard University's Human Flourishing Program. (2025). *Global Flourishing Study*. https://hfh.fas.harvard.edu/global-flourishing-study

Institute of Medicine (IOM). (2011). *The future of nursing: Leading change, advancing health*. National Academies Press. https://www.ncbi.nlm.nih.gov/books/NBK209881/

Kenny, D. J., & Kelley, P. W. (2019). Heavy burdens: Ethical issues faced by military nurses during a war. *OJIN, 24*(3), Manuscript 1.

Klein, C. (2025). *How Native Americans struggled to survive on the trail-of-tears*. https://www.history.com/articles/trail-of-tears/conditions.

Miller, N. (2018). *Women in the war: The sick suffered much for want of good female nurses*. Maryland State Archives. https://msamaryland400.com/2018/08/02/the-sick-suffered-much-for-want-of-good-female-nurses/

National Academies of Sciences, Engineering, and Medicine. (2009). *Informing the future: Critical issues in health* (5th ed.). National Academies Press.

National Academies of Sciences, Engineering, and Medicine. (2021). *The future of nursing 2020–2030: Charting a path to achieve health equity*. The National Academies Press.

National League of Nursing. (2025). *History of the National League for Nursing*. https://www.nln.org/about/about/history-of-nln

National Library of Jamaica. (2025). *Mary Seacole (1805–1881)*. https://nlj.gov.jm/project/mary-seacole-1805-1881/

National Park Service. (n.d.) *Archeology this month: Native American heritage*. https://www.nps.gov/articles/000/archeology-this-month-american-heritage.html

National Park Service. (n.d.). *William Garrison, US Department of the Interior.* https://www.nps.gov/people/william-lloyd-garrison.html

National Women's History Museum. (n.d.). *Mary Mahoney*. https://www.womenshistory.org/education-resources/biographies/mary-mahoney

Ngô, T. T. T., & Nguyễn, Đ. (2024). War dead, trauma, and care: The differential reintegration of Vietnamese former combatants. *War & Society*, 43(4), 382–397. https://doi.org/10.1080/07292473.2024.2375884

Nightingale F. In L. McDonald, The collected works of Florence Nightingale (Vol. 3) Wilfred Laurier University Press; 2002.

Nightingale, F. (1915). *Florence Nightingale to her nurses*. Macmillan and Co, Limited.

Nightingale, F. (1969). *Notes on nursing: What it is and what it is not*. Dover Publications, Inc. (Original work published 1859)

Nutting, A. A. (1912). Educational status of nursing. *ERIC Bulletin*, 1912 (No. 7). https://eric.ed.gov/?id=ED543002

Parry, M. S. (2006). Dorothea Dix (1802–1887). *American Journal of Public Health, 96*(4), 624–625. https://doi.org/10.2105/AJPH.2005.079152

Pollitt, P., & Reese, C. N. (1997). Nursing and the New Deal: We met the challenge. *Public Health Nursing, 14*(6), 373–382. https://doi.org/10.1111/j.1525-1446.1997.tb00307.x

Rosch, P. J. (2009). Bioelectromagnetic and subtle energy medicine: The interface between mind and matter. *Annals of the New York Academy of Sciences, 1172*, 297–311. https://doi.org/10.1111/j.1749-6632.2009.04535

Schramme, T. (2023). Health as complete well-being: The WHO definition and beyond. *Public Health Ethics, 16*(3), 210–218. https://doi.org/10.1093/phe/phad017

Spring, K. (2017). *Mary Eliza Mahoney*. National Women's History Museum. https://www.womenshistory.org/articles/evolution-nursing

The Commonwealth Fund. (2014). *Mirror, mirror.* https://www.commonwealthfund.org/publications/fund-reports/2014/jun/mirror-mirror-wall-2014-update-how-us-health-care-system

National Association of Social Insurance. (2025). *The history of Medicare.* https://www.nasi.org/learn/medicare/the-history-of-medicare/

Red Cross. (2025). *World War I and the American Red Cross.* https://www.redcross.org/content/dam/redcross/National/history-wwi.pdf

Thomas, L. (2025). *What is a well-being society?* News-Medical Life Sciences. https://www.news-medical.net/health/What-is-a-Well-Being-Society.aspx

University of Pennsylvania School of Nursing. (n.d.). *Nursing through time: 1700-1869.* https://www.nursing.upenn.edu/nhhc/nursing-through-time/1700-1869/

Wilson Center. (n.d.). *Korean War: Chinese perspective - Charles Kraus*. https://www.wilsoncenter.org/audio/korean-war-chinese-perspective-charles-kraus

The WWII Medical Research Center. (n.d.). *The Army Nurse Corps*. https://www.med-dept.com/about-us/

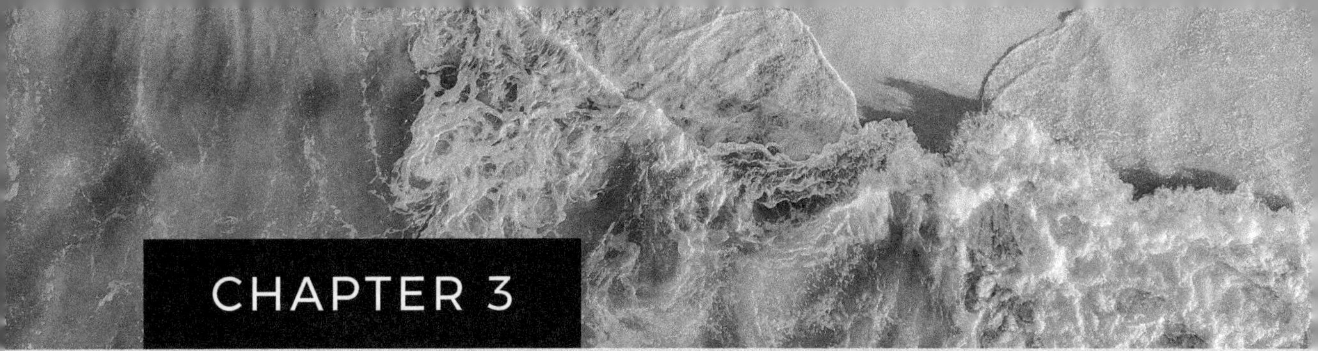

CHAPTER 3

Holistic Nursing: Scope and Standards of Practice

Carla Mariano and Caroline E. Ortiz

NURSE HEALER OBJECTIVES

Theoretical

- Describe the scope of holistic nursing.
- Describe the standards of holistic nursing.
- Discuss the five core values of holistic nursing.

Clinical

- Integrate the principles of holistic nursing into practice.
- Identify how you implement the standards of holistic nursing in your practice.
- Discuss the scope and standards of professional practice for holistic nursing with colleagues.

Personal

- Reflect on your worldview and how it is similar to or different from the philosophy of holism.
- Explore how the concepts of holistic nursing apply to your personal life.

DEFINITIONS[1]

Allopathic/conventional therapies: Medical, surgical, pharmacologic, and invasive and noninvasive diagnostic procedures; those interventions most commonly used in allopathic Western medicine.

Complementary/integrative health approaches (CIHA): A broad set of healthcare practices, therapies, and modalities that address the whole person—body, mind, emotion, spirit, and environment, not just signs and symptoms—and that may replace or be used as complements to or in conjunction with conventional Western medical, surgical, and pharmacologic treatments.

Critical thinking: An active, purposeful, organized cognitive process involving creativity, reflection, problem-solving, rational judgment, intuitive judgment, an attitude of inquiry, and a philosophical orientation toward thinking about thinking.

Culture: The beliefs, values, traditions, behaviors, communication ways, customs, and norms shared by a group that influence health behavior and the curing, healing, dying, and grieving processes of the person.

Disease: A disorder or state of unbalance that may produce signs or symptoms.

Healing: A lifelong journey into wholeness, seeking harmony and balance in one's own life and in family, community, and global relations. Healing involves those physical, mental, social, and spiritual or personally meaningful processes of recovery, repair, renewal, and transformation that increase wholeness and often (though not invariably) order and coherence. Healing is an emergent process of the whole system bringing together aspects of one's self and the body, mind, emotion, spirit, and environment at deeper levels of inner knowing, leading toward integration and balance,

---

[1] Many of the definitions in this chapter were adapted from *Holistic nursing: Scope and standards of practice,* 3rd ed. (ANA & AHNA, 2019) and from the previous edition of this book, *Holistic nursing: A handbook for practice*, 8th ed. (Helming et al., 2022).

with each aspect having equal importance and value. Healing can lead to more complex levels of personal understanding and meaning and may be synchronous but not synonymous with curing.

Healing process: A continual journey of change and the evolving of one's self through life that is characterized by the awareness of patterns that support or that are challenges or barriers to health and healing and that may be done alone or in a healing community.

Healing relationships: The quality and characteristics of interactions between one who facilitates healing and the person in the process of healing. Characteristics of such interactions involve empathy, caring, love, warmth, trust, confidence, credibility, competence, honesty, courtesy, respect, shared expectations, and good communication.

Healing system: A true healthcare system in which people can receive adequate, nontoxic, and noninvasive assistance in maintaining wellness and healing for body, mind, emotion, and spirit, together with the most sophisticated, aggressive curing technologies available.

Health: An individually defined state or process in which the individual (nurse, patient, family, group, or community) experiences a sense of well-being, harmony, and unity such that subjective experiences about health, health beliefs, and values are honored; a process of becoming an expanding consciousness.

Health promotion: Activities and preventive measures to promote health, increase well-being, and actualize the human potential of people, families, communities, society, and ecology; such activities and measures include immunizations, fitness and exercise programs, breast self-exams, appropriate nutrition, relaxation, stress management, social support, prayer, meditation, healing rituals, cultural practices, and promoting environmental health and safety.

Holistic communication: A free flow of verbal and nonverbal interchange between and among people and significant beings such as pets, nature, and God/Life Force/Absolute Being/Transcendent Being that explores meaning and ideas leading to mutual understanding and growth.

Holistic ethics: The basic underlying concept of the unity and integral wholeness of all people and of all nature, identified and pursued by finding unity and wholeness within the self and within humanity. In this framework, acts are not performed for the sake of law, precedent, or social norms but rather from a desire to do good freely to witness, identify, and contribute to unity.

Holistic healing: A form of healing based on attention to all aspects of an individual—physical, mental, emotional, sexual, cultural, social, spiritual, and energetic. The manifestation of right relationship at one or more levels of the body-mind-spirit-environment-energy system.

Holistic nurse: A nurse who recognizes and integrates body-mind-emotion-spirit-environment principles and modalities into daily life and clinical practice, creates a caring, healing space within themselves that allows the nurse to be an instrument of healing, shares authenticity of unconditional presence that helps to remove the barriers to the healing process, facilitates another person's growth (body-mind-emotion-spirit-environment-energetic connections), and assists with recovery from illness or transition to peaceful death.

Holistic nursing practice process: An iterative and integrative process that involves six steps that can occur simultaneously: (1) assessing; (2) diagnosing or identifying patterns, challenges, needs, and health issues; (3) identifying outcomes; (4) planning care; (5) implementing the care plan; and (6) evaluating.

Honor: An act or intention indicating the holding of self or another in high respect, esteem, and dignity, including valuing and accepting the humanity of people with regard for the decisions and wishes of another.

Human caring: The moral ideal of nursing in which the nurse brings one's whole self into a relationship with the whole self of the person being cared for to protect that person's vulnerability, preserve their humanity and dignity, and reinforce the meaning and experience of oneness and unity.

Human health experience: That totality of human experience including each person's subjective experience about health, health beliefs, values, sexual orientation, and personal preferences that encompasses health-wellness-disease-illness-death.

Illness: A subjective experience of symptoms and suffering to which the individual ascribes meaning and significance; not synonymous with disease; a shift in the homeodynamic balance of the person to disharmony and imbalance.

Intention: The conscious awareness of being in the present moment to help facilitate the healing process; a volitional act of love; conscious alignment of essence and purpose allowing the highest good to flow through a healing intervention.

Interdisciplinary/interprofessional: Conversation or collaboration across disciplines where knowledge is shared that informs learning, practice, education, and research; it includes individuals, families, community members, and various disciplines.

Meaning: That which is signified, indicated, referred to, or understood. Personal/individual meaning denotes symbolic value, significance, and purpose—an individual's perception of an experience. Philosophical meaning is meaning that depends on the symbolic connections that are grasped by reason. Psychological meaning is meaning that depends on connections that are experienced through intuition or insight.

Patient-centered care: Care that is respectful of and responsive to individual patient preferences, needs, and values and that ensures that patient values guide all clinical decisions. Patient-centered care encompasses identifying, respecting, and caring about patients' differences, values, preferences, and expressed needs; relieving pain and suffering; coordinating continuous care, effectively informing, engaging and communicating with, and educating patients; sharing decision making and management; and continuously advocating disease prevention, wellness, and promotion of healthy lifestyles, including a focus on population health (Institute of Medicine, 2001).

Person: An individual, patient, patient, family member, support person, or community member who has the opportunity to engage in interaction with a holistic nurse.

Person-centered care: The human caring process in which the holistic nurse gives full attention and intention to the whole self of a person, not merely the current presenting symptoms, illness, crisis, or tasks to be accomplished, and that also includes reinforcing the person's meaning and experience of oneness and unity; the condition of trust that is created in which holistic care can be given and received.

Presence: The essential state or core of healing; approaching an individual in a way that respects and honors their essence; relating in a way that reflects a quality of being with and in collaboration with rather than doing to; entering into a shared experience (or field of consciousness) that promotes healing potential and an experience of well-being.

Relationship-centered care: A process model of caregiving that is based on a vision of community where three types of relationships are identified: (1) patient–practitioner relationship, (2) community–practitioner relationship, and (3) practitioner–practitioner relationship. Each of these relationships is essential within a reformed integrative healthcare delivery system in a hospital, clinic, or community or in the home. Each component involves a unique set of responsibilities and tasks that addresses the three areas of knowledge, values, and skills (Tresolini & Pew-Fetzer Task Force, 1994).

Spirituality: The feelings, thoughts, experiences, and behaviors that arise from a search for meaning; that which is generally considered sacred or holy; usually, though not universally, considered to involve a sense of connection with an absolute, imminent, or transcendent force, however named, as well as the conviction that meaning, value, direction, and purpose are valid aspects of the individual and universe; the essence of being and relatedness that permeates all of life and is manifested in one's knowing, doing, and being; the interconnectedness with self, others, nature, and God/Life Force/Absolute/Transcendent; not necessarily synonymous with religion.

Transformational leadership: Leadership that creates valuable and positive change in individuals and systems, encouraging individuals to contribute to their fullest potential by enhancing the motivation, morale, and performance of followers.

Transpersonal: A personal understanding that is based on one's experiences of temporarily transcending or moving beyond one's usual identification with the limited biological, historical, cultural, and personal self at the deepest and most profound levels of experience possible; that which transcends the limits and boundaries of individual ego identities and possibilities to include acknowledgment and appreciation of something greater. From this perspective the ordinary biological, historical, cultural, and personal self is seen as an important, but only a partial, manifestation or expression of this much greater something that is one's deeper origin and destination.

Well-being: An inner attitude of feelings of comfort and harmony and acceptance to the wholeness of one's being. Integrated, congruent functioning aimed toward reaching one's higher potential.

Wellness: An active process through which people become aware of and make choices toward a more successful existence. It is a conscious, self-directed and evolving process of achieving full potential. Wellness is multidimensional and holistic, encompassing lifestyle, mental and spiritual or personally meaningful well-being, and the environment.

Scope and Standards of Holistic Nursing Practice

Extraordinary changes occurred in health care and nursing from 2010 to 2020. During this time, holistic nurses recognized that not only were they practicing a unique specialty within nursing, but also that they needed to develop and publish standards of practice to document and define that specialty practice. Holistic nursing was officially recognized as a distinct specialty within the discipline of nursing by the American Nurses Association (ANA) in November 2006.

Holistic nursing: Scope and standards of practice (3rd ed.) (ANA & AHNA, 2019) articulates the scope and standards of the specialty practice of holistic nursing and informs holistic nurses, the nursing profession, other healthcare providers and disciplines, employers, third-party payers, legislators, and the public about the unique scope of knowledge and the standards of practice and professional performance of a holistic nurse. *Holistic nursing: Scope and standards of practice* (3rd ed.) is the foundational document and resource for holistic nursing education at all levels (undergraduate, graduate, continuing education) and for holistic nursing practice, theory, research, advocacy, and certification.

Function of the Scope of Practice Statement of Holistic Nursing

The scope of practice statement describes the *who*, *what*, *where*, *when*, *why*, and *how* of the practice of holistic nursing. These elements provide a picture of the dynamic and complex practice of holistic nursing, its evolving boundaries, and its members.

Nursing: Scope and standards of practice (4th ed.) (ANA, 2021) applies to all professional registered nurses engaged in practice, regardless of specialty, practice setting, or educational preparation. With the *Code of ethics for nurses with interpretative statements* (ANA, 2015) and *Nursing's social policy statement: The essence of the profession* (ANA, 2010a), it forms the foundation of practice for all registered nurses. The scope of holistic nursing practice is specific to this specialty, but it builds on the scope of practice expected of all registered nurses.

Function of the Standards of Holistic Nursing

"The Standards of Professional Nursing Practice are authoritative statements of the actions and behaviors that all registered nurses, regardless of role, population, specialty, and setting, are expected to perform competently" (ANA, 2021, p. 73). "Standards reflect the values and priorities of the profession. Standards provide direction for professional nursing practice and a framework for evaluation of this practice. Written in measurable terms, these standards define the nursing profession's accountability to the public and the outcomes for which registered nurses are responsible" (ANA, 2004, p. 1).

The standards of holistic nursing practice are specific to this specialty but build on the standards of practice expected of all registered nurses.

Competencies accompany each standard of holistic nursing and articulate the "expected level of performance that integrates knowledge, skills, abilities, and judgment" (ANA, 2021, p. 74).

Holistic nursing: Scope and standards of practice (3rd ed.) presents a differentiation between practice at the basic and advanced practice levels. The scope and standards are organized according to the ANA criteria used to recognize a nursing specialty area and build on nursing knowledge, skills, and competencies required for licensure (ANA, 2010b; Mariano, 2006). The text reflects a consensus of the most current thinking in the specialty and provides a blueprint for holistic nursing philosophy, theory, principles, education, research, and practices. It incorporates the fundamental philosophical beliefs, theories, and practices as well as new developments and advancements in the field of holistic nursing. It is a foundational resource for holistic nursing and a key resource for certification in holistic nursing. The standards guide clinicians, educators, researchers, nurse leaders, and administrators in professional activities, knowledge, and performance that are relevant to basic and advanced practice, education, research, and advocacy in holistic nursing. The third edition is derived from values that are central to the specialty and are consistent with the philosophies and theories of holism.

Evolution of Holistic Nursing

Ancient cultures have defined holism within the healing arts in terms of the balance of forces in nature. These elements are foundational in the healing arts practiced today by traditional and Indigenous peoples around the globe. In 1835, American physician Dr. Jacob Bigelow encouraged physicians to rethink their practice of prescribing medicine for all diseases. He stated that "some diseases are controlled by nature alone" (Bigelow, 1859, p. 36). This holistic philosophy, emphasizing a relationship with nature and its elements, was deeply embedded in the sphere of American domestic medicine and family self-care and ascribed to by many physicians, community healers, and the professional midwives and nurses of the period. Holism and the relationship with the environment and the elements of care is a foundational philosophy of care that has endured throughout centuries of American nursing care.

Early 19th-century American nurses working in religious communities sought the balance of the humors and the elements, as did the ancient Greeks. In the United Kingdom, Florence Nightingale continued the holistic tradition. She believed that "Nature alone cures . . . and what nursing has to do in either case, is to put the patient in the best condition for nature to act upon him" (Nightingale, 1859, p. 133). Nightingale believed in care that focused on unity, wellness, and the interrelationship of human beings, events, and environment (Dossey, 2010). She, like her American predecessors, demonstrated an enduring commitment to a holistic philosophy and approach that incorporated the elements of care in response to people's physical, mental, emotional, and spiritual or personally meaningful needs.

Even Hippocrates, the father of Western medicine, espoused a holistic orientation when he taught physicians to observe their patients' life circumstances and emotional states. Socrates, too, promoted it, stating, "Curing the soul; that is the first and essential thing" (Plato, 2004). In holism, symptoms are believed to be an expression of the body's wisdom as it reacts to cure its own imbalance or disease.

The root of the word *heal* comes from the Greek word *halos* and the Anglo-Saxon word *haelan*, which means to be or to become whole. The word *holy* also comes from the same source. Healing means "making whole"—or restoring balance and harmony. It is a movement toward a sense of wholeness and completion. Healing, therefore, is the integration of the totality of the person in body, mind, emotion, spirit, and environment.

One of the driving forces behind the holistic nursing movement in the United States was the formation of the American Holistic Nurses Association (AHNA). In 1980, founder Charlotte McGuire and 75 founding members began the national organization in Houston, Texas. The national office is now located in Topeka, Kansas. The AHNA's mission is to advance the philosophy and practices of holistic nursing and unite nurses in healing with a focus on holistic principles of health, preventive education, and the integration of allopathic and complementary caring and healing modalities to facilitate care of the whole person and significant others. From its inception in 1980, the AHNA has been the leader in developing and advancing holistic principles, practices, and guidelines. The association predicted that holistic principles, caring and healing, and the integration of complementary and integrative therapies and approaches would emerge into mainstream health care.

The AHNA, the definitive voice for holistic nursing, has as its vision: "Every nurse is a holistic nurse" (ANA & AHNA, 2019, p. 5). The mission of the AHNA is "to illuminate holism in nursing practice, community, advocacy, research, and education" (ANA & AHNA, 2019, p. 5). It is committed to promoting wholeness and wellness in individuals, families, communities, nurses themselves, the nursing profession, and the environment. Through its various activities, AHNA provides vision, direction, and leadership in the advancement of holistic nursing; integrates the art and science of nursing into the profession; empowers holistic nursing through education, research, and standards; promotes research and scholarship in holistic nursing; encourages nurses to be models of wellness; honors individual excellence in the advancement of holistic nursing; and influences policy to change the healthcare system to a more humanistic orientation.

The goals and endeavors of the AHNA have continued to map conceptual frameworks and the blueprint for holistic nursing practice, education, and research, which is the most complete way to conceptualize and practice professional nursing. The relevance and validity of holistic nursing as a science and practice have been increasingly demonstrated in recent years, as noted here:

> While becoming more popular and more highly regarded, holism and holistic nursing have contributed to enhancing the human condition in many ways. Holism as a philosophy, concept, theory, and practice has been used to expand our understanding of human wellness and illness. Holistic nursing has become more systematized, refined, and diversified as strategies and practices have been shown to have an impact on health and well-being. Holistic nursing . . . has progressed . . . through the development of standards, endorsement of programs, and certification of beginning and advanced practitioners. Holistic nursing's contributions to human welfare have been increasingly recognized . . . as evidenced in their current standing in health care and appreciation by society. . . . Holism as a perspective and holistic nursing as a response may offer the world something that counteracts the fragmentation and isolation that exists so predominantly in our society. . . . Holistic nursing . . . provides a context in which nurses can consider, understand, and appreciate all the aspects of human experience that contribute to patterns of life, health, and illness. (Cowling, 2011, p. 5)

Scope of Holistic Nursing

Holistic nursing is defined as "all nursing practice that has healing the whole person as its goal" (AHNA, 1998). Holistic nursing is a specialty practice that draws on nursing knowledge, theories of nursing and wholeness, expertise, and intuition to guide nurses in becoming therapeutic partners with people in strengthening human responses to facilitate the healing process and achieve wholeness. Holistic nursing focuses on protecting, promoting, and optimizing health and wellness; assisting healing; preventing illness and injury; alleviating suffering; supporting people to find peace, comfort, harmony, and balance through the diagnosis and treatment of human response; and advocacy in the care of individuals, families, groups, communities, populations, and the planet.

Holistic nursing care is healing oriented and centered on the relationship with the person in contrast to an orientation toward diseases and their cures. Holistic nursing emphasizes practices of self-reflection and self-care, intentionality, presence, mindfulness, and therapeutic use of self as pivotal for facilitation of healing and patterning of wellness in others. In some sense, all nursing practice can be comprehensive—that is, all nursing practice may have a biopsychosocial perspective. What makes holistic nursing practice a specialty is that there is a philosophy, a body of knowledge, and an advanced set of nursing skills applied to practice that recognize the totality of the human being and the interconnectedness of body, mind, emotion, spirit, energy, society, culture, relationships, context, and environment. Philosophically, holistic nursing is a worldview, a way of being in the world, not just a modality. This philosophy honors the unique humanness of all people regardless of who and what they are.

Knowledge for holistic nursing practice derives not only from nursing but also from theories of wholeness, energy, and unity as well as from other healing systems and approaches. Holistic nurses incorporate both conventional nursing and integrative modalities and interventions into practice.

Through unconditional presence, mindfulness, and intention, holistic nurses create environments conducive to healing, using techniques that promote empowerment, peace, comfort, and a subjective sense of harmony and well-being for the person. The holistic nurse acts in partnership with the individual or family in providing options and alternatives regarding health and treatment. In addition, the holistic nurse assists the person to find meaning in the health and illness experience.

Holistic nursing focuses on simultaneously integrating as an iterative process all of these realms: a philosophy of being and living, using theories of nursing and wholeness with related knowledge and skills, focusing on the unity and totality of humans, incorporating healing approaches, creating healing environments, partnering with and empowering individuals, and assisting in the exploration of meaning in the care of people. In holistic nursing, the nurse is the facilitator of healing, honoring that the person heals themself. The holistic nurse assists individuals in identifying themselves as healers and accessing their own innate healing capacities.

The practice of holistic nursing requires nurses to integrate self-care and self-responsibility into their own lives and to serve as role models for others. Holistic nurses strive for an awareness of the interconnectedness of individuals to the human and global community. Thus, holistic nurses also attend to the health of the ecosystem.

Holistic nurses are instruments of healing and facilitators in the healing process. They honor the individual's subjective experience of health, health beliefs, and values. To become therapeutic partners with individuals, families, communities, and populations, holistic nurses draw on nursing knowledge, theories, research, expertise, intuition, and creativity, incorporating the roles of clinician, educator, consultant, coach, partner, role model, and advocate. Holistic nursing practice encourages peer review of professional practice in various clinical settings and provides care based on current professional standards, laws, and regulations that govern nursing practice. The major phenomena of concern to holistic nursing are listed in **Box 3-1**.

Box 3-1 Phenomena of Concern to Holistic Nursing

- The caring-healing relationship
- The subjective experience of and meanings ascribed to health, illness, wellness, healing, birth, growth and development, and dying
- The cultural values, beliefs, and folk and Indigenous practices of health, wellness, well-being, illness, healing, and death
- Spirituality in nursing care
- Energy and consciousness
- Reflective practice
- The use and evaluation of complementary and integrative health approaches (CIHA) in nursing practice
- Comprehensive health promotion, disease prevention, and well-being
- Self-reflection, self-care, and self-development processes
- Physical, mental, emotional, and spiritual or personally meaningful comfort, discomfort, and pain
- Empowerment, decision making, and the ability to make informed choices
- Social and economic policies and their effects on the health of individuals, families, and communities
- Diverse and alternative healthcare systems and their relationships to access and quality of health care
- The environment, ecosystem, and prevention of disease
- Healing environment

Philosophical Principles of Holistic Nursing

Holistic nurses express, contribute to, and promote an understanding of the following:

- A philosophy of nursing that values healing as the desired outcome

- A foundation of holistic nursing in the sciences of health, wellness, well-being, and healing
- Nursing as an art
- The human health experience as a complex, dynamic relationship of an individual's understanding of health, wellness, illness, and disease
- Environmental influences and cultural perspectives that inform an individual's health experience

Person

- There are unity, totality, and energetic interconnectedness of everyone and everything (body, mind, emotion, spirit, sexuality, age, environment, social/cultural, belief systems, relationships, context).
- Human beings are unique, diverse, and inherently good.
- People are able to find meaning and purpose in their own life, experiences, and illness.
- All people have an innate power and capacity for growth, development, and self-healing. Health/illness is subjectively described and determined by the view of the individual. Therefore, the person is honored in all phases of growth, development, and healing process, regardless of expectations or outcomes.
- People/persons/individuals are the recipients of holistic nursing services. They may be healthcare consumers, patients, families, significant others, populations, or communities, local to global. They may be well and moving toward personal betterment and enhanced well-being or ill within the healthcare delivery system.

Healing/Health

- Health and illness are natural and a part of life, learning, and movement toward growth, development, and potential change.
- Health is seen as balance, integration, harmony, right relationship, and the betterment of well-being, not just the absence of disease. Healing can take place without cure. The focus is on health promotion, disease prevention, health restoration, and lifestyle patterns and habits, as well as symptom relief.
- Illness and disease are seen as a teacher, an opportunity for self-awareness and growth, and part of the life process. Health challenges and symptoms are respected for their potential messages.
- Healing is multidimensional, can occur at any level of the human energetic system, and is creative, unfolding, and unpredictable.
- Healing is an experience defined by the individual and therefore is variable.
- People, as active partners in the healthcare and healing process, are empowered when they take some control of their own lives, health, and well-being, including personal choices and relationships.
- Treatment is a process that considers the root of the problem, issue, or illness, not merely treating the obvious signs and symptoms.

Practice

- Practice is a science (clinical reasoning, critical thinking, reflection, evidence/research/theory) as foundational to practice and an art (intuition, creativity, appreciation, presence, self/personal knowing) as integral to practice.
- The values and ethic of holism, caring, moral insight, dignity, integrity, competence, responsibility, accountability, and legality underlie holistic nursing practice.
- Intention for the well-being and highest good for the care of the recipient is the cornerstone of all holistic practice.
- Any and all interventions have an effect on the whole.
- There are various philosophies and paradigms of health, wellness, well-being, healing, and illness and approaches/models for the delivery of health care (both in the United States and in other cultures) that should be understood and utilized.
- Older adults represent the predominant population served by nurses.
- The health and well-being of society influence public policy, the healthcare delivery system, and professional nursing.

Environment

- The environment includes the surroundings and conditions in which persons/groups live and function; humans constantly interact with their environment.
- The World Health Organization defines *environment*, as it relates to health, as "all the physical, chemical, and biological factors external to a person and all the related behaviors" (ODPHP, 2025).
- Environment is physical, social, psychological, cultural, and spirituality-related characteristics; external and internal features; animate and inanimate objects; climate; seen and unseen vibrations, frequencies, and energy patterns not yet understood (Luck, 2022).
- Environmental health integrates numerous interacting factors such as safety, security, and violence; it is not a result of physical qualities (such as air quality and temperature).
- Holistic nurses advocate for environmental conditions and policies that foster health, wellness, well-being, and healing for all people.

Nursing Roles

- Utilizing warmth, compassion, caring, authenticity, respect, trust, and relationship as instruments of healing in and of themselves and as part of the healing environment.
- Utilizing conventional nursing interventions as well as CIHA that enhance body-mind-emotion-spirit-environment connectedness to foster the healing, health, wholeness, and well-being of people.
- Collaborating and partnering with all constituencies in the health process, including the person receiving care, family, significant others, community, peers, and other disciplines using principles and skills of cooperation, alliance, consensus, and respecting and honoring the contributions of all.
- Participating in the change process to develop more caring cultures in which to practice, learn, and live.
- Assisting everyone to nurture and heal themselves.
- Participating in activities that contribute to the improvement of local and global communities, as well as the betterment of public health, the environment, and the planet.
- Acting as an advocate for the rights of, equitable distribution of, and access to health care for all persons, especially vulnerable populations.
- Participating in and providing leadership in the positive transformation of systems.
- Participating in research of the human experience and improvement of the nursing process.
- Conducting independent and collaborative research and quality demonstration projects to contribute to the rapidly changing knowledge base for education and practices.
- Honoring the ecosystem and our relationship with and need to preserve it, as we are all connected.

Self-Reflection, Self-Development, and Self-Care

- Self-reflection—defined as turning inward to examine one's thoughts, values, beliefs, experiences, behaviors, and inner wisdom—enhances self-awareness and understanding and facilitates reflective practice.
- The nurse's self-reflection, self-assessment, self-care, healing, and personal development are necessary for support of others, as are growth and change in the nurse's own well-being and understanding of the nurse's own personal journey.
- The nurse values themself and their calling to holistic nursing as a life purpose through mobilizing the necessary resources to develop and care for themself.

Core Values of Holistic Nursing: Integrating the Art and Science of Nursing

Holistic nursing emanates from five core values summarizing the ideals and principles of the specialty. These core values are listed here and are then discussed:

1. Holistic philosophy, theories, and ethics
2. Holistic nurse self-reflection, self-development, and self-care
3. Holistic caring process
4. Holistic communication, therapeutic relationship, healing environment, and cultural care
5. Holistic education and research

Core Value 1: Holistic Philosophy, Theory, and Ethics

A nurse's philosophy is their personal approach to nursing. It is shaped by the nurse's reflection on their practice, beliefs, experiences, education, relationships, and the environment. Holistic nursing celebrates a way of being that values connection with others and the environment. Holistic nurses recognize the human health experience as a complicated, dynamic relationship of health, illness, and wellness, and they value healing as the desired outcome of the practice of nursing. Their practice is based on scientific foundations (theory, research, evidence-based practice, critical thinking, reflection) and art (relationship, communication, creativity, presence, caring).

Holistic nursing is grounded in nursing knowledge and skill and guided by nursing theory. Florence Nightingale's writings are often referenced as a significant precursor of the development of holistic nursing. Although each holistic nurse chooses which nursing theory to apply in any individual case, the following theories, listed with their developers, are most often used to support holistic practice:

- Theory of Human Caring and Caring Science (Jean Watson)
- Science of Unitary Human Beings (Martha Rogers
- Health as Expanding Consciousness (Margaret Newman)
- Theory of Cultural Care Diversity and Universality (Madeleine Leininger)
- Human Becoming School of Thought (Rosemarie Rizzo Parse)
- Humanistic Nursing Theory (Josephine Paterson and Loretta Zderad)
- Modeling and Role Modeling (Helen Erickson, Evelyn Tomlin, and Mary Ann Swain)

There has been significant development in the evolution of holism, healing, and caring conceptualization and theory, largely due to the work of holistic nurses. Prominent among those (with their theories in parentheses) are the following:

- Barbara Dossey (Theory of Integral Nursing)
- Anne Boykin (Theory of Nursing as Caring)
- Marlaine Smith (Theory of Unitary Caring)
- Marilyn Anne Ray (Theory of Bureaucratic Caring)
- Rozzano Locsin (Technological Competency as Caring and the Practice of Knowing Persons in Nursing)
- Mary Jane Smith and Patricia Liehr (Story Theory)
- Joanne Duffy (Quality Caring Model)

In addition to nursing theory, holistic nurses utilize philosophies and theories from other disciplines to guide and inform healing practice. Examples include but are not limited to the following:

- Theories of consciousness
- Systems theory
- Biofield theory
- Quantum physics
- Complexity science
- Chaos theory
- Coherence
- Complementarity
- Spirituality
- Self-in-relation
- Holographic theory
- Psychoneuroimmunology
- Morphic resonance
- Integral theory
- Rig Veda
- Four Directions
- Eastern contemplative orientations such as the following:
    - Zen Buddhism
    - Taoism
- Alternative medical systems such as the following:
    - Traditional Chinese medicine
    - Ayurveda
    - Native American and Indigenous healing

Holistic nurses further recognize and honor the ethic that each person is the authority on their own health experience. The holistic nurse is an option giver and helps the person develop an understanding of alternatives and implications of various health and treatment options. The holistic nurse first ascertains what the individual thinks or believes is happening to them and then assists the person to identify what will help the situation. The assessment begins from where the individual is. The holistic nurse then discusses options, including the person's choices across a continuum and the possible effects and implications of each. The holistic nurse acts as partner and co-prescriber versus sole prescriber. The relationship is a copiloting of the individual's health experience where the nurse respects the person's decision about their own health. It is a process of engagement versus compliance.

Client/patient narratives, whether they arise from individuals, families, or communities, provide the context of the experiences and are used as an important focus in understanding the person's situation. Holistic nurses hold the belief that people, through their inherent capacities, heal themselves. Therefore, the holistic nurse is not the healer but the guide and facilitator of the individual's own healing.

In the belief that all things are connected, the holistic perspective espouses that an individual's actions have a ripple effect throughout humanity. Holism places the greatest worth on individuals' developing higher levels of human awareness. This, in turn, elevates the whole of humanity. Holistic nurses believe in the sacredness of one's self and of all nature. One's inner self and the collective greater self have stewardship over not only one's body, mind, and spirit but also the planet. Holistic nurses focus on the meaning and quality of life deriving from their own character and from their relationship to the universe rather than that imposed from without.

Holistic nurses hold to a professional ethic of caring and healing that seeks to preserve the wholeness and dignity of the self and others. They support human dignity by advocating and adhering to the Patient Bill of Rights (JCAHO, 1992) and the AHNA *Position statement on holistic nursing ethics* (AHNA, 2012).

The *Code of ethics for nurses with interpretive statements* (ANA, 2015) provides a framework for the ethics of nursing. Each of the nine provisions of the code is applicable to and of distinct importance in guiding holistic nursing practice as defined in the Scope and Standards. These provisions are noted in **Box 3-2**.

Box 3-2 ANA Code of Ethics

Provision 1: The nurse practices with compassion and respect for the inherent dignity, worth, and unique attributes of every person.

Provision 2: The nurse's primary commitment is to the patient, whether an individual, family, group, community, or population.

Provision 3: The nurse promotes, advocates for, and protects the rights, health, and safety of the patient.

Provision 4: The nurse has authority, accountability, and responsibility for nursing practice; makes decisions; and takes action consistent with the obligation to promote health and to provide optimal care.

Provision 5: The nurse owes the same duties to self as to others, including the responsibility to promote health and safety, preserve wholeness of character and integrity, maintain competence, and continue personal and professional growth.

Provision 6: The nurse, through individual and collective effort, establishes, maintains, and improves the ethical environment of the work setting and conditions of employment that are conducive to safe, quality health care.

Provision 7: The nurse, in all roles and settings, advances the profession through research and scholarly inquiry, professional standards development, and the generation of both nursing and health policy.

Provision 8: The nurse collaborates with other health professionals and the public to protect human rights, promote health diplomacy, and reduce health disparities.

Provision 9: The profession of nursing, collectively through its professional organizations, must articulate nursing values, maintain the integrity of the profession, and integrate principles of social justice and equity into nursing and health policy.

Core Value 2: Holistic Nurse Self-Reflection, Self-Development, and Self-Care

Self-reflection, self-development, and self-care, as well as personal awareness and continual focus on being an instrument of healing, are significant requirements for holistic nurses. Holistic nurses reflect in and on action to become aware of values, beliefs, feelings, perceptions, and judgments that may affect actions, and they also reflect on their experiences to obtain insight for future practice and to become more authentic and mindful. Holistic nurses value themselves and mobilize the necessary resources to develop and care for themselves. They endeavor to integrate self-awareness, self-care, and self-healing into their lives by incorporating practices such as self-assessment, meditation, yoga, good nutrition, energy therapies, movement, creative endeavors, support, and lifelong learning. Holistic nurses honor their unique patterns and the development of the body, the psychosocial and cultural self, the intellectual self, the energetic self, and the self relating to spirituality. Nurses cannot facilitate healing unless they are in the process of healing themselves. Through continuing education, practice, and self-work, holistic nurses develop the skills of authentic and deep self-reflection and introspection to understand themselves and their journey. It is a lifelong process.

Holistic nurses strive to achieve harmony and balance in their own lives and assist others to do the same. They create healing environments for themselves by attending to their own well-being, letting go of self-destructive behaviors and attitudes, and practicing centering and stress-reduction techniques. By doing this, holistic nurses guide others on their healing journey and serve as role models to others, be they clients/patients, colleagues, or personal relations.

Holistic nurses have played instrumental roles in creating and implementing self-care programs to increase health and well-being for clients/patients and families, communities, healthcare staff, and nurses themselves. Recent research on the effects of holistic self-care programs for nurses and nursing students demonstrates that such programs foster good health behaviors; resilience; improved nurse–patient communication, care, and satisfaction; and improved work environments and may help sustain the nursing profession.

Core Value 3: Holistic Caring Process

Holistic nurses provide care that recognizes the totality of the human being (the interconnectedness of body, mind, emotion, spirit, society, culture, relationships, context, and environment). This is an *integrated* as well as a comprehensive approach. Although physical symptoms are treated, holistic nurses also focus on how the individual cognitively perceives and emotionally deals with the illness; the illness's effect on the person's family, social relationships, and economic resources; the person's values, culture, and spiritual or personally meaningful beliefs and preferences regarding treatment; and the meaning of this experience to the person's life. In addition, holistic nurses may also incorporate several modalities (e.g., cognitive restructuring, stress management, visualization, aromatherapy, therapeutic touch) with conventional nursing interventions. Holistic nurses focus on care interventions that promote healing, peace, comfort, and a subjective sense of well-being for the person.

The holistic caring process involves six often simultaneously occurring steps: assessment, diagnosis (pattern, problem, need identification), outcomes, therapeutic care plan, implementation, and evaluation. Holistic nurses apply the holistic caring process in all settings with individuals and families across the life span, population groups, and communities.

Holistic nurses incorporate a variety of roles into their practice, including expert clinician and facilitator of healing; consultant, coach, and collaborator; educator and guide; administrator, leader, and change agent; researcher; and advocate. Holistic nurses strongly emphasize partnership with individuals throughout the entire decision-making process. Holistic assessments include not only physical, functional, psychosocial, mental, emotional, cultural, and sexual aspects but also the spiritual or personally meaningful, transpersonal, and energy field assessments of the whole person. Energy assessments are based on the concept that all beings are composed of energy. Congestion or stagnation of energy in any realm creates disharmony and disease. Holistic nurses use understanding of energy anatomy and electromagnetic fields in both their assessments and the healing process. Assessments relating to spirituality not only glean religious beliefs and practices but also query a person's meaning and purpose in life and how that may have changed due to the present health experience. Assessments relating to spirituality also include questions about an individual's sense of serenity and peace, what provides joy and fulfillment, the meaningfulness of things, and the source of strength and hope.

Holistic assessment data are interpreted into patterns, challenges, and needs from which meaning and understanding of the health and disease experience can be mutually identified with the person. Holistic nurses first ask an individual, "What do you think is going on (happening) with you?" and then, "What do you think would help?" Another important responsibility of the holistic nurse is to help the person identify risk factors such as lifestyle, habits, beliefs and values, personal and family health history, and age-related conditions that influence health and then to find and use opportunities to increase well-being. The focus is on the individual's goals, not the nurse's.

Therapeutic plans of care respect the person's experience and the uniqueness of each healing journey. The same illness may have different manifestations in different individuals. A major aspect of holistic nursing practice, in addition to competence, is intention. That is, the nurse intends for the wholeness, well-being, and highest good of the person in every encounter and intervention. This intention honors and reinforces the innate capacity of people to heal themselves. Therefore, holistic nurses respect that outcomes may not be those expected and may evolve differently based on the person's individual healing process and health choices. Holistic nurses endeavor to detach themselves from the outcomes. The nurse does not produce the outcomes; the individual's own healing process produces the outcomes, and the nurse facilitates this process. An important focus of the holistic nurse is on guiding individuals and significant others to use their inner strength, wisdom, knowing, and resources through the course of healing.

Holistic nurses consistently provide appropriate and evidence-based information (including current knowledge, practice, and research) regarding the health condition and various treatments and therapies and their side effects. Holistic care always occurs within the scope and standards of practice of registered nursing and in accordance with state and federal laws and regulations.

A holistic nurse supports the integration of Complementary Integrative Health Approaches (CIHA) into conventional health care to enable the patient to benefit from the best of all treatments available. In their provision of holistic care, nurses employ practices and therapies from CIHA and conventional approaches, thus creating a focus on integrative health (Mariano, 2019). AHNA has developed a position statement on the role of nurses in the practice of CIHA (AHNA, 2016).

The National Center for Complementary and Integrative Health (NCCIH, 2025a) distinguishes complementary health approaches as falling into four general categories based on how they are delivered or implemented:

- Nutritional (e.g., special diets, dietary supplements, herbs, and probiotics)
- Psychological (e.g., mindfulness)
- Physical (e.g., massage, spinal manipulation)
- Combinations such as psychological and physical (e.g., yoga, tai chi, acupuncture, dance or art therapies) or psychological and nutritional (e.g., mindful eating)

Integrative care merges interventions from conventional and complementary fields with the aim of treating the person as a whole system versus separate, independent parts. This approach is contained within the concept of "whole person health" and makes reference to "helping individuals, families, communities, and populations improve and restore their health in multiple interconnected domains—biological, behavioral, social, environmental—rather than just treating disease" (NCCIH, 2025a). Further extending the science in whole person health includes studying the ways in which these multiple aspects of health are related and interconnected.

Holistic nursing practice incorporates a vast number and variety of CIHA, but because so many healthcare issues are related to or exacerbated by undue stress, holistic nurses highly empower individuals by teaching them stress-management techniques (NCCIH, 2025b). Many interventions used in holistic nursing elicit the relaxation response (e.g., breath work, meditation, relaxation, imagery, aromatherapy and essential oils, nature-based activities, and diet). People can learn these therapies and use them without the intervention of a healthcare provider. This allows people to take an active role in the management of their own health care. Holistic nurses also can teach families and caregivers to use these techniques for loved ones who may be ill (e.g., simple foot or hand massage for older patients/clients with dementia). In addition, individuals are taught how to evaluate their own responses to these modalities and respond accordingly.

Holistic nurses may prescribe as legally authorized. They instruct individuals regarding drug, herbal, and homeopathic regimens, and, just as important, they consult on the side effects and interactions between medications and herbs. They consult, collaborate, and refer, as necessary, to both conventional allopathic providers and to holistic practitioners. They provide information and counseling to people about alternative, complementary, integrative, and conventional healthcare practices. Importantly, holistic nurses facilitate negotiation of services as they guide individuals and families between conventional Western medicine and alternative systems. Holistic nurses, in partnership with the individual and others, evaluate whether care is effective and whether changes in the meaning of the health experience occur for the individual.

Holistic nurses also take a lead in incorporating a holistic caring perspective and integrating healing strategies into practice and systemwide programs and organizations.

Core Value 4: Holistic Communication, Therapeutic Relationship, Healing Environment, and Cultural Care

Creation of a therapeutic relationship through holistic communication, and the context for its expression—an optimal healing environment—is an enduring tradition in holistic nursing use of self in interacting with "another" (Thornton & Mariano, 2016, p. 465). Incorporating the processes and constructs of therapeutic communication, it acknowledges the infinite, spirituality-related, and energetic nature of being, the centrality of heart centeredness, and the incorporation of intention, self-knowledge, transcendent presence, and intuition in our interactions.

The holistic nurse's communication ensures that each individual experiences the presence of the nurse as authentic, caring, compassionate, and sincere. This is deep listening, or as some say, "Listening with the heart and not just the ears." It is done with conscious intention and without preconceptions, busyness, distractions, or analysis. It takes place in the now within an atmosphere of shared humanness—human being to human being. Through presence or being with in the moment, holistic nurses provide each person with an interpersonal encounter that the individual can experience as a connection with one who is giving undivided attention to their needs and concerns. Holistic nurses actively engage in the therapeutic use of self. Communication techniques used by holistic nurses to build therapeutic relationships include but are not limited to unconditional regard, respect, deep and active listening, active observing, demonstrating empathy and concern, instilling hope, mindfulness, relaxation, stress management, goal management, crisis intervention, negotiation, and problem-solving.

Using these techniques, holistic nurses convey to the individual receiving care the belief in their worth and value as a human being, not solely as a recipient of medical and nursing interventions. More about communication and relatedness in holistic nursing practice is discussed in the chapter titled "Holistic Communication for Caring–Healing Relationships."

The holistic nurse recognizes the importance of context in understanding the person's health experience, including family history and community relationships, culture, health, social roles, interdependence, and self-concept. Space and time are allowed for exploration. Each person's health encounter is truly unique and may be contrary to conventional knowledge and treatments. Therefore, the holistic nurse must be comfortable with ambiguity, paradox, and uncertainty. This requires a perspective that the nurse is not the expert regarding another's health and illness experience but is actually a learner.

Holistic nurses have a knowledge base of the use and meanings of symbolic language and use interventions such as imagery, creation of sacred space and personal rituals, dream exploration, narrative, story, journaling, and aesthetic therapies such as music, color, visual arts, and dance. They encourage and support others in the use of prayer, meditation, and other spiritual or personally meaningful and symbolic practices for healing purposes.

A cornerstone of holistic nursing practice is assisting individuals to find meaning in their experience. Regardless of the person's condition, the meaning that individuals ascribe to their situation can influence their response to it. Holistic nurses attend to the subjective world of the individual. They consider meanings such as the person's concerns in relation to health and family economics, as well as deeper meanings related to the person's purpose in life. Regardless of the technology or treatment, holistic nurses address the human spirit as a major force in healing. Each person's perception of meaning is related to all factors in health-wellness-disease-illness.

Holistic nurses realize that suffering, illness, and disease are natural components of the human condition and have the potential to teach us about ourselves, our relationships, and our universe. Every experience is valued for its meaning and lesson.

Holistic nurses have a particular obligation to create a therapeutic healing environment that values holism, caring, social support, and integration of conventional and complementary/integrative approaches to healing. They seek to create caring cultures and environments where individuals, both clients/patients and staff, feel connected, supported, and respected. A particular perspective of holistic nursing is the nurse as the healing environment and an instrument of healing. Holistic nurses shape the physical environment (e.g., light, fresh air, pleasant sounds or quiet, neatness and order, healing smells, earth elements), and they provide a relationship-focused environment by creating sacred space through presence and intention where another can feel safe, unfold, and explore the dimensions of self in healing. The focus on healing environments is extended to the creation of caring cultures and communities where families, populations, and nations can feel connected, supported, and respected. Holistic nurses have an integral role in revisioning and transforming organizational cultures into authentic healing healthcare systems and in trying to remove the political and financial barriers to the inclusion of holistic care in the healthcare system.

Culture, beliefs, and values are inherent components of a holistic approach. Concepts of health and healing are deeply rooted in culture and, consciously or not, influence people's actions to promote, maintain, and restore health. Culture also may provide an understanding of a person's concept of illness or disease and appropriate treatment. Holistic nurses nurture a curiosity and high regard for cultural traditions and healthcare practices from various racial, ethnic, and social backgrounds. However, holistic nurses honor the individual's understanding and articulation of their own cultural values, beliefs, and health practices, avoiding and actively discouraging stereotypical cultural classifications and descriptions. The nurse then uses these understandings to provide care that corresponds with the beliefs, values, traditions, language, and health practices of people. With cultural humility and appreciation, holistic nurses ask individuals and communities, "What do I need to know culturally in caring for you?" This understanding is then used in the creation of a healing environment and in promoting communication and cultural care that is responsive to the beliefs, values, traditions, and health practices of all people. The chapter titled "Transcultural Engagement" delves more deeply into culture and the ways it intersects with the work of holistic nurses.

Holistic healing is a collaborative approach. Of particular importance to holistic nurses is the human connection with ecology. Holistic nurses actively participate in building an ecosystem that sustains the well-being of all life. This includes raising the public's consciousness about environmental issues and stressors that affect not only the health of people but also the health of the planet.

Core Value 5: Holistic Education and Research

Holistic nurses possess an understanding of a wide range of norms and healthcare practices, beliefs, and values concerning individuals, families, groups, and communities from a variety of racial, ethnic, spirituality-related, and social backgrounds. This rich knowledge base reflects their formal academic and continuing education preparation. Their knowledge also includes a wide diversity of practices and modalities outside of conventional Western medicine. Because of this, holistic nurses have a significant effect on people's understanding of healthcare options and alternatives, thus serving as both educators and advocates.

In addition, holistic nurses provide much-needed information to individuals on health promotion, including such topics as healthy lifestyles, risk-reducing behaviors, preventive self-care, stress management, living with changes secondary to illness and treatment, and opportunities to enhance well-being.

Holistic nurses value all the ways of knowing and learning. They assess health literacy and individualize learning, appreciating that science, intuition, introspection, creativity, aesthetics, and culture produce different bodies of knowledge and perspectives. They help others to know themselves and access their inner wisdom to enhance growth, wholeness, and well-being.

Holistic nurses may offer guidance and support to individuals and families in their healthcare choices and decisions, especially regarding conventional biomedical and integrative health approaches. Therefore, they must be knowledgeable about the best evidence available for both conventional approaches and CIHA. In addition to developing evidence-based practice using research, practice guidelines, and expertise, holistic nurses strongly consider the person's values and healthcare actions, customs, behaviors, and beliefs.

The American Holistic Nurses Association embraces and supports all research that has holism as a foundation (AHNA, 2016). Holistic nursing research is based on a philosophy of holism, or belief in the union of body-mind-emotion-spirit-energy-environment. The focus of holistic nursing research is understanding holistic phenomena, determining the effectiveness of holistic interventions, and developing an evidence base for holistic nursing practice.

Holistic nurses conduct and evaluate research in diverse areas such as:

- Outcome measures of various CIHA (e.g., therapeutic touch, prayer, aromatherapy, imagery)
- Instrument development to measure holistic phenomena, caring behaviors and dimensions, spirituality, self-transcendence, cultural competence, intuition, presence, mindfulness, and more
- Client/patient responses to holistic interventions in health, illness, and wellness
- Explorations of client/patients' lived experiences with various health, illness, and life phenomena
- Health decision making
- Health and wellness promotion and illness prevention
- Theory development in healing, wholeness, caring, intentionality, well-being, compassion, social and cultural constructions, empowerment, and more
- Healing relationships and healing environment
- Teaching and evaluation of holism
- Identification of attributes and skills that influence health (e.g., presence)

It is critical that holistic nursing continue to advance the scientific knowledge base of evidence for holistic practice. Healthcare professionals need such quality information to provide comprehensive evidence and outcome-based care that promotes a focus on healing and recognizes the importance of compassion and caring. The varied settings in which holistic nurses practice offer many opportunities to conduct meaningful research to improve healthcare consumer outcomes. The AHNA has incorporated an active research agenda by assisting and mentoring members in research endeavors, granting research awards, identifying and reporting on research that focuses on holistic healing phenomena and modalities, and applying research in practice.

Standards of Holistic Nursing Practice

There are 17 standards in *Holistic nursing: Scope and standards of practice*—6 for practice and 11 for professional performance (ANA & AHNA, 2019). Each standard addresses competencies for both the registered nurse and the graduate level–prepared and advanced practice registered nurse (APRN). Because each standard has numerous competencies, *only one or two competency examples per standard are included in the following sections.*

Overarching Philosophical Principles of Holistic Nursing

Holistic nurses express, contribute to, and promote an understanding of the following: a philosophy of nursing that values growth, development, and healing as desired outcomes; the human health experience as a complex, dynamic relationship of health, wellness, illness, disease, and well-being; the scientific foundations of nursing practice; and nursing as an art. As discussed earlier in this chapter, the philosophical principles of holistic nursing are embedded in every standard of practice and standard of professional performance.

Standards of Practice for Holistic Nursing

Standard 1. Assessment

The holistic registered nurse collects comprehensive data pertinent to the healthcare consumer's health or the situation.

Competencies. The holistic registered nurse:

- Collects comprehensive data, including but not limited to demographics, social determinants of health, health disparities, and physical, functional, psychosocial, emotional, cognitive, sexual, cultural, age-related, environmental, spirituality-related or transpersonal, economic and energy field assessments in a systematic, ongoing process with compassion, unconditional acceptance, and respect for the inherent dignity, worth, and unique attributes of every person.
- Assesses the healthcare consumer's health and cultural practices, values, beliefs, preferences, meanings of health, wellness, illness, disease, well-being, lifestyle patterns, family issues, and perceived risk behaviors and context.

The graduate level–prepared holistic registered nurse:

- Explores the meanings of the symbolic language expressed in dreams, images, symbols, narratives, sensations, rituals, and prayers as part of the healthcare consumer's experience.
- Uses advanced assessments, knowledge, and skills to maintain, enhance, or improve health conditions and facilitate growth and development.

The advanced practice holistic registered nurse:

- Initiates diagnostic tests and procedures relevant to the healthcare consumer's current status.

Standard 2. Diagnosis

The holistic registered nurse analyzes assessment data to determine the actual or potential diagnosis or issues expressed as challenges, problems, or needs.

The holistic registered nurse:

- Formulates the diagnosis, health challenges, or issues from comprehensive holistic assessment data.
- Validates the diagnosis, health challenges, or issues with the healthcare consumer, family or significant other, group, community, population, and other healthcare providers when possible and appropriate.

The graduate level–prepared holistic registered nurse:

- Utilizes complex data and information obtained during interview, examination, and diagnostic procedures in identifying diagnoses.

The advanced practice holistic registered nurse:

- Formulates a differential diagnosis based on the holistic assessment, history, examination, and diagnostic test results.

Standard 3. Outcomes Identification

The holistic registered nurse identifies expected outcomes for a plan individualized to the healthcare consumer or the situation. (The holistic nurse values the evolution and the process of healing as it unfolds. Unfolding outcomes may not be immediately evident, due to the nonlinear nature of the healing process, so both expected or anticipated and evolving or emerging outcomes are considered.)

The holistic registered nurse:

- Defines expected outcomes in terms of the healthcare consumer's values and beliefs, preferences, culture, age, practices related to spirituality, ethical considerations, environment, or situation.
- Partners with the healthcare consumer to identify realistic goals based on the person's present and potential capabilities and quality of life.

The graduate level–prepared holistic registered nurse, including the APRN:

- Identifies expected outcomes incorporating healthcare consumer satisfaction, the person's understanding and meanings in their unique patterns and processes, quality of life, cost, practice effectiveness, and continuity and consistency among providers.

Standard 4. Planning

The holistic registered nurse develops a plan outlining primary strategies and suggested alternatives to attain expected outcomes.

The holistic registered nurse:

- In partnership with the healthcare consumer, family, and others, develops an individualized plan considering the characteristics or situation, including values, beliefs, knowledge and understanding, practices related to spirituality and health, preferences, choices, developmental level, coping style, culture and environment, and available technology.
- Establishes practice settings, safe space, and time for both the nurse and healthcare consumer, family, and significant others to explore suggested, potential, and alternative options.

The graduate level–prepared holistic registered nurse:

- Identifies assessment strategies, diagnostic strategies, therapeutic interventions, therapeutic effects, and side effects that reflect current evidence, including data, research, literature, expert practice-based knowledge, and the healthcare consumer's experiences.
- Uses linguistic and symbolic language, including but not limited to word associations, dreams, storytelling, and journals, to explore with individuals the possibilities and options.

The advanced practice holistic registered nurse:

- Integrates assessment strategies, diagnostic strategies, and therapeutic interventions reflecting current evidence-based knowledge and practice.

Standard 5. Implementation

The holistic registered nurse implements the identified plan. (Sometimes, the plan is not directed to clinical care but administrative, educational, or other foci.)

The holistic registered nurse:

- Partners with the healthcare consumer, family, significant others, and caregivers as appropriate to implement the holistic plan in a safe, realistic, effective, efficient, timely, person-centered, and equitable manner.
- Uses self as an instrument of healing.

The graduate level–prepared holistic registered nurse:

- Uses advanced knowledge of pharmacology, psychoneuroimmunology, nutritional supplements, homeopathic remedies, herbal remedies, and a variety of CIHA.
- Uses systems, organizations, and community resources to lead effective change and implement the plan.

The advanced practice holistic registered nurse:

- Uses prescriptive authority, procedures, referrals, treatments, and therapies in accordance with state and federal laws and regulations.

Standard 5A. Coordination of Care

The holistic registered nurse coordinates care delivery.

The holistic registered nurse:

- Organizes the components of the holistic care plan.
- Assists the healthcare consumer to identify options for conventional and/or alternative care.

The graduate level–prepared holistic registered nurse:

- Provides leadership in the coordination of interprofessional holistic health care for integrated delivery of healthcare consumer services to achieve safe, effective, efficient, timely, patient-centered, and equitable care.
- Synthesizes holistic data and information to prescribe and provide necessary system and community support measures, including modifications of environments.

The advanced practice holistic registered nurse:

- Serves as the healthcare consumer's primary care provider and coordinator of holistic healthcare services in accordance with state and federal laws and regulations.

Standard 5B. Health Teaching and Health Promotion

The holistic registered nurse employs strategies to promote holistic health and wellness and a safe environment.

The holistic registered nurse:

- Provides opportunities for the healthcare consumer to identify needed holistic healthcare promotion, disease prevention, and self-management topics.
- Uses health promotion and health teaching methods in collaboration with the healthcare consumer's values, beliefs, health practices, developmental level, learning needs, readiness and ability to learn, language preference, spirituality, culture, and socioeconomic status.
- Assists others to access their own inner wisdom that may provide opportunities to enhance and support growth, development, and wholeness.

The graduate level–prepared holistic registered nurse, including the APRN:

- Synthesizes empirical evidence on risk behaviors, societal roles, learning theories, behavioral change theories, motivational theories, translational theories for evidence-based practice, epidemiology, and other related theories and frameworks when designing holistic health education information and programs.

Standard 6. Evaluation

The holistic registered nurse evaluates progress toward attainment of goals and health outcomes.

The holistic registered nurse:

- Conducts a holistic, systematic, ongoing, and criterion-based evaluation of the goals and outcomes in relation to the structure, processes, and timeline prescribed in the plan.
- Determines, in partnership with the healthcare consumer and other stakeholders, the patient-centeredness, effectiveness, efficiency, safety, timeliness, and equitability of the strategies in relation to the responses to the plan and attainment of expected and unfolding outcomes. Other defined criteria (e.g., Quality and Safety Education for Nurses) may be used as well.

The graduate level–prepared holistic registered nurse, including the APRN:

- Synthesizes evaluation data from the healthcare consumer, community, population, and/or

institution to determine the effectiveness of the plan.
- Evaluates, in partnership with the healthcare consumer, the accuracy of the biomedical and nursing diagnoses and the effectiveness of the interventions in relationship to the client's/patient's attainment of expected and evolving outcomes and changes of meaning in the client's/patient's healing experience.

Standards of Professional Performance

Standard 7. Ethics

The holistic registered nurse practices ethically.

The holistic registered nurse:

- Integrates the *Code of ethics for nurses with interpretive statements* (ANA, 2015) to guide nursing practice and articulate the moral foundation of nursing.
- Advocates for equitable consumer healthcare, particularly regarding the rights of vulnerable or underserved populations, by such activities as:
    - Acting on behalf of individuals, families, groups, and communities as requested or required by law.
    - Seeking to eliminate barriers to care, such as affordability and accessibility.
- Commits to self-reflection, self-assessment, self-development, and self-care strategies to enhance physical, psychological, intellectual, sociological, and spirituality-related well-being.

The graduate level–prepared holistic registered nurse, including the APRN:

- Provides information on the risks, benefits, and outcomes of healthcare regimens to allow informed decision making by the healthcare consumer, including informed consent and informed refusal.
- Actively contributes to creating an ecosystem that supports well-being for all life.

Standard 8. Culturally Congruent Practice

The holistic registered nurse practices in a manner that is congruent with cultural diversity and inclusion principles.

The holistic registered nurse:

- Demonstrates cultural awareness and sensitivity by seeking knowledge of health beliefs and practices that are representative of the cultural values, beliefs, practices, and traditions of individuals, families, groups, and communities for whom they care.
- Understands that a lack of cultural awareness and a failure to provide care that is culturally congruent with the worldview of a person can greatly increase the stresses experienced by healthcare consumers and caregivers alike.
- Uses skills and tools that are appropriately vetted for the culture, literacy, and language of the population served.

The graduate level–prepared holistic registered nurse:

- Advances organizational policies, programs, services, and practices that reflect respect, equity, and the values of diversity and inclusion.
- Leads interprofessional teams to identify and act on the cultural and language needs of the consumer.

The advanced practice holistic registered nurse:

- Promotes shared decision-making solutions in planning, prescribing, and evaluating processes when the healthcare consumer's cultural preferences and norms may create incompatibility with evidence-based practice and the values, beliefs, and norms of the biomedical culture.

Standard 9. Communication

The holistic registered nurse communicates effectively in a variety of formats in all areas of practice.

The holistic registered nurse:

- Assesses one's own communication skills and effectiveness in encounters with individuals, families, significant others, and colleagues.

- Uses communication styles and methods that demonstrate intention, centering, presence, caring, respect, deep listening, authenticity, and trust.
- Contributes the holistic nursing perspective in interactions with others and discussions with the interprofessional team.

The graduate level–prepared holistic registered nurse, including the APRN:

- Provides leadership for establishing, improving, and sustaining collaborative relationships to achieve safe, quality care for healthcare consumers.
- Functions as a role model and leader in creating healthy work environments that facilitate and support effective communication and healing.

Standard 10. Collaboration

The holistic registered nurse collaborates with the healthcare consumer, family, and other key stakeholders in the conduct of holistic nursing practice.

The holistic registered nurse:

- Identifies the expertise and contribution of diverse disciplines, approaches to health care, and key stakeholders.
- Communicates the holistic nurse's role and responsibilities within the team.
- Engages in teamwork and team-building processes.

The graduate level–prepared holistic registered nurse, including the APRN:

- Facilitates the negotiation of holistic, complementary, alternative, integrative, and conventional healthcare services for continuity of care and program planning.

Standard 11. Leadership

The holistic registered nurse leads within the professional practice setting and the profession.

The holistic registered nurse:

- Mentors colleagues for the advancement of holistic nursing practice, the profession, and quality holistic health care.
- Engages at local, state, national, and international levels to expand the knowledge and practice of holistic nursing and awareness of holistic health issues.

The graduate level–prepared holistic registered nurse, including the APRN:

- Influences decision-making bodies to improve holistic integrative care, the professional practice environment, and holistic healthcare consumer outcomes.
- Articulates the ideas underpinning holistic nursing philosophy, placing these ideas in a historical, philosophical, and scientific context while projecting future trends in thinking.

Standard 12. Education

The holistic registered nurse attains knowledge and competence that reflect current nursing practice and promotes futuristic thinking.

The holistic registered nurse:

- Participates in ongoing educational activities related to nursing, holism, and interprofessional knowledge bases and professional topics.
- Demonstrates a commitment to lifelong learning through self-reflection and inquiry for learning and personal growth.

The graduate level–prepared holistic registered nurse, including the APRN:

- Uses current healthcare research findings and other sources of evidence to expand clinical knowledge, skills, abilities, and judgment; to enhance holistic role performance; and to increase knowledge of professional issues and changes in national standards for practice and trends in holistic care.

Standard 13. Evidence-Based Practice and Research

The holistic registered nurse integrates evidence and research findings into practice.

The holistic registered nurse:

- Utilizes the best available evidence, which includes nursing theories and research findings, to guide practice.

- Incorporates evidence from experience, intuition, research, and population responses to care when initiating changes in nursing practice.
- Participates in research related to holistic nursing.

The graduate level–prepared holistic registered nurse, including the APRN:

- Contributes to nursing knowledge by conducting or synthesizing research that discovers, examines, and evaluates current practice, knowledge, theories, philosophies, context, criteria, and creative approaches to improve holistic healthcare outcomes.
- Disseminates research findings through activities such as presentations, publications, consultations, and journal clubs for a variety of audiences (including nursing, other disciplines, and the public) to improve holistic care and further develop the foundation and practice of holistic nursing.

Standard 14. Quality of Practice

The holistic registered nurse contributes to quality nursing practice.

The holistic registered nurse:

- Ensures that holistic nursing practice is safe, effective, efficient, equitable, timely, patient centered, and grounded in holism.
- Uses creativity and innovation to enhance holistic nursing care.

The graduate level–prepared holistic registered nurse:

- Engages in development, implementation, evaluation and/or revisions of policies, procedures, and guidelines to improve holistic healthcare quality.
- Evaluates the practice environment and quality of holistic care rendered in relation to existing evidence and feedback from individuals, families, and significant others.

Standard 15. Professional Practice Evaluation

The holistic registered nurse evaluates one's own and others' nursing practice.

The holistic registered nurse:

- Engages in self-reflection and self-evaluation of practice on a regular basis, identifying areas of strength as well as areas in which professional development and personal growth would be beneficial.
- Reflects on their practice and how their own personal, cultural, and/or spiritual or personally meaningful beliefs, experiences, biases, education, and values may affect care given to individuals, families, and communities.

The graduate level–prepared holistic registered nurse:

- Applies knowledge obtained from advanced preparation, as well as current research and evidence-based information, to clinical decision making at the point of care to achieve optimal holistic health outcomes.

Standard 16. Resource Utilization

The holistic registered nurse utilizes appropriate resources to plan, provide, and sustain evidence-based nursing services that are holistic, safe, effective, and fiscally responsible.

The holistic registered nurse:

- Assists the healthcare consumer, family, significant other, and caregivers in identifying and securing appropriate and available services to address needs across the healthcare continuum.
- Addresses discriminatory healthcare practices and the impact on resource allocation.

The graduate level–prepared holistic registered nurse:

- Designs innovative solutions to use resources effectively and maintain quality.
- Engages organizational and community resources to formulate and implement interprofessional plans.

Standard 17. Environmental Health

The holistic registered nurse practices in an environmentally safe and healthy manner.

The holistic registered nurse:

- Assesses the practice environment for factors that support or threaten health and healing, such as sound, odor, vibration, light, clean air, shelter, water, and food to ensure that the basic health and safety needs within our own world and that of healthcare consumers are met.
- Promotes a safe and healthy practice environment that reduces environmental health risks for self, workers, and healthcare consumers to support resilience and protect them from harm.

The graduate level–prepared holistic registered nurse, including the APRN:

- Ascertains the impact of social, political, and economic influences on the environment and human health exposures.
- Acts as a leader, collaborator, consultant, and change agent in evaluating global health issues related to environmental health and safety; designing holistic plans of care that address all effects of environmental changes on the health and welfare of individuals, groups, and communities; and assisting in reducing or eliminating environmental hazards.

Settings for Holistic Nursing Practice

Holistic nurses practice in numerous fields and settings, including but not limited to:

Ambulatory outpatient settings

Acute care hospitals

Long-term and extended care facilities, nursing homes, and assisted living facilities

Home care settings

Complementary and integrative care centers

Women's health and birthing centers

Hospice palliative care

Psychiatric mental health facilities

Private practitioner offices

Schools

Rehabilitation centers

Religious parishes

Community health and primary care centers

Student and employee health clinics

Managed care organizations

Independent, self-employed private practice

Telehealth and cyber care services

Correctional facilities

International and travel nursing

Military

Professional nursing and healthcare organizations

Informatics

Administration

Staff development

Universities and colleges

There are increasing numbers of holistic nurses who hold leadership roles as clinicians, educators, authors, and researchers in university-based schools of nursing, practice environments, nursing, and other professional organizations. Holistic nursing practice also occurs when there is a request for consultation or when holistic nurses advocate for care that promotes health and prevents disease, illness, or disability for individuals, communities, or the environment. A holistic nurse may choose not to work in a critical care setting but provide consultation regarding self-care or stress management to nurses practicing in that area. Or holistic nurses may practice in preoperative and recovery rooms, instituting a pre- and postsurgical program for individuals that teaches them meditation and positive affirmation techniques while incorporating a homeopathic regimen for trauma and cell healing. Employment or voluntary participation of holistic nurses also can influence civic activities and the regulatory and legislative arenas at the local, state, national, or international levels.

Because holistic nursing focuses on the wellness, wholeness, and development of the whole person, holistic nurses also practice in health-enhancement settings such as spas, gyms, and wellness centers. With all populations and in any setting, nurses can empower patients/clients/families by teaching them self-care practices for a healthier lifestyle. In addition, there are numerous entrepreneurial possibilities for holistic nurses to develop integrative care programs in hospitals, home care, primary care practices, occupational and school settings, and the community.

Because holistic nursing is a worldview, a way of being in the world, and not just a modality, holistic nurses can practice in any setting and with individuals throughout the life span. As the public increasingly requests holistic and CIHA services and a comprehensive, humanistic emphasis on the whole person, there will be a greater need for holistic nurses in a wider array of settings, because "Holistic nursing takes place wherever healing occurs" (Mariano, 2009, p. 6).

Educational Preparation and Certification for Holistic Nursing Practice

Holistic nurses are registered nurses who are educationally prepared for practice from an approved school of nursing and are licensed to practice in their individual state, commonwealth, or territory. The American Holistic Nurses Credentialing Corporation (AHNCC) conducted an examination of nursing education from the basic to the advanced level. This process included reviewing state licensure requirements, exploring best practices in education, and analyzing the AACN Essentials of Baccalaureate, Master's and Doctorate of Nursing Practice education in nursing. The comparative analysis of these with the AHNA Core Values and *Holistic nursing: Scope and standards of practice* resulted in the development of the Foundations, Competencies, and Curricular Guidelines for Basic to Doctoral Holistic Nursing Education (Erickson et al., 2017). The holistic registered nurse's experience, education, knowledge, and abilities establish the level of competence. *Holistic nursing: Scope and standards of practice* identifies the scope of practice of holistic nursing and the specific standards and associated measurement criteria of holistic nurses at both the basic and advanced levels (ANA & AHNA, 2019). Regardless of the level of practice, all holistic nurses integrate the previously identified five core values.

A registered nurse may prepare for the specialty of holistic nursing in a variety of ways. Educational offerings range from associate's degree, baccalaureate, and graduate courses and programs to continuing education programs with extensive contact hours.

Basic Practice Level

The education of all nursing students preparing for registered nurse (RN) licensure includes basic content on physiological, psychological, emotional, and some spirituality-related processes with populations across the life span and conventional nursing care practices within each of these domains. In addition, basic nursing education incorporates experiences in a variety of clinical and practice settings from acute care to community. However, the educational focus is most frequently on specialties often emanating from the biomedical disease model and cure orientation. In holistic nursing, the individual across the life span is viewed in context as an integrated totality of body, mind, emotion, environment, society, energy, and spirit, with the emphasis on wholeness, well-being, health promotion, and healing using both conventional and complementary/alternative practices. Because of the lack of intentional focus on integration, unity, and healing, the educational exposure of most nursing students is not adequate preparation for assuming the specialty role of a holistic nurse.

Increasingly, schools of nursing are embracing holistic nursing practices and CIHA and adding them to their curricula, responding to consumer use of CIHA and consumer demand for health professionals who are knowledgeable about holistic practices. The most recent version of *The essentials: Core competencies for professional nursing education* (AACN, 2021) includes language on preparing the professional nursing graduate to practice from a holistic, caring framework; engage in self-care; develop an understanding of health within diverse cultural contexts; work from and contribute to the pillars of evidence-based practice; and incorporate patient teaching and health promotion, spirituality, and caring, healing techniques into their activities and interactions. This acknowledges that nursing recognizes the importance of healing principles and practices in health care and the need for nurses to learn them in the educational process.

Advanced Practice Level

As with the basic level, there are a variety of ways through both academic and professional development that registered nurses can acquire the additional specialized knowledge and skills that prepare them for advanced holistic nursing practice. These nurses are expected to hold a master's or doctoral degree and demonstrate a greater depth and scope of knowledge, a deeper integration of information, increased complexity of skills and interventions, and notable role autonomy. They provide leadership in practice, teaching, research, consultation, advocacy, and policy formation in advancing holistic nursing to improve the holistic health of people. Several schools of nursing that offer graduate programs in holistic nursing have a stable or growing number of applicants. Current advanced practice nurses are increasingly gaining specialized knowledge preparing them as holistic nurses through post-master's programs, continuing education offerings in holistic nursing care, and certificate programs throughout the country that focus on specific modalities and on the essence of holism.

Continuing Education for Basics and Advanced Practice Levels

The AHNA is a provider and approver of continuing education and is recognized by the American Nurses Credentialing Center (ANCC). Continuing educational programs, workshops, and lectures in holistic nursing and complementary/integrative medicine have been popular nationwide, with AHNA or other bodies granting continuing education units.

The AHNA endorses certificate programs in specific areas. These include Holistic Integrative Healing, Reflexology, Imagery, Aromatherapy, Healing Touch, Spirituality, Craniosacral Therapy, Holistic Stress Management, Integrative Healing Arts, Coaching, Whole Health Education, and RN Patient Advocate. It also approves continuing education offerings in holistic nursing as well as providing the AHNA home study course, Foundation of Holistic Nursing. Other programs in distinct therapies such as acupuncture, Reiki, homeopathy, massage, imagery, healing arts, holistic health, Chinese Oriental Medicine, nutrition, Ayurveda, therapeutic touch, healing touch, herbology, chiropractic, and so on are given nationally as degrees, certificates, or continuing education programs by centers, specialty organizations, or schools.

Certification

Competency mechanisms for evaluating holistic nursing practice as a specialty exist through a national certification and recertification process overseen by the AHNCC. The AHNCC offers four certifications: Holistic Nurse, Board Certified (HN-BC), which requires a minimum of a diploma or associate degree in nursing from an accredited school; Holistic Baccalaureate Nurse, Board Certified (HBN-BC), which requires a baccalaureate degree in nursing from an institution regionally accredited by the Association of Schools and Colleges; and Advanced Holistic Nurse, Board Certified (AHN-BC), and Advanced Practice Holistic Nurse (APHN-BC, APRN), which require a master's degree in nursing from an institution regionally accredited by the Association of Schools and Colleges. Further, the AHNCC provides endorsement for schools of nursing meeting the specifications put forth in *Holistic nursing: Scope and standards of practice* (ANA & AHNA, 2019). In addition, holistic nurses are often certified in specific complementary integrative modalities such as imagery, Reiki, aromatherapy, healing touch, biofeedback, and reflexology.

Implications

Self

1. What attributes do I have that reflect the core values of holistic nursing?
2. What contributions can I make as a holistic nurse to the wholeness and betterment of humankind?

Clinical Practice

1. Given their education and experience, holistic nurses are the logical leaders in holistic and integrative care and must advance that position.
2. Through monitoring state boards of nursing for evidence of their recognition and support of holistic, integrative nursing practice and requirements that include CIHA, holistic nursing has the challenge of working with the state boards to incorporate this content into the National Council Licensure Examination, thus ensuring the credibility of this practice knowledge.

Education

1. There is an urgent need for integration of holistic, relationship-centered, caring–healing philosophies into nursing curricula.
2. With the increased use of CIHA by the American public, both students and faculty need knowledge of these therapies and skill in their use.

Research

1. Exploration of research modalities and approaches that are congruent with the holistic paradigm.
2. Examination of how the standards of holistic nursing practice are being implemented in healthcare settings.
3. Secure funding for their holistic research to identify and describe outcomes of CIHA and therapies, such as healing, well-being, and harmony, and to develop instruments to measure these outcomes.

Policy

1. Working with Medicare and other third-party payers, insurance groups, boards of nursing, healthcare policy makers, legislators, and other professional nursing organizations to ensure that holistic nurses are appropriately reimbursed for services rendered.
2. Active participation in healthcare reform and the political arena as leaders in the movement to ensure quality, value, an increased focus on wellness, patient-centered humanistic care, and access and affordability for all.

Conclusion

The specialty practice of holistic nursing is generally not well understood. Therefore, each holistic nurse must educate other nurses, healthcare providers and disciplines, and the public about the role, value, and benefits of holistic nursing, whether it be in direct practice, education, management, or research. Holistic nurses communicate the ideas underpinning the holistic paradigm and the philosophy of the caring–healing relationship. Jean Watson reminds us that society and the public are searching for something deeper in terms of realizing self-care, self-knowledge, and self-healing potentials. Nurses need to acknowledge the human aspects of practice—attending to people and their experience rather than just focusing on the biomedical orientation and disease. Watson concludes that "nurses have a covenant with the public to sustain caring. It is our collective responsibility to transform caring practices into the framework that identifies and gives distinction to nursing as a profession" (Mariano 2005, p. 12). In a 2019 interview, Mariano expressed hope that eventually all nurses will be holistic nurses; holism will be introduced in all educational levels; and that all nurses will learn self-care, integrative approaches, energy work, and care of the whole person. "By incorporating holistic principles and practices, nurses will find more meaning and purpose in their work and life" (Hart, 2019, p. 2). *Holistic nursing: Scope and standards of practice* is a means through which holistic nurses are educating the profession and others about the values, principles, and practice requirements of this specialty.

Note: This chapter is derived from Carla Mariano, *Holistic nursing: Scope and standards of practice* (3rd ed.) (2019), also the Revision Workgroup member and primary contributor for the 1st and 2nd editions. Printed with permission of the American Holistic Nurses Association (AHNA).

References

American Association of Colleges of Nursing (AACN). (2021). *The essentials: Core competencies for professional nursing education*. AACN.

American Holistic Nurses Association (AHNA). (1998). *Description of holistic nursing*. American Holistic Nurses Association.

American Holistic Nurses Association (AHNA). (2012). *Position statement on holistic nursing ethics*. American Holistic Nurses Association.

American Holistic Nurses Association (AHNA). (2016). *White paper: Research in AHNA*. American Holistic Nurses Association.

American Holistic Nurses Association (AHNA). (2016). *Position on the role of nurses in the practice of complementary and integrative health approaches (CIHA). AHNA.* In M. A. B. Helming, D. A. Shields, K. M. Avino, & W. E. Rosa (Eds.), *Holistic nursing: A handbook for practice* (8th ed.). Jones & Bartlett Learning.

American Nurses Association (ANA). (2004). *Nursing: Scope and standards of practice*. American Nurses Association.

American Nurses Association (ANA). (2010a). *Nursing's social policy statement: The essence of the profession*. American Nurses Association.

American Nurses Association (ANA). (2010b). *Recognition of a nursing specialty, approval of a specialty nursing scope of practice statement, and acknowledgement of specialty nursing standards of practice*. American Nurses Association.

American Nurses Association (ANA). (2015). *Code of ethics for nurses with interpretive statements*. American Nurses Association. http://www.nursingworld.org/MainMenuCategories/EthicsStandards/CodeofEthicsforNurses/Code-ofEthics-For-Nurses.html

American Nurses Association (ANA). (2021). *Nursing: Scope and standards of practice* (4th ed.). American Nurses Association.

American Nurses Association & American Holistic Nurses Association (ANA & AHNA). (2019). *Holistic nursing: Scope and standards of practice* (3rd ed.). American Nurses Association and American Holistic Nurses Association.

Bigelow, J. (1859). Discourses and essays. In *Nature in disease: Illustrated in various discourses and essays* (pp. 2–63). Phillips Sampson & Co. Medical Communications of the MA Medical Society.

Cowling, W. R. (2011). Holism as a sociopolitical enterprise. *Journal of Holistic Nursing, 29*(1), 5–6.

Dossey, B. M. (2010). *Florence Nightingale: Mystic, visionary, healer* (Commemorative Edition). F. A. Davis.

Erickson, H., Erickson, M., Enzman-Hines, M., Sandor, M. K., Shields, D., & Southard, M. E. (2017). *Foundations, competencies, and curricular guidelines for basic to doctoral holistic nursing education*. American Holistic Nurses Credentialing Corporation with the American Holistic Nurses Association.

Hart, J. (2019). The expanding field of holistic nursing—A growing trend. Interview with Carla Mariano. *Alternative and Complementary Therapies, 25*(1), 53–55.

Helming, M. A. B., Shields, D. A., Avino, K. M., & Rosa, W. E. (Eds.). (2022). *Holistic nursing: A handbook for practice* (8th ed.). Jones & Bartlett.

Institute of Medicine. (2001). *Crossing the quality chasm: A new health system for the 21st century*. National Academies Press.

Joint Commission on Accreditation of Healthcare Organizations (JCAHO). (1992). Patient bill of rights. In *Accreditation manual for hospitals*. Joint Commission on Accreditation of Healthcare Organizations.

Luck, S. (2022). Environmental health. In M. A. B. Helming, D. A. Shields, K. M. Avino, & W. E. Rosa (Eds.), *Holistic nursing: A handbook for practice* (8th ed.). Jones & Bartlett Learning.

Mariano, C. (2005). Caring for our future: An interview with Jean Watson. *Beginnings, 25*(3), 12–14.

Mariano, C. (2006). *Proposal for recognition of holistic nursing as a nursing specialty* (Unpublished document submitted to the American Nurses Association).

Mariano, C. (2009). Holistic nursing: Every nurse's specialty. *Beginnings, 29*(4), 4–6.

Mariano, C. (2019). Holistic integrative therapies in palliative care. In M. Matzo & D. Sherman (Eds.), *Palliative care nursing quality care to the end of life* (5th ed., pp. 257–286). Springer Publishing Co.

National Center for Complementary and Integrative Health (NCCIH). (2025a, January 4). *Complementary, alternative, or integrative health: What's in a name?* https://www.nccih.nih.gov/health/complementary-alternative-or-integrative-health-whats-in-a-name

National Center for Complementary and Integrative Health (NCCIH). (2025b, September 8). *Stress*. https://www.nccih.nih.gov/health/stress

Nightingale, F. (1859). *Notes on nursing: What it is and what it is not*. Harrison of Pall Mall.

Office of Disease Prevention and Health Promotion (ODPHP). (2025, February 16). *Environmental health workgroup*. U.S. Department of Health and Human Services. https://odphp.health.gov/healthypeople/about/workgroups/environmental-health-workgroup#:~:text=The%20World%20Health%20Organization%20defines,to%20the%20interactions%20between%20people

Plato. (2004). *Essential Thinkers—Socrates*. Barnes & Noble Collector's Library.

Thornton, L., & Mariano, C. (2016). Evolving from therapeutic to holistic communication. In B. Dossey & L. Keegan (Eds.), *Holistic nursing: A handbook for practice* (7th ed., pp. 465–478). Jones & Bartlett Learning.

Tresolini, C. P., & Pew-Fetzer Task Force. (1994). *Health professions education and relationship-centered care: Report of the Pew-Fetzer Task Force on advancing psychosocial education*. Pew Health Professions Commission. http://www.futurehealth.ucsf.edu/pdf_files/RelationshipCentered.pdf

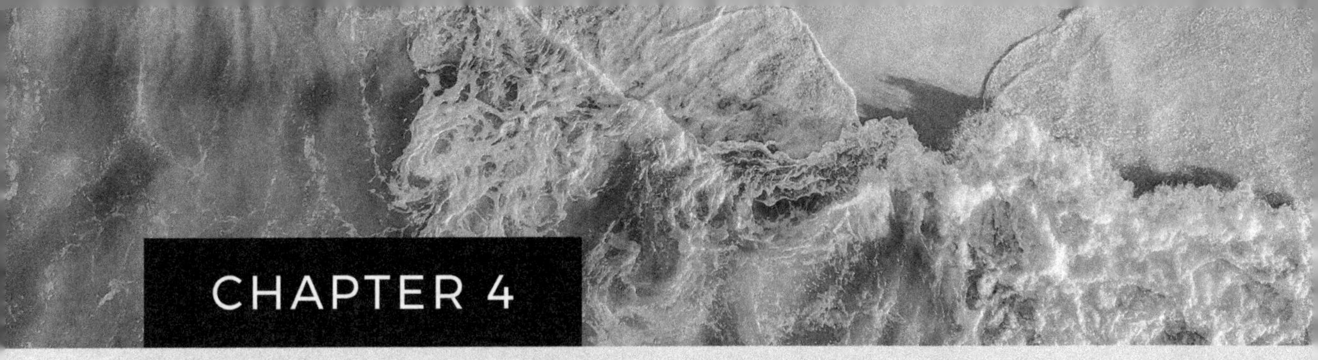

CHAPTER 4

The Theory of Integral Nursing

Barbara Montgomery Dossey

NURSE HEALER OBJECTIVES

- Define the theory of integral nursing (TIN).
- Explore the TIN components.
- Examine the TIN implications for clinical practice, education, research, and policy.

DEFINITIONS

Integral: A comprehensive way to organize multiple phenomena of human experience related to four perspectives of reality: (1) individual interior (subjective, personal/intentional); (2) individual exterior (objective, physiology/behavioral); (3) collective interior (intersubjective, shared/cultural); and (4) collective exterior (interobjective, systems/structures).

Integral dialogue: Transformative and visionary exploration of ideas and possibilities across disciplines where the four integral perspectives of reality are considered as equally important to dialogues and outcomes.

Integral healing process: The unitary whole person or persons interacting in mutual process with the environment that includes a four-quadrant perspective.

Integral health: A process through which we reshape basic assumptions and worldviews about well-being and see death as a natural process of living.

Integral health care: A patient-centered and relationship-centered caring process that includes the patient, family, and community and conventional, integrative, and integral healthcare practitioners and services and interventions.

Integral nurse: A 21st-century Nightingale who is engaged as a health diplomat and an integral health coach who is coaching from integral perspectives.

Integral nursing: A comprehensive integral worldview and process that enlarges our holistic understanding of body-mind-spirit-cultural-environmental connections and our knowing, doing, and being to more comprehensive and deeper levels.

Integral worldview: Process where values, beliefs, assumptions, meaning, purpose, and judgments are identified and related to how individuals perceive four perspectives of reality.

Note: The theory of integral nursing (TIN) has been published in *Holistic nursing: A handbook for practice* (5th ed., 2009; 6th ed., 2013; 7th ed., 2016, 8th ed., 2022). The TIN has also appeared in articles and in M. C. Smith. (2020). *Nursing Theories and Nursing Practice* (4th ed., 2015; 5th ed., 2020; 6th ed., 2025). F. A. Davis.

Introduction

The nursing profession asks nurses to wrap around all of life on so many levels with self and others that we can often feel overwhelmed. How do we get a handle on all of life? The question always arises: "How can overworked nurses and student nurses use an integral approach or apply the theory of integral nursing?" The answer is to start right now. By the time you finish reading this chapter, you will find answers to these questions that are about being and doing.

As you read about the theory of integral nursing (TIN), remember that the words *integral* and *integrally informed* are used often because this is a shift to a deeper level of understanding about being human as related to the four dimensions of reality. It is incorrect to substitute the word *holistic* because it does not mean the same thing. Begin to explore the integral process in your personal and professional projects, and endeavors. As nurses become more integrally aware in their personal and professional lives, it increases one's capacities to experience a journey of joy as one gains new perspectives and connections (Morrow & Dossey, 2024).

The Theory of Integral Nursing

The theory of integral nursing (TIN) is a grand theory in the integrative–interactive paradigm that presents the art and science of nursing (Dossey, 2008, 2025). Florence Nightingale's philosophy and legacy are woven within the theory (Dossey, 2010). It includes an integral process, integral worldview, and integral dialogues that are praxis—theory in action. Her work, like our work today, can be seen as sacred activism and radical action in the work (Harvey, 2009). Nursing incorporates existing theoretical work that builds on our solid holistic and multidimensional theoretical nursing foundation. This theory may be used with other holistic nursing and nonnursing caring concepts, theories, and research; it does not exclude or invalidate other nurse theorists who have informed this theory. This is not a freestanding theory because it incorporates concepts and philosophies from various paradigms including holism, multidimensionality, integral theory, chaos theory, spiral dynamics, complexity, systems theory, and many others.

TIN adapts the work of Ken Wilber, one of the most significant American new-paradigm philosophers, to strengthen the core concept of healing. Wilber's integral model is an elegant, four-quadrant model that has been developed over 35 years. In his eight-volume *Collected Works of Ken Wilber* (Wilber, 1999, 2000a), he synthesizes the ideas and theories of the best-known and most influential researchers and theorists to show that no individual or discipline can determine reality or have all of the answers (Wilber, 2000b, 2005). Within the nursing profession, other nurses are exploring integral theories (Dossey, 2015; Dossey et al., 2017; Shea et al., 2019; Shea & Frisch, 2014, 2016).

The TIN intentions are presented in **Box 4-1**. The philosophical assumptions are presented in **Box 4-2**. The interventions most frequently used in TIN are observed in **Table 4-1**.

Box 4-1 Theory of Integral Nursing Intentions

1. To embrace the unitary whole person and the complexity of the nursing profession and health care.
2. To explore the direct application of an integral process and integral worldview that includes four perspectives of realities—the individual interior and exterior and the collective interior and exterior.
3. To expand nurses' capacities as 21st-century Nightingales, health diplomats, and integral nurse coaches—local to global.
4. To embrace the unitary whole person and the complexity of the nursing profession and health care.
5. To explore the direct application of an integral process and integral worldview that includes four perspectives of realities—the individual interior and exterior and the collective interior and exterior.
6. To expand nurses' capacities as 21st-century Nightingales, health diplomats, and integral nurse coaches—local to global.

 Dossey, B. M. (2008). Theory of integral nursing. *Advances in Nursing Science, 31*(1), E52–E73.

Box 4-2 Theory of Integral Nursing Philosophical Assumptions

1. An integral understanding recognizes the individual as an energy field connected to the energy fields of others and the wholeness of humanity; the world is open, dynamic, interdependent, fluid, and continuously interacting with changing variables that can lead to greater complexity and order.
2. An integral worldview is a comprehensive way to organize multiple phenomena of human experience from four perspectives of reality: (a) individual interior (subjective, personal); (b) individual exterior (objective, behavioral); (c) collective interior (intersubjective, cultural); and (d) collective exterior (interobjective, systems/structures).
3. Healing is a process inherent in all living things; it may occur with curing of symptoms, but it is not synonymous with curing.
4. Integral health is experienced by a person as wholeness with development toward personal growth and expanding states of consciousness to deeper levels of personal and collective understanding of one's physical, mental, emotional, social, spiritual, cultural, and environmental dimensions.
5. Integral nursing is founded on an integral worldview using integral language and knowledge that integrates integral life practices and skills each day.
6. Integral nursing is broadly defined to include knowledge development and all ways of knowing that also recognizes the emergent patterns of not knowing.
7. An integral nurse is an instrument in the healing process and facilitates healing through their knowing, doing, and being.
8. Integral nursing is applicable in practice, education, research, and healthcare policy—local to global.

 Dossey, B. M. (2008). Theory of integral nursing. *Advances in Nursing Science, 31*(1), E52–E73.

Table 4-1 Interventions Most Frequently Used in the Theory of Integral Nursing

Affirmations	Humor, laughter, play	Presence
Appreciative inquiry	Intention	Probing questions
Aromatherapy	Journaling	Reflection
Art and drawing	Meditation	Relaxation modalities
Celebration	Mindfulness practice	Ritual
Cognitive reframing	Motivational interviewing	Self-assessments
Contracts	Movement	Self-care interventions
Deep listening	Music and sound	Self-reflection
Energy practices	Nature walks	Silence
Exercise	Open-ended questions	Somatic awareness
Goal setting	Patient assessments	Stories
Guided imagery	Prayer	Visioning

 Dossey, B. M. (2008). Theory of integral nursing. *Advances in Nursing Science, 31*(1), E52–E73.

Barnum's Content, Context, and Process

To present the theory of integral nursing, Barbara Barnum's framework to critique a nursing theory—content, context, and process—provides an organizing structure that is most useful (Barnum, 2005). The theory of integral nursing includes an integral process, integral worldview, and integral dialogues that compose praxis—theory in action (**Figure 4-1**).

Content

The content of a nursing theory includes the subject matter and building blocks that give a theory its form. It comprises the stable elements that are

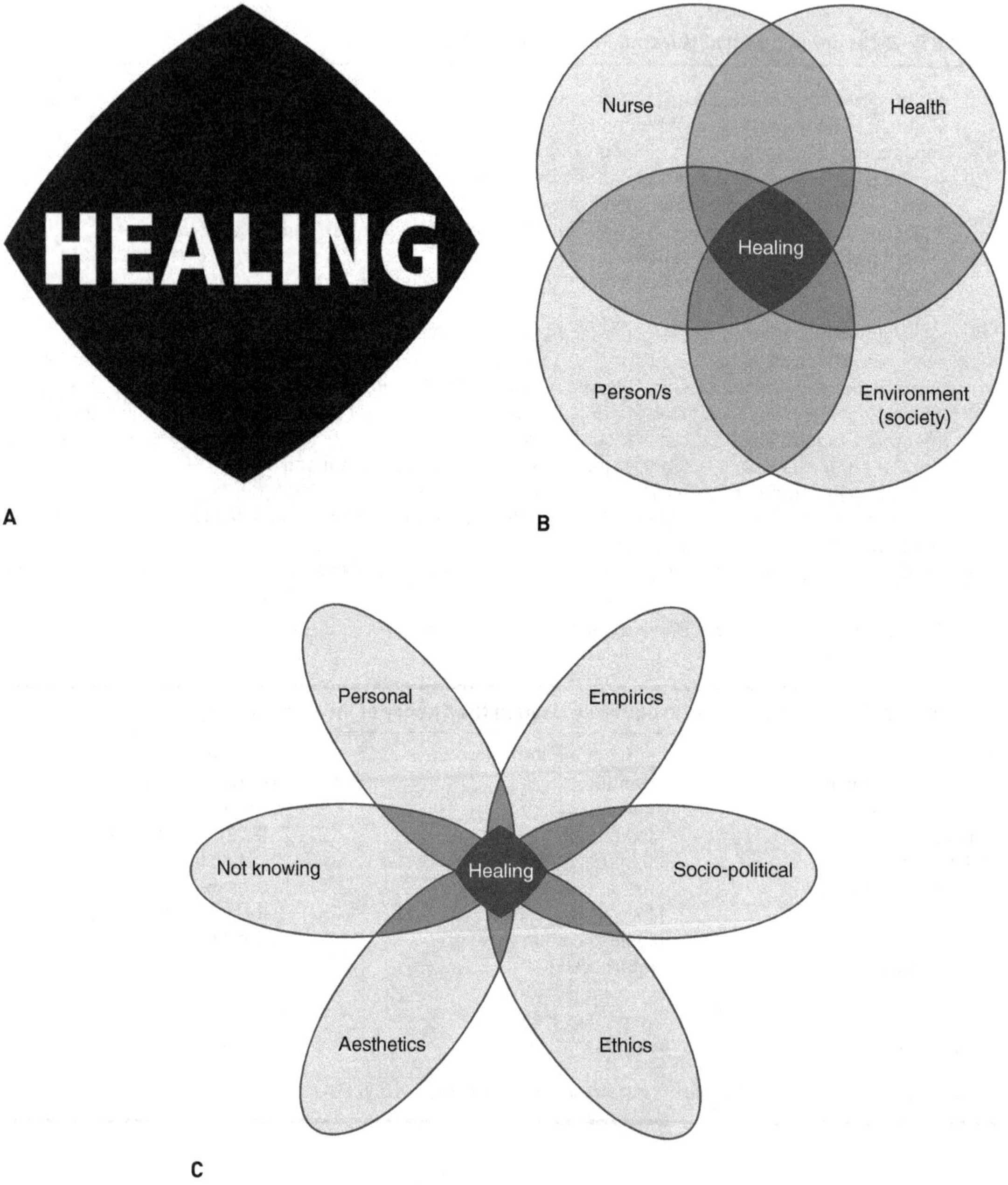

Figure 4-1 Theory of integral nursing: **A.** healing; **B.** healing and metaparadigm of nursing; **C.** healing and patterns of knowing in nursing;

A, B, C, and F. Dossey, B. M. (2008). Theory of integral nursing. *Advances in Nursing Science, 31*(1), E52–E73; **D and E.** Data from Wilber, K. (2000a). The collected works of Ken Wilber, Vols. 5–8. Shambhala. Used with permission.

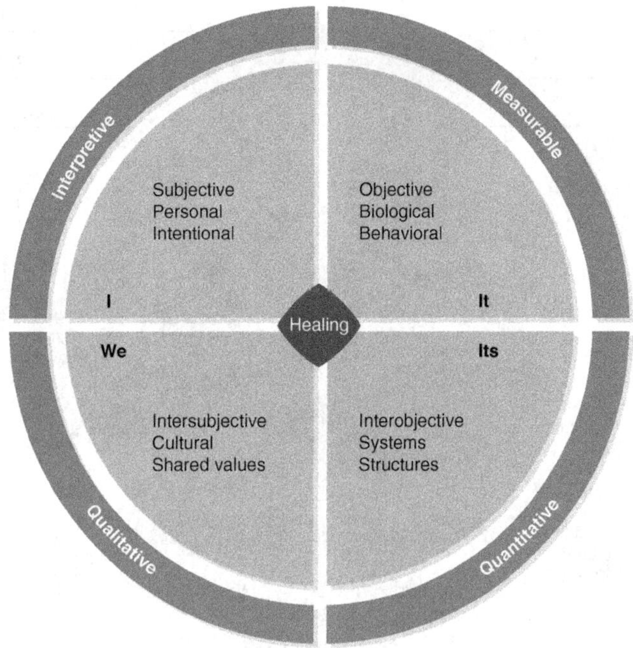

D

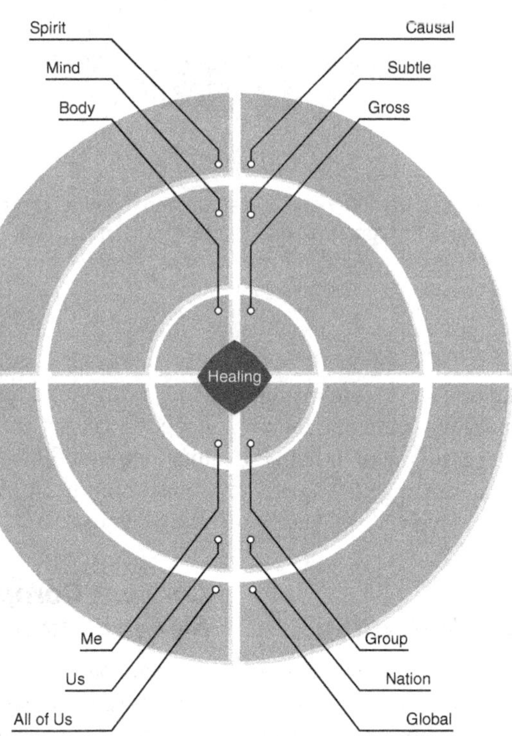

E

Figure 4-1 *(Continued)* **D.** healing and four quadrants (I, we, it, its); **E.** healing and all quadrants, all levels;

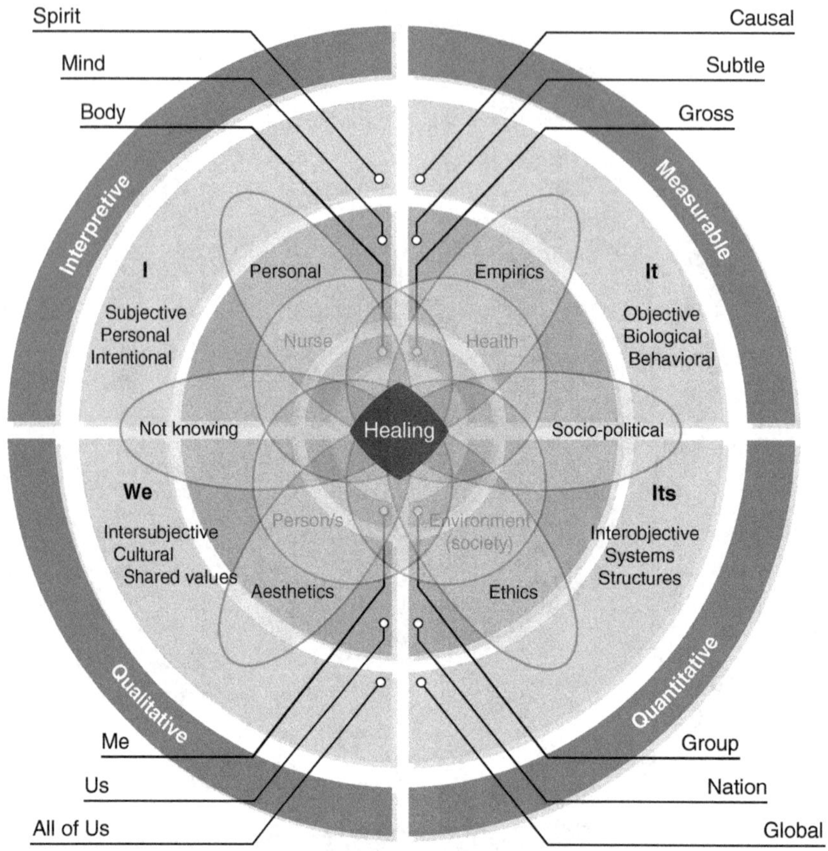

F

Figure 4-1 (*Continued*) **F.** theory of integral nursing (healing, metaparadigm, patterns of knowing in nursing, four quadrants, and all quadrants, all levels). Note: Although the patterns of knowing in **F** are superimposed as they are in the various quadrants, they can also fit into other quadrants.

acted on or that do the acting. The following five content components describe the subject matter and building blocks in the theory of integral nursing: (1) healing; (2) metaparadigm of nursing; (3) patterns of knowing in nursing; (4) quadrants; and (5) all quadrants, levels, lines, states, and types.

Content Component 1: Healing

Healing is at the core and includes knowing, doing, and being (**Figure 4-1A**). Healing is a lifelong journey of seeking harmony and balance in one's own life and in family, community, and global relations. It is an emergent process of the whole system bringing together aspects of one's self and the body-mind-spirit-culture-environment at deeper levels of inner knowing, leading toward integration and balance, with each aspect having equal importance and value. **Box 4-3** provides more details.

Content Component 2: Metaparadigm of Nursing

A metaparadigm in a nurse theory includes nurse, persons (patient, family members, significant others), health, and environment (internal and external) (society) (Fawcett, 1995). These areas are part of nurses' social contract with the public that

Box 4-3 Content Component 1: Healing

- Healing includes evolving one's state of consciousness to higher levels of personal and collective understanding that acknowledges the individual's interior and exterior experiences and the shared collective interior and exterior experiences with others where authentic power is recognized within each person.
- Disease and illness at the physical level may manifest for many reasons and variables. It is important *not* to equate physical health, mental health, and spiritual health, as they are not the same thing. They are facets of the whole jewel of health.
- Healing involves recovery, repair, renewal, and transformation that increase wholeness and often (though not invariably) order and coherence.
- Healing leads to more complex levels of personal understanding and meaning and may be synchronous but not synonymous with curing.
- Healing with self or another can happen until the moment of death.

is a "covenant" to work together for a common goal or outcome toward health and well-being. As nurses recalibrate their social contract with society, they embrace a more robust notion of a morally grounded social contract. Three factors, the nurses as human beings, nursing as relational, and nurses as linchpins, can inform why this shift is important (Fry-Bowers & Rushton, 2023).

Starting with healing at the center, a Venn diagram surrounds healing to illustrate the interrelation, interdependence, and effect of these domains as each informs and influences the others; a change in one will create a change in the others, thus affecting healing at many levels (**Figure 4-1B**). **Box 4-4** provides more details.

Content Component 3: Patterns of Knowing in Nursing

The third content component in a theory of integral nursing is the recognition of the patterns of knowing in nursing. These six patterns of knowing are personal, empirics, aesthetics, ethics, not knowing, and sociopolitical (**Figure 4-1C**). As a way to organize nursing knowledge, Carper (1978), in her now-classic article, identified the four fundamental patterns of knowing (personal, empirics, ethics, aesthetics) followed by the introduction of the pattern of not knowing by Munhall (1993) and the pattern of sociopolitical knowing by White (1995). All of these patterns continue to be refined and reframed with new applications and interpretations. These patterns of knowing assist nurses in bringing themselves into a full presence in the moment, integrating aesthetics with science, and developing the flow of ethical experience with our knowing, doing, and being (**Box 4-5**).

Content Component 4: Quadrants

The fourth content component in the theory of integral nursing examines four perspectives of reality (**Figure 4-1D**) that are adapted from Wilber's integral theory as demonstrated in **Table 4-2** (Wilber, 2000b, 2005).

Virtually all human languages use first-person, second-person, and third-person pronouns to indicate three basic dimensions of reality (Wilber, 2000b, 2005). First person is the person who is speaking, which includes pronouns like *I, me,* and *mine* in the singular and *we, us,* and *ours* in the plural (Wilber, 2000b, 2005). Second person means the person who is spoken to, which includes pronouns like *you* and *yours.* Third person is the person or thing being spoken about, such as *she, her, he, him, they, it,* and *its.* For example, if I am speaking to you about my new car, *I* am first person, *you* are second person, and the new car is third person. If you and I are communicating, the

Box 4-4 Content Component 2: Metaparadigm in a Nursing Theory

Nurse: A registered nurse that is a 21st-century Nightingale engaged in social action and sacred activism. The nurse is an instrument in the healing process where they bring one's whole self into relationship to the whole self of another or a group of significant others that reinforces the meaning and experience of oneness and unity.

Person: An individual (patient, family members, significant others) who engages with a nurse in a manner that is respectful of a person's subjective experiences about health, health beliefs, values, sexual orientation, and personal preferences. It also includes an individual nurse who interacts with nursing colleagues, other healthcare team members, or a group of community members, and concerned citizens around health issues.

Health: A state or process defined by an individual in which one experiences the growth, well-being, harmony, and unity. Each individual reshapes basic assumptions and worldviews about well-being and recognizes death as a natural process of living. Health places the patients at the center of care and addresses the bio-psycho-social-spiritual-cultural-environmental aspects that influence health.

Environment (society): An expanded consciousness to usher in the 22nd century for healthy people living on a healthy planet—local to global. Includes both interior and exterior aspects. The interior environment includes the individual's feelings, meaning, mental, emotional, and spiritual dimensions; it also includes a person's physiology that is an internal (inside) aspect of the exterior self. The exterior environment includes objects that can be observed and measured that are related to the physical and social in some form in any of the gross, subtle, and causal/infinite levels.

Box 4-5 Content Component 3: Patterns of Knowing in Nursing

Personal knowing: The nurse's dynamic process and awareness of wholeness that focuses on the synthesis of perceptions and being with self. It may be developed through art, meditation, dance, music, stories, and other expressions of the authentic and genuine self in daily life and nursing practice. This may be related to living and nonliving people and things, such as a deceased relative, animal, or a lost precious object through flashes of memories stimulated by a current situation (a touch may bring forth memories of abuse or suffering). Insights gained through dreams and other reflective practices that reveal symbols, images, and other connections also influence one's interior environment.

Empirical knowing: The science of nursing that focuses on formal expression, replication, and validation of scientific competence in nursing education and practice. It is expressed in models and theories and can be integrated into evidence-based practice. Empirical indicators are accessed through the known senses that are subject to direct observation, measurement, and verification.

Aesthetic knowing: The art of nursing that focuses on how to explore experiences and meaning in life with self or another that includes authentic presence, the nurse as a facilitator of healing, and the artfulness of a healing environment. It is the combination of knowledge, experience, instinct, and intuition that connects the nurse with a patient in order to explore the meaning of a situation about the human experiences of life, health, illness, and death. It calls forth resources and inner strengths from the nurse to be a facilitator in the healing process. It is the integration and expression of all the other patterns of knowing in nursing praxis.

Ethical knowing: The moral knowledge in nursing that focuses on behaviors, expressions, and dimensions of both morality and ethics. It includes valuing and clarifying situations to create formal moral and ethical behaviors intersecting with legally prescribed duties. It emphasizes respect for the person, the family, and the community that encourages connectedness and relationships that enhance attentiveness, responsiveness, communication, and moral action.

Not knowing: The capacity to use healing presence, to be open spontaneously to the moment with no preconceived answers or goals to be obtained. It engages authenticity, mindfulness, openness, receptivity, surprise, mystery, and discovery with self and others in the subjective space and the intersubjective space that allows for new solutions, possibilities, and insights to emerge. It acknowledges the patterns that may not be understood that may manifest related to various situations or relationships.

Sociopolitical knowing: Addresses the important contextual variables of social, economic, geographic, cultural, political, historical, and other key factors in theoretical, evidence-based practice and research. This pattern includes informed critique and social justice for the voices of the underserved in all areas of society along with protocols to reduce health disparities.

Data adapted from Carper, B. A. (1978). Fundamental patterns of knowing in nursing. *Advances in Nursing Science, 1*(1), 13–23; Dossey, B. M. (2008). Theory of integral nursing. *Advances in Nursing Science, 31*(1), E52–E73; Munhall, P. L. (1993). Unknowing: Toward another pattern of knowing in nursing, *Nursing Outlook, 41*(3), 125–128; White, J. (1995). Patterns of knowing: Review, critique, and update. *Advances in Nursing Science, 17*(4), 73–86. © Barbara M. Dossey (2008).

Table 4-2 Content Component 4: Quadrants

Upper Left	Upper Right
In this *I* space (subjective; the inside of the individual) can be found in the world of the individual's interior experiences. These are the nurse's thoughts, emotions, memories, perceptions, immediate sensations, and states of mind (imagination, fears, feelings, beliefs, values, esteem, cognitive capacity, emotional maturity, moral development, and spiritual maturity). Integral nursing requires development of the *I*.	In this *it* (objective; the outside of the individual) space can be found the world of the individual's exterior. This includes the material body (physiology [cells, molecules, neurotransmitters, limbic system], biochemistry, chemistry, physics), integral patient care plans, skill development (fitness, exercise, nutrition, etc.), behaviors, leadership skills, and integral life practices (refer to the "Process" section later in this chapter), as well as anything that we can touch or observe scientifically in time and space. Integral nursing with our nursing colleagues and healthcare team members includes the *it* of new behaviors, integral assessment and care plans, leadership, and skills development.
Lower Left	**Lower Right**
In this *we* (intersubjective; the inside of the collective) space can be found the interior collective of how we can come together to share our cultural backgrounds, stories, values, meanings, visions, languages, relationships, and how to form partnerships to achieve a healing mission. This can decrease our fragmentation and enhance collaborative practice and deep dialogue around things that really matter. Integral nursing is built on *we*.	In this *its* space (interobjective; the outside of the collective) can be found the world of the collective, exterior things. This includes social systems/structures, networks, organizational structures, and systems (including financial and billing systems in health care), information technology, regulatory structures (environmental and governmental policies, etc.), and any aspect of the technological environment and in nature and the natural world. Integral nursing identifies the *its* in the structure that can be enhanced to create more integral awareness and integral partnerships to achieve health and healing—local to global.

Modified by Barbara Dossey with permission of Ken Wilber (2000). *Integral psychology: Consciousness, spirit, psychology, therapy*. Boston, MA: Shambhala. Table adapted with permission of Ken Wilber. http://www.kenwilber.com

word *we* is used to indicate that we understand each other. *We* is technically first-person plural, but if you and I are communicating, then *you* as second person and *I* as first person are part of this extraordinary *we*. We represent first, second, and third person as *I*, *we*, *it*, and *its*.

The four quadrants describe the territory of our own awareness that is already present within us and an awareness of things outside of us. These quadrants help us connect the dots of the actual process to more deeply understand who we are and how we are related to others and all things. (*Note*: When working with various cultures, it is important to remember that within many cultures, the *I* comes last or is never verbalized or recognized, as the focus is on the *we* and relationships. However, this development of the *I* and an awareness of one's personal value, beliefs, and ethics is critical.)

These four quadrants show the four primary dimensions or perspectives of how we experience the world; these are represented graphically as the upper-left quadrant (UL), upper-right quadrant (UR), lower-left quadrant (LL), and lower-right quadrant (LR). It is essentially the inside and the outside of an individual and the inside and outside of the collective. It includes expanded states of consciousness where one feels a connection with something greater than the ego; it may be expressed as the divine and the vastness of the universe, the infinite that is beyond words. Integral nursing considers all these areas in our personal development and any area of practice, education, research, and healthcare policy—local to global. Each quadrant, which is intricately linked and bound to each other, carries its own truths and language (Wilber, 2000b).

We notice that the left-hand quadrants (UL, LL) describe aspects of reality as subjective, interpretive and qualitative (refer to Figure 3-1D). In contrast, the right-hand quadrants (UR, LR) describe aspects of reality as objective, measurable and quantitative. When we fail to consider these subjective, intersubjective, objective, and interobjective aspects of reality, our endeavors and initiatives become fragmented and narrow, inhibiting our ability to reach meaningful outcomes and goals.

Content Component 5: All Quadrants, Levels, Lines, States, and Types

The fifth content component in the theory of integral nursing is the exploration of Wilber's all quadrants, all levels, all lines, all states, all types, or AQAL (pronounced *ah-qwul*), as seen in **Figure 4-1E**. These levels, lines, states, and types are important elements of any comprehensive map of reality as seen in **Box 4-6** (Wilber, 2000b, 2005).

This part of TIN (refer to **Figure 4-1E**) starts with healing at the center surrounded by three increasing concentric circles with dotted lines of the four quadrants. This part of the integral theory moves to higher orders of complexity through personal growth, development, expanded stages of consciousness (permanent and actual milestones of growth and development), and evolution. These levels or stages of development can also be expressed as being self-absorbed (such as a child or infant), ethnocentric (which centers on group, community, tribe, or nation), or world centric (which exhibits care and concern for all peoples regardless of race or national origin, color, sex, gender identity, sexual orientation, or creed to the global level).

In the UL, the *I* space, the emphasis is on the unfolding awareness from body to mind to spirit. Each increasing circle includes the lower as it moves to the higher level.

In the UR, the *it* space is the external of the individual. Every state of consciousness has a felt energetic component that is expressed from the wisdom traditions as three recognized bodies: gross, subtle, and causal (Wilber, 2000b). We can think of these three bodies as the increasing capacities of a person toward higher levels of consciousness. Each level is a specific vehicle that provides the actual support for any state of awareness. The *gross body* is the individual physical, material, sensorimotor body that we experience in our daily activities. The *subtle body* occurs when we are not aware of the gross body of dense matter but of a shifting in energy, emotions, and fluid and flowing images. Examples might be in our shift during a dream, during different types of bodywork,

Box 4-6 Content Component 5: AQAL

Levels: Levels (also referred to as stages or waves) of development that become permanent with growth and maturity (e.g., cognitive, relational, psychosocial, physical, mental, emotional, spiritual) that represent a level of increased organization or level of complexity. Each individual possesses both the masculine and the feminine voice or energy. One is not superior to the other; they are two equivalent types at each level of consciousness and development.

Lines: Developmental areas that are known as multiple intelligences (e.g., *cognitive* line [awareness of what is]; *emotional* line [the full spectrum of emotions]; *somatic* line, awareness of body-mind; *interpersonal* line [how I relate socially to others]; *moral* line [awareness of what should be]; *spiritual* line [where spirit is viewed as its own line of unfolding, and not just as ground and highest state]; and *values* line [what a person considers most important]). These development lines are illustrated in **Figure 4-2** in the upper-right hand quadrant; they also apply to all quadrants. Each line appears differently to represent the dynamic developmental process, where one line of development may be more robust than others at different times depending on life's constantly changing circumstances.

States: Temporary changing forms of awareness (e.g., waking, dreaming, deep sleep, altered meditative states [such as occurs in meditation, yoga, contemplative prayer, etc.]; altered states due to mood swings, physiology and pathophysiology shifts with disease/illness, seizures, cardiac arrest, low or high oxygen saturation, or drug inducement]; peak experiences triggered by intense engagement with music, walks in nature, lovemaking, mystical experiences such as sensing a presence, hearing a voice, or receiving insight of god or of a deceased person, etc.

Types: Differences in personality and masculine and feminine expressions and development (e.g., cultural creative types, personality types, an enneagram).

Used with permission. Dossey, B. M. (2020). Theory of integral nursing. In M. C. Smith (Ed.), *Nursing theories and nursing practice* (pp. 211-234). Philadelphia: F. A. Davis. Data from Dossey, B. M. (2015). Theory of integrative nurse coaching. In B. M. Dossey, S. Luck, & B. G. Schaub (Eds.), *Nurse coaching: Integrative approaches for health and wellbeing* (pp. 29-49). North Miami, FL: International Nurse Coach Association; Wilber, K. (2007). *Integral spirituality: A startling new role for religion in the modern and postmodern world*. Boston: Shambhala.

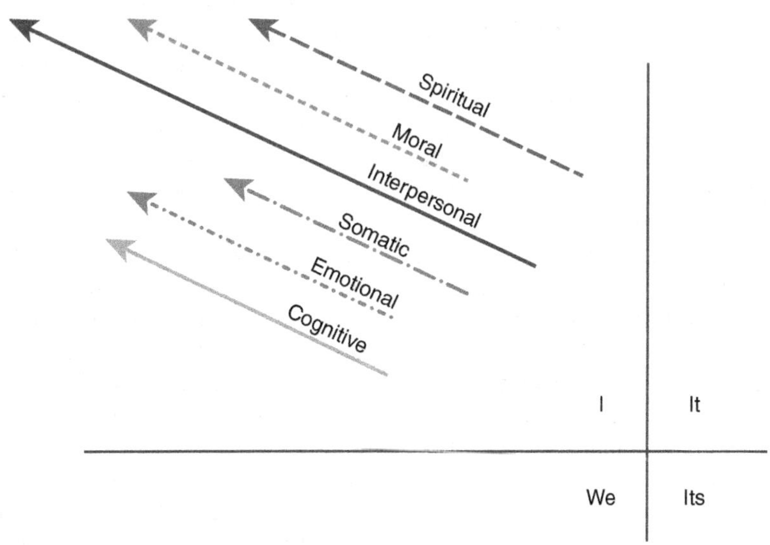

Figure 4-2 Six lines of development.

walks in nature, or other experiences that move us to a profound state of bliss. The *causal body* is the body of the infinite that is beyond space and time. Causal also includes nonlocality, in which minds of individuals are not separate in space and time (Dossey, 2013). When this is applied to consciousness, separate minds behave as if they are linked, regardless of how far apart in space and time they may be. Nonlocal consciousness may underlie phenomena such as remote healing, intercessory prayer, telepathy, premonitions, as well as so-called miracles. Nonlocality also implies that the soul does not die with the death of the physical body—hence, immortality forms some dimension of consciousness. Nonlocality can also be both upper and lower quadrant phenomena.

The LL, the *we* space, is the interior collective dimension of individuals that come together. The concentric circles from the center outward represent increasing levels of complexity of our relational aspect of shared cultural values, as this is where teamwork and the interdisciplinary and transpersonal disciplinary development occur. The inner circle represents the individual labeled as *me;* the second circle represents a larger group labeled *us;* the third circle is labeled *all of us* to represent the largest group consciousness that expands to all people. These last two circles may include people and animals, nature, and nonliving things that are important to individuals.

The LR, the *its* space, the exterior social system and structures of the collective, is represented with concentric circles. An example within the inner circle might be a group of healthcare professionals in a hospital clinic or department or the complex hospital system and structure. The middle circle expands in increased complexity to include a nation; the third concentric circle represents even greater increased complexity to the global level where the health of all humanity and the world are considered. It is also helpful to emphasize that these groupings are the physical dynamics such as the working structure of a group of healthcare professionals or the physical and technical structure of a hospital or a clinic versus the relational aspect that is an LL aspect. The LR also includes the family system and all its dynamics.

Integral nurses strive to integrate concepts and practices related to body, mind, and spirit (the all levels) in self, culture, and nature (the all quadrants part). The individual interior and exterior—*I* and *it*—as well as the collective interior and exterior—*we* and *its*—must be developed, valued, and integrated into all aspects of culture and society. The AQAL integral approach suggests that we consciously touch all these areas and do so in relation to self, to others, and the natural world. Yet to be integrally informed does *not* mean that we have to master all of these areas; we just need to be aware of them and choose to integrate integral awareness and integral practices. Because these areas are already part of our being in the world and cannot be imposed from the outside (they are part of our makeup from the inside), our challenge is to identify specific areas for development and find new ways to deepen our daily integral life practices.

Structure

The structure of the theory of integral nursing is indicated in **Figure 4-1F**. All content components are represented together as an overlay that creates a mandala to symbolize wholeness. Healing is placed at the center, followed by the metaparadigm of nursing, the patterns of knowing, the four quadrants, and all quadrants and all levels of growth, development, and evolution.

Using the language of Wilber (2000b, 2005), as well as Don Beck et al. (2018) and Beck (in Romischer, 2002) pertaining to Beck's spiral dynamics integral, individuals move through primitive, infantile consciousness to an integrated language that is considered first-tier thinking. As they move up the spiral of growth, development, and evolution and expand their integral worldview and integral consciousness, they move into second-tier thinking and participation. This is a radical leap into holistic, systemic, and integral modes of consciousness. Wilber also expands to a third tier of stages of consciousness that addresses an even deeper level of transpersonal understanding.

Context

Context in nursing theory is the environment in which nursing acts occur and is the nature of the world of nursing (Barnum, 2005). In an integral nursing environment, the nurse strives to be an integralist, which means that they strive to be integrally informed and is challenged to further develop an integral worldview, integral life practices, and integral capacities, behaviors, and skills. The term *nurse healer* is used to describe that a nurse is an instrument in the healing process and a major part of the external healing environment of a patient or family. An integral nurse values, articulates, and models the integral process, integral worldview, and integral life practices with self-care. Nurses assist and facilitate the individual persons (patient, family, and coworkers) to access their own healing process and potentials; they do not do the actual healing. An integral nurse recognizes themself as a healing environment interacting with a person, family, or colleague in being with rather than in doing to or doing for another person and enters into a shared experience (or field of consciousness) that promotes healing potentials and an experience of well-being. Relationship-centered care is valued and integrated as a model of caregiving that is based in a vision of community and partnerships.

Process

Process in a nursing theory is the method by which the theory works (Barnum, 2005). An integral healing process contains both nurse processes and patient/family and healthcare worker processes (individual interior and individual exterior), and collective healing processes of groups or individuals and of systems/structures (interior and exterior). Increased integral awareness also strengthens our moral resilience. This is the capacity of an individual to sustain or restore their integrity in response to moral complexity, confusion, distress, or setback (Rushton, 2023). This is the understanding of the unitary whole person interacting in mutual process with the environment. Refer to **Box 4-7** for an application of integral nursing principles. **Figure 4-3** illustrates the integral perspectives and reflective questions for each quadrant.

Integration

Clinical Practice

Using TIN assists nurses in assessment and care management in all clinical practice situations. By using an AQAL framework as a map, the nurse can see from multiple perspectives at once and better connect all aspects related to the complexity within a patient's care. To navigate the realities of racial and social injustice and the profound polarizing issues, the nurse can become more aware of their biases and educate themselves on the imbalances of inequalities and model cultural sensitivity in practice, education, research, policy, and global health (Mainwaring & Davis, 2022).

Education

A beginning level of understanding of TIN and integral concepts can support curriculum development and evaluation that is transferable beyond the classroom. The AQAL approach helps educators to design and revise curriculum to ensure there is not an overemphasis or reliance on the UR quadrant, and it brings us back into a more balanced approach of supporting students' evolution on their own healing path via the UL quadrant emphasis in order to best support others on their healing paths in the LL quadrant.

Darlene Hess uses the TIN in her Brown Mountain Visions business, where she provides clinical, education, and consulting services (Hess, 2016). She designed an RN-to-BSN curriculum based on the TIN that was adopted by Northern New Mexico College in Española, New Mexico. The RN-to-BSN program at the college is a truly integral holistic nursing education program that offers RNs the opportunity to delve deeply into integral theory and holistic nursing while completing requirements for a BS degree in nursing. Program learning outcomes, course

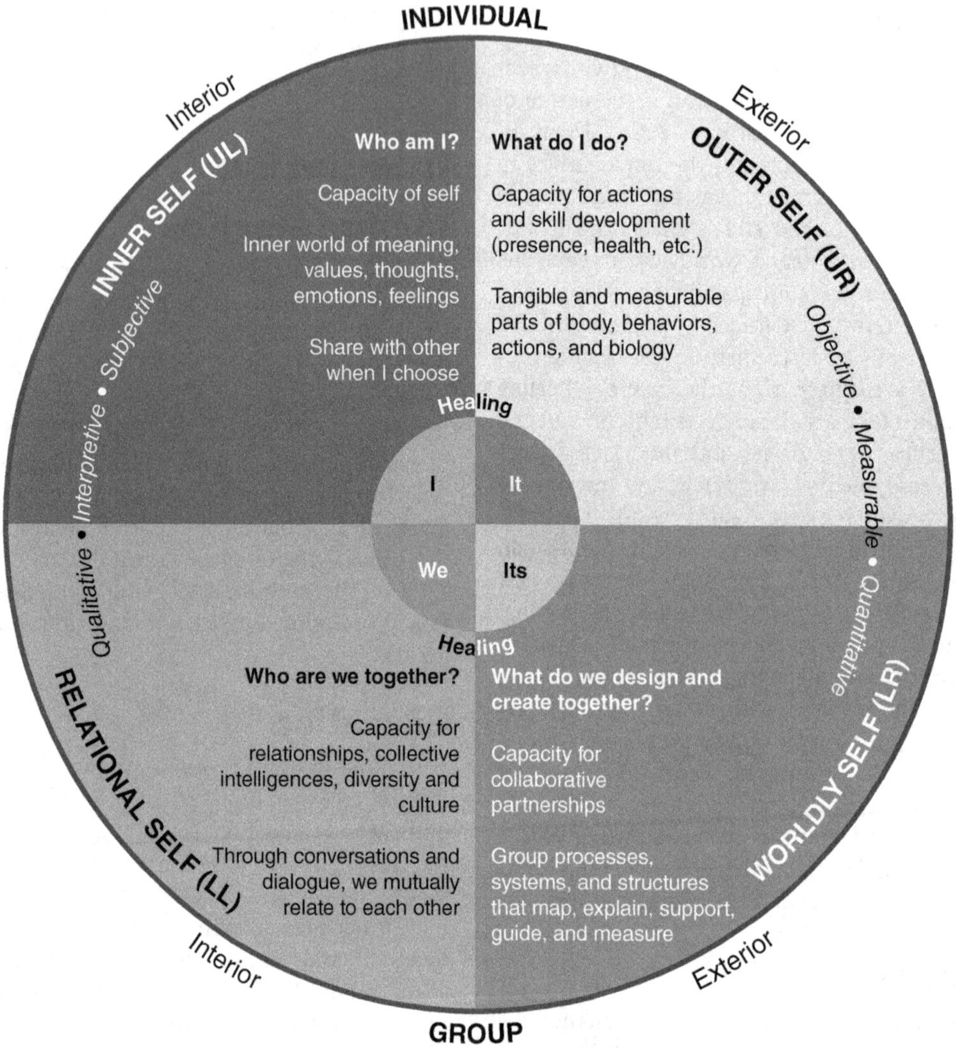

Figure 4-3 Integral perspective and reflective questions.

Box 4-7 Integral Nursing Principles

Integral Nursing Principle 1 (UL): *I* Capacity of Self. Integral nursing principle 1 recognizes the interior individual *I* (subjective) space. We ask, "Who am I?" "What is my capacity of self?" To deepen our state of beingness, our mindfulness about intentions, attitudes, and values helps us develop a conscious awareness about personal health and our role in creating a healthy world—local to global. We become aware of our personal challenges and parts of self that need healing. It also includes addressing one's own shadow as described by Jung (1981). We also recognize conscious dying and find time to contemplate one's own death and to increase awareness that there is no separation between our practice and actions in everyday life. This is a mature practice that is wise and empty of a separate self.

Integral Nursing Principle 2 (LL): *We* Capacity for Collective Intelligence. This principle recognizes the importance of the *we* (intersubjective) space. We explore "Who are we together?" "What is our capacity for collective intelligences?" We use deep listening, being present, and focused with intention to understand what another person is expressing or not expressing. Through authentic sharing of worldviews, beliefs, priorities, values, and concerns, we explore multiple perspectives.

This space also applies to the *we* with our family, friends, and communities. We engage in transpersonal dimensions moving from superficial conversations to a deeper dialogue that goes beyond the individual ego. This is the exploration of the sacred or holy that involves feelings, thoughts, experiences, rituals, meaning, value, direction, and purpose as valid aspects of the universe. It is a unifying force of a person with all that is—the essence of beingness and relatedness that permeates all of life and interconnectedness with self, others, nature, and God/life force/absolute/transcendent being.

Integral Nursing Principle 3 (UR): *It* Capacity for Actions and Skill Development. This principle recognizes the importance of the individual exterior *it* (objective) space. We ask, "What skills, behaviors, and action steps can assist me to achieve personal health?" "What personal actions can expand my awareness of my place with the health of my family, workplace, and community?" "How do my behaviors and actions lead to a healthy planet?" "What are the impacts of my behaviors and actions?" All behaviors and actions can be measurable and observable.

In this space, nurses and the healthcare team members compile the data around physiologic and pathophysiologic assessment, nursing diagnosis, outcomes, plans of care (including medications, technical procedures, monitoring, treatments, and traditional and integrative practice protocols), implementation, and evaluation. Nurses cocreate plans of care with patients, families, and community and integrate a caring-healing philosophy and interventions/modalities with traditional medical and surgical technology and treatment. Specific education is offered based on outcomes and evaluation, which also guides research questions and data collection.

Integral Nursing Principle 4 (LR): Its Capacity for Alignment in Systems/Structures. This nursing recognizes the importance of the exterior collective *its* (interobjective) space. Nurses and the healthcare team come together and ask, "How can we strengthen our capacity for alignment and collaboration in our work?" "What are the priorities?" They create exterior healing environments that incorporate nature and the natural world when possible. This principle also applies to the family system and structures and seeks ways to enhance all endeavors and gain a deeper understanding for what is working and what is not working, thus connecting all the other quadrant principles from an integral perspective.

Nursing Situation

Jan, a 58-year-old emergency room nurse, has decided to take charge of her life and become healthier as a result of engaging in the Healthy Nurse Healthy Nation initiative in her workplace (Healthy Nurse Healthy Nation, n.d.). She is 5 feet, one-half inch tall and weighs 168 pounds. At work she always feels stressed and does not take breaks and snacks on fast foods. She lives alone and also eats fast foods while watching television or movies most nights. She makes the commitment to see a nurse coach for the next 3 months with a session every 2 weeks. After completing the Integrative Health and Wellbeing Assessment, she has identified her top four goals as follows: (1) lose 1–2 pounds a week until her BMI is 25 (it is now 29); (2) start an exercise program of walking five times a week for 30 minutes with her neighbor; (3) learn mindfulness practices; and (4) reflect and explore new ways to think about who she is from a deeper perspective and find more moments of joy and compassion.

A nursing colleague introduced Jan to the TIN four quadrant integral perspectives and integral nursing principles as a way to explore her new goals (refer to **Table 4-2** and **Box 4-7**). They invited Jan to experience a reflective practice of being in the present moment and to shift her feelings and her interior awareness (and believe it!) to: "I am doing the best that I can in this moment," and "I have all the time needed to take a deep breath and relax my tight chest and shoulder muscles." Jan felt the shift and realized how she always carried tight muscles at work. Jan connect these four integral perspectives as follows: (1) the interior self (caring for yourself in this moment); (2) the exterior self (external action of breathing practice using a research-based relaxation and imagery integral practice to change their physiology); (3) the self in relationship to others (shifting their awareness and imagining engaging with a difficult patient with compassion); and (4) the relationship to the exterior collective of systems/structures (new ways to work with the emergency room team and department to improve patient care). Jan immediately grasps the quadrant perspectives and saw them as a map to help her "connect the dots" about all aspects of her life.

As Jan continued to think and apply the four integral perspectives and integral nursing principles in her life, she was able to make steady progress toward reaching her goals. Jan also developed a new awareness about her cognitive, emotional, somatic, moral, and spiritual lines of development and how they were always changing (refer to **Figure 4-2**). She noticed that she had expanded her capacities with moral resilience and was more balanced. When she explored reflective questions in each quadrant, she was thrilled to find that she had new joy in all aspects of her life (refer to **Figure 4-3**).

As her new integral awareness shifted, she felt a sense of deep gratitude. As she learned to have more compassion for herself, she began to listen to patients' stories from an integral perspective and to connect the dots to the patients and families.

competencies, and assignments are linked to the theory of integral nursing. In its short history, this innovative program has achieved national accreditation through the Center of Collegiate Nursing Education (CCNE), was endorsed by the American Holistic Nurses Credentialing Corporation from 2013 to 2017, and in 2015 received an excellence in holistic nursing education award from the American Holistic Nurses Association.

Research

TIN assists nurses to consider the importance of qualitative and quantitative research (Barrere & Delaney, 2022). Since knowledge emerges from all four quadrants, TIN assists us to connect all parts at a deeper level.

Policy

Compelling evidence in nursing and all healthcare professions shows that the origins of health and illness cannot be understood by focusing only on the physical body. Perceptions of health and illness within TIN and an AQAL approach provide limitless possibilities addressing nurse retention and nursing shortages now and in the future.

Global Health

Florence Nightingale in her times was confronted with the same environmental and social issues that we have in the 21st century. These issues are key in achieving global development and global health. TIN can guide global projects such as the Nightingale Initiative for Global Health (NIGH) (Beck & Dossey, 2025; Dossey, 2025; NIGH, n.d.). Global health awareness of being a global holistic nurse and a planetary citizen requires that we have a comprehensive integral worldview and process that enlarges our holistic understanding of body-mind-spirit-cultural-environmental connections and our knowing, doing, and being to more comprehensive and deeper levels. When we do this, we can account for one mind, one health, and one planet (Rosa, 2017).

Conclusion

The theory of integral nursing strengthens our 21st-century nursing endeavors and guides integral nurse self-development and expands our consciousness to recognize that all of us are engaged in global nursing. When we focus on improving our own health and that of our family and community at the local level, each small change connects me to us to all of us—that creates the ripple effect of healthy people living on a healthy planet—local to global.

References

Barnum, B. S. (2005). *Nursing theory: Analysis, application, evaluation* (6th ed.). Lippincott Williams & Wilkins.

Barrere, C. C., & Delaney, C. (2022). Holistic nursing research: Challenges and opportunities. In M. A. Helming, D. A. Shields, K. M. Avino, & W. E. Rosa (Eds.), *Dossey & Keegan's Holistic nursing: A handbook for practice* (8th ed., pp. 463-478). Jones & Bartlett.

Beck, D. E., Larsen, T. H., Solonin, S., Viljoen, R., & Johns, T. Q. (2018). *Spiral dynamics in action: Humanity's master code*. John Wiley and Sons Ltd.

Beck, D. M., & Dossey, B. M. (2025). Remembering Florence Nightingale in her turbulent times: Activating the theory of integral nursing in our turbulent times. *International Nursing Review*, 72(3), e13064. https://doi.org/10.1111/inr.13064.

Carper, B. A. (1978). Fundamental patterns of knowing in nursing. *Advances in Nursing Science, 1*(1), 13–23.

Dossey, B. M. (2008). Theory of integral nursing. *Advances in Nursing Science*, *31*(1), E52–E73.

Dossey, B. M. (2010). *Florence Nightingale: Mystic, visionary, healer* (Commemorative Edition). F. A. Davis.

Dossey, B. M. (2015). Theory of integrative nurse coaching. In B. M. Dossey, S. Luck, & B. G. Schaub (Eds.), *Nurse coaching: Integrative approaches for health and wellbeing* (pp. 29–49). International Nurse Coach Association.

Dossey, B. M. (2025). Theory of integral nursing. In M. C. Smith (Ed.), *Nursing theories and nursing practice* (6th ed., pp. 167–187). F. A. Davis.

Dossey, B. M., Beck, D. M., Oerther, S., & Manjrekar, P. (2017). Florence Nightingale's legacy: The rationale for an integral worldview in achieving the sustainable development goals. In W. Rosa (Ed.), *A new era in global health: Nursing and the United Nations 2030 agenda for sustainable development* (pp. 149–178). Springer Publishing Company.

Dossey, L. (2013). *One mind: How our individual mind is part of a greater mind, and why it matters*. Hay House International.

Dossey. B. M. (2025). *Theory of integral nursing*. https://nursology.net/nurse-theorists-and-their-work/theory-of-integral-nursing/

Fawcett, J. (1995). *Analysis and evaluation of conceptual models of nursing* (3rd ed.). F. A. Davis.

Fry-Bowers, E., & Rushton, C. H. (2023). Re-imaging nursing's social contract with the public. *American Nurse Journal*, 18(9). https://doi.org/10.51256/ANJ092314

Harvey, A. (2009). *The hope. A guide to sacred activism*. Hay House.

Healthy Nurse Healthy Nation. (n.d.). *Homepage*. https://www.healthynursehealthynation.org

Hess, D. R. (2016). Curriculum for an RN-to-BSN program using the theory of integral nursing. In B. M. Dossey & L. Keegan (Eds.), *Holistic nursing: A handbook for practice* (7th ed., pp. 40–46). Jones & Bartlett Learning.

Jung, C. G. (1981). *The archetypes and the collective unconscious* (2nd ed., Vol. 9, part I). Bollingen.

Mainwaring, J., & Davis, R. (2022). Cultural humility and allyship: Enhancing nursing education. *International Journal for Human Caring*, 26(4), 248-253.

Morrow, M. R., & Dossey, B. M. (2024). A journey of joy: Dr. Barbara M. Dossey's evolution in nursing. *Nursing Science Quarterly*, 37(2), 125-133.

Munhall, P. L. (1993). Unknowing: Toward another pattern of knowing in nursing, *Nursing Outlook, 41*(3), 125–128.

Nightingale Initiative for Global Health. (n.d.). *The Nightingale Declaration for a Healthy World*. http://www.nighvision.net /nightingale-declaration.html

Romischer, J. (2002). The never-ending upward quest: The practical and spiritual wisdom of spiral dynamics: An interview with Dr. Don Beck. *What is enlightenment* (Fall/Winter Special Issue), 105–126.

Rosa, W. (2017). One mind, one health, one planet—A pledge to planetary citizenship. In W. Rosa (Ed.), *A new era in global health: Nursing and the United Nations 2030 agenda for sustainable development* (pp. 517–527). Springer Publishing Company.

Rushton, C. H. (2023). Transforming moral suffering by cultivating moral resilience and ethical practice. *American Association of Critical-Care Nurses*, 32(4), 238-248. https://doi.org/10.4037/ajcc2023207.

Shea, L., & Frisch, N. C. (2014). Application of integral theory in holistic nursing practice. *Holistic Nursing Practice, 28*(6), 344–352.

Shea, L., & Frisch, N. C. (2016). Wilber's integral theory and Dossey's theory of integral nursing: An examination of two integral approaches in nursing scholarship. *Journal of Holistic Nursing, 34*(3), 244–252.

Shea, L., Reimer-Kirkham, S., & Frisch, N. C. (2019). Nursing perspectives on integral theory in nursing practice and education: An interpretive descriptive study. *Nursing Inquiry*, *26*, e12276. https://doi.org/10.1111/nin.12276

White, J. (1995). Patterns of knowing: Review, critique, and update. *Advances in Nursing Science, 17*(4), 73–86.

Wilber, K. (1999). *The collected works of Ken Wilber*, Vols. 1–4. Shambhala.

Wilber, K. (2000a). *The collected works of Ken Wilber* (Vols. 5–8). Shambhala.

Wilber, K. (2000b). *Integral psychology: Consciousness, spirit, psychology, therapy*. Shambhala.

Wilber, K. (2005). *Integral operating system*. Sounds True.

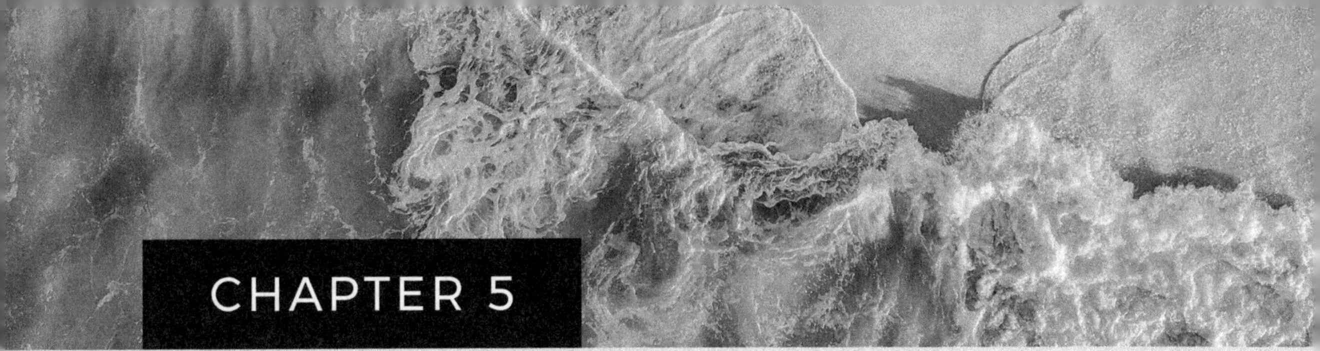

CHAPTER 5

Transpersonal Human Caring and Healing

Janet F. Quinn

NURSE HEALER OBJECTIVES

- Define transpersonal human caring.
- Define healing and contrast it with curing.
- Discuss the nature of right relationship as it relates to healing.
- Explore the ways that holistic nurses facilitate healing for patients, self, and systems.

DEFINITIONS

Habitats for Healing: Healthcare practice environments that provide a context of caring, for the purpose of healing, which may include curing (Quinn, 2010).

Healing: The emergence of right relationship at one or more levels/dimensions of the whole system (Quinn, 1989).

Healing healthcare system: A true healthcare system in which people can receive adequate, nontoxic, and noninvasive assistance in maintaining wellness and in healing for body, mind, and spirit, together with the most sophisticated, sometimes invasive curing technologies available.

Human caring: The moral ideal of nursing in which the nurse brings his or her whole self into relationship with the whole self of the patient, to protect the vulnerability and preserve the humanity and dignity of the one caring and the one cared for (Watson Caring Science Institute, 2024).

Right relationship: A process of connection among or between parts of the whole that increases energy, coherence, and creativity in the whole system (Quinn, 1989).

Transpersonal: That which transcends the limits and boundaries of individual ego identities and possibilities to include acknowledgment and appreciation of something greater and beyond the belief in/sense of a separate self. *Transpersonal* may refer to consciousness, intrapersonal dynamics, interpersonal relationships, and lived experiences of connection, unity, and oneness with the larger environment, cosmos, or Spirit/God/Ultimate Reality.

Introduction

Healing is at the heart of holistic nursing, and the transpersonal caring–healing relationship is at the heart of healing. The various alternative, complementary, and integrative modalities used by holistic nurses, while important, do not alone define nursing practice as holistic. The tools are secondary and, perhaps more importantly, when alternative, complementary, and integrative modalities are used without a holistic intention, a focus on healing for the whole bodymindspirit, and a caring–healing relationship, they are no more holistic than conventional treatments—perhaps even less so. Evidence from current placebo research suggests that it is the quality of the therapeutic relationships that turns out to be one of the most important and often the most important variable in positive health-caring outcomes (Pardo-Cabello et al., 2022, Saueressig et al., 2024; Wampold, 2021).

Transpersonal Human Caring

The term *transpersonal human caring* is most often associated with Jean Watson's theory of nursing as the art and science of human caring (Watson Caring Science Institute, 2024). Watson defines *human caring* as the moral ideal of nursing, in which the relationship between the whole self of the nurse and the whole self of the patient protects the vulnerability and preserves the humanity and dignity of both. This emphasis on the whole self—the whole person of both nurse and patient—requires the addition of the term *transpersonal* in Watson's framework and in the discussion of human caring as it relates to holistic nursing practice. Within a transpersonal perspective, people are more than the body physical and the mind as contained in that body. A transpersonal perspective acknowledges that all people are body, mind, and spirit or soul (represented in this chapter as *bodymindspirit*) and that interactions between people engage all/each of these aspects of the self. A nurse with a transpersonal perspective recognizes that this is a fact of human interaction, not an optional event. A holistic nurse recognizes, as Watson suggests, that there is something beyond the personal, separate selves of the nurse and the patient involved in the act of caring.

When nurses enter caring–healing relationships with patients, bringing with them an acknowledgment and appreciation of the holistic nature of their own bodymindspirit, they are engaged in a transpersonal human caring process. In this type of relationship, nurses know themselves to be interconnected with their patients and with the larger environment and cosmos. They know that they are walking on sacred ground when they walk this path with their patients, and they recognize that neither one will be the same afterward. For that moment, they are joined with the other who is patient and so become part of something larger than either alone. In this transpersonal healing process, they are each changed.

Watson calls these healing encounters *caring occasions* and suggests that they actually transcend the bounds of space and time (Watson Caring Science Institute, 2024). The field of consciousness created in and through the caring–healing relationship has the potential to continue healing the patient long after the physical separation of nurse and patient. Moreover, the nurse, following engagement in a true caring occasion, will also continue to benefit from the mutual process. When nurses can engage their full, caring selves in the art of nursing, it is both energizing and satisfying.

It is often assumed that nurses burn out as a result of caring too much. However, today's nurses are far more likely to burn out for a different reason: the difficulty in finding the time and institutional support to care for patients with their whole selves within healthcare systems that do not value caring.

Healing: The Goal of Holistic Nursing

Although caring is the context for holistic nursing, healing is the goal. There is no universal definition for healing in the nursing or related healthcare literature. Within the biomedical model, the word *healing* generally refers to processes of wound or lesion repair, while the term is used in alternative and complementary medicine literature as representing particular interventions, processes, outcomes, and sometimes all these at once (Levin, 2017, p. 244). Roots of the word *heal* can be found in Old English (*haelan*), German (*heilen*), Dutch (*helen*), and Old Saxon (*helian*) languages, where it means *to make whole*.

But what constitutes *whole* or *wholeness* in the context of holistic nursing? Is wholeness a goal, an end point that is something to work toward but is rarely achieved? Is wholeness a state of perfection of body, mind, and spirit? Is wholeness something that people either have or do not have, something that people can obtain and hold onto, or something that comes and goes? Is it a state or a process? Is wholeness dependent on the structure and functioning of the body? Can one ever be not whole—that is, can one ever be other than wholly who or what one is at any point in space and time? If one cannot be not whole, then how is it possible to talk about becoming whole? Each holistic nurse is invited to spend some time thinking about what healing and wholeness mean to them because a nurse's perspective on these concepts will influence everything that they do.

Healing as the Emergence of Right Relationship

Wholeness is frequently described as harmony of body, mind, and spirit. Thus, wholeness must involve more than the intactness of physical structure and function, or the status of isolated parts of a person. If wholeness depended on these factors, then every person who has a dysfunctional organ or has lost a body part would be viewed as inherently unwhole, a perspective that is entirely unacceptable from a holistic nursing perspective. If wholeness—and therefore healing—are about harmony, then it is necessary to expand our ways of knowing about them to include the aesthetic, the subjective, the ethical/moral, and the way of unknowing, in addition to the scientific/empirical ways of knowing.

Healing has been defined (Quinn, 1989) as the emergence of right relationship at, among, or between multidimensional aspects of the whole person/system. According to Nobel physicist David Bohm (1992), increasing the wholeness of a system is about establishing a pattern of relationships among its elements "that increases coherence." This increase in coherence results in increased order, energy, creativity, and freedom in the whole system—that is, the whole bodymindspirit and beyond—regardless of which elements or parts of the person/system shifted into new patterns of being. Healing, as a process of being or becoming whole, is an emerging pattern of relationships among the elements of the whole system. This new pattern of relationship can be called *right relationship*, not because it is good or moral or correct or even conscious but because it contributes to greater wholeness in the system, whether that be an individual person, a family, an institution, or beyond. It is a dynamic and unpredictable process rather than a fixed state.

Several principles related to the nature of systems are fundamental and have direct implications for the understanding of healing. The first and most basic is that a system is more than and different from the sum of its parts because the pattern of relationships among the parts of the whole gives the system its own unique identity. Knowing the properties of sodium (Na) and the properties of chlorine (Cl), for example, tells us nothing about the properties of sodium chloride (NaCl; table salt)—the new whole system that emerges from the combination of the parts.

A second principle is that a change in the part always leads to a change in the whole. Because human beings are living systems governed by these principles, any shift, no matter how small or at which level it appears, will always affect the whole bodymindspirit and the systems in which the person is embedded.

The third principle that relates directly to healing is that the nature of the change in the whole cannot be predicted by the nature of the change in the part. "The new state [of a system] is decided neither by initial conditions in the system nor by changes in the critical values of environmental parameters; when a dynamic system is fundamentally destabilized, it acts indeterminately" (Laszlo, 1987, p. 36). This is why sometimes the tiniest shifts in one family member's behavior, for example, can lead to almost miraculous healing for the whole family.

All living systems, as complex adaptive systems, possess an innate, inner evolutionary thrust toward becoming the fullness of what they intrinsically are, toward increasing complexity and diversity in the language of nurse theorist Martha Rogers or toward integration (of form and function) and transcendence, to use Ken Wilber's framework. Healing, as increasing wholeness/coherence through the emergence of right relationship, is part of that inherent life force directionality. Therefore, healing is not and cannot be done to or for a person/system. Healing emerges from within the whole system. This natural, emergent pattern of being in the direction of greater wholeness/healing has been called the *haelan effect*, the elicitation of which can be seen as the goal of holistic nursing practice (Quinn, 1989). The haelan effect is what underlies what has traditionally been called the *placebo effect*—the positive healing response to interventions with no known therapeutic benefits—and dismissed as a nuisance to researchers who are trying to find "real" therapies.

Because of its inherently creative nature, moving in the direction of actualizing the fullness of individual being, true healing is always a process of emergence into something new, rather than a simple return to prior states of being. Holistic nurses do not limit the focus of their care to recovery alone but rather expand their focus to helping patients integrate their illness experience and transcend their former selves toward new patterns of self-actualization. This is the growth process that is inherent in nature, as noted by Nightingale when she reminds us that the goal of nursing is to put the patient in the best condition so that nature can act on him.

Healing as the emergence of right relationship may occur at any level of the bodymindspirit. For example, when an organ is transplanted, the emergence of right relationship between the new organ and the surrounding cells and tissues of the recipient's bodymindspirit signals healing. If that right relationship does not occur, if the cells of the new organ do not become integrated into the existing bodymindspirit structure, if rejection rather than acceptance happens, then the patient may die from a lack of right relationship, and thus healing, at the cellular level. When broken bones knit together, or when the edges of a wound begin to approximate, right relationship is emerging at the physical level. Each of these emerging right relationships has an effect on the whole, as noted earlier.

The effects on the whole person of a shift toward right relationship at the emotional level are evident in a moment of forgiveness or a release of a long-held resentment. At such a time, the way in which a person stands in relationship to an event or a person from the past changes. The letting go of resentment carries with it an often almost overwhelming release of energy that becomes available for new growth and an expanded consciousness and creative unfolding. The bodymindspirit of one who is experiencing forgiveness moves toward integration and transcendence of previous patterns and forms. Forgiveness of one's self or another has profound effects at every level of being.

Sometimes, right relationship emerges at the spiritual level before it manifests itself anywhere else. In moments of deep, positive emotion—such as gratitude, unconditional love, or the sudden awareness that one is not alone but in fact connected to everything and everyone else in the cosmos—individuals have come into right relationship with the transcendent dimensions of life: God, the One, Ultimate Reality, the Ground of Being, etc. The language is not as important as the recognition of change. Those who have this experience are more whole, more coherent, freer to become who they are most deeply meant to be; in other words, more healed. Experiences of this kind of life-transforming healing are often reported by those who experience psychedelic-assisted psychotherapy.

Healing Versus Curing

Healing, as we have been discussing it, and curing are clearly different yet related processes. Curing is the elimination of the signs and symptoms of disease, which may or may not even correspond to the end of the patient's disease or distress. The diagnosis and cure of disease provide the focus of the modern healthcare (sickness–cure) system. This is not a wrong focus, only an incomplete one. When it is estimated that at a minimum 85 percent of health problems are either self-limiting or chronic, it becomes clear that something in addition to a focus on the curing of diseases is required.

What is required is healing, which is different from curing in several key ways, the most important of which is that healing may occur without curing. Because healing is the emergence of right relationship at any or all levels/dimensions of the bodymindspirit system, it can happen even when there is no possibility for physical cure. Indeed, for some people, the very fact that they are facing an incurable disease or situation provides enough instability in the system to catalyze tremendous healing shifts. This is a fact that most nurses who have worked in hospice, for example, have observed. So much deep and profound healing—of relationships, of self-identity, of regrets, of spiritual connections, etc.—may occur as people are facing the imminent end of their time on this planet. Their bodies continue to decline and shut down; they are decidedly not cured. Yet beautiful healing emerges and may continue right up to (and after, some would say) the moment of physical death. Thus, even when there is no physical cure, healing of the whole bodymindspirit is always possible.

Another difference between curing and healing relates to the expectations of the sick–cure system that the course of disease, illness, and recovery is predictable, in fact, so predictable that discharge plans can be written as part of a hospital admission process. Healing, as an emergent phenomenon, is always creative and unpredictable in both process and outcome (Quinn, 1997). The nature, direction, and end point of a healing change—as the emergence of right relationship at one or more levels and dimensions of the whole—cannot be predicted or prescribed. It can only be observed and named as it emerges.

The Healer

> It is often thought that medicine is the curative process. It is no such thing; medicine is the surgery of functions as surgery proper is that of limbs and organs. Neither can do anything but remove obstructions; neither can cure. Nature alone cures. (Nightingale, 1969, p. 133)

This same perspective applies to healing: Nature alone heals. Healing is completely unique and creative and may not be coerced, manipulated, or controlled, even by the one healing. The nurse healer is a facilitator of this process—a sort of midwife—but is not the one doing the healing. Neither is the locus of the healing an isolated part of the patient (i.e., the mind or the spirit). All healing and curing could be thought of as self-healing because it emerges from within the totality of the unique bodymindspirit of the one healing, sometimes with the assistance of therapeutic interventions but not because of them. Therapeutics (drugs; surgery; holistic, integrative, or complementary therapies) may be *necessary* for the patient to be cured or healed, but they are *not sufficient* causes of outcomes. Every nurse has cared for patients who "should have" gotten better but did not, as well as patients who "should have" died but went on to live long, healthy lives. Why? Because we cannot impose or create healing from the outside and because the nature of whole-person healing is creative and unpredictable.

Caution is necessary when considering the assumption that all healing and curing is self-healing. It does not mean that the patient can control all healing and curing or create it as desired. The causes of illness, cure, and/or healing are so complex and multidimensional (including the transpersonal) that no simple statement of cause and effect is appropriate to describe either. Holistic nurses can participate knowledgeably in the healing process, using all forms of knowing, formulating a healing intention and doing what they believe is best in the situation, but the outcome of that process remains categorically indeterminate. At least part of the healing process will always be an unfolding mystery, because there are always elements, dimensions, and processes of the whole person (interconnected with all that is) about which we can know nothing as patients or providers. Believing otherwise may contribute to a terrible sense of failure for patients (and for the nurses who care for them) when they are unable to cure themselves of their diseases despite all their best efforts. True caring is a moral commitment to protect the vulnerability of self and other. My first Therapeutic Touch teacher, healer and clairvoyant Dora Kunz, once reminded all of her students that "the destiny of any human being is not in your hands. There are too many variables that you know nothing about" (1993). Understanding and acknowledging the fundamental mystery that we are called to serve, to witness, and to partner with and helping patients to do the same is part of ethical holistic care.

A True Healing Healthcare System

As noted previously, the current healthcare system continues to focus almost exclusively on the curing process, thus making it more akin to a sickness–cure system. The use of new tools of care, including alternative, holistic, integrative, or complementary therapies, without a fundamental shift in the philosophy of care with which they are used, will not transform the sickness–cure system into a true, healing healthcare system. The error of confusing the tools of care with the philosophy of care may lead to serious consequences for both healthcare practitioners and their patients.

The fundamental orientation of a holistic practitioner is toward an appreciation of and attention to the wholeness and uniqueness of every person. Holistic nurses remember that, in effect, there is nothing that is not holistic. There is no intervention that does not affect the whole bodymindspirit of the patient because the bodymindspirit is integral and cannot be divided. There are natural and nonnatural modalities, for example, but both affect the whole bodymindspirit.

For this reason, simply adding new tools of care will not transform the sickness–cure system. The way in which practitioners use the tools available (whether the tools are conventional or alternative, complementary, and integrative) and their willingness to become midwives to nature and self-healing, rather than the heroes of success stories, are what make the care holistic. The true healing healthcare system will emerge when both curing and healing processes are equally valued, sought after, and facilitated for all and when the full range of curing, caring, and healing modalities is available to all.

Holistic nurses have a key role to play in facilitating this level of change in the existing systems and in revisioning and recreating hospitals and clinics, wellness centers, and hospices as *Habitats for Healing*, optimal healing environments in which nurses thrive and patients heal. Habitats for Healing are characterized by autonomy of the nursing staff; a holistic, caring–healing relationship-centered framework that guides practice; and the integration of complementary and alternative healing modalities into regular nursing care (Quinn, 2010).

Facilitating Healing: Nurse as Healing Environment

The sickness–cure system is characterized almost exclusively by an approach that might be abbreviated as "getting the job done," while facilitating whole-person healing requires quite a different approach that I have labeled "holding sacred space."

Table 5-1 suggests some differences between the two approaches to being with people who are seeking health and healing and even curing (Quinn, 1992, p. 33).

One of the most powerful tools for facilitating healing is the presence of the nurse in the patient's environment. In fact, the nurse has the greatest effect of all the elements in the patient's environment, for better or sometimes, sadly, for worse. Simply by virtue of the role, a nurse has all the ritual power of the shaman of other cultures. The nurse is guardian of the patient's journey through illness and healing; the keeper and bestower of information, medicines, and treatments; and the mediator of the system and the comings and goings of others in the system.

In recent years, there has been a rapidly growing increase in research about the placebo effect (more accurately, the *haelan effect,* as noted earlier), particularly as it relates to the therapeutic relationship (Bayoumy et al., 2020; Cadorin et al., 2020; Colloca et al., 2023; Kelley et al., 2014; Ko et al; 2024; Montag et al., 2023; Palese et al., 2019; SmithBattle et al., 2016). In reviewing more than 200 papers published between 1995 and 2013, Jubb and Bensing (2013) suggested that "it is the quality of the patient–practitioner interaction that accounts for a sizeable chunk of the effect seen in placebo responses" (p. 2712), while Pardo-Cabello et al. (2022) concluded in their placebo review paper that "the factors associated with the occurrence of placebo effect are multiple, but in addition to those that depend on the placebo itself, the doctor-patient relationship would be the most important" (p. 1343).

Table 5-1 Ways of Being with People Seeking Help

Getting the Job Done	Holding Sacred Space
Authority vested in the external expert	Authority vested in the individual one healing
Source of healing: what the expert provides	Source of healing: the bodymindspirit of the one healing
Gathering, collecting, taking in information	Receiving information
Problem-solving/fixing	Life unfolding/facilitating
Making something happen, where something is	Allowing something to happen, where something is
■ defined by the external expert	■ defined mutually
■ defined ahead of time	■ defined in the moment
■ meeting the goal	■ an emergence of mystery
Directing/taking over to make it happen	Guiding/helping to allow it to happen
Doing to or for	Being with
Leading	Walking with
Power over	Power with
Expert is accountable and responsible for the outcome	Facilitator is accountable and responsible for competent practice
Failure is the nonachievement of predetermined outcome	Failure is giving up on the unfolding process

Aspects of holistic nursing such as delivering therapies in a warm and caring way; incorporating reassurance, relaxation, suggestion, and anxiety reduction; listening; providing empathy and understanding; and touching the patient have all been identified as having the potential to elicit patients' innate healing capabilities and thus enhance the effects of all therapies (Walach & Jonas, 2004). This evidence supports holistic nurses in reclaiming time and attention for their fundamental role as healers, experts in the offering of genuine, authentic healing presence that is essential to positive outcomes for patients.

In a universe that includes the nonlocal nature of consciousness and the existence of a human energy field that extends beyond the skin, the nurse is not simply part of the patient's environment, but rather the nurse *is* the patient's environment (Quinn, 1992). The healing environment of the patient may be optimized when the nurse intentionally shifts consciousness into a centered, present or meditative state. This is holding sacred space for healing operationalized. The interconnectedness of the energy fields of the nurse and the patient can facilitate relaxation, rest, or healing in the patient. When a nurse is centered in the present moment and has the intention to be an instrument for healing, he or she becomes a healing environment; this intention is carried in the nurse's energy field and manifests in the voice, the eyes, the general atmosphere of the nurse, and the quality of his or her touch. Nurses should ask themselves:

- Do patients hear in my voice that I am fully here and present and that I care? That I have time for them? That they are safe with me? What else can be communicated through the voice? The voice is vibrational, and the quality of the whole bodymindspirit of the nurse is conveyed in just the vibration of the voice, often well beyond what one is conscious of. The vibration of the voice can be a healing instrument or can be disturbing and disruptive to healing.
- What is the quality of my facial expression? Of my eyes? Do they communicate care and compassion, or are they perfunctory and distant? Does the patient feel seen by me, or does she feel overlooked? If the eyes are the windows to the soul, what is my soul saying to the soul of my patient? What is the patient's soul saying in response? In some spiritual traditions, it is understood that it only takes the gaze of the teacher for the student to become

fully realized or enlightened. Might our gaze also be healing?

- How am I touching this sacred other? Am I focused on the task at hand and simply touching the patient to get the job done? Or does my touch convey care, dignity, support, nurturance, and competence? Does my touch communicate that I know I am touching this person's spirit with my spirit as I contact his or her skin, because where else is the spirit located but in the body? Do I speak of love and kindness and respect through my hands?

Learning how to hold sacred space, how to shift consciousness into a healing state, is a basic skill for the holistic nurse. Nurses are not simply separate selves *doing to* the patient but an integral part of the patient's environment, *being with* them on the healing journey. The quality of the energy with which the patient is interacting is part of what nurses attend to, and this means attending to their own state of consciousness and well-being before, during, and after their interactions with patients. Thus, taking time for themselves to learn and practice relaxation, meditation, centering, or other self-care strategies becomes essential in this model and serves both nurses and patients. Nurses are not being selfish by taking this time. They are recognizing that unless they are energized, relaxed, and centered, they will be trying to give what they do not have to give. This results in less than optimal care for patients and burnout for nurses. Thus, self-care is a moral and ethical responsibility for the holistic nurse.

Nursing Situation

Georgia was dying of metastatic colon cancer at 49 years of age; she had been semicomatose for several days. The nurse sat quietly by Georgia's bedside and initiated Therapeutic Touch, but as an act of inner intentionality rather than through the outward use of her physical hands. Knowing that her intentions and thoughts could be conveyed through the energy field that she, Georgia, and the universe shared, she centered herself and silently made the intention to be an instrument for unconditional love and compassion, thus explicitly becoming a healing environment. In her mind's eye, she moved her hands over Georgia's body as if she were doing physical Therapeutic Touch, head to toe, while visualizing Georgia surrounded in a beautiful cobalt blue light and projecting an energy of deep peace, wholeness, and healing. After a few minutes, Georgia opened her eyes and turned her head toward the still unmoving, silent nurse, and said, "You make it so much easier." She smiled softly and closed her eyes again. Those were her last words to the nurse, her daughter, this writer. Clearly, while there would be no curing, while disease was slowly but surely claiming Georgia's body, her healing continued, up to the moment of her death.

Integration/Implications

There are many implications for the integration of transpersonal human caring and healing in nursing, including those for clinical practice, education, and research, as follows.

Clinical Practice

- Include goals related to caring and healing and not just curing in patient care plans.
- Ask patients what they think would help them to be in the best condition for their healing to happen.
- Recognize and/or create opportunities in providing nursing care to hold sacred space for healing in addition to getting the job done.

Education

- Include findings from current placebo research as part of the evidence base that supports the importance of transpersonal caring and the caring–healing relationships in creating positive healthcare outcomes.
- Include content on the intrinsic potential for self-healing and the haelan effect in multiple courses, such as pathophysiology and pharmacology.
- In clinical rotations, include questions such as "how will you (or how did you) put the patient in the best condition for nature to act on him or her today?" in care plans and post-conferences.

Research

- Collect personal stories and narratives that provide exemplars of caring occasions.
- Conduct interviews with patients who see themselves as healing, even in the absence of curing, to search for patterns that may facilitate this shift for other patients.
- Participate in conducting, publishing, and disseminating nursing and interdisciplinary research about the importance of the haelan effect/placebo effect in healing outcomes.

Policy

- Include content on the importance of transpersonal caring and the caring–healing relationship in all new nurse orientations.
- Create pilot units within existing institutions as Habitats for Healing, allowing staff to self-select these units.
- Offer continuing education in centering, meditation, and caring–healing presence and their importance to nurse well-being and patient clinical outcomes.

Conclusion

Transpersonal human caring provides the context for holistic nurses to facilitate healing—the emergence of right relationship—in patients, self, and systems. Using centering and intentionality, the holistic nurse may become a healing environment and participate in the creation of a true, healing healthcare system that integrates both masculine and feminine principles. *Holding sacred space* for healing is a skill of the holistic nurse that requires learning and practice. This skill does not replace *getting the job (of curing) done*, but it enhances and completes it. When we master this integration, we may have the capacity to make the way easier for our patients, our colleagues, our communities, and our world as we walk the most beautiful way of the healer.

References

Bayoumy, H. M. M., Almuwallad, G. E., & Eissa, A. O. (2020). Investigating knowledge, attitude, and beliefs regarding placebo interventions in clinical practice: A comparative study of nursing and medical university students. *Advances in Medical Education and Practice, 11*, 619–635.

Cadorin, L., Rossettini, G., Testa, M., Geri, T., & Palese, A. (2020). The awareness of contextual factors, placebo and nocebo effects among nursing students: Findings from a cross-sectional study. *Nurse Education in Practice, 42*, 102670.

Bohm, D. (1992). Response to a question raised at the International Transpersonal Association meeting, Prague, Czechoslovakia.

Colloca, L., Noel, J., Franklin, P. D., & Seneviratne, C. (eds.). (2023). *Placebo effects through the lens of translational research.* Oxford University Press.

Jubb, J., & Bensing, J. M. (2013). The sweetest pill to swallow: How patient neurobiology can be harnessed to maximize placebo effects. *Neuroscience Biobehavioral Review, 37*(10, part 2), 2709–2720.

Kelley, J. M., Kraft-Todd, G., Schapira, L., Kossowsky J, & Riess H. (2014). The influence of the patient–clinician relationship on healthcare outcomes: A systematic review and meta-analysis of randomized controlled trials. *PLoS ONE, 9*(4), e94207.

Ko, S. J., Kim, K., Kaptchuk, T. J., Napadow, V., Kuo, B., Gerber, J., Ha, N. Y., Lee, J., Kelley, J. M., Park, J. W., & Kim, J. (2024). Influence of patient-clinician relationship style on acupuncture outcomes in functional dyspepsia: A multi-site randomized controlled trial in Korea. *Patient Education and Counselling, 121*, 108133.

Kunz, D. (1993). Interview comment in Quinn, J., *Therapeutic touch: Healing through human energy fields. Video II: The method* [Videotape series]. National League for Nursing.

Laszlo, E. (1987). *Evolution: The grand synthesis*. Shambhala.

Levin, J. (2017). What is "healing"? Reflections on diagnostic criteria, nosology, and etiology. *Explore, 13*(4), 244–256.

Montag, L. T., Bisson, E. J., Duggan, S., Gregory, T., Murphy, G., Gilron, I., Wilson, R., & Salomons, T. V., (2023). Patient expectations and therapeutic alliance affect pain reduction following lidocaine infusion in an interdisciplinary chronic pain clinic. *The Journal of Pain, 25*(6),104443.

Nightingale, F. (1969). *Notes on nursing: What it is and what it is not*. Dover.

Palese, A., Rossettini, G., Colloca, L., & Testa, M. (2019). The impact of contextual factors on nursing outcomes and the role of placebo/nocebo effects: A discussion paper. *PAIN Reports, 4*, e716.

Pardo-Cabello, A. J., Manzano-Gamero, V., & Puche-Cañas, E. (2022). Placebo: A brief updated review. *Naunyn-Schmiedeberg's Archives of Pharmacology, 395*(11), 1343-1356.

Quinn, J. F. (1989). On healing, wholeness and the haelan effect. *Nursing and Healthcare, 10*(10), 552–556.

Quinn, J. F. (1992). Holding sacred space: The nurse as healing environment. *Holistic Nursing Practice, 6*(4), 26–36.

Quinn, J. F. (1997). Healing: A model for an integrative health care system. *Advanced Practice Nursing Quarterly, 3*(1), 1–7.

Quinn, J. F. (2010). Habitats for healing: Healthy environments for healthcare's endangered species. *Beginnings, 30*(2), 10–11.

Saueressig, T., Owen, P. J., Pedder, H., Arora, N. K., Simons, M., Kaczorowski, S., Miller, C. T. Donath, L., & Belavy, D. L. (2024). Boosting treatment outcomes via the patient-practitioner relationship, treatment-beliefs or therapeutic setting. A systematic review with meta-analysis of contextual effects in chronic musculoskeletal pain. *Journal of Orthopaedic and Sports Physical Therapy, 54*(7), 440–456.

SmithBattle, L., Pohlman, S., Palmer, J. L., Lorenz, R. A., & Cibulka, N. J. (2016). Placebo and the healing process. *Clinical Nursing Research, 25*(6), 587–589.

Walach, H., & Jonas, W. (2004). Placebo research: The evidence base for harnessing self-healing capacities. *Journal of Alternative and Complementary Medicine* (10, Suppl. 1), S-103–S-112.

Wampold, B.E. (2021). Healing in a social context: The importance of clinician and patient relationship. *Frontiers in Pain Research, 2*, 1-11.

Watson Caring Science Institute. (2024). *Caring science theory*. https://www.watsoncaringscience.org/jean-bio/caring-science-theory

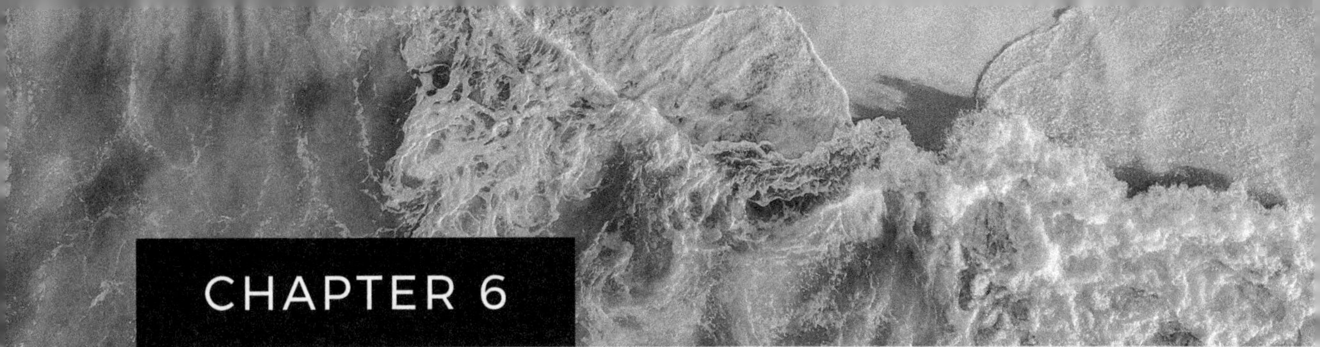

CHAPTER 6

Holistic Ethics

Margaret A. Burkhardt and Lorrine Hall

NURSE HEALER OBJECTIVES

- Explore the concept of holistic ethics.
- Relate self-reflection to holistic ethical practice.
- Discuss Earth ethics as an integral component of holistic ethics.
- Relate holistic ethics to clinical situations.
- Describe processes for ethical decision making in clinical situations.

DEFINITIONS

Earth community: A community that includes all beings of the Earth, nonhuman as well as human.

Earth ethics: A code of behavior that incorporates the understanding that the Earth community has core value in and of itself, includes ethical treatment of the nonhuman world and the Earth as a whole, and influences how we interact with the environment and all beings of the Earth.

Holistic ethics: The basic underlying concept of the unity and integral wholeness of all people and of all nature, which is pursued by finding unity and wholeness within oneself and within humanity and includes the desire to do good freely, to witness, identify, and contribute to unity.

The Nature of Ethical Problems

Ethical questions and issues arise from all areas of life, reflecting diverse values and perspectives; thus they are extremely complex. Examples of the myriad of ethical issues in health care include the ramifications of life-sustaining technology, the population explosion, assisted death, human trafficking, genetic engineering, environmental degradation, equitable treatment and access to health care for all people, social justice, and allocation of increasingly scarce resources. Ongoing developments in our society such as advances in medical technology, greater recognition of patients' rights, limited access to health care for some populations, health disparities, and end-of-life decisions, call nurses to increase their ethical awareness. Another factor that becomes increasingly important in holistic ethics is the ethical treatment of the nonhuman world—indeed the Earth as a whole—the health of which is intricately connected to human health.

Ethical dilemmas are characterized by the fact that there is no right answer. There are often two or more unsatisfactory answers or conflicting responses. Ethical dilemmas are made more complex when expectations of employers, physicians, patients, or other nurses are in conflict with each other and the best interests of the patient (Burkhardt & Nathaniel, 2025). Advances in health care and changes in the knowledge that forms the basis of our values are leading to new sources of ethical dilemmas. For example, technologies related to electronic health records, communications, and social media have affected patient confidentiality. Life-support technology may prolong living but may also increase suffering and prolong the dying process. Amid dealing with sophisticated technology, nurses often find that their focus is more on the machines than on the patient. Although advances provide new possibilities for extending or prolonging life, they also prompt a critical ethical question: Does having the technology always mean it should be used?

Morals and Principles

Ethical principles serve as a guide for dealing with ethical issues. These principles are basic and obvious moral truths that offer guidance for both deliberation and action. Principles found in major ethical theories include autonomy, beneficence, nonmaleficence, veracity, confidentiality, justice, caring, and fidelity. All these ethical principles presuppose respect for persons. These principles represent many obligations: to respect the wishes of competent persons, to not harm others, to take actions that benefit others, to produce a net balance of benefits over harms, to distribute benefits and harms fairly, to keep promises and contracts, to be truthful, to disclose information, and to respect privacy and protect confidential information (Beauchamp & Childers, 2019; Burkhardt & Nathaniel, 2025).

Orentlicher (2001), a physician, lawyer, and ethicist, suggests that there are two basic ways to guide proper behavior: rules and precedents. He notes that rules are designed to support underlying values (e.g., speed limits are set to promote public safety). Rules are attractive because they provide seemingly clear lines of conduct that prevent metaphorical slippery slopes. They can also help to avoid the capriciousness of personal discretion and the obtrusiveness of governmental intrusion in decision making. He voices concern, however, with the unintended consequences of rules. He argues that rules sometimes work to the detriment of the value that prompted implementation of the rule in the first place (known as the law of unintended consequences). For example, a medicolegal question might ask whether pregnant women should be forced to undergo treatment to help their fetuses. If forced treatments were endorsed, then some women might avoid prenatal care. This might result in the unintended consequence of harming their fetuses. The ethical response might depend on whether forced treatment would help more fetuses than would be harmed by women who would avoid prenatal care. This is but one example of the complexity of ethical decision making. Another moral concern is the political difficulty of having explicit rules when life-and-death decisions are being made, such as the allocation of scarce organs. Here, society tends to adopt a system of vague precedents that operate under the guise of rules. The appearance of objectivity, which is inherent to general rules, can hide the vagueness of the processes that are being used.

Within natural law ethics, the principle of double effect has special importance for nurses. Often, nurses are involved in actions that have untoward consequences. For example, administering a drug to relieve a cancer patient's pain may shorten the patient's life. In double-effect situations, four conditions must be met before an act can be justified (McIntyre, 2014):

1. The act itself must be morally good, or at least indifferent.
2. The good effect must not be achieved by means of the bad effect.
3. Only the good effect must be intended, even though the bad effect is foreseen and known.
4. The good effect intended must be equal to or greater than the bad effect.

Moral problems incorporate a mix of values, risks, benefits, and harms. They are as complex as they are important, include elements of uncertainty and conflict, and defy easy solutions. One must take care with moral decision making because many such decisions are irreversible. Ethics addresses different types of moral issues, including the following:

- Moral uncertainty (unsureness about moral principles or rules that may apply, or the nature of the ethical problem itself)
- Moral dilemma (conflict of moral principles that support different courses of action)
- Moral distress (inability to take the action known to be right because of external constraints)

- Practical dilemmas (a situation where moral claims compete with nonmoral claims)
- Moral courage (willingness to stand up for personal and professional ethical values even when this stance is unpopular and may mean standing alone)

Ethical debate helps to relieve moral uncertainty by clarifying questions and illuminating the ethical features of a situation. Discussion and reflection with others help to clarify moral dilemmas by revealing general and specific obligations and values. Adhering to ethical obligations and personal values and facing fears related to standing up for what is ethically right regardless of consequences supports the ability to act with moral courage. Awareness of factors that contribute to the complexity of ethical problems enables nurses to see the dilemma from a broader perspective. These factors include:

- Context (a person's unique life circumstances)
- Uncertainty (a lack of predictability of the outcome of a given act)
- Multiple stakeholders with potentially strong and diverse preferences
- Power imbalance within the healthcare institution
- Variables outside of the direct patient care setting, such as institutional policies
- Urgency (situations in which a decision must be made before one has a chance to deliberate as much as one would like) (Burkhardt & Nathaniel, 2025)

Holistic nurses need to know the language of ethics and have the courage to act ethically and participate fully in ethical decision making. This requires using principles and theory to deal with issues of relationships as well as healthcare concerns. A holistic approach to ethical problems incorporates both thinking and feeling as credible ways of knowing and recognizes a legitimate role for both in ethical decision making. Heart, mind, reason, and emotion need to be attended to when making ethical decisions, appreciating that what one feels in relation to the circumstances of the situation is as important as what one thinks is right or wrong.

Commitment to Care

Holistic nursing is grounded in the moral commitment to care for all patients. The Ethic of Care addresses holistic nursing's concern for relational caring. A fundamental directive of the ethic of care is to meet the needs of *particular* others, appreciating that gaining clarity about these needs occurs within the context of intentional caring relationships (Lee et al., 2017; Watson, 2018, 2024). Moving beyond personal biases and prejudices, opening to another's perspective, and being with persons as individuals enables nurses to support processes that help them figure out what they need. Developing a caring heart is fundamental in this process, recognizing that emotions are integral to the moral life.

Holistic nursing ethics is incomplete without embracing the values of Equity, Equality, Inclusion, Diversity, and Social Justice. These values are embedded in nursing codes of ethics and standards of practice (American Nurses Association [ANA], 2015; American Holistic Nurses Association [AHNA] & ANA, 2019). Nurses need to develop the moral courage to promote and uphold these professional core values, which can be facilitated through reflective practice(s). An absence of judgment for ourselves and others is essential in order to develop awareness of various perspectives. This enables the nurse to engage with others with an absence of judgment supported by true listening with one's heart through a lens of compassion.

Development of Holistic Ethics

Ethics is the study of the paths of practical wisdom. It is concerned with judgments of good and bad and right and wrong, based on a philosophic view of the nature of the universe. The holistic view of reality reopens vistas of thought that were dominant in the pretechnologic era, when people were generally closer to their environment and the Earth. The allure of new science and technology sidetracked many into primarily linear, rational, unidirectional thought. Furthermore, although technology has provided conveniences and easy solutions, it has also contributed to a tendency to objectify the universe.

Holistic ethics is a philosophy that couples both reemerging and rapidly evolving concepts of holism and ethics that reflect elements of Eastern and Western philosophies and spiritual and ethical beliefs of people from contemporary and Indigenous cultures. It involves a basic underlying concept of the unity and integral wholeness of all people, and of all nature, which is identified and pursued by finding unity and wholeness within one's self, within humanity, and within the larger Earth community. Within the framework of holistic ethics, acts are not performed solely for the sake of law, precedent, or social norms; they are performed from a desire to do good freely, to witness, identify, and contribute to unity of the self and of the universe, of which the individual is a part. Encompassing traditional ethical views, the holistic view is characterized by the balance and integration evident in the Eastern monad of the yin–yang mode and in the Western concept of masculine–feminine.

Holistic ethics originates in the individual's own character and relationship to the universe. In some way, the universe is present totally in each individual; paradoxically, the person is just a small part of that same universe. Gregorios (1987) believed that wisdom is a condition in which the self and the world are in communion with one another, within the larger communion, and with the infinite totality of being in its integrity. Albert Einstein, in the course of a serious illness, was asked if he feared death. He replied, "I have such a feeling of solidarity with every living being, that it does not matter to me where the individual begins and ends" (Born, 1971, p. 91).

Holistic ethics is grounded not so much in the act performed or in the distant consequences of the act as in the conscious evolution of an enlightened individual who performs the act. Understanding that all things are connected, the primary concern is the effect of the act on the individual and their larger self (the unity of which the individual is a part, including the entire Earth community). Unethical acts are those that degrade or brutalize the individual who performs the act and that detract from their conscious evolution, which, in turn, degrades the whole. The effect of an unethical act is to make us aware of the deprivation of divinity within humanity and of humanity itself. The unethical act dissolves the unity of matter and takes away wholeness. Acts must be judged in this setting to determine whether they promote wholeness and integration of either an individual or the collective whole. By evolving our own individual consciousness, we assess and direct the evolution of our species' consciousness and contemplatively examine our relationship with the universal being.

An a priori belief for a holistic person is likely "I believe in being" or, even more simply, "I am." In this belief system, no act, principle, or person is independent, but all are interrelated; all are *I*. Every action is a moral action, either contributing to the unity of being or diminishing it. It is the enlightened and completely expanded *I* that creates a holistic view of ethics.

Moral acts may be judged not solely in terms of their intrinsic nature or solely in terms of their ends but in both ways. The act may affect the nature of the person performing the act (the *I*) and their relationships, as well as affect the object of the act and the object's relationships. In addition, it can be helpful to explore the relationship of the act to the present and future of humanity and the Earth as a whole. Through this construct, holistic ethics is both deontologic (the rightness or wrongness of an action determines its morality) and teleologic (the consequences of an act determine its morality).

As a philosophic design for living, holistic ethics is a system for the individual. It appeals to the emotions, senses, aesthetic appreciation, and the inner self as revealed by meditative techniques. Such techniques may be active (e.g., the body movements of tai chi or jogging), passive (e.g., a sitting, meditative posture), or traditional prayer. The educative process of holistic ethics is not merely a matter of memorizing facts or historical perspectives but is instead a process of developing an attitude of awareness of the sacredness of ourselves and of the entire Earth community. It is a process in which there is an expanded view that, for both internal and external transformation, our inner self and the collective greater Self have stewardship not only of our bodies, minds, and spirits but also of our planet and the total universe.

Based on this emergent ethical theory, AHNA developed a position statement on holistic nursing ethics (**Box 6-1**).

Holistic ethics embraces and strives for the fusion between self and others. In the process, it becomes a cosmic ecology, a flowing with the universal tide of events, and a cocreator of celestial harmony. All events and ethical decisions become part of the unfolding of a harmonious order and

Box 6-1 **AHNA Position Statement on Holistic Nursing Ethics**

Code of Ethics for Holistic Nurses

We believe that the fundamental responsibilities of the nurse are to promote health, facilitate healing and alleviate suffering. The need for nursing is universal. Inherent in nursing is the respect for life, dignity and right of all persons. Nursing care is given in a context mindful of the holistic nature of humans, understanding the body-mind-spirit. Nursing care is unrestricted by considerations of nationality, race, creed, color, age, sex, sexual preferences, politics, or social status. Given that nurses practice in culturally diverse settings, professional nurses must have an understanding of the cultural background of clients in order to provide culturally appropriate interventions.

Nurses render services to clients who can be individuals, families, groups or communities. The client is an active participant in health care and should be included in all nursing care planning decisions.

In order to provide services to others, each nurse has a responsibility toward themself. In addition, nurses have defined responsibilities towards the client, coworkers, nursing practice, the profession of nursing, society, and the environment.

Nurses and Self

The nurse has a responsibility to model health behaviors. Holistic nurses strive to achieve harmony in their own lives and assist others striving to do the same.

Nurses and the Client

The nurse's primary responsibility is to the client needing nursing care. The nurse strives to see the client as a whole, and provides care that is professionally appropriate and culturally consonant. The nurse holds in confidence all information obtained in professional practice, and uses professional judgment in disclosing such information. The nurse enters into a relationship with the client that is guided by mutual respect and a desire for growth and development.

Nurses and Coworkers

The nurse maintains cooperative relationships with coworkers in nursing and other fields. Nurses have a responsibility to nurture each other, and to assist nurses to work as a team in the interest of client care. If a client's care is endangered by a coworker, the nurse must take appropriate action on behalf of the client.

Nurses and Nursing Practice

The nurse carries personal responsibility for practice and for maintaining continued competence. Nurses have the right to utilize all appropriate nursing interventions and have the obligation to determine the efficacy and safety of all nursing actions. Wherever applicable, nurses utilize research findings in directing practice.

Nurses and the Profession

The nurse plays a role in determining and implementing desirable standards of nursing practice and education. Holistic nurses may assume a leadership position to guide the profession toward holism.

(continues)

Box 6-1 AHNA Position Statement on Holistic Nursing Ethics *(continued)*

Nurses support nursing research and the development of holistically oriented nursing theories. The nurse participates in establishing and maintaining equitable social and economic working conditions in nursing.

Nurses and Society

The nurse, along with other citizens, has responsibility for initiating and supporting actions to meet the health and social needs of the public.

Nurses and the Environment

The nurse strives to manipulate the client's environment to become one of peace, harmony, and nurturance so that healing may take place. The nurse considers the health of the ecosystem in relation to the need for health, safety, and peace of all persons.

a realization of potentials. Even tragic events can be analyzed within this harmonious spectrum with full realization of the fusion of relationships. One's own actions can become courageous; full of truth, being, and beauty; assured; detached; and virtuous.

Earth Ethics

Ethical discussions and deliberations most often refer to principles and practices related to human experiences, values, and ways of being in the world. Such discussions seldom include consideration of ethical treatment of the nonhuman world. Our awareness of relationship with the natural world flows from our worldview or cosmology. The worldview that underlies the Western scientific perspective holds that there is a radical distinction between humans as subjects and the natural world as object (Swimme & Tucker, 2011). A belief that the human experience is separate from and in opposition to nature has engendered and permitted a destructive attitude toward Earth and a belief that all species and resources of the Earth have been put here primarily for human use. A shift, which began emerging in the 17th century, from an organic understanding of reality in which everything is alive, to a mechanistic view of reality, engendered the belief that humans have a right to do anything they want with nature. This attitude promotes little regard for ethical responsibility toward the nonhuman world. Instead, it has allowed us to disregard our complicity in the exploitation of the planet. After several centuries of demoting the natural world to a collection of material objects available for human exploitation, we are now realizing that this complete disregard for the realities of ecological systems and the limited capacity of the natural world to sustain this exploitation and destruction are contributing to the ill health of humans and to the planet itself. (Refer to **Chapter 20**.)

There is an urgent need for holistic nurses and all of humanity to move beyond a human-centered focus in ethical concerns and begin to relate to all parts of the Earth community as having core value. Indeed, holistic nurses have a responsibility to address the health of the planet (AHNA, 2021). We need to incorporate Earth ethics into our understanding and practice of holistic ethics. Remembering that we are part of the interconnected web of life, we recognize that what we do to the Earth we do to ourselves. Indigenous peoples, mystics of many traditions, and contemporary scholars teach us that the world is a seamless garment in which there is no separation between humans and nature, the sacred and the secular. We cannot have healthy minds, bodies, spirits, or communities without healthy land and environment. When we destroy the source of our life and sustenance, our health (physical, mental, emotional, and spiritual) suffers. When we understand that, as humans, we are only one part of the interconnected Earth community, and we recognize the interdependence and unity of all in the natural world, we appreciate that all species have an intrinsic right to exist. Within this understanding, our ethical principles must address the integrity and health of the entire community of life. The moral imperative of holistic ethics then directs us to apply principles of beneficence, nonmaleficence, caring, and justice to our treatment of the whole Earth community, not only to its human members.

Self-Reflection

Nurses are expected to act in principled ways in all areas of practice. Principled behavior flows from personal and professional values that guide our behaviors and decisions. Holistic nurses engage in self-reflection to promote awareness of personal and professional values and how they influence relationships with self, others, and the Earth community.

Values include beliefs, codes of conduct, ideals, and qualities that are highly prized by individuals, groups, and society. They develop over time and have cultural, familial, environmental, and educational components. Core values that underlie the ethical practice of nursing are found in nursing codes of ethics and include caring, integrity, honesty, respect for persons, advocacy, accountability, autonomy, reducing health disparities, equity, equality, inclusion, diversity, and social justice. Internalizing the ethical values and norms of holistic nursing is foundational to taking on the professional identity as a holistic nurse. Self-reflection is an ongoing process through which holistic nurses become increasingly aware of both personal and professional values. The process enables nurses to articulate personal beliefs and values, reflect on how they are congruent with those of the profession, and to more consciously integrate the two. Through self-reflection, nurses become more aware of personal thoughts, judgments, feelings, beliefs, biases, and perceptions. Appreciating one's own perspective offers insight into personal responses and reactions and helps one acknowledge similarities and differences of values and beliefs in interactions with others. Self-reflection enhances a holistic nurse's ability to act ethically, promoting positive outcomes for patients by basing actions and decisions on internalized values and norms. Often, patients must clarify their values to participate fully in ethical decision making. Holistic nurses can assist patients in this process in a variety of ways. One way is for nurses to listen carefully and reflect back what patients communicate as personally important to them. Another might be to list several health behaviors or values, such as happiness, good relationships with family, health, and independence, and ask patients to rank them or to identify how they incorporate them into their lives.

Integrity and Empowerment

Personal integrity and a sense of empowerment are cornerstones of ethical behavior that are espoused throughout *Holistic nursing: Scope and standards of practice* (AHNA & ANA, 2019). Both are grounded in self-awareness and personal reflection and are essential to the holistic caring process. Identifying personal values strengthens the ability to make choices that reflect these values. Integrity implies trustworthiness; wholeness; and consistency of values, emotions, and behaviors, as well as adherence to moral norms over time. Empowerment implies having the ability to choose; being responsible and accountable for personal actions; having the courage to take risks; and having the desire, ability, and resources to make decisions. When faced with ethical issues, personal empowerment enables us to be true to ourselves, make choices based on our core values, and allow our actions to flow from our essence. Having the moral courage to do what is right despite fear of reprisal, such as rejection, ridicule, anxiety, shame, and even potential unemployment, reflects a high degree of personal integrity and empowerment.

Self-care reflects personal integrity and empowerment. Being honest with and caring for ourselves and treating ourselves with respect are ways we demonstrate congruence between our values and behavior. Knowing that the energy of the self is interconnected with the energy of the Earth community, holistic nurses understand that the growth of personal strength and power unfolds within the context of love and respect for all forms of life.

Transcultural Considerations

Cultural values and beliefs guide our way of being in the world and our reaction to life experiences in patterned ways. Culture guides choices regarding when and where to go for health care, what kind of care to seek, and how long to participate in care. Patterns influenced by culture that are significant in providing holistic health care include beliefs about health and practices related to health and healing. These beliefs and practices manifest in both direct and subtle ways, and sensitivity to them can affect patient outcomes and satisfaction with the care. When considering definitions of health and values such as autonomy, beneficence, justice, or the right to self-determination, it is important to ask from whose perspective these values are understood—that of the nurse or that of the patient. For example, some cultures place a higher emphasis on loyalty to the group than on Western values of individual autonomy. Healthcare decisions in these cultures may require input and agreement from groups such as the family, community, or society rather than relying primarily on the individual.

The diversity in our global society impels holistic nurses to understand the influence of culture on moral development and ethical decision making (Andrews & Boyle, 2020; Jensen, 2015). Transcultural ethical issues arise when nurses, patients, and families are guided by different moral paradigms and hold differing views of what is important or necessary regarding health, recovery, illness, or the dying process. Ethical or legal dilemmas may arise from lack of understanding of language, procedures, expectations, and other elements of the culture that lead to miscommunication, unclear decisions, and a sense of powerlessness or lack of control. Dealing with transcultural issues requires self-awareness on the part of the nurse. A good starting point for becoming sensitive to the culture of another is to understand one's own culture and its influence on personal perceptions and behaviors. Similarly, incorporating cultural assessment into care with patients facilitates better understanding of sometimes overlooked factors that influence a patient's health behaviors and decisions (Andrews & Boyle, 2020; McFarland & Wehbe-Alamah, 2015). Cultural assessment provides insight into the congruence, or lack thereof, between patients' and nurses' values, understandings of health, and how healthcare decisions are made. Nurses who provide culturally congruent care are better able to facilitate the process of ethical decision making.

Ethical Decision Making

Nurses are confronted daily with the need to make personal and professional ethical decisions, yet many of them feel unprepared to be equal participants in ethical decision making. Some decisions nurses face are minor, and others are fraught with long-term, multifaceted ramifications. As noted previously, in order to make decisions appropriately, holistic nurses need to be grounded in an understanding of the integral wholeness of all beings and do their best to articulate and examine their core values and their relationship to nursing and institutional standards. Participation in decision-making groups necessitates that nurses become fluent in the language of nursing and bioethics and that they learn to appreciate the diverse moral perspectives of patients and colleagues. It is necessary as well that nurses operate from a stance of moral integrity and have facility with processes that help sort out and classify the elements of the issue. There are many well-established guidelines for analyzing individual cases in ethics that may be helpful to nurses. Two such processes are summarized here.

Five-Step Process of Ethical Decision Making

Burkhardt and Nathaniel approach ethical decision making from a nursing frame of reference that includes sensitivity to the human story (Burkhardt & Nathaniel, 2025). They suggest that, although the steps of an ethical decision-making process may seem linear on paper, the process is nonlinear in practice. They note that the ethical decision-making process overlies other dynamic biological, psychological, and social processes—layer on layer. Because nothing in the human sphere is static, nurses need to appreciate that physical conditions and opinions change, knowledge evolves, and time passes. In light of the changing nature of human experience, decision making is spiral in nature. This process requires an ongoing evaluation and assimilation of key facets and information, with each step being revisited as often as is required and molded by the dynamics of changing facts, evolving beliefs, unexpected consequences, and participants who move in and out of the process. This five-step process of ethical decision making includes:

1. Articulating the problem
2. Gathering data and identifying conflicting moral claims
3. Exploring strategies
4. Implementing the strategy
5. Evaluating outcomes of the action

1. Articulating the Problem

Ethical decision making begins when there is concern that a moral problem exists. Carefully articulating and identifying the undesirable situation enables one to also clarify the goal because a problem consists of a discrepancy between the current situation and a desired state or goal. A goal must be identified before moving toward strategies (refer to step 3).

2. Gathering Data and Identifying Conflicting Moral Claims

Clarify the issues by gathering information that provides evidence of conflicting goals, obligations, principles, duties, rights, loyalties, values, or beliefs. In this process, nurses must pay attention to the societal, religious, and cultural values and beliefs of all involved. Data gathering should include information about facts as well as feelings that seem important, such as expectations, preferences, quality-of-life issues, understanding of the situation, relationships and supports, and projected outcomes of available options. Gaps in the information also need to be identified. Key participants (which include healthcare providers) need to be identified, including who is affected and how; who is legitimately empowered to make the decision; issues of conflict and agreement among participants and what is most important to each; the level of competence of the person most affected; and the rights, duties, authority, and capabilities of all participants. These data can help those involved to understand the ethical components, principles of concern, and various perceptions of issues and principles of all involved in the situation.

3. Exploring Strategies

Through the assessment process, possible alternative strategies that address the desired outcomes begin to emerge. In consideration of legal and other consequences, participants need to determine which alternatives best meet the identified goals and fit their basic beliefs, lifestyles, and values. By reviewing options with both head and heart, participants need to eliminate unacceptable alternatives and begin the process of listing, weighing, prioritizing, and sensing the energy of those that are considered acceptable, recognizing that there is rarely a perfect solution. Once an option is chosen, the decision makers must be willing to act on the choice.

4. Selecting and Implementing the Strategy

Although taking action is a major goal of the process, it can be one of the most difficult parts of the process. Emotions that are laced with both certainty and doubt about the rightness of the decision often emerge. Empowering patients and families to make difficult decisions requires special attention to the emotions that often manifest at this point of the process.

5. Evaluating Outcomes and Revising the Plan as Needed

Once the action step is taken, participants begin a process of response and evaluation that sheds light on the effectiveness and validity of the process. In evaluating the action, it is important to determine whether the original ethical problem has been effectively resolved and whether other problems have emerged related to the action. As new data emerge and the situation changes, participants may identify subsequent moral problems that require adjusting the course of action based on both new information and responses to the previous decision.

Four Components of the Ethical Case Analysis Process

Jonsen et al. (2015) divide the ethical case analysis process into the following four components:

1. Medical indications
2. Patient preferences
3. Quality of life
4. Contextual issues

Present in every clinical, ethical case, these four topics are necessary for a thorough analysis. The holistic approach adds relationship questions: Who am I? What is my relationship to others and to the whole? What other factors are contributing to my decisions? Am I wise and courageous enough to perceive and respect others' differences and honor them as I would honor my own beliefs?

Medical Indications

The underlying ethical principle in considering medical indications is beneficence—be of benefit—and do no harm. Discussion should focus on discerning the relationship between the pathophysiology and the diagnostic and therapeutic interventions (both conventional and integrative) available to remedy the patient's pathologic condition. Questions regarding the overall goal of the care are important considerations in this component. For example, for the patient who is terminally ill, there may be discussions about the time to switch from further medical treatment to palliative care.

Patient Preferences

In all interventions, patient preferences are relevant. There are many questions to be asked. What does the patient want? Does the patient comprehend their choices? Is the patient being coerced? In some cases, there is no certainty because the patient is incapable of self-expression. Whenever possible, it is essential to ensure that the patient's right to self-determination based on their personal values and evaluation of risks and benefits is honored. However, it is necessary to be clear about what is realistically feasible in relation to the patient's wishes. In the case of a child, nurses must ask the questions: Do the parents understand the situation? Do the parents appear to have the best interests of the child at heart? Are the parents in agreement or discord? At which level can a child have input into the discussion?

Quality of Life

A patient enters a health crisis with an actual or potential reduction in quality of life, manifested by the signs and symptoms of the illness. The objective of healthcare interventions is to improve quality of life. In each case, multiple questions surround quality-of-life issues. What does quality of life mean, in general and in particular? How are others responding to their perceptions of it? How do particular levels of quality impose obligations, if any, on providers? Although this component may be a difficult part of the analysis, it is indispensable.

Contextual Issues

Every case has a patient at its center. The patient exists in a social, psychological, spiritual, economic, and relational environment. All decisions must be considered in the light of this expanded conceptual and holistic view of personhood and personality. The major factors affected are psychological, emotional, financial, legal, scientific, educational, and spiritual.

Supporting Holistic End-of-Life Decisions

Many ethical dilemmas relate to end-of-life care options and choices. Supporting a patient's right and ability to make choices is an essential element of holistic nursing practice and holistic ethics (refer to **Chapter 17** also). The Patient Self-Determination Act, effective December 1, 1991, requires that institutions receiving Medicare or Medicaid funds provide adult patients written information about their right to accept or refuse medical or surgical treatment and their right to initiate advance directives. Advance directives are instructions that indicate healthcare interventions to initiate or withhold or that designate someone who will act as a surrogate in making such decisions if decision-making capacity is lost. Advance directives support people in making decisions on their own behalf and help to ensure that patients have the kind of end-of-life care they want. These directives are of two types: *treatment directives* (often referred to as living wills) and *appointment directives* (often referred to as powers of attorney or health proxies). A living will specifies the medical treatment that a patient wishes to refuse in the event that they are terminally ill and cannot make those decisions. A durable power of attorney for health care appoints a proxy or surrogate, usually a relative or trusted friend, to make medical decisions on behalf of the patient if they can no longer make such decisions. It has broader applications than a living will and can apply to any illness or injury that causes the patient to lose decision-making capacity temporarily or long term. The authority of the surrogate is effective only for the duration of the loss of decision-making capacity. An advance directive applies only if a patient is incapacitated. Individuals can cancel advance directives at any time. An advance directive may be simple or complex. Individuals should give a copy of the advance directive to their family members and healthcare provider and should carry a copy if hospital admission is necessary.

As part of patient assessment, a holistic nurse may consider asking the following questions to help determine if the patient has advance directives or to empower them to consider their preferences:

- Have you discussed your end-of-life choices with your family and/or designated surrogate and healthcare team workers?
- Do you have basic information about advance medical directives, including living wills and durable powers of attorney?
- Do you wish to initiate an advance medical directive?
- If you have already prepared an advance medical directive, can you provide it now?

Legal Aspects

Healthcare providers must adhere to the law. All nurses are responsible and accountable to comply with the nursing practice act as well as the rules and regulations of the board of nurse examiners in the state or province where they are licensed and work. Standards of professional nursing practice require that each nurse practice to the level of their knowledge and skills. In this regard, holistic nurses need to know and adhere to the standards of practice for holistic nurses. Whatever an individual nurse's personal ethic, they must still adhere to professional standards of practice and to the law.

Implications

Education

Because nursing is inherently a moral endeavor, the study of ethics and its application to all areas of nursing should be key content in educational programs at all levels. Students need to become well versed in the *Code of ethics for nurses with interpretive statements* (ANA, 2015) and professional scope and standards for care since these documents ground all nursing practice.

Practice and Research

Holistic nursing care and research require awareness of, respect for, and congruence with the culture and needs of individuals and communities that are the focus of holistic nursing services or research (McFarland & Wehbe-Alamah, 2015). Broad principles and concepts guiding practice or research include beneficence, respect for persons and communities, equity, diversity, honoring the unity and wholeness of all beings, justice, contextual caring, fidelity to one's professional code of ethics, and advocating for patients' rights to self-determination.

Ensuring legal and ethical protection of a patient's right to personal autonomy includes obtaining informed consent regarding medical, holistic/integrative, and other treatments, as well as participation in research studies. Informed consent in clinical practice provides the opportunity for the patient to choose a course of action regarding plans for health care, including the right to refuse treatment recommendations and to choose from available therapeutic alternatives. An informed consent must include the following:

- The nature of the health concern and prognosis if nothing is done
- Description of all treatment options, even those that the healthcare provider does not favor or cannot provide
- The benefits, risks, and consequences of the various treatment alternatives (or the research protocol), including nonintervention

Because listing alternative treatments is part of an informed consent, a question to ponder is whether it is an ethical duty for conventional healthcare practitioners to include holistic/integrative modalities in discussion of therapeutic alternatives. Nurses also need to ask whether practitioners of other healing modalities should ensure that their clients are aware of biomedical alternatives. Holistic nurses who provide integrative therapies should explain the intervention and discuss risks, expected effects and benefits, and treatment options prior to initiating therapy. Because holistic/integrative therapies may affect conventional interventions in varying ways, it is important to inform other health team members of the use of these therapies.

The principles that underlie the ethical conduct of research include respect for human dignity (i.e., the rights to full disclosure and self-determination or autonomy), beneficence (i.e., the right to protection from harm and discomfort, as in balancing between the benefits and risks of a study), and justice (i.e., the rights of fair treatment and privacy, including anonymity and confidentiality). These principles provide the basis for informed consent related to participation in research studies (U.S. Department of Health and Human Services, n.d.). Informed consent in research refers to freely choosing to participate in a research study after the research purpose, expected commitment, risks and benefits, any invasion of privacy, and ways that anonymity and confidentiality will be addressed have been explained. Nurses who work in clinical areas where research is being conducted must ensure that these principles are followed. Nursing's advocacy role is especially important when research studies focus on vulnerable populations such as children; persons with disabilities; persons who are challenged, institutionalized, or incarcerated; older adults; pregnant women; and those who are dying. Nurses who are involved in research are accountable to professional standards for reporting research findings, including the ethical treatment of data, assuring the integrity of research protocols, and honesty in reporting data.

Policy

The ethic of care and politics of caring directs nurses to advocate for a healthcare system that values caring and supports equity, diversity, inclusivity, social justice, and mitigation of health disparities. This means creating caring environments in institutions and supporting and justly compensating nurses and others who do the work of caring.

Conclusion

The holistic view of reality reopens vistas of thought that were dominant in the pretechnologic era, when people were generally closer to their environment and the Earth. Holistic ethics is a philosophy that couples both reemerging and rapidly evolving concepts of holism and ethics. It involves a basic underlying concept of the unity and integral wholeness of all people, and of all nature, that is identified and pursued by finding unity and wholeness within the self, within humanity, and within the Earth community. The complexity of ethical issues relates to the diverse values and perspectives involved. Skills in cultural assessment can help nurses to more effectively deal with ethical issues. Understanding the nature of ethical problems requires holistic nurses to be familiar with ethical theories, concepts, and various ethical paradigms and to be able to integrate this knowledge with holistic theory and practice. Attentiveness to equity, diversity, inclusivity, social justice, and mitigation of health disparities in all healthcare settings is an ethical imperative for holistic nurses. An increasingly important factor in holistic ethics is the ethical treatment of the nonhuman world and the Earth as a whole, the health of which is intricately connected to human health. Awareness of personal values, beliefs, and understanding of health grounds the ability to deal effectively with ethical situations. The principles and processes of holistic ethics apply to research as well as to clinical practice situations. Holistic nurses need to know the language of ethics, be familiar with processes of ethical decision making, be attentive to cultural differences, and have the courage to participate fully in ethical decision making. Caring relationships and incorporating both thinking and feeling as credible ways of knowing in ethical decision making are essential to this process.

References

American Nurses Association. (2015). *Code of ethics for nurses with interpretive statements*. https://codeofethics.ana.org/home

American Holistic Nurses Association & American Nurses Association. (2019). *Holistic nursing: Scope and standards of practice* (3rd ed.). Nursesbooks.org.

American Holistic Nurses Association. (2021). *Position statement: Planetary health*. https://www.ahna.org/Portals/66/Docs/Press%20Releases/AHNA%20Planetary%20Health%20Position%20Statement%20March%202021%20Final.pdf?ver=dBuX3QToJOK7pcHMlZO5BQ%3d%3d

Andrews, M. M., & Boyle, J. S. (2020). *Transcultural concepts in nursing care* (7th ed.). Wolters Kluwer.

Beauchamp, T. L., & Childers, J. (2019). *Principles of biomedical ethics* (8th ed.). Oxford University Press.

Born, M. (1971). *The Born–Einstein letters: Friendship, politics and physics in uncertain times*. Macmillan Press.

Burkhardt, M. A., & Nathaniel, A. K. (2025). *Ethics and issues in contemporary nursing*. Elsevier.

Gregorios, P. M. (1987). *Science for sane societies*. Paragon House.

Jensen, A. (2015). *Moral development in a global world: Research from a cultural-developmental perspective*. Cambridge University Press.

Jonsen, A. R., Siegler, M., & Winslade, W. J. (2015). *Clinical ethics. A practical approach to ethical decisions in clinical medicine* (8th ed.). McGraw-Hill.

Lee, S., Palmieri, P., & Watson, J. (2017). *Global advances in human caring literacy*. Springer Publishing.

McFarland, M. R., & Wehbe-Alamah, H. B. (Eds.). (2015). *Leininger's culture care diversity and universality: A worldwide nursing theory* (3rd ed.). Jones & Bartlett Learning.

McIntyre, A. (2014). Doctrine of double effect. In E. N. Zalta (Ed.), *Stanford encyclopedia of philosophy*. https://plato.stanford.edu/entries/double-effect/

Orentlicher, D. (2001). *Matters of life and death: Making moral theory work in medicine and the law*. Princeton University Press.

Swimme, B., & Tucker, M. E. (2011). *Journey of the universe*. Yale University Press.

U.S. Department of Health and Human Services. (n.d.). *About ORI*. https://ori.hhs.gov/

Watson, J. (2018). *Unitary caring science: Philosophy and praxis of nursing*. University of Colorado Press.

Watson, J. (2024). *Metaphysics of Watson's unitary caring science: A cosmology of love*. Springer Publishing.

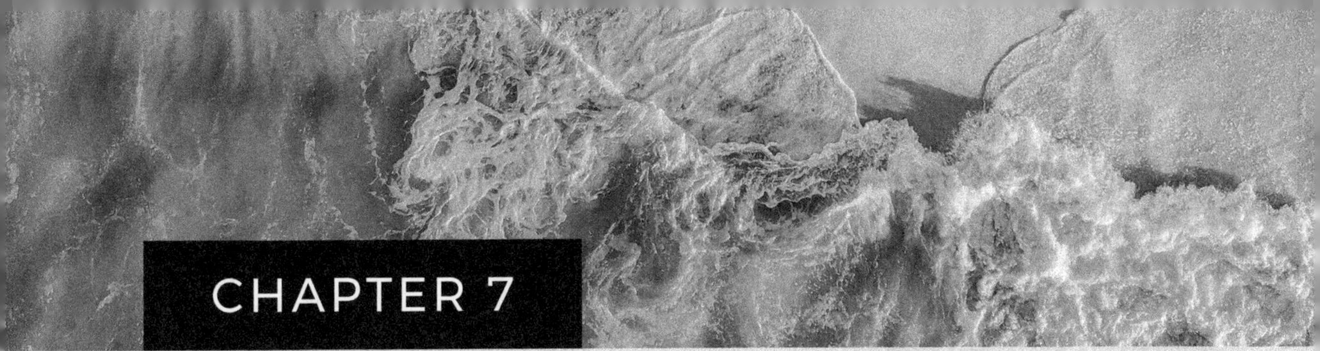

CHAPTER 7

Spirituality and Health

Margaret A. Burkhardt, Mary Gail Nagai-Jacobson, and Jennifer Reich

NURSE HEALER OBJECTIVES

- Describe spirituality and how spirituality relates to religion.
- Explore common facets of spirituality and how they manifest in different people.
- Recognize expressions and experiences of spirituality such as mystery and miracles, suffering, love, compassion, hope, forgiveness, peace and peacemaking, grace, joy, and prayer.
- Discuss the role of listening, intentional presence, story, and prayer in spiritual care.
- Identify approaches to spiritual caregiving integral to holistic care.
- Acknowledge the need for nurses to nurture their own spirits and ways to do so.

DEFINITIONS

Religion: An organized system of beliefs and associated practice regarding the cause, purpose, and nature of the universe that is shared by a group of people. Religion connects persons through shared beliefs, values, and practices, distinguishing one belief system, and group, from another.

Spirituality: The essence of our being that permeates our living in relationships and infuses our unfolding awareness of who we are, our purpose in being, and our inner resources. Inherent in the human condition, spirituality is expressed and experienced through living our connectedness with the Sacred Source, the self, others, and nature.

Introduction

We join spokes together in a wheel,
but it is the center hole
that makes the wagon move.
We shape clay into a pot,
but it is the emptiness inside
that holds whatever we want.
We hammer wood for a house,
but it is the inner space
that makes it livable.
We work with being,
but non-being is what we use (Lao Tzu)

Spirituality is the cornerstone of holistic nursing, health, and healing. It is woven into the physical, mental, emotional, and energetic aspects of one's being, infusing every aspect of life. Understanding spirituality and its role in health and healing and developing competence in spiritual caregiving are essential to holistic nursing. Scholarship related to spirituality in nursing practice and education has grown significantly since the 1990s. Studies explore spiritual expressions, understandings, and care approaches across religious and spiritual traditions cultures, ages, ethnic and socioeconomic groups, and nursing populations. While emphasis on different elements of spirituality may vary, the core aspects of spirituality remain consistent. This chapter discusses these key elements and how to approach spirituality and spiritual caregiving within a holistic framework.

Spirituality—The Cornerstone of Holistic Nursing

Spirituality is perhaps the most basic, yet least understood, aspect of holistic nursing. Being intangible and difficult to measure, it eludes the cognitive mind. While definitions highlight key aspects of spirituality, the mystery and experience itself defies full explanation. Language for spirit or soul is limited; thus, people often express spirituality through symbols, metaphor, and story (Burkhardt & Nagai-Jacobson, 2002). Recall that the term *spirituality* derives from the Latin *spiritus* and Greek *pneuma*, both meaning breath. Spirituality is the essence of who we are and how we are in the world and, like breathing, is integral to our existence as human beings.

All people, at all ages, are bio-psycho-social-spiritual beings. Attending to spirituality across the life span implies an understanding of the developmental aspects of spirituality, particularly an awareness that expressions of spirituality may vary with age and other factors.

Some may not see themselves or others as spiritual if they do not attend religious services or believe in God, reflecting the common confusion between religion and spirituality. Because of this, nurses often link spiritual caregiving with determining a patient's religion and related health beliefs. While this is valuable, holistic nurses understand that spirituality is broader than religion and that all persons are spiritual even if not religious.

Spirituality and Religion

Holistic nurses appreciate that spirituality and religion are not synonymous. Spirituality is a manifestation of each person's wholeness and being that is not subject to choice but simply is. Being spiritual is integral to the human experience in the same way that being physical, emotional, and sexual are part of being human. Religion per se is not essential to existence. Religion is chosen. Spirituality is expressed and experienced in many ways, both within and beyond the context of religion.

Religion refers to an organized system of beliefs shared by a group of people and the practices related to that system. Ritual, worship, prayer, meditation, style of dress, and dietary observances are examples of such practices. Because culture influences a person's values and beliefs, religious and other spiritual expressions often relate to personal culture. Religions reflect approaches to, and understandings of, spirituality. For some people, spirituality is deeply intertwined with their religious tradition. Religious precepts and practices often assist persons in attending to their spiritual selves; at times, however, these actions do little to nurture a person's true spirituality. Life experiences that are spiritual in nature may or may not relate to religion. Knowledge of the histories, symbols, beliefs, practices, and languages of various religious traditions increases the nurse's ability to hear, recognize, and address the religious needs of patients. However, information alone about religious affiliation and practices offers only a glimpse into a person's spiritual self. Information about numerous religious traditions is available on websites such as Britannica.

Because religion offers a particular structure for expressing spirituality, nurses may be more comfortable discussing spiritual concerns when they arise within an identifiable religious context than when they occur within a broader perspective of spirituality. However, satisfying the rites and rituals of a religion may or may not meet all of a patient's spiritual needs. Spiritual care and interventions need to be individualized and reflect the patient's personal beliefs, cultural perspectives, and worldview (Michaelson et al., 2023; Murgia et al., 2022; Yeşilçınar et al., 2018). This is of special concern when a patient's spiritual expression is not aligned with the practices of a religion or when their religious, cultural, and spiritual perspectives differ from the nurse's. Holistic nurses recognize that religion and spirituality are distinct and honor diverse expressions and ways of nurturing the spiritual self.

Spirituality: Language and Expression

One of the barriers to incorporating spirituality into holistic nursing care is the paucity of language within Western societies for discussing and expressing matters of the spirit or soul. In Western cultures, the language used for describing and expressing spirit is generally that of science or of religion derived from the Judeo-Christian tradition. Research related to spirituality in different cultures has increased in past years. However, much of the discussion of spirituality within nursing and other healthcare literature continues to reflect Judeo-Christian values and perspectives regarding the Divine, relationships with others and the world, experience of suffering, prayer, and the like. Understandings of spirituality and language describing spiritual values and experience may be different for many people in the world who do not adhere to the Judeo-Christian tradition. Because spirituality is the essence of every person and is not limited to a particular religious perspective, holistic nurses strive to be open to or to create a language that allows room for each person's unique expression of spirituality.

Approaching spirituality primarily from a Western cultural perspective can lead to misinterpretation of spiritual expression and concerns. When spiritual issues do not fit into a familiar paradigm, the spiritual nature of the situation may not be recognized. If expressions of spirituality are misunderstood, there is a risk of labeling the spiritual issue as pathology.

Engebretson (2016) noted that not all assumptions of Western Judeo-Christian-Islamic traditions (e.g., monotheism, transcendence, dualism) are shared with Eastern and Nature religious traditions. Monotheism is the belief in one God that is above and beyond Nature, contrasted with the belief in the existence of many gods (polytheism) or the existence of the sacred in all living things (pantheism) found in Eastern and Nature religions. Transcendence, which means to exist above material existence, is implied in the Western view of God as separate from humanity. People from such Western traditions often seek connection with the Divine by focusing outward through ritual and prayer. Eastern and Nature traditions focus on immanence, or the experience of the Divine within each person. Looking inward through meditation and spiritual exercises is a way of connecting with the Divine in these traditions. Dualism (the separation of spirit and matter) is a familiar concept in Western traditions. In contrast, reality is conceived of as a unified whole in the Eastern metaphysical traditions of monism. The polarization of science and religion generally found in the West reflects the impact of the assumptions of dualism on perceptions, definitions, and expectations of the spiritual experience within health care. In contrast, nursing theories such as Martha Rogers's *science of unitary human beings* and Jean Watson's *unitary caring science* offer nurses both language and framework for recognizing and giving voice to spiritual experiences.

Facets of Spirituality: Interconnectedness

Increased interest in spirituality and health since the 1990s has generated many definitions and descriptions of spirituality within the healthcare literature, examples of which are found in **Box 7-1.** In many ways, however, trying to define spirituality is like trying to lasso the wind. The wind can be felt and its effect on things observed, but it cannot be contained within imposed boundaries, conceptual or otherwise. This elusive nature of spirituality requires opening up to multiple ways of knowing, including cognitive, intuitive, aesthetic, experiential, and deep inner sensing or knowing. Willis and Leone-Sheehan (2019) discussed *spiritual knowing* as an essential pattern of knowing in nursing. These authors posited that nurses engage in spiritual knowing when they recognize and address nonmaterial or spiritual qualities and experiences that relate to a greater reality, meaning, caring, humanization, and facilitation of healing and wholeness for self, others, and humanity.

Facets of spirituality found in broad descriptions of the concept include the essence of being, a unifying and animating force, the life principle of each person, a sense of meaning and purpose, transcendence, mystical, intangible, connectedness,

Box 7-1 Evolving Descriptions/Definitions of Spirituality in Nursing

The definition of *spirituality* in nursing literature continues to evolve as noted in these quotations.

- Spirituality is the essence of our being and unifying force which permeates our living in relationship with Self, Others, Nature and God or Higher Power, infuses our unfolding awareness of who and what we are, our purpose in being and our inner resources, and shapes our life journey (Burkhardt & Nagai-Jacobson, 2002, p. 21).
- Spirituality is an aspect of humanity that refers to the way individuals seek and express meaning and purpose, the way they experience their connectedness to the moment, to self, to others, to nature, and to the significant or sacred (Puchalski et al., 2009, p. 887).
- Spirituality is an innate feature of being human reflected in the human spirit, whereby human beings experience meaning and purpose, awareness of a greater reality, and connection with others, nature, and/or to the infinite/sacred/divine, Source, or a Supreme Being, which may or may not involve religion (Willis & Leone-Sheehan, 2019, p. 62).
- Spirituality is a dynamic and intrinsic aspect of humanity through which persons seek ultimate meaning, purpose, and transcendence, and experience relationship to self, family, others, community, society, nature, and the significant or sacred. Spirituality is expressed through beliefs, values, traditions and practices (Southard, 2020, p. 4).
- Spirituality is a personal construct . . . a mystical and self-transcendent experience that allows an individual to go beyond personal boundaries, create a broader worldview to find meaning and purpose in one's life's experiences, and often results in personal or spiritual transformation and growth (Lalani & Chen. 2021, p. 209).

Data from Burkhardt, M. A., & Nagai-Jacobson, M. G. (2002). *Spirituality: Living our connectedness. Delmar*; Puchalski, C., Ferrell, B., Virani, R., Otis-Green, S., Baird, P., Bull, J., Chochinov, H., Handzo, G., Nelson-Becker, H., Prince-Paul, M., Pugliese, K., & Sulmasy, D. (2009). Improving the quality of spiritual care as a dimension of palliative care: The report of the Consensus Conference. *Journal of Palliative Medicine, 12*(10), 885–904. https://doi.org/10.1089/jpm.2009.0142, Willis, D. & Leone-Sheehan, D. (2019). Spiritual knowing: Another pattern of knowing in the discipline. *Advances in Nursing Science, 42*(1), 58–68; Southard, M. E. (2020). Spirituality: The missing link for holistic health care. *Journal of Holistic Nursing, 38*(1), 4–7; Lalani, N., & Chen, A. (2021). Spirituality in nursing and health: A historical context, challenges, and way forward. *Holistic Nursing Practice, 35*(4), 206–210.

values, and awareness of and a commitment to something greater than the self (Blasdell, 2015; Burkhardt & Nagai-Jacobson, 2002; Healthcare Chaplaincy Network & Spiritual Care Association, 2017; Lalani & Chen, 2021; Smith-Trudeau, 2019; Southard, 2020; Victor & Treschuk, 2020; Yeşilçınar et al., 2018). Spirituality permeates life, shapes our life journey, and is vital to the process of discovering purpose, meaning, and inner strength. Although matters of spirit transcend culture, a person's cultural perspective influences personal expressions of spirituality. Personal values are rooted in and flow from spirituality and are reflected in a cultural perspective. Spirituality helps to ground one's sense of place and fit in the world. Being practical and relevant to daily life, spirituality is experienced in the mundane and secular as well as in the profound and sacred.

Research continues to demonstrate that people express and experience spirituality through relationships with the body/mind/spirit self, with others, with nature/cosmos, and with the Sacred Source/Mystery/Greater Reality (Blasdell, 2015; Healthcare Chaplaincy Network & Spiritual Care Association, 2017; Lalani & Chen, 2021; Michaelson et al., 2023; Stephenson & Hebeshy, 2017; Victor & Treschuk, 2020; Yeşilçınar et al., 2018). Attentiveness to these interconnections enables holistic nurses to integrate spirituality into a holistic plan of care.

Connectedness with Sacred Source/Sacred Mystery

The Sacred Source may be experienced as a person, a presence, or a mystery that is beyond words. The inadequacy of language is especially apparent when we try to discuss or describe that power that is greater than us, yet is within, among, and still beyond us. Humanity has always searched and sought to understand the mystery of the Sacred Source. Names such as Life Force, Source, God, Allah, Lord, Goddess, Absolute, Higher Power, Spirit, Vishnu, Inner Light, Tao, Great Mystery, Tunkasila, the Way, Universal Love, and the One with No Name refer to this Sacred Being or Presence. For this discussion, we refer to this Being/Presence or Sacred Mystery as *God* or the *Sacred Source*.

Connection with the Sacred Source is at the heart of one's being. Our rational minds cannot think or grasp God, and any descriptions or words used to refer to the Sacred Source are lacking. God is far more than anything the human mind can conceptualize. Words and descriptions are, however, tools of the rational mind that can point us toward God or the Sacred Source. Concepts of God may be personal or shared within a group. Persons find and name the Sacred Source in ways that are authentic to them, using terms and language that reflect their experiences and perspectives. Connecting with the Sacred Source may involve such things as prayer, ritual, reconciliation, and stillness. Receptive openness to Love, Light, Life, and the Sacred Source is a spiritual stance. Teachings of various religious traditions offer their own perspectives and guidance on how to be in relationship with the Sacred Source. Understanding how persons seek and experience connection with the Sacred Source and the obstacles they may encounter is important in spiritual caregiving.

The concepts of reverence and awe are often associated with experiences of the Sacred Source or something greater than oneself. Reverence arises from a deep appreciation of human limitations and a sense of awe in relation to what is beyond understanding and outside our control—God, truth, the natural world, and even death. Awareness that the sacred is intrinsic and omnipresent engenders reverence toward the Sacred Source and all of life (Berry & Tucker, 2009). Reverence acknowledges that we are in and of God; yet, as Woodruff (2001) noted, it also keeps human beings from trying to act like gods. "Awe is the feeling of being in the presence of something vast that transcends your current understanding of the world" and "is about our relation to the vast mysteries of life" (Keltner, 2023, pp. 7, 8). Relationship with the Sacred Source is one of many ways that people experience awe. Although some persons do not claim a religion or give a name to that which they hold most sacred, they may experience a sense of mystery, awe, and reverence in relation to that which is beyond their own understanding.

Connectedness with Nature/Cosmos

Spirituality is frequently expressed and experienced in and through a sense of connectedness with Nature, the environment, and the universe. Relationship with creatures of the Earth, both wild and domesticated, provides meaning and joy for people of all ages and cultures. Awareness of all beings of the Earth, and their belonging within the natural order, is a way of connecting with the spiritual in all of life (Vaughan-Lee, 2016). Ocean waves, red rock canyons, or bees among the flowers reflect the wonder of nature that may provide deeply spiritual experiences.

Awareness of a connectedness with the Earth and, indeed, the entire cosmos is particularly evident within Indigenous spiritual traditions. These traditions emphasize that all things are connected, that we are each a strand in the web of life. What we do to the web, we do to ourselves. Thus, what happens to the Earth and the environment affects us, and conversely, our choices and actions in all levels of our being affect the Earth. Understanding that spirit and matter are interconnected is basic to many traditions and known at some level in all spiritual traditions, particularly among the mystics.

Many people, particularly those who live close to the land, experience a sense of connection with the Sacred Source through Nature, regardless of their religious background. Paying close attention to the natural world and living in conscious relationship with the nonhuman beings of the world is a way of attuning more to one's own soul and spirit. People often express a feeling of closeness to their spiritual selves while walking on a beach; sitting by a favorite tree; viewing a sunset; listening to flowing water; tending plants/crops, animals, the land; and otherwise experiencing the natural order. Nature can be a source of strength, inspiration, awe, and comfort, all of which are attributes of spirituality. A sense of awe at the wonder of life and a feeling of connectedness with all things, with or without a belief in a divine being, is an experience of spirituality. Connection with Nature may flow from a sense of finding God in all things or experiencing a relationship with the Earth and all creatures at an energetic level. Appreciating, respecting, and caring for the Earth are spiritual practices that ground responses to environmental concerns (refer to **Chapter 24**).

Connectedness with Others

Spirituality is known and experienced in and through relationships with others. People express and experience spirituality through an appreciation of a common bond with all humanity and in their personal relationships with others, with the comfort, support, conflict, and strife that mark these connections. Cultural norms and traditions inform both how one understands and how one expresses connectedness. Formal and informal communities (including family) shape and nurture spiritual expression and development, providing a space to share spiritual journeys.

The formation, work, nurture, and healing of relationships are important parts of one's spirituality. Being with others in loving and supportive ways is an expression of spirituality, as is struggling with painful and difficult relationships with family, friends, and acquaintances. Relationships that need healing are as important to spiritual care as those that provide support and comfort. Spirituality embraces both the joys and sorrows of relationships and prompts reconciliation where connections have been frayed. Lack of connections often produces a dispiriting sense of isolation that may lead to spiritual crisis.

Spiritual connectedness with others involves both giving and receiving. Although it is common to think of spirituality in terms of giving, being able to receive from others, both the gift of who they are and the things they offer and share, is also an expression of spirituality. Indeed, the genuine shared presence between two people, with its implicit loving honesty and intimacy, is a manifestation of spirituality (Watson, 2018, 2024). Spirituality is evident in common experiences of daily living and in special times shared with others: times of joy, sorrow, ritual, loving sexuality, prayer, play, encouragement, anger, and reconciliation. Relationships as a source of growth and change are integral to spirituality.

Advances in technology have brought both individuals and distant countries and cultures together into a world community. As a result, understanding factors that create and support community has become essential. The ability to connect with people around the globe enables better understanding of how personal and collective decisions affect the larger human family. Social structures that provide a context for relationships with others often are instrumental in nurturing the spiritual dimensions of community life. Structures such as health care, educational institutions, faith-based services, social organizations, informal affiliations, social media, and various internet links are often spaces that mediate and support the spiritual dimensions of life.

Connectedness with Self

Spirituality infuses the ever-unfolding awareness of who one is—of self-becoming. The ability to be in the place of awareness that flows from spirit or soul is a pivotal element of connectedness with self. Awareness opens people to the experience of living in the moment, present to their own body-mind-spirit, and it allows them to receive all aspects of themselves without judgment. They experience awareness through Being—the art of stillness and presence with self, others, the Sacred Source, and Nature. Being is bringing one's whole self—alert and aware—to an experience, allowing one to pay attention to the quiet place inside and find inner peace, synchrony, harmony, and openness. Attentiveness to being allows a person to attune to sources of inner strength and deepest knowing.

Spirituality is manifested in and experienced through knowing, with its cognitive, intuitive, and energetic dimensions. Knowing provides ways of understanding our multidimensional nature and our relationships to the Sacred Source, self, others, Earth, and the cosmos. Knowing flows from a stance of openness and attuning to an inner source. It involves actively seeking knowledge and insights and maintaining an openness and receptivity to the lessons that life offers. Spirituality reflected in one's knowing includes appreciation of life as a gift and a sense of connectedness to all creation.

Doing, the outward and more visible aspect of spirituality, flows from being and knowing. Because doing is more tangible and measurable, it is the manifestation of spirituality that is most often addressed in healthcare literature. Generally, the concept of doing brings to mind activities such as attendance at religious services or ceremonies, scripture study, prayer or meditation, participation as student or teacher in religious education, and spiritual reading. Spirituality also can be demonstrated through actions such as assisting others, involvement in environmental concerns, attending to the sick, caring for family, spending time with friends, taking a walk, making time to nurture one's own spirit, and creating sacred space for self and others.

The concept of sacred space applies both to one's inner being and to places in one's environment. Although to create sacred space suggests doing something, inner sacred space is often the result of being aware and still. Buildings such as religious edifices or monuments represent sacred space for many. Special places in Nature are often experienced as sacred. Any place can become sacred space if one intentionally brings awareness of the spirit into the setting. Words, actions, sounds, scents, colors, and objects may shape such spaces. A sacred space is a home for the spirit, providing rest, stillness, nurture, and opportunities for opening to various connections. A sunlit space filled with special plants, a garden or workshop, a room for prayer or meditation, a corner of a porch with a rocking chair, a hospital bed with family surrounding a loved one—each touched by the intention of those who arrange it—are sacred spaces.

Facets of Spirituality: Expressions and Experiences

Life experiences such as mystery, love, suffering and compassion, hope and trust, forgiveness, peace and peacemaking, grace, joy, and prayer are inherent in the spiritual domain. They are not quantifiable and are more authentically expressed as questions, tentative definitions, or mysteries that cannot be fully explained. They often draw people to explore the deepest places in their beings and challenge them to experience life at its highest heights and deepest depths.

Mystery and Miracles

Discovering with others the personal and unique ways that mystery and experiences of miracles are encountered on their spiritual journeys is an important part of spiritual care. Mystery and miracle are "a complex enigma stretching beyond commonly held expectations and explanations" (Cowling, 2024, p. 228). Mystery is inherent to human experience and thus is inherent to spirituality. Mystery may be described as a truth that is beyond understanding and explanation. Miracles arise from the mystery of life and illuminate the hidden possibilities residing within each person (Cowling, 2024). Many life experiences prompt questions of why and what if. As people encounter that which may be troubling or unexplainable, appreciation of the mystery inherent in life events can sustain them in the unknowing and hold space for miracles both subtle and profound. Spirituality supports and encourages them in the questioning and seeking that often emerge when they are faced with mystery and experiences of miracles. The spiritual self helps them embrace both the darkness and the light, enabling them to appreciate the challenges and gifts of both.

Love

Loving presence is a key component of spiritual care. Love, which many recognize as the source of all life, fuels spirituality, prompting each person to live from the heart, the center where the ego is detached from outcomes. As the universal source of energy, love is a cosmic force and the highest level of consciousness (Watson, 2018, 2024). Like the spirit, love is nonlocal, transcending place and time, enabling its energy to be shared for healing at many levels. The relationship of love to healing is a continuing source of exploration and wonder (Costello, 2018; Watson, 2018, 2024). In its truest sense, love is a mystery that involves both choice and emotion. It infuses caring and compassion and often underlies acts of courage and compassion that defy explanation. Love is both personal and universal, and is experienced and expressed in both giving and receiving care. Flowing from and prompting interconnectedness, love includes dimensions of self-love, divine love, love for others, and love for all of life.

Suffering and Compassion

In both its presence and its meaning, suffering is one of the core issues and mysteries of life. It occurs on physical, mental, emotional, and spiritual levels. Suffering may be linked to a crisis of meaning (Eustache et al., 2014). Attempts to make sense of suffering have shaped cultural and religious traditions. Suffering may be a transformative experience—the nature of the transformation varying with each individual. For some, suffering enhances spiritual awareness; for others, suffering appears meaningless and engenders feelings of anger and frustration. Compassion, meaning *to suffer with*, is a response that calls us to recognize our kinship with another as we accompany them through their experience of suffering. Grounded in love, compassion is a component of spiritual care that requires nurses to tend to their own spirits as they address the spiritual needs of another. One interpretation of burnout among healthcare professionals is that it represents the inability to find ways to tend one's own spirit as one suffers the suffering of another. This was evident in the experiences of many nurses during the COVID-19 pandemic.

Sociocultural, religious, familial, and environmental factors influence an individual's response to suffering. Knowledge of personality, culture, religious traditions, and family background helps us to understand the nature and meaning of suffering for a particular person. Nurses who are aware of their own responses to and understanding of suffering are less likely to confuse their perceptions with those of the patient and are able to be more fully present in an intentional, healing way with those who are suffering. Such presence allows nurses to discern whether honoring another's suffering requires action, presence, absence, or a combination of these. The ability to be with another who is suffering is crucial, particularly when nurses confront suffering that cannot be alleviated and must be borne. Such presence supports a person's spiritual journey toward discovering transcendent meaning within the experience (Costello, 2018; Watson, 2018, 2024). Listening with one's whole being as another wonders aloud and expresses deep feelings regarding some of life's unanswered questions is a critical part of being with those who suffer.

Hope and Trust

Hope, a desire accompanied by an expectation of fulfillment, goes beyond believing or wishing. Hope is future-oriented yet grounded in the present moment. The saying "hope springs eternal" reflects this energy of the spirit and prompts the anticipation that tomorrow things will be better, or at least different. There are two levels of hope: specific and general. Specific hope implies a goal or desire for a particular event or outcome. A more general sense of hope holds that the future is somehow in safekeeping. Hope is a significant factor in overcoming illness and in living through difficult situations (Eustache et al., 2014; Stewart et al., 2016). It helps people deal with fear and uncertainty and to envision positive outcomes.

Spirituality can manifest as a sense of trust in life in general and that one has, or is given, the resources needed for dealing with whatever comes their way—expected or not. These resources include both strength and guidance from within and support from sources beyond themselves. Through encountering obstacles along their life path, learning through experiences, and developing new awareness, people gain appreciation for the ways that spirituality shapes and gives meaning to their unfolding life journey. Reaching this point may require reconciling new experiences with previously held values, resulting in new values and understandings. Often, the pattern of the journey and the meaning of life events become clear only in retrospect.

Forgiveness

Ultimately a matter of self-healing, forgiveness is a deep need and hunger of the human experience.

Religious beliefs, cultural traditions, family upbringing, and personal experience all help to shape an individual's attitudes about forgiveness, both given and received. Beliefs about the nature of God or the Sacred Source influence one's ability to offer and receive forgiveness. Difficulties with forgiving others, forgiving oneself, and accepting forgiveness from others often relate to a misunderstanding of the nature of forgiveness. Forgiveness is something one does for oneself, not for others. Forgiveness does not necessarily mean forgetting, condoning, absolving, or sacrificing; rather, it is a process of extending love and compassion to self and others (Biley & Giovannoni, 2018; Stewart et al., 2016; VanderWeele, 2018). An act of the heart, forgiveness is an internal process of releasing intense emotions attached to incidents from the past, releasing any need to carry grudges, resentments, hatred, self-pity, or desire to punish people who have done hurtful acts, and accepting that no punishment of others will promote internal healing. Principles of the Unitary Caring Science paradigm include the understanding that we live in and belong to a universe in which past, present, and future are contained in the ever-present NOW (Watson, 2018, 2024). Within the context of this paradigm, forgiveness is an act of compassion that, when extended to others, is also extended to self. Forgiveness, a sign of positive self-esteem, allows one to put the past in proper perspective. This frees energy once consumed by grudges and resentments and allows an individual to nurse unhealed wounds and use the freed energy for healing and moving on with life.

Self-forgiveness—releasing the desire or need to berate or punish oneself for past actions—is an important part of forgiveness and is essential for spiritual growth and healing (Biley & Giovannoni, 2018; Davis et al., 2015). Self-forgiveness is not about regret or guilt but rather concerns acknowledgment of responsibility for one's choices and actions. Self-forgiveness is an act of self-compassion that provides an opportunity to remove the energetic consequences from past actions and thoughts. Acknowledging personal responsibility for past thoughts and actions and being willing to let go of any energetic attachment to these thoughts and actions enables the cumulative energy of these actions to be released so that they will not adversely affect the self. The notion of free will—that the actual or energetic result of one's actions and thoughts cannot be bypassed by God or the universe—is basic to self-forgiveness.

The following analogy illustrates the self-forgiveness process: If you go for a walk and along the way get a sharp pebble in your shoe, every step from that point on is painful. The more you walk, the more it hurts. The pebble will cause pain and potential harm to the foot as long as it is in the shoe. Healing cannot take place as long as the pebble is irritating the foot; however, once the pebble is removed, the healing process can begin. Self-forgiveness, like taking the pebble out, enables the natural self-healing energy that is a part of the universe to begin and gives all of God's grace room to provide comfort.

Peace and Peacemaking

A sense of peace, often described as inner peace, is a spiritual attribute. Peace in this context implies a deep confidence and an ability to remain calm during the storm, to know somehow that all is well. Spiritual peace is experienced in the space of the heart and may not make sense to the cognitive mind. In the Judeo-Christian tradition, references to *a peace which passeth understanding* flow from an awareness of life beyond immediate circumstances and unbounded by the past. In the Zen tradition, practices of mindfulness foster connection with the peace that is available in every moment within every life experience. Peace is a product of living in relationship with the Sacred Source, others, and all creation in a way that acknowledges and nurtures the soul in the midst of all that life brings.

Peace, for many people, is inseparable from justice. Inner peace reflects a way of being, a space from which one can live and be in ways that nurture and heal. This peace does not depend on external circumstances; it flows from the connections that sustain us. Spiritual practices from many traditions sustain people and help them align with an inner peace amid trials and hardships. Today, as in the past, many people throughout the world are experiencing brutal trials. Living as peacemakers in times and places of uncertainty, fear, injustice, and war is a spiritual challenge facing all citizens of the world, and it demands courageous and creative solutions. The work of peacemaking is grounded in the following awareness:

> There is an inherent power in rightness, in goodness in love, and in love of peace, and that if even a single individual chooses to act rightly and truthfully and peacefully in the midst of tempting and contrary choices, the power of that act and aspiration can change the world. By extension, if untold numbers of single individuals love peace enough, seek peace enough, stand for peace enough, are themselves persons of peace, the ideal of peace will become the world's transforming reality. (Arnold et al., 2002, p. xv)

As persons appreciate and live in the reality of their connection with others and all creation across distance, time, and space, the possibility of peace with justice grows.

Grace

Experiences of grace contain elements of surprise, awe, mystery, and gratitude. Grace is often experienced as a support that is unplanned and unexpected. An experience of grace may touch one's spirit in deep and profound and life-changing ways. Grace opens one's awareness to the experience of wholeness, healing, and connectedness. Grace is reflected in statements such as:

- He just showed up at the door right when I needed him.
- I don't know why my spirits lifted that morning; perhaps it was the rain after such a long drought.
- I didn't think I could stand another bout of chemotherapy, but my friend said she will go with me and we'll take one day at a time.

Although some perceive such happenings as coincidence or chance, others sense something deeper that connects persons within the web of life and enables us to find acceptance, courage, peace, and endurance beyond our own making or understanding. Grace is often spoken of as a gift from the Sacred Source, or from Life itself, that enables, assists, and empowers a person in difficult and sometimes seemingly overwhelming circumstances. The experience of grace as a blessing that comes into one's life unearned calls forth a response of gratitude.

Joy

Joy is an expression of spirituality that flows from our deepest spiritual nature. Experienced alone or with others, joy brings one into the present moment where one encounters the sacred in self and others. Joy may show up as a serene inner sense, an exuberance that cannot be contained, an unexpected gift or blessing. Arnett (2023, p. 1) described joy as "the elation of right relationship," noting that it is a state in which there is a match between one's identity and one's experience. The many faces of joy include laughter, lightheartedness, play, and gratitude. Moments of joy can show up even in the midst of experiences such as suffering and sorrow. Experiences of joy may include senses of freedom and ease, harmony within self and with others and the world, vitality or aliveness, transcendence, the rightness of the moment, and connection with one's true self (Arnett, 2023; Johnson, 2019). Sources of joy include connecting with family, friends, and other groups, engaging in meaningful activities, connecting with nature, faith, spiritual practices, and religious support (Arnett, 2023; Goodwin et al., 2023).

Prayer

An expression of the spirit, prayer is a deep human instinct that flows from the core of one's being where the longing for and awareness of one's connectedness with the source of life are blended. Prayer represents a longing for communion or communication with God or the Sacred Source. It is a conscious relationship and conversation with God that involves both the mind and the heart (Martin, 2021). The most fundamental, primordial, and important language that humans speak, prayer is an endeavor that starts and ends without words. In this sense, prayer flows from yearnings of the soul rising from places too deep for words and moving to a space beyond words. Larry Dossey's classic work on the practice and effect of praying for healing reminds us of our nonlocal, unbounded nature, that prayer is infinite in space and time, and that we are not alone (Dossey, 1996).

That prayer is an appropriate consideration for nursing is grounded in the writings of Florence Nightingale (Dossey, 2000). Forms and expressions of prayer are as varied as the people who pray. Prayer is intrinsic to many religious traditions and rituals and may be public or private, individual or communal. It is not always a fully conscious activity. Speaking (sometimes silently), singing, chanting, listening, waiting, moaning, being attuned to what is going on in the present moment, and being silent can all be elements of prayer. Prayer includes petition, intercession, confession, lamentation, adoration, invocation, thanksgiving, being, and showing care and concern for others. Some people incorporate processes and techniques such as relaxation, quieting, breath awareness, focusing, imagery, and visualization into their prayer. Movement such as walking, dancing, or drumming may be expressions of prayer.

Spiritual and Psychological Dimensions

The term *psyche* means soul or spirit, reflecting the relationship between the spiritual and the psychological that is evident even in the spoken language. Before the time of Sigmund Freud, phenomena of the sentient realm that could not be explained physically often were considered matters of the spirit and viewed in religious terms. With the advent and ongoing development of psychology, matters of the soul often have been subsumed into psychological theory and frequently interpreted as pathology. Within a holistic paradigm, spiritual and psychological elements are interconnected because the body-mind-spirit is an integrated whole. Failing to differentiate the spiritual and psychological dimensions, however, can lead nurses to miss cues regarding spiritual concerns and thus inappropriately label spiritual issues as psychopathology. Consider, for example, a 90-year-old deeply spiritual man who was active and independent until sustaining a compression fracture of his lower spine. He exhibits obvious distress related to pain and his limited mobility. When he says he is praying for God to take him home, a holistic nurse recognizes the need to differentiate between spiritual concerns related to meaning, purpose, and suffering and psychological concerns such as depression or even suicide risk. Although spiritual awakening and deepening may be accompanied by elements of psychological distress, the "dark night of the soul" may be a significant aspect of the process of moving to greater awareness, spiritual deepening, and healing. Fortunately, many contemporary psychological models address the spiritual dimension.

Unlike Eastern and Indigenous traditions around the world, Western traditions have only a limited familiarity and comfort with the spiritual nature of different levels of awareness. The misinterpretation of behaviors, emotions, and reactions associated with individual experiences and expressions of the spiritual is keenly evident in the life of Florence Nightingale and the many interpretations of her life (Dossey, 2000, 2010). Some have interpreted the behaviors and health issues evident throughout her life after her return from Crimea as psychological pathology, such as anxiety, neurosis, malingering, depression, and stress burnout. Approaching Nightingale's life from a spiritual as well as psychological perspective enabled Dossey to recognize the spiritual nature of many of Nightingale's experiences and behaviors, including ways that Nightingale's spiritual journey reflected the phases of spiritual development of other mystics (Dossey, 2000, 2010). In a similar vein, appreciating the difference between spiritual and psychological domains enables nurses to assess spiritual cues and spiritual crises more effectively, as well as to recognize opportunities to foster spiritual growth.

Spirituality in Nursing Theories

Addressing the spiritual dimension of persons is a key component of major nursing theories (refer to **Chapter 5**). One example is the ongoing development and evolution of Jean Watson's transpersonal caring theory (Watson, 2018, 2024). Elements of spirituality and spiritual caregiving discussed throughout this chapter are evident in the core Caritas Processes of her caring theory summarized here:

- Sustaining humanistic-altruistic values by practicing loving-kindness with self and others.
- Being authentically present, fostering faith and hope, and valuing others.
- Nurturing sensitivity to self and others by evolving spiritual practices, transcending ego.
- Fostering and maintaining loving, trusting–caring relationships.
- Allowing for expression of positive and negative feelings—authentically listening to another person's story.
- Creatively problem-solving through the Caritas Process—full use of self and artistry of caring–healing practices via use of all ways of knowing, being, doing, and becoming.
- Engaging in transpersonal teaching and learning within the context of caring relationships.
- Creating a healing environment at all levels; subtle environment for energetic authentic caring presence.
- Reverentially assisting with basic needs as sacred acts, touching mind, body, and spirit of others; sustaining human dignity.
- Opening to spiritual, mystery, unknowns—allowing for miracles.

https://www.watsoncaringscience.org/jean-bio/caring-science-theory/

Spiritual Care in Holistic Nursing

Recalling that the words *healing*, *whole*, and *holy* derive from the same root: Old Saxon *hal* or *haelan*, meaning whole, we understand that healing is a spiritual process that attends to the wholeness of a person. Within a holistic perspective, providing spiritual care is an ethical obligation that, if ignored, deprives patients of their dignity as human beings. Nurses must become competent with spiritual caregiving by expanding their skills in attending to the spiritual domain. A persistent barrier to incorporating spirituality into clinical practice is the fear of imposing religious values and beliefs on others. Holistic nurses recognize that although each person is informed by personal spiritual perspectives, acting from this foundation is not the same as imposing these beliefs and values on another. Nurses who are grounded in an awareness of their own spiritual journeys are less likely to impose their values and beliefs on others. Because spirituality permeates every encounter, attentiveness to the spiritual dimension of each person, including the healer, is essential.

At the heart of caring for the spirit of self and others are *intention* (to be fully present, receptive and authentic), *attention* (alert and aware with all senses to verbal, nonverbal, environmental, and energetic cues), *loving/caring presence* (being in the moment with one's whole being), and *intentional listening* (with eyes, ears, heart, and undivided attention). Key ways of attending to Spirit with self and others are briefly included here, with references to practices and processes that nurture the spirit and are integral to spiritual caregiving found in other chapters in this book.

Nurturing the Spirit

Care of one's own spirit is a professional nursing responsibility and an intrinsic part of holistic nursing. The way that nurses care for and nurture themselves influences their ability to function effectively in a healing role with another. Appreciating oneself as a spiritual being and attentiveness to one's own spirit are key components of living in a healing way and recognizing that the spiritual path is a life path. They are also foundational to integrating spirituality into clinical practice. Care of the spirit or soul calls nurses to pause to reflect on and absorb what is happening within and around them; to take time for themselves, for relationships, and for things that animate them; and to be mindful about nourishing their spirits. The many ways that nurses nurture their spirits and respond to their spiritual concerns are the same as those that they suggest to their patients. Regular practices of prayer, centering, mindfulness, or meditation assist nurses in both maintaining and drawing from their own wholeness and ground their practice of intentional presence with each patient encounter (refer to **Chapters 10, 11, 13, 15, 16**).

Listening and Intentional Presence

Attentive listening and focused presence are at the heart of caring for the spirit (refer to **Chapter 5**). Exploring spiritual issues requires good therapeutic communication skills (refer to **Chapter 18**). Listening for language that connotes the spiritual, creating sacred space in which spirituality can be expressed, and maintaining clarity about one's own spiritual perspective enhance a nurse's facility with spiritual caregiving. The nurse's healing–caring presence is enhanced by the ability to focus on the relationship with a particular person in a particular moment (refer to **Chapter 18**). One of the gifts of intentional, active listening is that the patient, in sharing with an open-hearted and fully present listener, often hears themself with greater clarity and understanding. A hospice patient illustrated an experience of intentional listening and presence in describing their relationship with one of the hospice workers on their team:

> It feels good to see him come in. One day he and I both fell asleep, kind of took a nap for a bit. He probably knows as much about me as anyone—because he's the kind of guy who's interested in everything I talk about, my family, my worries, my sickness. Sometimes he asks a question, but mostly he just listens—but I mean really listens, like he wants to know about whatever is on my mind.

Considering personal experiences of listening and presence, nurses might ask themselves the following questions: When have I been intentionally present for another, listening with my whole being and with an open heart? Which factors, internal and external, help me to listen attentively or make listening difficult for me? When have I been in the presence of one who was fully present for me? How did I recognize that full presence? How did that affect me? According to Bruchac, "It all begins with listening. There are stories all around us, but many people don't notice those stories because they don't take the time to listen" (1997, p. 1). **Box 7-2** lists important considerations for nurses as they strive to listen in healing ways to their patients.

Box 7-2 Listening in Healing Ways

- Be intentionally present.
- Maintain focus on the patient as a whole person.
- Set aside the need to fix, answer, or correct.
- Interrupt as little as possible, recognizing that even what is not said has meaning and that the way and sequence in which a story is told are part of the story.
- View the other as embodied spirit, an ongoing and unfinished story.
- Hear the journey, the relationships, and the meanings in the story.
- Listen with all your senses.
- Do not prematurely diagnose.
- Let the conversation flow, being with silence as well as words.
- Breathe!

Story and Metaphor

Recognizing all persons, including themselves, as ongoing and unfolding stories offers nurses a valuable perspective from which to approach spiritual caregiving as an integral part of holistic nursing (Burkhardt & Nagai-Jacobson, 2002; Liehr & Smith, 2018). More broadly, such a perspective recognizes that each person's life story contains information about the meaning of their life. Story and metaphor often provide a language and form that conveys the richness of one's spirituality better than merely sharing facts about an experience. Stories bring people enjoyment, teach them to solve problems, help them form identities, and are wonderful teachers. Sharing stories helps people to understand themselves and their world, learning to know self and others from many perspectives. Stories reveal experiences of relationships, emotions, conflicts, struggles, and responses that are at once personal and universal. Nurses become part of the life stories of those for whom they care. Nurses' own life stories inform and form them, and understanding those stories deepens the awareness with which they hear another's story.

Stories make it possible to move beyond physical symptoms, diagnoses, and theoretical constructs, which may be similar for any number of patients. Attentiveness to story allows nurses another glimpse into the wholeness and uniqueness of each person and the way they fit into the family and community. Story and metaphor provide insight into spiritual concerns such as supportive and disruptive relationships, questions of meaning, values and purpose, issues of forgiveness, hope and hopelessness, and experiences of grace. Listening is a reminder that life stories are ongoing and unfinished.

In sharing with a fully present listener, patients hear their own stories with new insights and appreciation for their own lives—affirmations and validations, conflicts and struggles, questions of meaning and dark times—life in its variety and fullness. In a safe space, patients can express fears and perceived failures, hopes and wonderings, and disappointments and achievements as they consider pages of their life stories. Through this process, patients come to a deeper understanding of themselves in an atmosphere of acceptance, and acknowledge themselves in their full humanity. From such a stance, patients can participate more consciously in the present situation. The case of Mr. M. is an example of the power of the story:

> Mr. M. has been diagnosed with probable cancer of the lungs and is scheduled for exploratory surgery in a few days. Several times he has asked the nurse, "How serious do you think this is?" After he asks once again, the nurse says, "Mr. M., you seem to be asking me more than how serious this is. Can you tell me more about what is concerning you?" He responds, "Well, to be honest, I've been thinking about telling the kids . . . especially my son in Chicago. You see, we haven't been on very good terms."
>
> And so begins an important story for Mr. M. to tell and for the nurse to hear. The medical information about Mr. M.'s illness is but one piece of the greater fabric of his life as a family man and father. The nurse now hears Mr. M. talk about his concerns for his family and the relationships within the family as his upcoming surgery and uncertain future affect them. In telling his story, Mr. M. participates in both the assessment and intervention related to his spiritual care. The nurse learns about his relationships and his concerns surrounding them, and Mr. M. begins to understand what the most important aspects of his situation are from his unique perspective. With that understanding, he can begin to plan what he will do and what help he will seek. The nurse becomes a partner in his plan, which will be revised and updated as his story continues to unfold.

Sharing a story brings the listener face to face with quandaries, insights, struggles, joy, suffering, pain, and healing moments. Stories may make the listener feel helpless in the face of perceived hopeless situations or help the listener recognize the hope that lies in such a situation. Stories challenge nurses to understand the wholeness of a person and to listen for the meaning of a life. One nurse commented:

> I used to think that people who told me stories about their lives were just wasting my time and theirs, but now I realize that they are telling me about what is really important. I've learned to listen and to use what they say to help them see who they really are, what they

can really do. When they tell me things that are really hard to hear, or even to understand, it seems like they just want me to know that it is part of their life, too.

Stories allow the nursing process to fit the patient rather than requiring the patient to fit the process. Some shared inquiries that may help others express their stories include the following:

- If you were writing your life story, what would be the title?
- What is the title of the current chapter?
- Who are some of the heroines and heroes of your story?
- How would you like this chapter to turn out?
- Tell me more about how you handled your child's accident.
- I wonder where you get your spunk.
- I wonder what it is like to live with your physical limitations.
- You've mentioned several times that your sister is ill, and you seem worried.

Nurses can affirm the sharing of stories through statements such as, "Your sharing has helped me see this in a different light." As nurses encourage patients to share their stories, it is helpful to encourage the significant people in the patients' lives to participate in the process. The exercises presented in **Box 7-3** may increase attentiveness to story, both among nurses and with patients.

Box 7-3 Exercises to Facilitate Awareness of Story

1. Take a few moments to become quiet, perhaps using some breath awareness. In this quiet space, allow yourself to remember, in as much detail as possible, something about yourself, some event or incident that comes to mind. How has this experience or event become a part of who you are? What meaning does it have for your life at this moment?
2. Keep a journal in which you record events, feelings, experiences, insights, and questions in your life. Periodically review your writings, noting themes that flow through your story. Reflect on your story as it keeps evolving.
3. Think about books, stories, songs, fairy tales, movies, plays, or works of art that have special meaning for you. Take time to consider why and how they hold that meaning for you. Think about the images, characters, colors, and sounds that are found in each of these and how they are reflective of your own story. What meanings do you find that provide insight into your own unfolding journey?
4. Write an autobiography for your eyes only. Take your time. Reread and reflect on it. Are there parts you want to share? With whom would you share? What new awareness and insights into yourself and your life journey have come to you?
5. Look at some old family photos or photos of friends. What story do they tell? What memories and feelings come with these pictures? Do you want to tell someone else about them? What do you want to say? Would you like to hear someone else's story about these same photos?

Rest and Leisure

Rest and leisure are integral aspects of holistic living and care of the spirit that enhance growth, creativity, and renewal. Leisure is an attitude of the heart that facilitates connection with the inner self and the Sacred Source and opens one to reflect on and envision a life of doing to allow for more Being. Authentic leisure implies an approach to living that allows one to relax into a level of being that deepens self-awareness, nourishes one's wholeness, and enriches connections with the Sacred Source and other people. In an increasingly busy society—where filling each moment is viewed in terms of productivity, where even leisure time is scheduled—the notion of rest and leisure deserves thoughtful consideration. Taking stock of how one integrates rest and leisure into one's life is a spiritual practice and a necessary part of self-care for nurses. Assisting patients to consider the place of rest and leisure in their lives is part of spiritual caregiving.

Spiritual Caregiving: Questions, Cues, and Actions

Holistic nurses recognize that providing spiritual care is an on going, nonlinear process that is incorporated into every patient encounter and interaction. Spiritual caregiving does not require more time; rather, it requires the nurse to be authentically present in every encounter with patients, attentive to cues, listening with one's whole being, asking meaningful questions, and recognizing the sacred dimension of every nursing action (Southard, 2020; Watson, 2018, 2024). Appreciating the sacredness of every encounter, holistic nurses create sacred space that honors diversity in perspectives and beliefs and invites patients to reflect on the spiritual dimension of their life journeys. Within the context of routine care, nurses can encourage patients to more deeply explore what gives meaning to their lives; attend to important connections with the self, the Sacred Source, others, and nature; and reflect on, and perhaps give voice to, current spiritual needs and concerns.

Spirituality assessment guides may help nurses to begin to feel more confident with spiritual caregiving. When incorporated into a clinical setting, these guides can be a means of gaining a deeper understanding of a person from a holistic perspective. Rather than considering the completion of an instrument as an end point, the questions of an assessment guide can be openings or reference points for discussing spirituality with patients and thus come to know and understand them better as unique persons. Knowledge obtained about a person through any process of assessment is not an end in itself; rather, it is useful inasmuch as it adds to understanding and knowing more of the essence of the person. Many spirituality assessment scales have been developed for use in clinical and educational settings and in research. Some scales have been translated from English and evaluated for use in different cultural, religious, and ethnic groups, and some scales have been developed specifically for use in different groups. Examples of these scales are listed in **Table 7-1**. Readers are encouraged to review these and other assessment guides in the literature. Some scales focus more on religious beliefs and practices while others reflect a broader understanding of spirituality. Cultural sensitivity and cultural humility are essential to spirituality assessment in both practice and research. Factors to consider when utilizing spirituality assessment scales include whether the scale is holistic, whether the language related to spirituality is implicit or explicit, how the scale was developed, whether the scale is intended for research or clinical practice, characteristics (including ethnocultural, religious, and practice perspectives) of the population within which the scale was developed and is to be used, appreciation that many people do not express their spirituality within a religious tradition, and awareness of any bias within the scale toward particular traditions or beliefs that may suggest that those who do not ascribe to these traditions may not be spiritual.

Asking Meaningful Questions

As previously noted, a goal of holistic nursing is to know a person in the fullness and complexity of their wholeness. Appreciating the elusive nature of spiritual phenomena, nurses recognize that an individual's spiritual journey has many facets and meanings. Providing opportunities for a patient to explore their own spiritual terrain is essential to effective spiritual caregiving. This process can help patients recognize ways that their spiritual terrain is holding firm or may be shifting in relation to their current health issues, life challenges, and changes.

Incorporating open-ended reflective questions into interactions with patients assists them to become more aware of and attentive to spiritual needs, concerns, supports, and direction at the present time (refer to **Chapter 18**). Questions may focus on areas such as the role and influence of important connections in both present and past circumstances; issues related to meaning and purpose; important beliefs, values, and practices; prayer or meditation styles; and desire for connection with religious groups or rituals. Such prompts encourage patients to identify spiritual

Table 7-1 Examples of Spirituality Assessment Scales and Guides

Assessment Guides	Scales
T—Traditions **R**—Reconciliation **U**—Understandings **S**—Searching **T**—Teachers (Barss, 2012)	Spirituality Assessment Scale ■ Purpose and meaning in life ■ Innerness or inner resources ■ Unifying interconnectedness ■ Transcendence (Howden, 1992)
H—Source of hope, meaning, strength, love, connection **O**—Organized religion **P**—Personal spirituality practice **E**—Effects on health care (Anandarajah & Hight, 2001)	Spirituality Scale ■ Meaning and purpose ■ Relationships ■ Eco-awareness (Delaney, 2005)
F—Faith, spiritual beliefs **A**—Application (in daily life) **I**—Influence, importance in life and on healthcare decisions **T**—Talk (about spiritual issues) **H**—Help (support with spiritual concerns) (Neely & Minford, 2009)	FACIT-SP-Ex ■ Meaning, purpose, reason for living ■ Spiritual beliefs, faith, connection to higher power ■ Connection with others ■ Love, hope, forgiveness, gratitude ■ Inner harmony, peace ■ Appreciation of nature (Agil et al., 2017)
F—Faith, beliefs, meaning **I**—Importance and influence (in life and on health) **C**—Community (important people or groups) **A**—Address (how person would like spiritual issues to be addressed) (Puchalski et al., 2009)	Spiritual Care-Giving Scale ■ Attributes for spiritual care ■ Spiritual perspectives ■ Defining spiritual care ■ Spiritual care attitudes ■ Spiritual care values (Cruz et al., 2017; Tiew & Creedy, 2012)

Agil, O., Bailly, N., & Ferrand, C. (2017). Validation of the Functional Assessment of Chronic Illness Therapy—Spiritual Well-being (FACIT-sp12) on French old people. *Journal of Religion and Health*, *56*, 464–476. http://www.jstor.org/stable/44158327

Anandarajah, G., & Hight, E. (2001). Spirituality and medical practice: Using the HOPE questions as a practical tool for spiritual assessment. *American Family Physician*, *63*(1), 81–89.

Barss, K. S. (2012). T.R.U.S.T.: An affirming model for inclusive spiritual care. *Journal of Holistic Nursing: Official Journal of the American Holistic Nurses' Association*, *30*(1), 24–34. https://doi.org/10.1177/0898010111418118

Cruz, J. P., Alshammari, F., & Colet, P. C. (2017). Psychometric properties of the Spiritual Care-Giving Scale–Arabic version in Saudi nursing students. *Journal of Holistic Nursing*, *35*(2), 175–184. https://doi.org/10.1177/0898010116647804

Delaney, C. (2005). The Spirituality Scale: development and psychometric testing of a holistic instrument to assess the human spiritual dimension. *Journal of Holistic Nursing: Official Journal of the American Holistic Nurses' Association*, *23*(2), 145–167. https://doi.org/10.1177/0898010105276180

Howden, J. W. (1992). *Development and psychometric characteristics of the Spirituality Assessment Scale* (doctoral dissertation). Texas Woman's University, Denton.

Neely, D., & Minford, E. (2009). FAITH: spiritual history-taking made easy. *Clinical Teacher*, *6*(3), 181–185. https://doi.org/10.1111/j.1743-498X.2009.00317.x

Puchalski, C., Ferrell, B., Virani, R., Otis-Green, S., Baird, P., Bull, J., Chochinov, H., Handzo, G., Nelson-Becker, H., Prince-Paul, M., Pugliese, K., & Sulmasy, D. (2009). Improving the quality of spiritual care as a dimension of palliative care: The report of the Consensus Conference. *Journal of Palliative Medicine*, *12*(10), 885–904. <https://doi.org/10.1089 /jpm.2009.0142>

Tiew, L. H., & Creedy, D. K. (2012). Development and preliminary validation of a composite Spiritual Care-Giving Scale. *International Journal of Nursing Studies*, *49*(6), 682–690. https://doi.org/10.1016/j.ijnurstu.2011.11.014

Box 7-4 **Asking Meaningful Questions: Some Examples**

- Tell me about a time when you felt a sense of meaning or purpose in your life (or a time you felt really engaged with life). What would give your life more meaning at this time?
- What things are important in your life right now?
- What gives you hope? Can you describe a time you felt hopeful (or without hope)?
- What are some things you are grateful for?
- Tell me about times you have felt discouraged. What keeps you going in these times?
- What sustains you in difficult or challenging times?
- What do you feel are your inner strengths?
- Can you recall a time of special joy or happiness? Where do you find joy in life now?
- What is most sacred for you (consider objects, relationships, places, literature, etc.)?
- How do you connect with God/Sacred Source/Higher Power?
- Who or what do you look to for spiritual support?
- Are you part of a religious or spiritual tradition? Are there aspects of this tradition that are especially meaningful and supportive?
- Is prayer, meditation, or another practice important to you? What is prayer for you?
- Tell me about important persons in your life. Are pets among your significant relationships?
- Who do you rely on for support and to help you get through challenging times?
- Are there places in nature that nurture or enliven you?

strengths and supports, needs and concerns, processes or actions, and questions about life, meaning, suffering, forgiveness, regret, death, or reason for being in the world that can assist and support them on the spiritual journey. Intentional presence and attentive listening (including listening for story) noted previously are essential to this process. Responses, needs, and insights to a question may vary with each encounter. **Box 7-4** notes examples of areas to explore. As nurses become more at home with the concept of spirituality and its language, they will form their own questions and make their own observations in understanding another person as a whole being whose essence is spirit.

Fostering Connectedness

Relationships are a major aspect of spirituality (refer to **Chapters 5, 18, 20**). Awareness and an appreciation of important relationships in the patient's life enable the nurse to help strengthen meaningful and supportive bonds. Visits from pets may be as spiritually uplifting for some people as those from humans. Imagery, pictures, and stories can foster connection with important places, people, and experiences.

The patient's sense of connection with the environment may be an important source of comfort and strength. Being able to feel the wind, see the stars, smell the flowers, touch the trees, and simply experience the world may be significant aspects of healing. Considerations for bringing nature to patients include a window with a view of nature, spending some time outside perhaps in a healing garden, a photograph of a scene from nature or of a special place, a plant or flowers, and audio recordings of music or nature sounds. Spiritual uplifting can occur when visitors share the progress of the vegetable garden or the news of a recent fishing trip.

Supporting a person's relationship with the sacred includes attentiveness to the patient's unique and personal understandings and experiences of the sacred and the language used when talking about this aspect of spirituality. Nurses recognize that some people who are comfortable with the Judeo-Christian tradition of God or Lord or the Islamic Allah may find themselves less comfortable with understandings expressed as Higher Power, Tao, Universal Light, or Absolute. The reverse may also be true. For some people, *new age* is a relevant term that connotes spiritual growth and expansion; for others, however, anything new age is suspect and can be spiritually distressing. Listening beyond specific words to hear what is most sacred for this person and how their relationship with the sacred may be nurtured is important in addressing spiritual concerns. Are particular words of importance to this person? What is the place of formal religion and a person's own rabbi, priest, shaman, minister, imam, or spiritual leader in their spiritual journey? What is the role of music, prayer, sacred texts, books, particular objects, foods, or rituals in nurturing the spirit of this person?

Sensitivity to and appreciation of persons who profess atheism (i.e., disbelief in the existence of a supreme being) or agnosticism (i.e., doubt surrounding the existence of God or ultimate knowledge) involve moving beyond what is not believed. Instead, the nurse listens for that which gives meaning and purpose to the patient's life, including that which brings joy and satisfaction, the nature of hopes and fears, and the recognition of important relationships. How does this health crisis fit into the patient's understanding of their life, and how they are dealing with it? For example, an astronomer who noted that they were not religious and did not believe in God described their understanding and awe in regard to the evolution of the universe as a cause of deep wonder to themself that all that had gone before led to this particular time. This sense gave them a feeling that they belonged. The words voiced were not traditionally religious language, but their expressions of appreciation, awe, wonder, and meaning spoke of spirituality.

Nurses who attend to spiritual concerns are willing to be present with mystery, uncertainty, pain, or suffering. They seek not to fix this suffering or to answer uncertainty but to be in the mystery with the patient. Nurses demonstrate holistic care by letting the patient know that they are willing, with their whole being and intention, to stay the course through times of difficulty, pain, and mystery. Patients may feel support when nurses are willing to say, "I don't understand this either." This willingness on the part of the nurses may help family and friends to understand that, when they feel that there is nothing they can do, their presence and expressions of love and care are important and valuable components of their healing support.

Touching

Physical contact through touch in its myriad forms may foster connection and a sense of presence. Sensitivity to the meaning, comfort with, and appropriateness of touch for each person is essential in using touch therapeutically. When appropriate, a hand on the shoulder can provide support, a handclasp can convey understanding and presence, an arm around the waist can literally and figuratively give a lift. One patient described a nurse's support in saying, "When the doctor came in to give me the news, she was standing beside me and I could feel her hand on my arm the whole time the doctor was talking. I was so glad that she was just there with me." At times when words cannot be found, or in circumstances where persons are more comfortable with physical expression than with words, touch is a powerful expression of spirit and an instrument of healing.

Praying and Meditating

Holistic nurses clarify the patient's understanding of and need for prayer by asking if they would like to pray, to whom they wish to pray, and how they pray. Some patients want others to pray with or for them, while others do not believe in prayer. The nurse can facilitate the patient's desire for shared prayer, for participation in religious worship, or for quiet, uninterrupted periods of time for personal spiritual practices. Sacred or inspirational readings, music, drumming, movement, light or darkness, aromas, and time of day are among the many factors that may be important considerations in one's prayer life. The process of listening and appreciating the prayer life of another nurtures the spirit and acknowledges the spiritual dimension of that person.

Implications

Spirituality infuses every aspect of life, is the cornerstone of holistic nursing, health, and healing, and grounds holistic nursing practice, education, and research.

- Holistic nurses recognize that spiritual caregiving honors a person's wholeness, is essential to promoting health and well-being of patients, and is an essential aspect of self-care and all holistic nursing care.
- Both didactic and experiential processes that assist students in learning how to integrate spirituality into self-care and incorporate spiritual caregiving into holistic nursing care need to be integral components of nursing education.
- Research is needed to deepen the understanding of spirituality within diverse ethnocultural, religious and spiritual traditions and further explore the influence of spirituality in health and illness across cultures, spiritual traditions, and age groups.
- Holistic nurses need to advocate for the inclusion of spiritual caregiving as a priority in all aspects of patient care, including nursing self-care.

Conclusion

Because all persons, nurses as well as patients, are spiritual beings, care of the spirit is integral to holistic nursing care. Care of the spirit requires the evolution of language to express this dimension of ourselves better and an approach to the nursing process that is integrative rather than linear. Spiritual caregiving requires an understanding of the integrative holistic caring process in which assessment and intervention may well be the same process, and where description is more useful than labeling. Identification of needs in the area of spirituality does not necessarily indicate pathology or impairment; rather, it provides a way of understanding a person in their wholeness and a glimpse into what provides meaning. Nurses facilitate this process when they promote an atmosphere that is accepting and encouraging of spiritual expression in its many and varied forms. Research on spirituality and health continues to highlight the importance of describing the human spirit in the language of each person's unique experience and expression and exploring individual meaning within the context of the person's life story. Spiritual caregiving requires intention, attention, intentional listening, presence, and a willingness to hear another's story. Nurses offer spiritual support as they are able to be present with mystery and the life questions of others, understanding that people express and experience their spirituality in and through relationships with the Sacred Source, others, Nature, and themselves. Tending to matters of the spirit may include incorporating ritual, prayer, meditation, rest, art, and any activity that enhances awareness of oneself and one's place in the world.

References

Agil, O., Bailly, N., & Ferrand, C. (2017). Validation of the Functional Assessment of Chronic Illness Therapy—Spiritual Well-being (FACIT-sp12) on French old people. *Journal of Religion and Health*, *56*, 464–476. http://www.jstor.org/stable/44158327

Anandarajah, G., & Hight, E. (2001). Spirituality and medical practice: Using the HOPE questions as a practical tool for spiritual assessment. *American Family Physician*, *63*(1), 81–89.

Arnett, J. J. (2023). Joy: An integrative theory. *Journal of Positive Psychology*, *18*(1), 1–14. https://doi.org/10.1080/17439760.2022.2053878

Arnold, M., Ballif-Spanvill, B., & Tracy, K. (Eds). (2002). *A chorus for peace—A global anthology of poetry by women*. University of Iowa Press.

Barss, K. S. (2012). T.R.U.S.T.: An affirming model for inclusive spiritual care. *Journal of Holistic Nursing : Official Journal of the American Holistic Nurses' Association*, *30*(1), 24–34. https://doi.org/10.1177/0898010111418118

Berry, T., & Tucker, M. E. (2009). *The sacred universe: Earth, spirituality, and religion in the twenty-first century*. Columbia University Press.

Biley, A. M., & Giovannoni, J. (2018). Pondering forgiveness in a unitary science paradigm: A reflection. *International Journal for Human Caring*, *22*(3), 140–146.

Blasdell, N. D. (2015). The evolution of spirituality in the nursing literature. *International Journal of Caring Science*, *8*(3), 756–764.

Bruchac, J. (1997). *Tell me a tale*. Harcourt, Brace.

Burkhardt, M. A., & Nagai-Jacobson, M. G. (2002). *Spirituality: Living our connectedness*. Delmar.

Costello, M. (2018). Watson's Caritas Processes® as a framework for spiritual end of life care for oncology patients. *International Journal of Caring Sciences, 11*(2), 639–644.

Cowling, W. R. (2024). Mystery and miracle: A preliminary unitary appreciative study. *Advances in Nursing Science, 47*(2), 218–230. https://doi.org/10.1097/ANS.0000000000000531

Cruz, J. P., Alshammari, F., & Colet, P. C. (2017). Psychometric properties of the Spiritual Care-Giving Scale–Arabic version in Saudi nursing students. *Journal of Holistic Nursing, 35*(2), 175–184. https://doi.org/10.1177/0898010116647804

Davis, D. E., Ho, M. Y., Griffin, B. J., Bell, C., Hook, J. N., Van Tongeren, D. R., DeBlaere, C., Worthington, E. L., Jr., & Westbrook, C. J. (2015). Forgiving the self and physical and mental health correlates: A meta-analytic review. *Journal of Counseling Psychology, 62*(2), 329–335. https://doi.org/10.1037/cou0000063

Delaney, C. (2005). The Spirituality Scale: development and psychometric testing of a holistic instrument to assess the human spiritual dimension. *Journal of Holistic Nursing: Official Journal of the American Holistic Nurses' Association, 23*(2), 145–167. https://doi.org/10.1177/0898010105276180

Dossey, B. M. (2000). *Florence Nightingale: Mystic, visionary, healer*. Springhouse.

Dossey, B. M. (2010). Florence Nightingale: A 19th-century mystic. *Journal of Holistic Nursing, 28*(1), 10–35.

Dossey, L. (1996). *Prayer is good medicine*. Harper.

Engebretson, J. C. (2016). Cultural diversity and care. In B. M. Dossey & L. Keegan (Eds.), *Holistic nursing: A handbook for practice* (7th ed., pp. 439–463). Jones & Bartlett Learning.

Eustache, C., Jibb, E., & Grossman, M. (2014). Exploring hope and healing in patients living with advances non-small cell lung cancer. *Oncology Nursing Forum, 41*(5), 497–508.

Goodwin, V. A., Hall, A. J., Bethel, A., Taylor, E., Tatnell, L., Turner, M., & Frost, J. (2023). Understanding joy amongst older people: A scoping review. *Archives of Gerontology and Geriatrics, 115*, 105118 https://doi.org/10.1016/j.archger.2023.105118

Healthcare Chaplaincy Network & Spiritual Care Association (2017). *Spiritual care and nursing: A nurse's contribution and practice*. https://www.healthcarechaplaincy.org/docs/about/nurses_spiritual_care_white_paper_3_3_2017.pdf

Howden, J. W. (1992). *Development and psychometric characteristics of the Spirituality Assessment Scale* (doctoral dissertation). Texas Woman's University, Denton.

Johnson, M. K. (2019). Joy: A review of the literature and suggestions for future directions. *The Journal of Positive Psychology, 15*(1), 5–24. https://doi.org/10.1080/17439760.2019.1685581

Keltner, D. (2023). *Awe: The new science of everyday wonder and how it can transform your life*. Penguin Books.

Lalani, N., & Chen, A. (2021). Spirituality in nursing and health: A historical context, challenges, and way forward. *Holistic Nursing Practice, 35*(4), 206–210.

Liehr, M. P. R., & Smith, M. J. (2018). Story theory. In M. J. Smith & P. R. Liehr (Eds.), *Middle range theory for nursing* (4th ed., pp. 241–264.). Springer.

Martin, J. (2021). *Learning to pray: A guide for everyone*. HarperOne.

Michaelson, V., Smigelskas, K., King, N., Inchley, Malinowska-Cieslik, M., & Picketts, W. (2023). Domains of spirituality and their importance to the health of 75 533 adolescents in 12 countries. *Health Promotion International, 38*, 1–11. https://doi.org/10.1093/heapro/daab185

Murgia, C., Notarnicola, I., Caruso, R., De Maria, M., Rocco, G., & Stievano, A. (2022). Spirituality and religious diversity in nursing: A scoping review. *Healthcare, 10*(9), 1661. https://doi.org/10.3390/healthcare10091661

Neely, D., & Minford, E. (2009). FAITH: spiritual history-taking made easy. *Clinical Teacher, 6*(3), 181–185. https://doi.org/10.1111/j.1743-498X.2009.00317.x

Puchalski, C., Ferrell, B., Virani, R., Otis-Green, S., Baird, P., Bull, J., Chochinov, H., Handzo, G., Nelson-Becker, H., Prince-Paul, M., Pugliese, K., & Sulmasy, D. (2009). Improving the quality of spiritual care as a dimension of palliative care: The report of the Consensus Conference. *Journal of Palliative Medicine, 12*(10), 885–904. https://doi.org/10.1089/jpm.2009.0142

Smith-Trudeau, P. (2019). Spirituality: A very misunderstood work. *Vermont Nurse Connection, 22*(2), 2–3.

Southard, M. E. (2020). Spirituality: The missing link for holistic health care. *Journal of Holistic Nursing, 38*(1), 4–7.

Stephenson, P., & Hebeshy, M. (2017). The delivery of end-of-life spiritual care to Muslims by non-Muslim providers. *Medsurg Nursing, 27*(5), 281–285.

Stewart, W. C., Reynolds, K. E., Jones, L. J., Stewart, J. A., & Nelson, L. A. (2016). The source and impact of specific parameters that enhance well-being in daily life. *Journal of Religion and Health, 55*(4), 1326–1335. https://doi.org/10.1007/s10943-015-0076-8

Tiew, L. H., & Creedy, D. K. (2012). Development and preliminary validation of a composite Spiritual Care-Giving Scale. *International Journal of Nursing Studies, 49*(6), 682–690. https://doi.org/10.1016/j.ijnurstu.2011.11.014

Tzu, L. *Tao Te Ching*. Goodreads. https://www.goodreads.com/quotes/search?utf8=%E2%9C%93&q=lao+tzu+and+spokes&commit=Search

VanderWeele, T. J. (2018). Is forgiveness a public health issue? *American Journal of Public Health, 108*(2), 189–190.

Vaughan-Lee, L. (Ed.). (2016). *Spiritual ecology: The cry of the earth* (2nd ed.). The Golden Sufi Center.

Victor, C. G. P & Treschuk, J. (2020). Critical literature review on the concept of faith, religion, and spirituality. *Journal of Holistic Nursing, 38*(1), 107–113.

Watson, J. (2018). *Unitary caring science: Philosophy and praxis of nursing*. University of Colorado Press.

Watson, J. (2024). *Metaphysics of Watson's unitary caring science: A cosmology of love*. Springer Publishing.

Willis, D. & Leone-Sheehan, D. (2019). Spiritual knowing: Another pattern of knowing in the discipline. *Advances in Nursing Science, 42*(1), 58–68.

Woodruff, P. (2001). *Reverence: Renewing a forgotten virtue.* Oxford University Press.

Yeşilçınar, İ., Acavut, G., İyigün, E., & Taştan, S. (2018). Eight-step concept analysis: Spirituality in nursing. *International Journal for Human Caring, 22*(2), 34–42. https://doi.org/10.20467/1091-5710.22.2.34

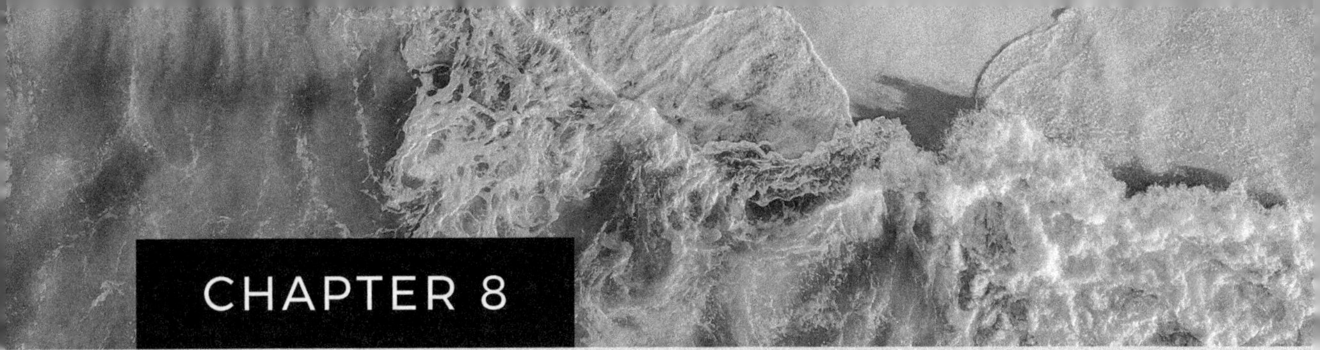

CHAPTER 8

Nursing Theory in Holistic Nursing Practice

Diane L. Gullett, Charlotte D. Barry, and Shirley C. Gordon

NURSE HEALER OBJECTIVES

- Understand nursing as a discipline of knowledge and professional practice.
- Describe the role of theory in guiding holistic nursing practice.
- Define common terms associated with theory.
- Select a nursing theory or theories that provide a framework and philosophy consistent with your nursing values.
- Apply nursing theory to guide your holistic nursing practice.

DEFINITIONS

Concept: A description and name of an abstract idea or phenomenon that gives it meaning.

Conceptual model: A construction of the relationship of concepts. Abstract set of concepts and propositions that are integrated into a meaningful configuration and represent an involvement in theoretical formulations by describing nursing phenomena and their interrelationships in abstract terms (Smith, 2020).

Discipline: A field of study, grounded in higher education, that delineates unique phenomena of concern, the context in which they are viewed, relevant questions, and method of inquiry (Fawcett, 1984).

Framework: A group of related ideas that promotes the understanding of theory and can guide research within the theory.

Nursing theory: Interrelated concepts that give meaning to experiences and practice, help organize thinking and guide the discovery of new knowledge through research (Fawcett, 1984). Theories are not discovered but are created from practice.

Paradigm: The concept of a paradigm as a global framework or worldview made of assumptions held by members of a discipline that illuminates its focus and boundaries and guides the development of knowledge (Kuhn, 1970). A paradigm is not static but reflects unfolding ideas and knowledge.

Nursing Theory Introduction: Nursing as a Discipline and Profession

The study of theory in nursing is grounded in the belief that nursing is both a discipline of knowledge and professional practice. Boykin and Schoenhofer describe this beautifully. They write, "the discipline of nursing and profession of nursing are inextricably bound and exquisitely woven aspects of the single unity of nursing. Each aspect illuminates particular duties, privileges and practices relevant to nursing as an entity" (Boykin & Schoenhofer, 2001, p. 6).

The classic work of Donaldson and Crowley (1978) outlines eight attributes of a discipline and helps to illustrate nursing as a discipline of knowledge grounded in theory. The attributes are as follows:

1. **An expression of human imagination**: This is exemplified in the unique interactions nurses create to describe, explain, and respond to unique calls for humanization and betterment of those for whom we care.
2. **A domain**: A domain is the central focus and boundaries of the discipline. Donald and Crowley identify three, each one focused on concern for the well-being and optimal functioning of human beings in sickness or health. Other scholars identify the central domain as caring, caring in the human health environment, health and wholeness, the nurse–patient relationship, facilitating humanization, and quality of life. Although there are numerous ideas about the domain of nursing, each one describes the intention of creating nursing interactions that nurture the well-being, more being, healing, or peaceful death of those cared for.
3. **Syntactic or conceptual structures**: The syntactical structures and concepts are explained in nursing theories, which are used to guide the development and use of knowledge in research and practice.
4. **Specialized language and symbols**: The language of nursing expresses the sacredness of those we care for and provides a means of communication among the members of the discipline.
5. **Heritage of literature and networks of communication**: The members of the discipline have created a myriad of theories to guide practice as well as books, journals, conferences, presentations, videos, and other forms of traditional and social media. Each of these modes of knowing communicates the emphasis on understanding the nature of the discipline.
6. **Tradition**: The tradition of the discipline in caring for others has had historical and sustained recognition through the theoretical underpinnings of the works of Florence Nightingale, Clara Barton, Mary Seacole, Mary Eliza Mahoney, Lillian Wald, Margaret Sanger, and so many others who have transformed nursing care for the betterment of humankind.
7. **Values and beliefs**: The deeply held values and beliefs of nursing are foundational to nursing theories. Theories are grounded in values, and each describes a unique response to a phenomenon of care and concern for persons, understood as cultural beings, nursed.
8. **Systems of education**: A hallmark of a discipline is the educational preparation of its members. Nursing education programs abound at colleges and universities and provide gateways to understand the substantive theoretical knowledge of the discipline and professional practice of nursing.

The knowledge based in the discipline is related to its general domain or focus. A discipline offers a unique perspective–a specific and distinct way of viewing phenomena–and through networks of philosophies, theories, concepts, cultures, approaches to inquiry, research findings, and practices, discovers ways to illuminate this distinct perspective (Smith & Parker, 2015). Development of nursing knowledge is a result of theory-based nursing inquiry (Smith & Parker, 2015).

Role of Theory in Knowledge Development

Theories are part of the knowledge structure of any discipline, while the metaparadigm or the domain of inquiry/focus of the discipline is the foundation of this knowledge structure. Fawcett (1984) described nursing's metaparadigm as the interrelationship between the four concepts of nursing, persons, environment, and health, and what distinguished nursing from other disciplines. Historically, many other nursing scholars have suggested modifications and alternative concepts to nursing's metaparadigm; for example, suggesting the focus of the discipline as the life process of unitary human beings (Rogers, 1970), caring (Boykin & Schoenhofer, 2001, pp. 8–10), caring in the human health experience (Newman et al., 1991), human-universe-health interrelationships

(Parse, 1998), and healing (Dossey, 2008). In 2024, Fawcett expanded the nursing's metaparadigm to include culture (Fawcett, 2024). The inclusion of culture highlights its importance in understanding and respecting the knowledge of nursing within and across global communities.

Smith (2019) conducted a historical analysis of the literature on the focus of the discipline with the purpose of regenerating the disciplinary perspective of nursing. Her analysis identified human wholeness; health, healing, and well-being; the human-environment-health relationship; and caring as the major themes most reflective of nursing's disciplinary perspective. Additionally, Smith (2019, pp. 12–13) suggested that developing knowledge of the discipline should include inquiry into the following nine areas: (1) promoting health, well-being, and quality of living and dying; (2) stress, coping, and adaptation throughout the life process; (3) transitions in the life process; (4) cultural care; (5) human-environment energy field patterning; (6) consciousness and health; (7) health-related lived experiences; (8) caring relationships, processes, and practices; and (9) environments that facilitate health, healing, and well-being.

Theories serve as the lenses that color and shape how the phenomena of interest to the discipline of nursing are understood. In essence, nursing theories are patterns that guide thinking about nursing and serve to guide knowledge development in nursing. Theories have both empirical and abstract dimensions and are used as tools for conceptualizing and studying practice problems, proposing explanations and interventions, and testing and refining ideas (Reed & Crawford Shearer, 2018). Theories link the everyday world of practice and the philosophical perspectives of reality (Reed & Crawford Shearer, 2018). There are various definitions of *theory*; however, each definition recognizes theory as an organizing framework of concepts and their relationships to one another providing descriptions, explanations, and predictions about phenomena (Smith, 1994, p. 7). Theories are composed of concepts connected to the phenomenon of concern for a discipline and are classified as *descriptive* (focused on observing a phenomenon and identifying its elements or events) or *exploratory* (focused on cause-and-effect relationships, correlations, or interactions among a theory's component parts).

Nursing theories are used to guide education, research, and practice. Nursing theories vary in scope or level of abstraction. They range from grand theories as the most abstract and broad, followed by middle-range theories, which are narrower in scope and appropriate for empirical testing, and practice-level theories representing the lowest level of abstraction and developed for use within a specific range of nursing situations. Often there is no distinction made between conceptual models and grand theory as they both focus on the metaparadigm of nursing. However, Fawcett (1984) differentiates a conceptual model as one that addresses her definition of nursing's metaparadigm (persons, health, environment, and nursing), while grand theories address alternative concepts of the metaparadigm—for instance, caring. Ideally, middle-range theories are interrelated with concepts and/or frameworks from grand theories while practice level theories are interrelated with concepts from middle-range theories or from the framework of grand theories (Fawcett, 1984).

Holistic Nursing

Background

Historically, nursing has been understood as a holistic practice. Nightingale is credited with being the mother of modern nursing, and her emphasis on care focused on unity, wellness, and the interrelationship of human beings, events, and the environment embodies holism as recognized by holistic nursing practice. Her beginning conceptualizations about health, caring, nursing, person, and environment, originating in observation and scientific discovery, served as the foundation for further theoretical development in nursing as a holistic practice and professional discipline. Since 2000, holistic nursing has emerged as a specialty in professional nursing practice and was officially recognized by the American Nurses Association (ANA) in 2006 (American Holistic Nurses Association & American Nurses Association, 2019).

Theory Guiding Holistic Nursing Practice

Holistic nursing is a science and an art, with a body of knowledge grounded in a philosophical and theoretical framework that assists nurses in remembering the heart of their nursing practice (Andrus, 2000). The core of holistic nursing practice is the quality of the relationship between the nurse and person(s) being nursed; a way of entering and being in relationship. The art of practicing nursing is to apply the philosophy and theory of professional caring relationships consciously and creatively in day-to-day practice.

Holistic nursing characteristics as outlined in *Holistic Nursing: Scope and Standards of Practice* (American Holistic Nurses Association & American Nurses Association, 2019) encompass all nursing practice whose goal is healing of the whole person. A holistic nurse recognizes the interconnectedness of self, others, nature, and spirituality, as well as the integration and healing of a person's body-mind-emotion-spirit-energy-environment principles, modalities, and connections, as a unified whole human being in which the whole is greater than the sum of its parts. The standards establish the criteria for the practice while the core values provide the philosophical context necessary to guide practice.

The art and science of holistic nursing emanates from the five core values, representing the essence of holistic nursing (American Holistic Nurses Association & American Nurses Association, 2019). Each core value is necessary for holistic practice; therefore, recognizing which theories are congruent with these values provides a guide for choosing a theory whose concepts, relationships, and philosophies are situated within holistic nursing practice. Additionally, choosing a theory consistent with holistic nursing requires recognition of how said theory aligns with the ontology of one's own practice as a holistic nurse. It is the responsibility and expectation that all holistic nurses be informed by theory to ensure knowledgeable theory-guided practice.

Table 8-1 provides an overview of the core values and implications for choosing a

Table 8-1 Linking Holistic Core Values to Nursing Theory

Core Value (CV) (American Holistic Nurses Association & American Nurses Association, 2019; Andrus, 2000)	Definition/Descriptions (American Holistic Nurses Association & American Nurses Association, 2019; Andrus, 2000)	Implications for Practice (American Holistic Nurses Association & American Nurses Association, 2019; Andrus, 2000)
CV 1: Holistic philosophy, theories, and ethics	Philosophical, theoretical, and ethical foundations define the *who* and *why* of holistic nursing. Holistic nurses embrace a professional ethic of caring and healing that seeks to preserve the wholeness and dignity of self and others. Holistic practice uses presence, intentionality, compassion, and authenticity throughout the holistic nursing process.	Holistic nursing is grounded in nursing knowledge and skill and guided by nursing theory. Holistic nurses utilize theories and perspectives of wholeness and healing to guide their practice. Theories grounded in unity such as integral theory (Dossey), science of unitary human beings (Rogers), as well as caring (Watson) align with holistic nursing practice.
CV 2: Holistic nurse self-reflection, self-development, and self-care	The nurse's self-reflection, self-assessment, self-care, healing, and personal development are essential to serve others as well as to facilitate growth in personal well-being (American Holistic Nurses Association & American Nurses Association, 2019, p. 25).	Phenomena of interest to holistic theory include self-care strategies, self-awareness, self-reflection, self-development, self-healing, empowerment, resiliency, creating healthy environments, holistic nourishment, and growth.

Core Value (CV) (American Holistic Nurses Association & American Nurses Association, 2019; Andrus, 2000)	Definition/Descriptions (American Holistic Nurses Association & American Nurses Association, 2019; Andrus, 2000)	Implications for Practice (American Holistic Nurses Association & American Nurses Association, 2019; Andrus, 2000)
	Self-reflection is a turning inward to examine one's own beliefs and thoughts which enhances self-awareness and facilitates reflective practice (American Holistic Nurses Association & American Nurses Association, 2019, p. 15). Self-development involves valuing self and holistic nursing as a life purpose through mobilization of resources essential for self-care. Self-care includes self-assessment, personal development, and conscious empowerment. Self-reflection is both a self-care strategy and a professional practice integrating critical thinking of the mind and compassion of the heart (American Holistic Nurses Association & American Nurses Association, 2019, p. 25).	Holistic theory demonstrates a commitment to practice holistic self-care strategies to manage stress and enhance well-being
CV 3: Holistic caring process	The holistic caring process identifies *what* holistic nurses do—i.e., the practice of holistic nursing. Holistic nurses provide care that recognizes the totality of the human being (the interconnectedness of body, mind, emotion, spirit, social/cultural relationships, context, environment, and energy). Holistic nurses integrate complementary and integrative approaches into conventional health care. Holistic health is a multidimensional state of well-being as perceived by the individual. Holistic health elicits the patient's story to reveal the context and complexity of the human health experience.	Theories utilized must be congruent with holism as recognized by the holistic nurse. Holistic nursing responds to the following two views of holism, believing that the goals of nursing can be achieved within either framework. Holism involves identifying the interrelationships of a person's bio-psycho-social-spiritual dimensions, recognizing that the whole is greater than the sum of its parts. Holism involves understanding the individual as a unitary whole in mutual process with the environment. Theory development surrounding concepts of healing, wholeness, caring, intentionality, well-being, compassion, social and cultural constructions, empowerment, healing relationships and environments is consistent with holistic nursing (American Holistic Nurses Association & American Nurses Association, 2019, p. 20).

(continues)

Table 8-1 Linking Holistic Core Values to Nursing Theory *(continued)*

Core Value (CV) (American Holistic Nurses Association & American Nurses Association, 2019; Andrus, 2000)	Definition/Descriptions (American Holistic Nurses Association & American Nurses Association, 2019; Andrus, 2000)	Implications for Practice (American Holistic Nurses Association & American Nurses Association, 2019; Andrus, 2000)
		Holistic nurses use theories and philosophies grounded in holism to help integrate one's knowing, doing, and being in practice.
CV 4: Holistic communication, therapeutic relationship, healing environment and cultural care	Through holistic communication, therapeutic relationships, healing environments, and cultural care, holistic nurses transform their beliefs into practice, highlighting the *how* of holistic nursing (American Holistic Nurses Association & American Nurses Association, 2019, p. 34). Holistic nurses create therapeutic relationships using holistic communication, which finds expression within the context of optimal healing environments. Inherent to creating healing environments is the holistic nurse's ability to promote cultural care responsive to beliefs, traditions, and healthcare practices of all persons. Holistic nurses provide culturally competent care. Holistic nurses integrate authentic presence, active listening, being in the moment shared humanness, and interpersonal encounter to create unique health encounters.	The patient is valued as a person, and the holistic nurse assists individuals to find meaning in their experience (American Holistic Nurses Association & American Nurses Association, 2019, p. 16). The holistic nurse chooses theories grounded in cultural diversity that are culturally and ethnically sensitive, such as Madeleine Leininger's (1987) theory of culture care diversity and universality. Theories and philosophies centered around healing environments, therapeutic use of self, reflective practice, energy, and consciousness in which healing is the outcome are consistent with holistic nursing. Recognition of suffering, illness, and disease are natural components of the human condition and have the potential to teach about oneself, one's relationship, and the universe.
CV 5: Holistic education and research	Holistic nursing is further realized through education and research (American Holistic Nurses Association & American Nurses Association, 2019, p. 18). Holistic nurses value all ways of knowing and learning. Holistic health integrates current trends, research, and evidence-based interventions specific to the patient's needs, problem, or situation. Holistic nursing research is focused on developing and expanding the knowledge base of holism and healing for education and practice (Freysteinson et al., 2023).	Holistic nurses support theoretical development by exploring the context in which phenomena occur and the meaning of patterns that emerge.

Core Value (CV) (American Holistic Nurses Association & American Nurses Association, 2019; Andrus, 2000)	Definition/Descriptions (American Holistic Nurses Association & American Nurses Association, 2019; Andrus, 2000)	Implications for Practice (American Holistic Nurses Association & American Nurses Association, 2019; Andrus, 2000)
	Educators need to familiarize themselves with the American Association of Colleges of Nursing (AACN) Essentials, core competencies for professional nursing education as a way to prepare nurses to practice from a holistic perspective (AACN, 2021). Holistic nurses consider alternative philosophies of science and research methods that are compatible with investigations of humanistic and holistic occurrences.	Holistic nurses explore various health/illness/life phenomena within context of lived experiences (Erickson & Sandor, 2017). Five nursing research priorities for 2023–2026 consistent with holistic theory development include enhancing the well-being of all nurses; innovative holistic nursing care practices and interventions; gleaning insight into and mitigating biophysical, psychosocial, and spiritual pain across the lifespan; understanding, intervening in, and reducing health inequities; and exploring nature and environmental factors on the impact of health (Freysteinson et al., 2023).

theory consistent with holistic nursing practice (American Holistic Nurses Association & American Nurses Association, 2019; Andrus, 2000).

Holistic nurses select theories to inform their professional practice that align with the competencies embedded in the core values established for all holistic nurses (American Holistic Nurses Association & American Nurses Association, 2019; Andrus, 2000). The scope and practice of holistic nurses as outlined by the American Holistic Nurses Association suggest that practice is built on both the science (theory, research, evidence-based/informed practice, critical thinking, reflection) and the art (relationship, communication, creativity, presence, caring) of nursing (Cowling, 2016). Without a fundamental understanding of the core values of holistic nursing, holistic nursing theory cannot be developed, advanced, or fully practiced.

Choosing and Evaluating a Theory for Practice

There are theories whose specific purpose is to guide holistic nursing and many others that can be applied easily to holistic nursing practice. Smith (2020) offers guidelines for selecting a theory for nursing practice. This process involves choosing a theory that is congruent with one's beliefs and values and congruent with the values of holistic practice while being focused on a specific phenomenon of interest, health situation, environment or setting and on determining if there is evidence of the usefulness of the theory to guide nursing practice and research. Selecting a theory to guide practice is not a static, once-in-a-lifetime decision but rather an everchanging motion that happens over time with emerging contemporary issues and concerns as well as personal changes in ideas and practice.

Choosing a theory begins by reading and thinking about the various nursing theories, and then reflecting on your own practice, ideas about nursing, and interests. What beliefs and values do you hold about nursing? Is nursing a discipline and professional practice with unique substantive knowledge that guides your practice, teaching, and research? What is the purpose or focus of the theory? Are these congruent with your practice? How are the concepts of nursing's metaparadigm—person, nursing, health, and environment—described within the theory? Are other concepts of the metaparadigm defined, such as well-being, caring, or nurse–patient relationships? Are the descriptions of these concepts congruent with yours? Will the theory ground your practice and keep you intentionally focused on specific outcomes? Will practicing from this theory advance your care of your patients? Will research findings and evidence on the usefulness of the theory inspire your practice to new and innovative interactions?

Choosing and evaluating a theory for practice is a circular activity. Theories emerge from practice and are then refined in research and translated for implementation in practice. Nursing theories are an essential component of nursing as a discipline and are an essential component of nursing as a professional practice.

Table 8-2 provides selected nursing theories used to guide holistic nursing practice and research.

Other sources to assist holistic nurses in identifying nursing theories consistent with holistic nursing practice include the American Holistic Nurses Association (American Holistic Nurses Association and American Nurses Association, 2019, p. 16–17) text, which offers a list of nursing theories most frequently used to support holistic nursing practice, as well as describing theories grounded in holism, healing, and caring. Additionally, there are websites with specific sections addressing holistic nursing theory: https://nursing-theory.org/theories-and-models/holistic-nursing.php; MRM Foundations—Society for the Advancement of Modeling & Role-Modeling, mrm-nursingtheory.org; https://nurseslabs.com/nursing-theories; Nursology.net; and Dr. Margaret A. Newman Center for Nursing Theory, https://www.uthsc.edu/nursing/community-partnerships/nursingtheorycenter.php

Advancements in holistic nursing knowledge development and application to research, education, and practice continue to be disseminated through peer-reviewed journals, such as the *International Journal of Human Caring, Journal of Holistic Nursing*, and *Holistic Nursing Practice*. The frontier of knowledge development is the production of new knowledge and theory within the patient-centered context of nursing practice (Reed & Crawford Shearer, 2018). Key recommendations for educating nurses emphasize more deliberative strategies to link theory with practice and are recognized through emerging holistic middle-range theory.

Emerging Middle-Range Theories for Holistic Practice

Grand theories or conceptual models may be applied in any setting and situation while middle-range theories address specific phenomena of interest in nursing that are directly linked to practice (Fawcett, 1984). It is important to acknowledge knowledge development as dynamic rather than static, making disciplinary knowledge important to ensure the current and future needs of the discipline are being met. Growth, development, and survival of nursing knowledge will require further explications of emerging conceptual models and theories moving into the 21st century. The nursing theories in the following sections address concepts and identify various phenomena of interest to holistic nursing practice including caring, culture, humanism, and the usefulness of artificial intelligence (AI) in the expanding global community of nursing.

The Theory of Unitary Caring

Smith (2015), a scholar of unitary science, caring science, theory-guided practice, and holistic practice, developed the theory of unitary caring. She describes the theory as grounded in the following

Table 8-2 Selected Nursing Theories Used to Guide Holistic Nursing Practice and Research

Theory Year First Published	Theorist Practice Settings	Major Concepts/Ideas	Practice Application/ Research
Environmental theory (Nightingale, 1975) 1860	Florence Nightingale Used in all practice settings.	The nurse's role is to manipulate the patient's environment to maximize healing, care for nutritional needs, and provide comfort. The nurse promotes healing by "the proper use of fresh air, light, warmth, [and] cleanliness" (Nightingale, 1975, p. 8).	Nagata and Lienr (2024), concept of vital power.
Interpersonal relations theory (Peplau, 1952) 1952	Hildegard Peplau Used in all practice settings.	Focuses on the importance of the nurse–patient relationship. Nurses can provide better care for their patients if they build a strong relationship based on mutual respect. Peplau's theory evolves in three phases: orientation, working, and termination.	Mersha et al. (2023), therapeutic communication between nurses and patients in Ethiopia. Sundean et al. (2021), understanding interpersonal relationships among board members.
Science of unitary beings (Rogers, 1970) 1970	Martha Rogers Middle-range theory that can be applied in all practice settings, especially those concerned with psychiatric/behavioral health settings.	Major concepts include unitary human beings, human energy field, and environmental energy field. Argues for evolution of people in irreversible and unidirectional ways.	Mygatt et al. (2023), adolescent relatedness. Smith and Reed (2023), development of the theory of healing through touch. Phillips (2021), beauty as a concept for advancement of nursing science.
Theory of transpersonal caring and caring science (Watson, 1979) 1979	Jean Watson Used in all practice settings.	Emphasizes caring relationships between nurse and patient. Describes multiple truths, physical and nonphysical realities, relativity of time and space. Caring ethic is foundational to all health care.	Dong et al. (2023), role of workplace stress and nurse's humanistic caring ability. Walker et al. (2023), using nursing theory to support sexual and reproductive health education. Bagheri et al. (2023), caring science–based health promotion for caregivers of people with schizophrenia.

(continues)

Table 8-2 Selected Nursing Theories Used to Guide Holistic Nursing Practice and Research *(continued)*

Theory Year First Published	Theorist Practice Settings	Major Concepts/Ideas	Practice Application/ Research
Modeling and role modeling (Erickson, 2015) 1983	Helen Erickson, Evelyn Tomlin, Mary Ann Swain Used in all practice areas and settings. Particularly useful in environments where the expectation is that the patient will be in charge of their own health decisions.	Describes adaptation (striving for equilibrium) and assessment of adaptive potential. Five aims of intervention: build trust; promote positive orientation; promote perceived control; promote strengths; and set mutual health-directed goals. Nurse models the patient's world (building a model of the world from the patient's perspective). Role modeling healthy behaviors from within the patient's worldview.	Jeddi et al. (2023); the effect of self-care nurturance on self-efficacy in stroke clients. Ordouni et al. (2023), the effect of self-care nurturance on quality of life for individuals with upper gastrointestinal cancer.
Theory of self-transcendence (Reed, 1991) 1991	Pamela Reed Middle-range predictive theory that can be applied in all settings.	Focuses on self-transcendence as a human capacity to expand personal boundaries intrapersonally, interpersonally, and transpersonally. Other key concepts include vulnerability and well-being.	Garcia et al. (2024), psychedelic-assisted therapy to facilitate healing relating to spirituality and existential healing.
Comfort theory (Kolcaba, 1991) Theory of holistic comfort (Kolcaba, 1994) 1991/1994	Katherine Kolcaba Middle-range predictive theory that can be applied in all practice settings where comfort is a patient concern.	Comfort is a holistic phenomenon. Comfort reflects holistic well-being. People experience comfort as feelings of relief, ease, and/or transcendence.	Bilgiç and Pamuk Cebeci (2022), stressors and comfort level in patients receiving hemodialysis. Hojjatoleslami et al. (2023), nurses' healing presence for patients with acute coronary syndrome.
Theory of health as expanding consciousness (Newman, 1999) 1999	Margaret Newman Used in all practice settings.	Nursing is caring—a moral imperative. Health is expanding consciousness that includes an individual's total pattern. Health–illness is a unitary process. People are open systems. Research is praxis.	Tang et al. (2022), psychology of nursing students during the pandemic.
Theory of integral nursing (Dossey, 2008) 2008	Barbara Dossey Used in all practice settings	The core concept is healing. Nursing is a healing process of knowing, doing, and being. The theory has three intentions: embrace the unitary whole person; explore fully the integral process; expand the nurse's capacities to heal.	Garmy (2023), holistic theory to guide teaching of academic nursing education.

concepts: manifesting intention, appreciating pattern, attuning to dynamic flow, experiencing the infinite, and inviting creative emergence. The concepts come alive in the intentional caring–healing hands therapies such as massage, therapeutic touch, and hand massage that offer healing and well-being by the simple, yet complex, touch of compassionate nurses. This theory has been advanced in palliative care, care of older adults, at a community-based primary care center, as well as globally in both small villages and large healthcare institutions.

The Community Nursing Practice Model

The community nursing practice model (CNPM) (Parker et al., 2015) emerged from a theoretical perspective of caring and analysis of years of community nursing practice exemplars, called "nursing situations." The CNPM is grounded in the values of respect for the wholeness and dignity of each person/family. The CNPM continues to evolve as its usefulness guides practice and research in various settings. One example is the inclusion of Ubuntu philosophy into the CNPM by Nambozi (2014) who asserted that many community nurse practice models employed in resource-limited communities were not designed to fit communities grounded in a non-Western culture, thereby posing challenges to implementation. The Ubuntu philosophy enhances the CNPM approach to community care as an essential way of caring for another, fostering belonging and obligation to one another, as well as caring for the welfare of the whole community. Additionally, nursing practice is intentionally actualized in the values of the World Health Organization's approach to primary health care: empowerment, multi-intersectoral collaboration, access, essentiality, and community participation. The CNPM is depicted as a watercolor of three concentric circles of community, expertise, and support surrounding the core: a nursing situation. The fluidity of the watercolor illustrates the interconnectedness of persons and families with communities. The model has been advanced using participatory action approaches and qualitative methods of study.

Shared Vulnerability

The theory of shared vulnerability (Gordon, 2007) emerged from a grounded theory study of caring for children with persistent head lice and many years of providing home visits to families with head lice infestations. Holistic values guiding the theory included a focus on the whole person and honoring relationship-centered care, as well as protecting and promoting the well-being of caregivers, children, and families. Parents caring for children were experiencing a stigmatized, chronic condition of shared vulnerability. This shared vulnerability is "conceptualized as the experience of suffering the same openness to injury as their child" (Gordon, 2007, p. 286), which creates perceived caregiver strain. Caregivers manage strain through a four-stage process of shared vulnerability: (1) being ostracized; (2) losing integrity of the self; (3) struggling with persistence; and (4) managing strain. Understanding the impact of caring for a child with a chronic stigmatized condition supports holistic nursing practice. Further research is needed to determine the usefulness of the theory in caring for persons experiencing other stigmatized conditions.

The Transactive Relationship Theory of Nursing

The transactive relationship theory of nursing (TRETON) (Tanioka, 2017) is a middle-range theory that advances not only the usefulness of AI in nursing practice but inspires engagement in the process of developing the capacity of humanoid healthcare robots as adjunctive to nursing practice. TRETON is grounded in the values of technological caring and mutual engagement in nursing encounters. Nursing encounters are described as the intentional transactional relationship between healthcare robots and human persons in the healthcare environment. Nursing encounters have three components including human engagement between the nurse and patient, technological engagement between the robot and the nurse, and engagement between the robot and the patient.

AI in health care is here now and advancing in nursing practice. King and Barry (2019) bring

AI to life in the description of the usefulness of a healthcare robot called Robin in assisting with deep breathing and relaxation techniques. Further, Osaka (2020) described the role of nursing as an intermediary, facilitating the implementation of AI pets with persons with Alzheimer disease. When the nurse prompted engagement with the AI pet, persons who had been nonverbal spoke and even laughed. Holistic nursing practice has always been on the leading edge of innovative healing practices: energy work, meditative practices, visualization processes, music, and movement therapies. Now, AI provides new and creative opportunities to heal.

The Theory of Compassion Energy

The theory of compassion energy (Dunn, 2009) provides a theoretical approach to the everydayness of nursing practice. Dunn, founder of the theory and a scholar of unitary and caring science, is a Reiki healer and is certified in holistic nursing. This theory emerged from years of reflective practice and the study of what kept nurses in nursing. Dunn (2009) described compassion energy as an intersubjective gift that awakens caring consciousness and inspires the nurse to know the patient as a whole. It is composed of compassionate presence, patterned nurturance, and intentionally knowing the one nursed and self as whole beings, and it aligns with holism as recognized by the holistic nurse. Intentional compassion energy is thus defined as the regeneration of the nurse's capacity to foster interconnectedness when the nurse activates the intent to nurse. Compassion energy provides an opening that uncovers what keeps nurses in nursing.

The Human Energy Model

The Human Energy Model (HEM), developed by Susan Leddy (2004), is grounded in Rogers' (1970) unitary nursing science and the concepts of energy field, mutual human-environment process, and pattern; Newman's (1994) and Rogers' (1970) health as a synthesis with illness; and Parse's (1995) idea of complementary opposites or paradox. Within the HEM, "knowledge-based consciousness in a goal-directed relationship with the client is the basis for nursing" (Leddy, 2004, p. 20) and "the purpose of nursing is to facilitate harmonious pattern manifestations of both the client and nurse" (Leddy, 2004, p. 20). Descriptive theories derived from the model include the Theory of Health in Illness and the Theory of Participation. In addition, the Theory of Energetic Patterning is an explanatory, practice theory based on the HEM construct of patterning. As the nurse facilitates harmonious health pattern manifestations, health pattern appraisal and recognition inform energetic nursing practice interventions. Two instruments consistent with the HEM have been developed to measure nursing outcomes in practice and facilitate research: the Leddy Healthiness Scale (Leddy, 1996) and the Person-Environment Participation Scale (Leddy, 1995).

Holistic Healing Environment Framework

The Holistic Healing Environment (HHE) Framework, developed by Gordon and France (2024), is grounded in the unitary–transformative paradigm. "The purpose of the framework is to guide the nurse in co-creating a HHE where healing emerges within and through caring" (Gordon & France, 2024, p. 25). Within the framework, a HHE is defined as the "dance of alternating rhythms with intentional knowing participation to co-create an environment through which holistic healing emerges for Nurse and persons(s)" (Gordon & France, 2024, p. 25). *Healing* is described as the unique focus of nursing with well-becoming understood as a manifestation of healing. *Healing* is defined as a personal experience of transcending suffering. The call for nursing is to co-create a holistic healing environment through authentic presence, integral presence, and compassionate unity. Compassionate unity emerges through mutual process, knowing participation, and *knowing-doing-becoming* (Gordon & France, 2024, p. 27). From this perspective, nurses are understood as healers and soul whisperers. The HHE does not stand alone, it is designed to be used in concert with holistic, caring theories of nursing within the unitary–transformative paradigm.

Box 8-1 Exemplar of Holistic Nursing Practice

The usefulness of theory to guide holistic nursing practice is illuminated in the following nursing situation describing Dunn's Reiki practice of healing energy as an intentional caring interaction between Dunn and a group of nursing students (Dunn, 2012).

Accelerated nursing students in the United States learn the art and science of nursing over one year. These intense cognitive, affective, and motor pathways during the year of their professional education can be extremely stressful. Teaching holistic nursing to students is about uncovering the heart while opening the mind to support and celebrate knowledge. Guided by Dunn's three assumptions (Dunn, 2012)—compassionate presence, patterned nurturance, and intentionally knowing the self as a whole—she guided an educational and practice experience using the healing energy of Reiki during office hours. Knowing that nursing students were experiencing stress and self-identifying feelings of being overwhelmed, the instructor offered the art and science of balance and harmony to the mind-body-spirit of both instructor and students. Four nursing students from a clinical group accepted the invitation to participate in 30-minute sessions over a semester.

The students who participated in the theory-guided Reiki sessions reflected upon their personal experience and how they were able to transform the energy-healing experience gained during the Reiki sessions from themselves to their patients. This creative educational offering was an intentional healing experience for students and advanced holistic nursing knowledge through philosophy (Reiki), practice (caring), and education (advancing knowledge). Reminding students of the importance of compassionate presence with self and other, being aware of patterned nurturance, and intentionally knowing self and other gives meaning in the nursing situation of caring compassionately (Dunn, 2012).

Implications

This chapter offers a review of theory-guided holistic nursing practice from an Eurocentric Eastern perspective (**Box 8-1**) (Suárez-Baquero, 2024). What we call *holistic nursing* has deep Indigenous and folkloric roots in knowledge that have inspired the theories described in this chapter. The authors acknowledge that other middle-range theories are emerging across the globe that may not be readily available at this time. As the discipline of nursing continues to grow, so too will nurses, bringing the usefulness of theory guided practice to holistic nursing, The usefulness of nursing theory is described within the milieu of contemporary holistic practice, education, research, and policy development. The following statements highlight the key components of the chapter:

- Guidance in choosing a theory consistent with a holistic nurse's own personal and professional values as well as beliefs that, in turn, positively influence client patient–nurse interactions in practice.
- Holistic nursing concepts and theories capable of guiding data collection, research, and evidence-based practice.
- A framework to choose and evaluate theory to determine congruence with holistic nursing's core values as well as convergence with the cultural beliefs of those cared for.
- The importance of nursing theory to guide holistic nursing practice and research.
- Emerging middle-range theories grounded in holistic nursing that could be expanded in practice and research, and applied in education.

Conclusion

Nursing theories provide a means for nurses to discern and evaluate their essential role in the healthcare setting and provide the organizing framework necessary for understanding the phenomena that are of importance to the discipline of nursing. Holistic nurses need to recognize current trends and examples of phenomena of concern within the discipline of nursing to inform holistic nursing research, education, practice, and theory development. This chapter provides a foundation by which holistic nurses can advance their practice using existing and emerging nursing theories consistent with the scope and standards of holistic nursing (American Holistic Nurses Association & American Nurses Association, 2019; Andrus, 2000).

References

American Association of Colleges of Nursing (AACN). (2021). *The essentials: Core competencies for professional nursing education*. AACN. https://www.aacnnursing.org/Portals/0/PDFs/Publications/Essentials-2021.pdf

American Holistic Nurses Association and American Nurses Association. (2019). *Holistic nursing practice: Scope and standards of practice* (3rd ed.). Nursesbooks.org.

Andrus, V. (2000). Holistic nursing: Remembering our nursing roots. *Newsletter of the Nurse Healers-Professional Associates International*, *XXI*(4), 1–3.

Bagheri, S., Zarshenas, L., Rakhshan, M., Sharif, F., Sarani, E. M., Shirazi, Z. H., & Sitzman, K. (2023). Impact of Watson's human caring-based health promotion program on caregivers of individuals with schizophrenia. *BMC Health Services Research*, *23*(1), 711. https://doi.org/10.1186/s12913-023-09725-9

Bilgiç, Ş., & Pamuk Cebeci, S. (2022). Relationship between stressors and comfort level in hemodialysis patients. *Archives of Health Science and Research*, *9*(2), 105–109. https://doi.org/10.54614/archealthscires.2022.21146

Boykin, A., & Schoenhofer, S. (2001). *Nursing as caring: A model for transforming practice*. Jones and Bartlett Publishers.

Cowling, W. R. (2016). Theoretical grounding of holistic nursing scholarship. *Journal of Holistic Nursing*, *34*(4), 316–317. https://doi.org/10.1177/0898010116677090

Donaldson, S., & Crowley, D. (1978). The discipline of nursing. *Nursing Outlook*, *26*(2), 113–120.

Dong, F., Huang, W., Chu, C., Lv, L., & Zhang, M. (2023). Influence of workplace stress and social support on humanistic caring ability in Chinese nurses. *Nursing Open*, *10*(6). https://doi.org/10.1002/nop2.1606

Dossey, B. M. (2008). Theory of integral nursing. *Advances in Nursing Science*, *31*(1), E52–E73. https://doi.org/10.1097/01.ans.0000311536.11683.0a

Dunn, D. J. (2012, June). *Empowering nursing students to practice holistically*. Poster presented at the 32nd American Holistic Nurses Association Annual Conference: Holistic Nurses: Catalyst for Conscious Change, Snowbird, UT.

Dunn, D. J. (2009). The intentionality of compassion energy. *Holistic Nursing Practice*, *23*(4), 222–229. https://doi.org/10.1097/hnp.0b013e3181aecebb

Erickson, H. (2015). Helen Erickson, Evelyn Tomlin and Mary Ann Swain's Theory of Modeling and Role Modeling. In M. Smith & M. Parker (Eds.). *Nursing Theories and Nursing Practice* (pp. 185–205). F.A. Davis.

Erickson, M., & Sandor, K. (2017). *Core essentials for the practice of holistic nursing*. American Holistic Nursing Credentialing Corporation. https://www.ahncc.org/wp-content/uploads/2018/01/2017-BASIC-HN-CORE-ESSENTIALS-Final.pdf

Fawcett, J. (1984). The metaparadigm of nursing: Present status and future refinements. *Image: The Journal of Nursing Scholarship, 16*(3), 84–87. https://doi.org/10.1111/j.1547-5069.1984.tb01393.x

Fawcett, J. (2024). More thoughts about the evolution of the metaparadigm of nursing: Addition of culture as another metaparadigm concept and definitions of all the concepts. *Nursing Science Quarterly*, *37*(2), 183–184. https://doi.org/10.1177/08943184231224409

Freysteinson, W. M., Enzman Hines, M., Wind Wardell, D., Friesen, M. A., Conrad, S., Zahourek, R., Gallo, A. M., & Prather, J. G. (2023). Identifying holistic nursing research priorities for 2023–2026. *Journal of Holistic Nursing*, *42*(2). https://doi.org/10.1177/08980101231213725

Garcia C. A., Maia, L. O., & Reed, P. G. (2024). Exploring psychedelics for alleviating existential and spiritual suffering in people with serious illnesses: Links to the theory of self-transcendence. *Journal of Holistic Nursing*. Published online May 29, 2024. https://doi.org/10.1177/08980101241257836

Garmy, P. (2023). Teaching the subject of nursing—Academic teaching based on Dossey's holistic nursing theory. *SAGE Open Nursing*, *9*, 237796082311678. https://doi.org/10.1177/23779608231167817

Gordon, S. C. (2007). Shared vulnerability: A theory of caring for children with persistent head lice. *The Journal of School Nursing*, *23*(5), 283–292. https://doi.org/10.1177/10598405070230050701

Gordon, S., & France, N. (2024). *Co-creating a holistic healing environment in nursing practice*. Cognella.

Hojjatoleslami, S., Sadeghi, A., Negarandeh, R., Soltanian, A. R., & Borzou, S. R. (2023). Nurses' healing presence: A panacea for the comfort of acute coronary syndrome patients in CCU, a qualitative study. *Nursing Open*, *10*(6). https://doi.org/10.1002/nop2.1631

Jeddi, H., Aghebati, N., Ghavami, V., & Rezaeitalab, F. (2023). The effect of self-care nurturance using the theory of modeling and role-modeling on self-efficacy in stroke patients. *Holistic Nursing Practice*, *37*(2), E24–E35. https://doi.org/10.1097/hnp.0000000000000567

King, B. M., & Barry, C. D. (2019). "Caring between" the nurse, the one nursed, and the healthcare robot: An interpreted nursing situation using the Barry, Gordon, King framework. *International Journal for Human Caring*, *23*(2), 168–177. https://doi.org/10.20467/1091-5710.23.2.168

Kolcaba, K. Y. (1991). A taxonomic structure for the concept comfort. *Image: The Journal of Nursing Scholarship*. *23*(4), 237–240. https://doi.org/10.1111/j.1547-5069.1991.tb00678.x

Kolcaba, K. Y. (1994). A theory of holistic comfort for nursing. *Journal of Advanced Nursing*, *19*(6), 1178–1184. https://doi.org/10.1111/j.1365-2648.1994.tb01202.x

Kuhn, T. (1970). *The structure of scientific revolutions*. University of Chicago Press.

Leddy, S. (1995). Measuring mutual process: Development and psychometric testing of the Person-Environment Participation Scale. *Visions: The Journal of Rogerian Nursing Science*, *3*, 20–31.

Leddy, S. (2004). Human energy: A conceptual model of unitary nursing science. *Visions: The Journal of Rogerian Nursing Science*, *12*(1), 14–27.

Leddy, S. K. (1996). Development and psychometric testing of the Leddy Healthiness Scale. *Research in Nursing & Health*, *19*(5), 431–440. https://doi.org/10.1002/(sici)1098-240x(199610)19:5%3C431::aid-nur7%3E3.0.co;2-r

Leininger, M. (1987). *Transcultural nursing*. Wiley.

Mersha, A., Abera, A., Tesfaye, T., Abera, T., Belay, A., Melaku, T., Shiferaw, M., Shibiru, S., Estifanos, W., & Wake, S. K. (2023). Therapeutic communication and its associated factors among nurses working in public hospitals of Gamo zone, southern Ethiopia: Application of Hildegard Peplau's nursing theory of interpersonal relations. *BMC Nursing*, *22*(1). https://doi.org/10.1186/s12912-023-01526-z

Mygatt, M. G., Smith, M. C., & Opalinski, A. (2023). Adolescent relatedness through the lens of unitary caring theory. *Nursing Science Quarterly*, *37*(1), 48–55. https://doi.org/10.1177/08943184231207372

Nagata, M., & Liehr, P. (2024). An evolving structure of nature immersion: Roots in Nightingale's vital power. *Creative Nursing*, *30*(1), 41–50. https://doi.org/10.1177/10784535241226494

Nambozi, G. (2014). *An evaluation of community based university nursing education programme and stakeholders' experiences* (Doctoral dissertation). The University of Hull. https://hull-repository.worktribe.com/output/4218898

Newman, M. A. (1994). *Health as expanding consciousness*. National League for Nursing Press.

Newman, M. A. (1999). *Health as expanding consciousness* (2nd ed.). National League for Nursing.

Newman, M. A., Sime, A. M., & Corcoran-Perry, S. A. (1991). The focus of the discipline of nursing. *Advances in Nursing Science*, *14*(1), 1–6. https://doi.org/10.1097/00012272-199109000-00002

Nightingale, F. (1975). *Notes on nursing: What it is and what it is not*. Dover Publications. (Originally published 1859)

Ordouni, K., Aghebati, N., Ghavami, V., & Movahed, S. (2023). The effect of self-care nurturance based on Erickson's modeling and role-modeling theory on quality of life of patients with upper gastrointestinal cancer: A randomized clinical trial. *Holistic Nursing Practice*, *37*(3), E36–E50. https://doi.org/10.1097/HNP.0000000000000578

Osaka, K. (2020). Development of the model for the intermediary role of nurses in transactive relationships with healthcare robots. *International Journal for Human Caring*, *24*, 265–274.

Parker, M., Barry, C., & King, B. (2015). The community nursing practice model. In M. Smith & M. Parker (Eds.). *Nursing Theories and Nursing Practice* (pp. 435–447). F.A. Davis.

Parse, R. (1995). The human becoming theory. In R. Parse (Ed.), *Illuminations: The human becoming theory in practice and research* (pp. 5–8). National League for Nursing.

Parse, R. (1998). *The human becoming school of thought: A perspective for nurses and other health professionals*. SAGE Publications.

Peplau, H. E. (1952). *Interpersonal theory in nursing practice*. G. P. Putnam's Sons.

Phillips, J. R. (2021). The revelation of beauty in nursing. *Nursing Science Quarterly*, *35*(1), 46–53. https://doi.org/10.1177/08943184211051362

Reed, P. G. (1991). Self-transcendence and mental health in oldest-old adults. *Nursing Research*, *40*(1), 5–11. https://doi.org/10.1097/00006199-199101000-00002

Reed, P. G., & Crawford Shearer, N. M. (2018). *Nursing knowledge and theory innovation: Advancing the science of practice*. Springer Publishing Company, LLC.

Rogers, M. E. (1970). *An introduction to a theoretical basis of nursing*. F.A. Davis.

Smith, M. (2015). Theory of unitary caring. In M. Smith & M. Parker (Eds.). *Nursing Theories and Nursing Practice* (pp. 435–447). F.A. Davis.

Smith, M. C. (1994). Arriving at a philosophy of nursing. In J. F. Kikuchi & H. Simmons (Eds.), *Developing a philosophy of nursing* (pp. 43–60). SAGE Publications.

Smith, M. C. (2019). Regenerating nursing's disciplinary perspective. *Advances in Nursing Science*, *42*(1), 3–16. https://doi.org/10.1097/ans.0000000000000241

Smith, M. C. (2020). *Nursing theories and nursing practice* (5th ed.). F.A. Davis.

Smith, M. C., & Parker, M. E. (2015). Nursing theory and the discipline of nursing. In M. C. Smith & M. E. Parker (Eds.), *Nursing theories and nursing practice* (pp. 1–18). F.A. Davis.

Smith, M. C., & Reed, S. M. (2023). A unitary theory of healing through touch. *Advances in Nursing Science*, *46*(2). https://doi.org/10.1097/ANS.0000000000000487

Suárez-Baquero, D. F. M. (2024). Decolonizing nursing knowledge: Challenging Eurocentrism centering global south voices. *Nursing Outlook*, *72*(4). https://doi.org/10.1016/j.outlook.2024.102197

Sundean, L. J., Fawcett, J., & Prybil, L. D. (2021). Board culture and the role of interpersonal relations. *Nursing Economic$*, *39*(4), 161–161. https://doi.org/10.62116/nec.2021.39.4.161

Tang, L., Lu, S., Lai, Y., & Deng, R. (2022). Health as expanding consciousness: Change of psychological situation in nursing students. *Nursing Open*, *10*(3):1923–1930. https://doi.org/10.1002/nop2.1444

Tanioka, T. (2017). The development of the Transactive Relationship Theory of Nursing (TRETON): A nursing engagement model for persons and humanoid nursing robots. *International Journal of Nursing & Clinical Practices*, *4*(1). https://doi.org/10.15344/2394-4978/2017/223

Walker, C. M., Anderson, J. N., Clark, R., & Reed, L. (2023). The use of nursing theory to support sexual and reproductive health care education in nursing curricula. *Journal of Nursing Education*, *62*(2):69-74. https://doi.org/10.3928/01484834-20221213-01

Watson, J. (1979). *Nursing: The philosophy and science of caring*. University Press of Colorado.

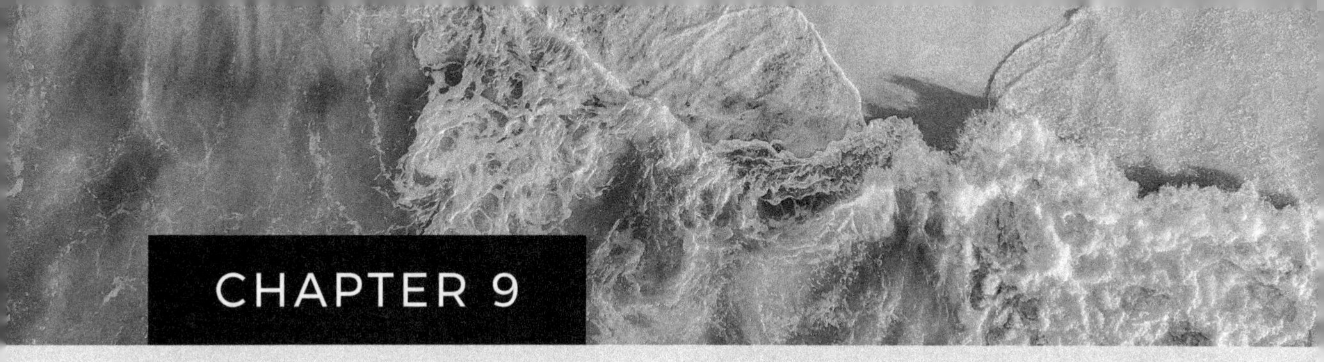

CHAPTER 9

Holistic Leadership

Veda L. Andrus and Marie M. Shanahan

NURSE HEALER OBJECTIVES

- Develop strategies to link the caring case and business case of healthcare transformation.
- Develop strategies to incorporate the principles of holistic leadership into practice.
- Identify the seven core characteristics of a holistic leader.

DEFINITIONS

Appreciative inquiry: An asset-based approach built on the assumption that every organization has positive elements and processes and that these strengths can be the starting point for positive change.

Cultural transformational agent: An individual who holds the vision for and works to actualize a plan to transform the culture of an organization to become a caring, healing environment.

Holistic leadership: A participative leadership model in which people, regardless of formal titles, engage in a constructive process as equal partners to influence an affirming, sustainable, and humanistic outcome.

Human-centered leadership: A leadership model that focuses on the fulfillment and effectiveness of the leader who simultaneously focuses on others through establishing cultures of caring, excellence, and trust.

Nurse empowerment: The ability to motivate self and others to accomplish positive outcomes of professional nursing practice.

Nurse engagement: A positive state of fulfillment and satisfaction experienced by nurses at work. When nurses are engaged, they feel energetic and dedicated to their work and become immersed in work activities.

Structural empowerment: Work environment structures and processes designed to promote innovative, high-performance, and professional practice.

Therapeutic healing environment: A milieu consciously created by a holistic healthcare professional(s) to promote the outcomes of health, healing, and well-being.

Transformational leadership: A style of leadership in which the individual identifies the needed change and creates a clearly articulated vision to guide the change through inspiration, integrity, and mutual respect. The change is accomplished with the commitment of the group members and by maximizing human potential and mentorship.

Visionary: Having or marked by foresight and imagination (Merriam-Webster, 2024c).

General Leadership Frameworks and Leadership Assumptions

> I define a leader as anyone who takes responsibility for finding the potential in people and processes, and who has the courage to develop that potential. (Brown, 2018, p. 4)

The holistic leadership model draws its inspiration from two general progressive leadership frameworks that have informed its development. Subsequently, a series of evolutionary leadership assumptions have influenced its continuing evolution. These frameworks and assumptions have, at their roots, common conceptual perspectives that focus on principles that serve as the container and guiding light for leader actions. The principles become the foundation and springboard for the leader's relationship with self, others, and the organization and then, by extension, become the keys to influence and manifest change.

Transformational Leadership

The concept of *transformational leadership* was introduced by James MacGregor Burns in 1978. It is a leadership style in which the formal leader influences high performance by developing and articulating a compelling vision that inspires, motivates, and empowers colleagues-as-partners to work toward fulfillment of a common goal.

Transformational leadership in nursing fosters a supportive, empowering healthcare environment. A transformational leadership style in nursing motivates teams to work together to deliver exceptional patient care and outcomes. Transformational nurse leaders build a culture of respect and open collaboration (American Nurses Association, 2023).

The following are the core characteristics of transformational leadership (Broome & Marshall, 2020):

- **Charisma or idealized influence**: The leader possesses and models self-confidence, inspires trust and encouragement for partners/colleagues to bring forth their best selves, and provides mentorship that enhances nurse engagement.
- **Inspiration and vision**: The leader develops, articulates, and models a compelling vision that inspires others to passionately execute the vision.
- **Intellectual stimulation**: The leader respects their colleagues' creativity through identification of cocreated goals, encourages identification and actualization of innovative solutions, and guides others to find meaning and purpose in their work.
- **Individual consideration**: The leader maintains open, clear, and effective communication; fosters quality relationships with their colleagues; and offers support, encouragement, and recognition.

Transformational leadership is one of the five components of the American Nurses Credentialing Center's Magnet Recognition Program model (American Nurses Credentialing Center, 2023). This component was selected with the understanding that nurse leaders today must provide the necessary leadership to prepare organizations to meet the current and future demands of healthcare reform.

Human-Centered Leadership

This innovative approach to leadership was introduced by Kennedy, Campis, and Leclerc in 2020 with the intention of providing a model of leadership specifically designed for healthcare professionals. Human-centered leaders establish cultures of excellence, trust, and caring through demonstrating attributes in the domains of an awakener, a connector, and an upholder:

Awakener: Motivates and ignites individuals to be their best selves by establishing a learning environment for individual growth and team innovation. Acting as a coach, mentor, advocate and engaged team member, the human-centered leader contributes to building a *culture of excellence*.

Connector: Recognizes and encourages independent thought, collective wisdom in problem-solving, and self-organization to allow for innovation to emerge. Through building a collaborative community, the human-centered leader contributes to building a *culture of trust*.

Upholder: Creates and promotes a healthy work environment that nurtures human interactions. The human-centered leader engages in and models personal well-being through self-care, self-compassion, self-awareness, and mindfulness—and encourages and supports these work–life balance practices in others to build team resiliency. Through building collaborative community, the human-centered leader contributes to building a *culture of caring*.

All three domains—awakener, connector, and upholder—collectively support sustainable paradigmatic change within an ever-evolving healthcare environment. "It is, in fact, a revolution within the history of nursing's evolution as a profession" (Kennedy et al., 2022, p. 210).

Evolutionary Leadership Assumptions

The evolutionary leadership assumptions presented by William Rosa in *Nurses as leaders: Evolutionary visions of leadership* provide overarching leadership qualities that serve as a container to guide clinical practice. The following insightful assumptions are beacons of light, shining the way for leaders to begin or continue their journey as nurse leaders:

- Evolutionary leadership embraces vulnerability.
- Evolutionary leadership calls for a state of openness and self-awareness.
- Evolutionary leadership requires self-renewal and self-reflection.
- Evolutionary leadership implies a willingness to mature in ways of being, doing, thinking, seeing, and knowing.
- Evolutionary leadership acknowledges the difference between striving and perfectionism.
- Evolutionary leadership is *both/and* and not *either/or*.
- Evolutionary leadership respects all voices in the room.
- Evolutionary leaders rehumanize work environments to promote ethical engagement and meaningful partnerships.
- Evolutionary leaders work to unveil and promote the truth.
- Evolutionary leaders allow for the transformation of self and systems (Rosa, 2016, p. 9).

As leaders consciously bring alive these qualities within their practice and allow them to take a place in their hearts, minds, and souls, there is great possibility for nursing leadership, from bedside to boardroom, to evolve into its full potential and to allow nursing to take its rightful place in health care and in the world at large.

Professional Practice Models

Professional practice models provide a container to operationalize theoretical frameworks within a course of action. Most practice models encompass an amalgam of theories that serve as an anchor to support nursing practice. The BirchTree Center model has been selected as a professional practice model that supports holistic leadership as a leadership model.

BirchTree Center Model

The BirchTree Center model was developed by Marie Shanahan and Veda Andrus in 2005. It is an integrative, interdisciplinary, progressive practice model of personal and professional transformation that promotes consistent and sustainable holistic practice in nursing and health care (refer to **Figure 9-1**). In this model, as individuals build the capacity for developing a caring, healing ethic to transform their practice, organizations build the capacity for developing a caring, healing work environment to transform the organizational culture.

Engagement with the BirchTree Center model begins with the relationship one has with self. Through self-reflection, individuals come to realize that self-care and renewal are essential to their effectiveness in therapeutic relationships. Engagement in self-renewal practices expands and enhances their ability to *be* a healing presence with others, and caring for oneself is thus properly reframed as integral with compassionate, professional care for others. Holistic leaders model self-awareness and renewal in professional settings and identify them as an essential leadership competency, indicating the importance of these behaviors in contributing to a therapeutic healing environment.

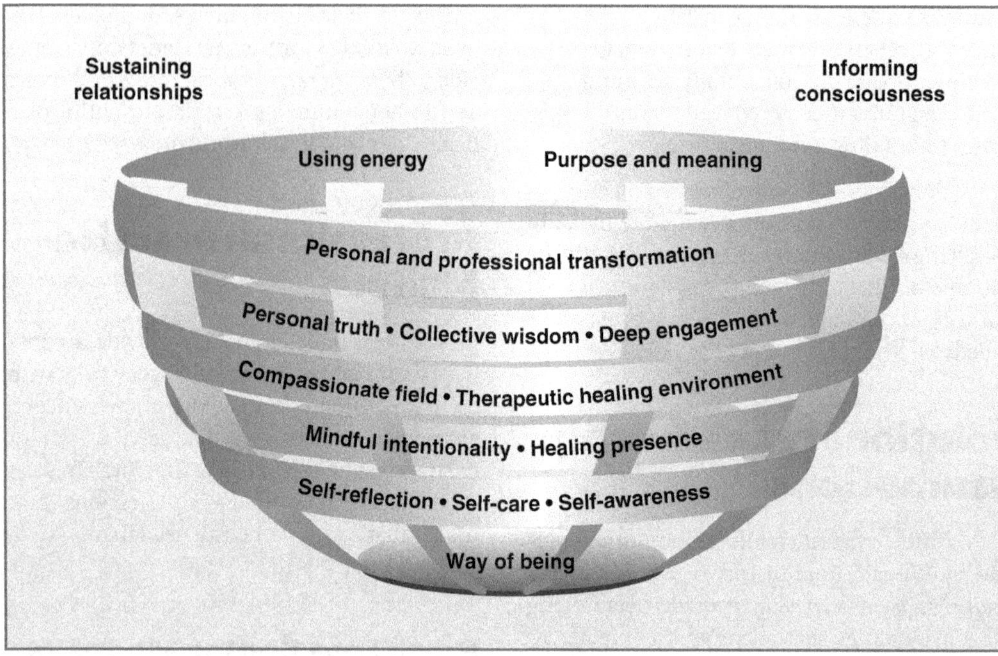

Figure 9-1 The BirchTree Center model.
BirchTree Center Press

The model is used within healthcare settings to reorient the values, behaviors, actions, and practice ethic toward healing and caring, through greater awareness of a shared humanity, diversity, equity, inclusion, and justice for all. When compassion is appropriately linked with organizational excellence, the intrinsic motivation to be or provide caring creates deeper engagement with the mission of the organization. As the field of compassion expands, the shift in organizational identity begins. The identification of compassion as a cultural anchor linked to performance fosters a sustainable transformation.

The model is represented in the image of an open basket. The open basket imagery holds space for the care provider and the organization to recognize, develop, and allow an ever-increasing capacity to heal and be healed; to receive new gifts, knowledge, and understanding; to let go of that which no longer is needed; and to transform and lead transformation with others. The concept of an open basket is intended to challenge the long-held image of a care provider's tool kit. The open basket of the BirchTree Center model invites the concept of holding all possibilities for a healing process, going well beyond a care provider tending to the person to encompass such notions as the care provider's own well-being and potential for influencing organizational and community health. By shifting to the image of an open basket, the potential to hold healing energy for ourselves, our patients, our coworkers, and the healthcare system is engaged (Shanahan, 2014).

Research

The concept and language of holistic leadership are on the cutting edge of a new paradigm of leadership. There is ample research available in the literature that substantiates the implementation of transformational leadership; however, holistic leadership, as presented in this chapter, currently does not have a research base that substantiates outcomes. Inclusion of various research methodological models (e.g., quantitative, qualitative, narrative inquiry) that reflect the principles of holistic leadership must be considered.

Appreciative Inquiry

Appreciative inquiry is an asset-based approach built on the assumption that every organization has things that work well and that these strengths can be the starting point for positive change. Appreciative inquiry is an energizing and inclusive process that fosters creativity through the art of positive inquiry (Center for Appreciative Inquiry, 2024b). This is a shift from the traditional deficit-based problem-solving approach to change and group engagement by studying what *does* work, building strategies and solutions from this knowledge base, unlocking innovation, and yielding greater creativity.

The 5-D process of appreciative inquiry includes the following cycle processes (Center for Appreciative Inquiry, 2024a):

1. **Definition**: Reframed focus of the inquiry in the affirmative and on topics valuable to the people involved.
2. **Discovery**: A collaborative search for the best of what is that already provides optimal performance. Discovery involves meaningful conversations.
3. **Dream**: Dialogue, reflection, envisioning. An exploration of what might be, where people collectively explore their hopes and dreams.
4. **Design**: Co-constructing the vision created in the *dream* phase into specific changes to create a preferred future.
5. **Destiny**: Focuses on personal commitments and implementation of innovation.

Appreciative inquiry is a cycle: When *destiny* is implemented, the cycle starts again with *definition*. The process of appreciative inquiry fosters excitement, enthusiasm, and commitment among nursing personnel through inclusivity of those who may have the best insights into solutions. This enhances nurse engagement, encourages identification of strengths and resources, stimulates optimal performance, and assists in recognizing what the organization does best.

Characteristics of a Holistic Leader

> To manage is to control; to lead is to liberate. (Owen, 1999, p. 53)[1]

Holistic leadership is a synthesis of participative leadership models with the recognition that it is imperative to redefine and expand the concept of leadership to meet the future directions within nursing and health care. Nurses hold the potential to play key roles in the continued evolution of healthcare reform and must assume leadership roles that align with a new model of holistic leadership. When approaching leadership roles from a holistic–integrative perspective, nurses, as holistic leaders, will position themselves to assume innovative roles as the edge runners of healthcare change.

There is one assumption to embrace: Everyone is a leader. This means that every nurse, whether holding a formal leadership title or not, has a responsibility to influence the advancement of the nursing profession. A shift in language from *follower*, as often articulated in the transformational leadership model, to *partner*, as presented in the holistic leadership model, is essential to authentically demonstrate that everyone is, indeed, a leader. It is critical not to underestimate the compelling value proposition of nursing as being a prime contributor of healthcare transformation.

There are seven core characteristics of a holistic leader:

1. Visionary
2. Inspirational presence
3. Role model

---

1 Quote reprinted with permission of the publisher. From *The spirit of leadership: Liberating the leader in each of us*, copyright 1999 by H. Owen, Berrett-Koehler Publishers, Inc., San Francisco, CA. All rights reserved. Available at www.bkconnection.com

4. Mentor
5. Champion for clinical excellence
6. Courageous advocate
7. Cultural transformational agent

Although these seven characteristics will be presented individually, it is important to recognize that they are interrelated and integral to one another. The thread that weaves them together radiates from a foundation of competence, heart-centered collaboration, and self-awareness as the essence of a leader's way of being, personally and professionally.

Holistic Leader as Visionary

> There are two ways of spreading light—to be the candle or the mirror that reflects it. (Wharton, 1902, p. 631)

A visionary is conventionally defined as "having or marked by foresight and imagination" (Visionary, 2024). When defined in concert with the concept of holistic leadership, the future is cocreated in a collaborative manner through the recognition that everyone is a leader and that drawing out each person's creative potential calls forth the best in people, bringing them together around a shared sense of purpose. The holistic visionary leader is open to learning from other points of view through evolving the art of full presence, deep listening, self-reflection, and a nonjudgmental attitude.

There is an inherent need on the part of human beings for their work to fulfill purpose and meaning. A visionary leader understands the deeper spiritual needs of people by caring for the souls of individuals as well as the soul of the organization. It is through this awareness that leaders align with a higher purpose for themselves, their coworkers, the organization, and the greater community.

As architects of change (change agents), holistic leaders see the big picture and utilize out-of-the-box thinking that allows for innovative co-participative strategic actions. This is not done in isolation. The visionary leader is often a catalyst for innovation, working with imagination, insight, and boldness through a partnership approach with other nurse colleagues and in concert with the interdisciplinary team.

Holistic Leader as Inspirational Presence

> Leaders cannot demand inspiration from others; they must create the environment that encourages such inspiration. (Secretan, 1999, p. 152)

The holistic leader has a role in creating a vibrant environment that *inspires* people to be their best selves through inclusion, respect, caring, and acknowledgment. The physical environment in which many nurses work may not be particularly inspiring in design and function; however, the culture of the work environment can always foster creativity, insight, and engagement. The holistic leader, through their very presence, can cultivate commitment and passion in the workplace where nurses and members of the interdisciplinary team are encouraged to grow, learn, and develop as care providers and as human beings.

As an inspirational presence, the holistic leader performs an important role in creating a positive and engaging environment. *Inspiration* is described as "emotions and behaviors determined by powers from within. Inspired people arouse the hearts of others" (Secretan, 1999, p. 51). When the heart is aroused, people become enthusiastic, knowing their participation is invited as a contribution to the developing landscape of their work environment.

The holistic leader understands that an expression of positive energy and vitality has an affirming correlation with indicators such as productivity and job performance. Although the primary focus may not be on these specific indicators, through an inspiring environment that fosters collaboration, teamwork, and shared information, the holistic leader conveys an air of confidence that the right energetic environment will support greater productivity and improved job performance.

An inspirational leader embodies a sense of personal integrity that radiates to others as respect; kindness; and genuine, authentic caring.

The words *genuine* and *authentic* are essential because words and actions, including genuine celebration of accomplishments and successes, that come from the place of true caring are acknowledged and appreciated by others.

Holistic Leader as Role Model

The responsibility of a role model is to set standards of excellence in clinical nursing in concert with exemplifying both the vision and values that are fundamental within the organization. The central intention of being a role model is to serve as a positive example for other nurses to follow and emulate.

Core Principles

There are four core principles that serve as pillars for role modeling holistic leadership: maintaining integrity, upholding ethical standards, demonstrating bold and courageous actions, and being visible–approachable–accessible.

1. **Integrity**: The role model adheres to superior moral principles and professional standards and is not willing to trade integrity for personal advancement. Holistic leaders choose not to compromise their integrity with behaviors that do not align with their sense of right action.
2. **Ethical**: The role model models a professional code of holistic nursing ethics that includes being a therapeutic, caring presence; facilitating healing and wholeness; practicing loving kindness; and sustaining honesty. "Holistic nurses [may] assume a leadership position to guide the profession toward a holistic philosophy of practices" (American Holistic Nurses Association & American Nurses Association, 2019, p. 256) through integration of holistic nursing Core Value 1: Holistic Philosophy, Theories, and Ethics (American Holistic Nurses Association & American Nurses Association, 2019, p. 9).
3. **Bold and courageous**: The role model stands firmly in their own truth and knowing and is confident and bold in speaking out in support of holistic nursing practice. Holistic leaders access their courage and assume the responsibility to take risks to advance nursing excellence.
4. **Visible–approachable–accessible**: The role model values meaningful connection with nurse colleagues and other care providers and intentionally maintains an open heart and mind, without judgment, to enhance engagement, communication, and exploration. Holistic leaders demonstrate a passion for nursing and a love of the profession, igniting the soul of nursing and exhibiting excitement for what the future will bring for the profession.

Artistry of Authentic Communication

Holistic leaders must be aware of and sensitive to the diversity of communication styles and present information in a manner that is clear, direct, and genuine. Presenting information in a way that others can best receive it is an art that takes practice and reflection. The practice of taking a breath as a momentary pause prior to presenting information can demonstrate role modeling as an authentic communication style.

Holistic leaders model respectful holistic communication through the following ways:

- Making no assumptions (creating a culture where asking questions is an acceptable practice).
- Fostering nonjudgmental behavior and actions.
- Choosing to be compassionate and sincere.
- Drawing information from a broad range of sources.
- Engaging in deep listening (heart/mind) through full presence.
- Acting in a manner that is reflective and responsive, rather than reactive.
- Modeling transparency through open and honest dialogue.

Self-Reflection and Self-Care

Core Value 2: Holistic Nurse Self-Reflection, Self- Development, and Self-Care is foundational to holistic nursing practice (American Holistic Nurses Association & American Nurses Association, 2019, pp. 25–27). Engaging in self-care practices, both personally and professionally, can be a challenge for many nurses because affirming models for self-care in their families and within the practice environment are frequently absent.

It is the responsibility of holistic leaders to model self-reflection and self-care on a regular and consistent basis with the intention of building their own resiliency and demonstrating support and encouragement for others to care well for themselves.

In a professional work environment, self-reflective and self-care practices may include taking lunch breaks, utilizing reflective time for decision making, and departing the workplace in a timely manner at the end of the day. Participating in these and other self-care activities demonstrates that the holistic leader values these practices, and, through role modeling, provides permission for others to do the same.

The use of grounding and centering techniques, such as taking a few deeps breaths prior to attending meetings, during all interactions, and in transitions from one activity to the next, models a process to help others cope with workplace stressors.

Holistic Leader as Mentor

Mentorship consists of "individualized, tailor-made, one-on-one environments for giving and receiving the gift of wisdom (Huang & Lynch, 1999, p. xi). Holistic leaders view mentorship as a mutually beneficial shared, rather than hierarchical, process where both people, as partners, learn and grow from one another's insights, ideas, experiences, and wisdom.

Through cultivation of a mentorship culture, holistic leaders guide and facilitate projects for skill development that demonstrate a commitment to lifelong learning. This environment fosters ongoing professional growth and continued career advancement in nursing leadership, strengthens confidence and competence, and enhances nurse engagement through a co-participative model.

Giving and receiving and working together as partners become the acceptable norm, allowing for acceptance, cooperation, appreciation, and inclusivity—a circle of influence.

Holistic Leader as Champion for Clinical Excellence

Serving as a champion for clinical excellence is a critical role for holistic nursing leaders in today's healthcare climate. This has always been an important role for nurse leaders and has become even more critical for holistic leaders to concentrate on clinical excellence and view this as a central construct for a new value proposition for nursing.

To begin, holistic leaders must become articulate in linking the *caring case* of bedside care with the *business case* of healthcare transformation—and require clinical nurses to do the same. This can be accomplished by promoting education and learning at every level, where nurses understand how their role as care providers has a direct relationship with the business case. The next step is to hold nurses accountable for clinical excellence as demonstrated by exceptional quality patient care, purposeful nurse–patient engagement, genuine peer-to-peer caring, personal self-care practices to enhance resiliency, and appreciation for the larger role their organization plays as an instrument of change within the community and the broader healthcare environment.

Innovative Strategies for Clinical Excellence

Holistic leaders are intentional about selecting and implementing progressive, innovative strategies that will achieve clinical excellence within a healthy, supportive work environment. The American Association of Critical-Care Nurses' synergy model for patient care states that "a patient's needs drive the nurse competencies required for patient care. When nurse competencies stem from patient needs, and the characteristics of the nurse and patient match, synergy occurs. This synergy enables optimal outcomes" (American Association of Critical-Care Nurses, 2024). Accessible provision of relevant professional development education to improve competency levels in knowledge development, clinical skills expertise, and critical thinking is an avenue that supports and fosters optimal clinical outcomes.

Cultivation of true collaboration among clinical nurses, across the interdisciplinary team, with inclusion of patients and their families, promotes clinical excellence when creative opportunities for communication and learning are employed. In this integrative approach, the knowledge and abilities of each professional and patient are respected to achieve safe, quality care. Implementation of initiatives such as bedside shift report and interprofessional rounds are examples of true collaboration that can enhance the quality of the patient experience and outcomes.

The Broader Context of Professionalism

Holistic leaders elevate the professionalism of nurses by encouraging and supporting ongoing professional development and clinical competence through advanced degrees and certifications. As a result of advancing their education and career, nurses are recognized and rewarded in a manner that demonstrates how this personal accomplishment also advances nursing within the specific healthcare organization and, by extension, within the overall profession.

Membership in professional organizations is promoted, viewing this as essential to support professional growth and serving as an avenue to effect change through a reshaping of the broader healthcare environment. This involvement empowers clinical nurses to find their voice and discover what they can do to further the profession.

Holistic Leader as Courageous Advocate

> **Courage**: Mental or moral strength to venture, persevere, and withstand danger, fear, or difficulty (Merriam-Webster, 2024b).
>
> **Advocate**: One who pleads the cause of another (Merriam-Webster, 2024a).

As courageous advocates, holistic leaders exhibit an unwavering commitment to support and enrich all dimensions of holistic nursing practice, from bedside to boardroom, for nurses, for the nursing profession, and for the planet. This is a tall order. However, the realm of advocacy must be inclusive of all areas in which nurses are influential. This must include listening, self-reflection, and learning about all inequities, discrimination, and social injustices. It takes courage to be a progressive thinker and innovative change agent to facilitate nursing in achieving its full potential.

For the Advancement of Holistic Nursing and the Nursing Profession

Holistic leaders are visible and vocal advocates for holistic nursing. They are active (visible) in professional organizations (e.g., American Holistic Nurses Association, American Organization of Nurse Executives, Sigma Theta Tau International), not only as members but also as vocal spokespersons for framing nursing practice in holistic nursing principles, philosophy, and theory. They choose to be informed on healthcare policy and financing with an intention of aligning current models to a holistic paradigm—building a business *and* a caring case for nursing and health care.

For Nurses

Creating a work environment and culture that fosters caring for nurses is foundational to holistic leaders who regard nurse self-care as a clinical competency. Inclusion of a self-care reflection on the annual performance review demonstrates that self-care within the work environment is valued and viewed as a benchmark of clinical excellence.

Holistic leaders endorse nurses taking their breaks and choose to fund the creation of workplace renewal spaces for rest, rejuvenation, and reflection. There is a reinforcement of unit-based, self-care activities (e.g., afternoon tea time, hand/foot massage) along with the development of nurse-initiated wellness-related activities (e.g., stair-climbing for aerobic exercise, aromatherapy for stress reduction).

For Patients

First and foremost, holistic leaders uphold a culture of quality and safety through reduction of interruptions and noisy, distracting work environments. Quiet time, when lights are lowered and a restful and healing environment is designated, creates a healing healthcare environment that benefits both patients and care providers (Hedges et al., 2019). It serves as an opportunity for patients to rest and for nurses to have a respite from continuous activity.

An innovative culture and workplace environment that enhances the patient experience and patient satisfaction that embraces enrichment of the nurse–patient engagement is developed. One way in which this can be demonstrated is through the delivery of integrative therapies at the bedside. Also, a subtle shift in language from *patient-centered care* to *person-centered care* assists in viewing patients (persons) as whole human beings with rich life stories and serves to include them as partners in their plan of care.

For Holistic Nursing

Finding one's voice as a holistic nurse leader holds great potential to influence nursing and health care in a broader context by advancing the profession and enhancing the safety and quality of patient care. Articulating the principles of holistic nursing in a concise and direct manner is critical, as is providing education to promote the value of holistic nursing for improved patient outcomes and delivery of cost-effective care.

The American Holistic Nurses Association (AHNA) board of directors adopted the *AHNA Advocacy Policy Platform & Purpose Statement*, which "guides our responses towards proposed federal statutory or regulatory initiatives and national policy movements that impact nursing and specifically holistic nursing" (Roberts, 2019). The AHNA provides holistic nurses with the necessary information, tools, and resources to act as ambassadors and influential champions for AHNA and holistic nursing—from the boardroom, to social media, to developing local and national strategies for holistic nursing implementation.

For the Community

Holistic leaders envision beyond the borders of their healthcare organization by building collaborative relationships and partnerships with community organizations. This is done by recognizing the importance of forming networks with other organizational leaders to promote community-based health and wellness educational programs and services.

For the Earth

The AHNA, with an eye on population health, includes an environmental standard in the *Scope and Standards of Practice*, stating that "the registered nurse integrates the principles of environmental health for nursing in all areas of practice" (American Holistic Nurses Association & American Nurses Association, 2019, p. 57). Holistic leaders demonstrate awareness of the influence their organization has on the health of the community and planet Earth by taking the bold, progressive stance of including environmental health as a nurse competency. For example, clinical nurses are expected to promote "a practice environment that reduces environmental health risks of workers and healthcare consumers" and participate "in strategies to promote healthy communities" (American Holistic Nurses Association & American Nurses Association, 2019, p. 110).

The Alliance of Nurses for Healthy Environments calls on nurses from around the world to unite to address climate justice: "Climate justice nursing addresses the social, racial, economic, environmental, and multi-species justice issues of the climate crisis through centering the experiences and knowledges of frontline and fenceline communities and safeguarding the rights of Nature to achieve planetary health" (Alliance of Nurses for Healthy Environments, 2024). For nursing, climate justice actions demand meaningful involvement of all voices in addressing environmental threats.

Holistic Leader as Cultural Transformational Agent

> Moving from a "chain of command" to a "web of influence." (Andrus, 2011, p. 55)

A cultural transformational agent, as defined at the start of this chapter, is an individual who holds the vision for and works to actualize a plan to transform the culture of an organization to become a caring, healing environment. An embodiment and actualization of all of the identified core characteristics of a holistic leader are critical to effect organizational culture change: being visionary, an inspirational presence, a role model, a mentor, a champion for clinical excellence, and a courageous advocate—all with the intention of cocreating an inspiring and engaging work environment that supports nurse well-being, nurse–patient engagement, and a collaborative partnership among healthcare providers.

The overarching key to cultural transformation is the cultivation of a therapeutic healing environment for nurses and patients in which fostering quality relationships becomes the primary focus: the relationship nurses have with themselves, their colleagues, their patients, and with the profession of nursing.

Nursing Situation

Holistic Caring Process

Dana has been a nurse manager on a busy medical-surgical unit in a 450-bed inner-city hospital for the past 2 years. She has been slowly, and intentionally, building team cohesiveness since her arrival and introducing holistic leadership as the leadership style for the unit.

An innovative hospital-wide initiative has been introduced to improve HCAHPS (Hospital Consumer Assessment of Healthcare Providers and Systems) scores with a rollout time of 3 months. The unit nurses are feeling stressed about implementing the new initiative and are complaining about having something else to add to their already busy work assignments.

Dana views the new initiative as an avenue to continue to strengthen her team and to practice the key principles of holistic leadership. Prior to introducing it to her staff, she prepared herself by taking quiet time to reflect on how best to present the initiative, understanding that how it is presented will make all the difference in receptivity. She chose to introduce the initiative in an affirming manner, inspiring everyone to approach it as an opportunity to enhance engagement and improve the quality of patient care.

This nursing situation will be presented from the perspective of the conventional nursing process (assessment, identification of patterns/challenges/needs, outcome identification, therapeutic care plan and interventions , implementation, and evaluation) and viewed through the lens of the holistic caring process. The 5-D model of appreciative inquiry will be woven throughout to demonstrate an asset-based approach to the caring process.

Holistic Assessment

- Engage in an inclusive, collaborative reflection and assessment:
    - Include full-time, part-time, day/night shift clinical nurses and nursing assistants as colleagues, partners, and community members in the process.
    - Yield a shared sense of purpose.
- Facilitate a time-regulated opportunity for colleagues to express concerns about the initiative and rollout time frame (reacting) and redirect to a proactive approach to identify a creative process for the rollout (responding).
- Empower the community to infuse the initiative with loving kindness, viewing it in a positive light and as an opportunity for professional growth and development.
- Set a team-inspired intention for the project:
    - Experience as an opportunity for grounding and centering rather than approaching the initiative only as a task to be completed.
- Envision a successful process/outcome.
- Complete the rollout plan on time.
- Work collaboratively together with ease, support, and joy.
- Review/assess past and current unit HCAHPS scores, without judgment, with rekindled interest in identifying new strategies to enhance engagement and improve quality of patient care.
- Inspire colleagues to view the initiative as an opportunity for change, not as a criticism of their practice.

- Collaboratively apply the *definition* step of the 5-D model of appreciative inquiry:
  - Define/describe the purpose and content of the initiative in commonly understood language.
  - Frame the initiative in an affirming light.
- Assess elements of structural empowerment:
  - Review policies, programs, and organizational structure that will support fulfillment of the initiative.
- Align with the care model and theory to provide a framework for assessing the initiative.

Identification of Patterns/Challenges/Needs

- Collaboratively apply the *discovery* step of the 5-D model of appreciative inquiry:
  - Discover or rediscover what already provides optimal performance.
  - Acknowledge strengths and challenges as growing edges.
- Foster inspired engagement through inclusivity of reflections and insights:
  - Creatively include all colleagues.
- Cocreate questions that inspire courageous conversations.
- Value the experience, contribution, and insight from each person.
- Identify resources/infrastructure (people, services, technology) that will support the initiative:
  - Require attendance at the professional holistic nurse practice council meeting to network with other clinical nurses.
- Select/mentor unit representatives: one registered nurse from the day shift, one registered nurse from the night shift, and one nursing assistant.
  - Select/mentor a three-person team to review the National Database of Nursing Quality Indicators data for quality improvement nurse-sensitive indicator information to inform the rollout plan.

Outcome Identification

- Collaboratively apply the *dream* step of the 5-D model of appreciative inquiry:
  - Reflection, dialogue, envision.
- Invite storytelling to inspire new creativity.
- Explore evidence-based and evidence-informed best practices:
  - Select/mentor a four-person team for research (webinars, hospital library).
- Provide unit coverage to support research process.
- Utilize out-of-the-box creative and critical thinking:
  - Record ideas and insights: storyboards, vision boards.

Therapeutic Care Plan and Interventions

- Collaboratively apply the *design* step of the 5-D model of appreciative inquiry:
  - Seek co-participation in shared decision making of the unit-based rollout plan.
- Unit representatives present to the professional holistic nurse practice council for feedback.
- Caring and business cases are identified, and both are considered integral within the rollout plan.
- Cocreate a project-based vision statement:
  - Vision statement posted in strategic locations on the unit.

Nursing Situation (Implementation)

- Collaboratively apply the *destiny* step of the 5-D model of appreciative inquiry:
  - Implementation of the rollout plan.
- Implement with enthusiasm, confidence, and commitment.
- Model and uphold self-care practices for resiliency:
  - Breaks, hand massages, tea time, aromatherapy.
  - Grounding and centering practices.
- Foster engagement, partnership, and personal/professional empowerment.

Evaluation

- Collaboratively reflect on the process, remaining open to revision as needed.
- Acknowledge and celebrate the process and outcome.

- Recognize each person for their valuable contribution.
- Include an exemplar in the mentorship program.
- Consider the possibility for unit-based research, poster presentation, and publication.
- Apply the *definition* step of the 5-D model of appreciative inquiry:
  - Begin the cycle again with intention of refining the process and preparing for future initiatives.

Holistic leaders create avenues and opportunities for *nurse empowerment* by encouraging autonomy through shifting the outmoded language of viewing nurses as *followers* to relating to them as *partners* who are vibrant contributors in evolving the culture of the organization. Participatory management through active involvement in a shared governance professional practice model is promoted to empower nurses and to enhance nurse satisfaction.

Holistic leaders develop an infrastructure for an innovative, collaborative practice environment by providing *structural empowerment* (American Nurses Credentialing Center, 2023). When nurses have a positive perception of organizational support and the work environment inspires caring and healing, they are able to place their attention on intentional engagement with their patients and colleagues. When highly engaged, nurses become partners in workforce transformation, which reignites their passion for nursing.

Implications

Holistic leadership, within the context of the work presented in this chapter, demonstrates exciting possibilities and unique opportunities for how nurses can be key contributors to the transformation of health care today. Whether as a clinical nurse, an educator, a researcher, or a policy maker, these are remarkable times to find our collective nursing voice and become involved as visionaries and agents of change.

- **Clinical practice**: Utilize the principles of holistic leadership to increase nursing structural empowerment, autonomy, and collegiality in clinical practice.
- **Education**: Provide opportunities for holistic leadership skill development to enhance readiness to demonstrate holistic leadership behaviors for new practice settings.
- **Research**: Explore the effect of the integration of the characteristics of holistic leadership and nurse satisfaction, nurse retention, and nurse–partner–colleague communication and engagement.
- **Policy**: Develop holistic leadership policies that recognize the growing influence of compassionate care and therapeutic healing environments within healthcare organizations and enhance leadership consciousness and policies that support an evolving caring–healing human–planetary paradigm.

Conclusion

Becoming a holistic leader is a process that takes practice, patience, and reflection. Although the core characteristics of holistic leadership, as identified in this chapter, are fundamentally interrelated and integral with one another, consider selecting one of these characteristics each week, and focus on strategic integration of that characteristic within nursing practice. At the end of the week, create the opportunity for reflection, considering what went well, what needs change, and how to best enrich the practice environment with creative approaches. Then, the next week, select another characteristic and continue through all the core characteristics, repeating the cycle with the intention to develop a felt experience of holistic leadership as a progressive leadership model and framework.

The development of an innovative and compelling value proposition for nursing requires nurses to play key roles in healthcare transformation. Nurses, as holistic leaders, are catalysts and architects of change, who, through the cultivation of true collaboration, contribute to the creation of an enlightened therapeutic healing environment.

References

Alliance of Nurses for Healthy Environments. (2024). *Climate Justice Agenda for Nursing.* https://envirn.org/climate-justice-agenda-for-nursing/

American Association of Critical-Care Nurses. (2024). *The AACN synergy model for patient care.* https://www.aacn.org/nursing-excellence/aacn-standards/synergy-model

American Holistic Nurses Association and American Nurses Association. (2019). *Holistic nursing: Scope and standards of practice* (3rd ed.). Nursesbooks.org.

American Nurses Association. (2023). *What is transformational leadership in nursing?* https://www.nursingworld.org/content-hub/resources/nursing-leadership/transformational-leadership-in-nursing/

American Nurses Credentialing Center. (2023). *ANCC Magnet Model–Creating a magnet culture.* https://www.nursingworld.org/organizational-programs/magnet/magnet-model/programs/magnet/magnet-model/

Andrus, V. L. (2011). Transformational leadership for organizational change. In *The integrative healing arts program training manual: Session one* (p. 55). BirchTree Center Press.

Broome, M. E. & Marshall, E. S. (2020). *Transformational leadership in nursing: From expert clinician to influential leader.* Springer.

Brown, B. (2018). *Dare to lead.* Random House.

Center for Appreciative Inquiry. (2024a). *5-D process of appreciative inquiry.* https://centerforappreciativeinquiry.net/resources/what-is-appreciative-inquiry-ai/

Center for Appreciative Inquiry. (2024b). *What is appreciative inquiry (AI)?* www.centerforappreciativeinquiry.net/more-on-ai/what-is-appreciative-inquiry-ai/

Hedges, C., Hunt, C. & Ball, P. (2019). Quiet time improves the patient experience. *Journal of Nursing Care Quality, 34*(3), 197–202.

Huang, C. A., & Lynch, J. (1999). *Tao mentoring.* Marlowe.

Kennedy, K., Leclerc, L. & Campis, S. (2022). *Human-centered leadership in healthcare: Evolution of a revolution.* Morgan and James Publishing.

Merriam-Webster. (2024a). Advocate. In Merriam-Webster.com dictionary. https://www.merriam-webster.com/dictionary/advocate

Merriam-Webster. (2024b). Courage. In Merriam-Webster.com dictionary. https://www.merriam-webster.com/dictionary/courage

Merriam-Webster. (2024c). Visionary. In Merriam-Webster.com dictionary. https://www.merriam-webster.com/dictionary/visionary

Owen, H. (1999). *The spirit of leadership: Liberating the leader in each of us.* Berrett-Koehler.

Roberts, T. (2019). Advocacy–shaping the policies that impact holistic nursing. *AHNA Beginnings, 39*(2), 4.

Rosa, W. (Ed.). (2016). *Nurses as leaders: Evolutionary visions of leadership.* Springer Publications.

Secretan, L. (1999). *Inspirational leadership: Destiny, calling and cause.* MacMillan Canada.

Shanahan, M. (2014). The BirchTree Center model: Transforming the healthcare system with heart! *Beginnings, 34*(3), 6–9, 30.

Wharton, E. (1902, November). Vesalius in Zante (1564). *North American Review, 175,* 631.

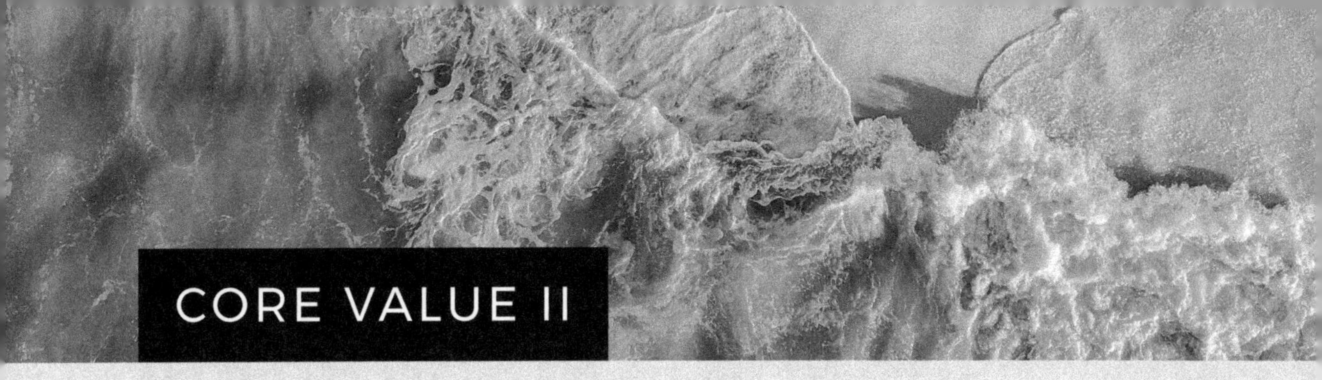

CORE VALUE II

Holistic Nurse Self-Reflection, Self-Development, and Self-Care

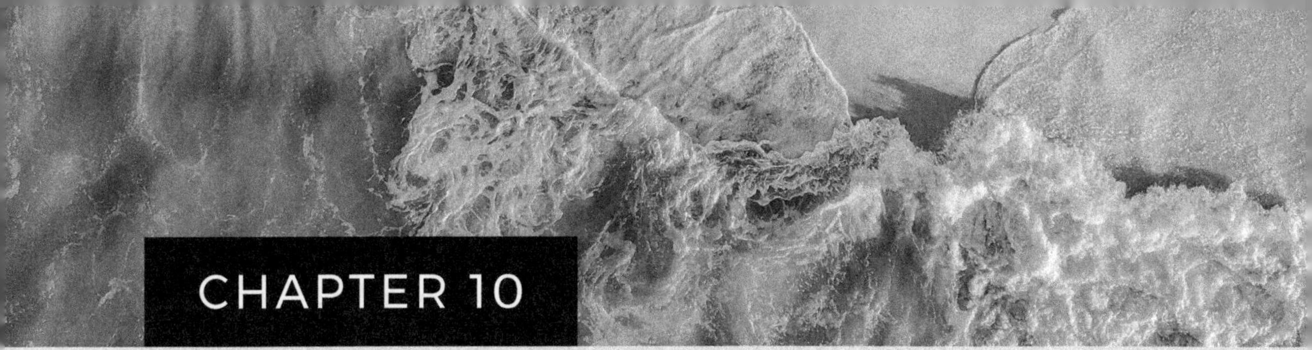

CHAPTER 10

Self-Development: The Foundation of Holistic Self-Care

Sharon Stout-Shaffer, Deborah A. Shields, and Heather Janiszewski Goodin

NURSE HEALER OBJECTIVES

- Value self-development as a moral imperative that includes caring for self, diverse populations, and the planet.
- Discuss how theory supports nurse self-development as foundational to the holistic caring process.
- Define the relationship among self-care, self-development, and use of self as an instrument of healing.
- Engage in contemplative practices required for evolving self-development, including intentional centering, attentional observation, reflective dialogue, and pattern identification/repatterning.
- Discuss how the practice of self-development informs relationships with self and relationships with others.

DEFINITIONS

Caring (healing) consciousness: An intentional state of consciousness where the being of the nurse is expressed as stable, heart-centered, and authentically present to another (achieved through centering) (Watson, 2018).

Centering: The process of being present to oneself; it involves quieting the mind and going inside to that still place within, where we are attuned to an expanded, conscious awareness of our being; it is essential for engaging in healing encounters (Waters & Daubenmire, 1997); a mind-body-spirit activity (breathing, exercise, meditation) that prepares the body to enter into caring consciousness in relationships.

Contemplation: A variety of experiential, integrated, and immersive forms of learning that lead to deep reflection, personal integration, transformative understanding and the cultivation of skills applicable to all domains of human life and constitute a critical pathway for individual and social flourishing (Center for Contemplative Mind in Society, n.d.).

Healing: Healing is an inner experience, a human potential and function, expressed as a shift in consciousness in which the practitioner and healing partner experience transformation or change; emerges when another recognizes an individual's wholeness (Hanley et al., 2017).

Health: An individually defined state or process in which the individual experiences a sense of well-being, harmony, and unity; a process of expanding consciousness (Mariano, 2022).

Inner wisdom: The innate inner knowledge or knowing that one can access through meditation, mindfulness, and other methods that expand conscious awareness.

Intention: Focusing the mind (thought) with the purpose of directing universal energy to help another. Behavior that can move one into conscious relationships; the active part of attention; using one's focused will (Hanley et al., 2017; Waters & Daubenmire, 1997).

Patterning: The continual expression of one's unique personal field in relationship with the universal energy field (Hanley et al., 2017).

Self: An individual expression or hologram of the whole; an interface between part (individual being) and whole (universal being), between personal and universal consciousness (Assagioli, 1965, 1973).

Self or *I*: A personal center of pure conscious awareness and will that act as a unifying center to integrate parts of the self into more wholeness; the core of one's being serves to connect personal consciousness and universal consciousness (Assagioli, 1965, 1973).

Self-care: Attention to specific activities such as creative expression, physical exercise, time in nature, mindfulness, and healthy eating that promote health.

Self-development: A lifeway pattern of intentional contemplative practice that integrates self-care as a means of self-healing and development of higher levels of conscious awareness of the "Beingness of the nurse"; connection to a higher purpose, and expression of higher states of consciousness such as lovingkindness, gratitude, forgiveness and compassion; development of a caring consciousness and ability to flourish; an ethical commitment of holistic nurses.

Stillpoint: The experience or inner awareness of a deep sense of openness, peace, calmness, and choice when one becomes consciously aware of the Self.

Transpersonal: A personal experience that transcends the boundaries of an individual ego identity to acknowledge and appreciate something greater than the personal self (Schaub & Schaub, 2015; Waters & Daubenmire, 1997).

Wellbecoming: Our multitude of potential life journeys toward meaning and purposefulness; a continuous process, not some steady state of managed contentment or state with a desired end point (Bartzak et al., 2023).

Well-being: An inner attitude of acceptance of the wholeness of one's being. Integrated, congruent functioning to achieve one's highest potential; may be classified as *objective* well-being (satisfaction of physical needs), and *subjective* well-being (emotional and psychological support needed to flourish) (Bartzak et al., 2023; National Academies of Sciences, Engineering, and Medicine; National Academy of Medicine; Committee on the Future of Nursing 2020–2030, 2021).

Introduction

The stressors associated with caregiving and the need to enhance nurse wellness are recognized as a national priority. Evidence clearly shows that nurse well-being is critical to the quality and safety of care, a fact underscored by the COVID-19 pandemic, which highlighted the vulnerability of clinicians working in high-stress environments. Various organizations, including the American Nurses Association (ANA), the American Holistic Nurses Association (AHNA), the American Association of Critical Care Nurses (AACN), and the National Academy of Medicine (NAM), have acknowledged the serious effects of caregiver stress and are developing policies and tools to support nurse well-being at individual, educational, and institutional levels. Additionally, *The Future of Nursing 2020–2030* emphasizes that nurses' capacity to thrive is crucial for addressing health equity, social determinants of health, and improving the overall health of the nation (American Holistic Nurses Association and American Nurses Association, 2019; Blake, 2022; National Academy of Medicine, 2021).

The ANA/AHNA Scope and Standards of Holistic Practice emphasize the importance of self-care for nurses to support the healing of others. These standards provide a foundation for nurses to promote their own well-being and, in turn, the well-being of the nation. Core Value 2: Holistic Nurse Self-Reflection, Self-Development, and Self-Care emphasizes commitment to personal self-healing and well-being practices that build our capacity to act with compassion, communicate effectively, and create healing environments. Holistic nurses view the commitment to developing their well-being as an ethic of care. Self-development is essential for effective practice within a caring science/unitary philosophy.

Self-care is commonly thought of as specific actions taken to maintain a level of personal health (physical, mental, or spiritual). While this is necessary, it is not sufficient from a holistic standpoint. This chapter defines self-development as developing a lifeway that integrates specific self-care activities with mindful reflection to deepen our understanding of ourselves. Personal self-care activities become a necessary dimension of self-healing required for self-development. Self-development leads to more conscious awareness of the Beingness of the nurse, connection to a higher purpose, and expression of higher states of consciousness such as lovingkindness, gratitude, forgiveness, and compassion in interaction with others; it expands one's caring capacity that enables self and others to flourish. It is more than personal; it is interpersonal.

Self-Development: Understanding Self-Care and Reflection from a Unitary Science Worldview

Self-development, as informed by unitary science, is based on the following theoretical assumptions:

> **Assumption 1:** There is a core essence to our being experienced as a point of stillness (stillpoint) that connects us directly to expanded levels of consciousness.
>
> **Assumption 2:** Connecting with this core essence allows us to connect with and actualize the authentic purpose of our lives.
>
> **Assumption 3:** A discipline of contemplative practice is required for self-development.

From a unitary worldview, there is no separation between us and the environment in which we exist; boundaries are nonexistent. We are not physical beings who have conscious awareness; instead, we are conscious, energetic beings embodied in physical form and at the same time connected with the energetic fields of others and the environment; thus, there is no separation between self and other. Caregiving, from this view, is a dynamic, reciprocal process rooted in compassion and responsiveness to the suffering of others; it requires intentional development of our healing consciousness through practices that build patterns of thought and the energetic frequencies with innate compassion, empathy, and felt experience of being connected to others.

Self-care can be viewed as behaviors that we do for ourselves to support overall health. This is important for holistic practice. When viewed from the lens of unitary science (holism), it requires intentional development of self-awareness, reflection, and ongoing integration of who we are, our being (Self) with our doing (self), to nurture the well-being of the whole. In other words, the quality of one's being leads the doing for self and others; there is no separation of self/other. Without this perspective, specific self-care behaviors might be good for us in some ways (e.g., daily running, weight management), but there is a risk that they become a habit pattern that provides only a superficial nurturing and does not lead to deepening levels of self-healing and well-being. Self-development means that we deepen awareness of and reflect upon our inner personal and ethical knowledge and choose intentional action from our stillpoint where we are aware of our felt senses and possibilities. The ability to consciously connect with our inner, authentic self, to hold sacred space, and to act from that level of awareness is no less important than empiric, measurable knowledge for professional nursing practice (Chinn & Kramer, 2018). Please take some time now to complete **Reflective Exercise 10-1**.

Reflective Exercise 10-1

Reflect on these words and allow their meaning to deepen in your awareness.

> *For holistic nurses, self-care is something we Want and Choose to do as a means of developing a deeper and deeper sense of well-being, growth of our potential and connection to a larger purpose—you are caring for your own being and, as you do so, you develop your capacity to care for others.*

Now, for a moment, gently close your eyes, take a deep breath, and just sense into or imagine what it feels like to be living with an ever-deepening sense of well-being. What emotions are there? Where do you feel this sense of well-being in your body? What color is it? Can you draw an image that describes it?

Reflective Exercise 10-2

Before reading further, you are invited to pause, breathe deeply, and relax. Allow yourself to just begin breathing, using a practice that helps you be aware of your breath. If you do not have regular breathing practice that is okay—just notice and pay attention to the gentle in, gentle out—the flow. Observe your breath as you notice your body relaxing; drop your awareness into your body. As your bodymind begins to relax, allow yourself to imagine the following script. When you finish, make some notes on your experience of this centered state of awareness.

Path to Center

Get in a comfortable position and take a moment to just look around the room. Really see the light, the colors, and the people. Now, take a deep breath, close your eyes, and let the visual awareness go . . .

As your visual awareness fades, be aware of the sounds in the room. Attend only to the sounds that surround you, noticing what you hear. Now, take a deep breath and let go of all sounds as you move your awareness more deeply into center.

Lightly scan your body from head to toe . . . very gently . . . and if you need to move to be more comfortable, do that now. With the next breath, let go of your body awareness and pay attention only to the breath. Just be aware of your breathing without trying to change it.

As you focus on the breath, notice any thoughts or feelings that arise and let them go. Do not hold onto them. Just let them pass through and breathe more deeply into your center of silence. Breathe into your stillpoint. Breathe in the peace and silence of this center . . . still . . . calm . . . deepening. . . sacred spaciousness.

Now notice how it feels to be you in this moment.

Self-development requires an inward journey to deepen insight and connection to the caring, energetic beings that we are. The exercises in this chapter invite you to enter a new, lifelong process to uncover those energetic patterns of thought, attitude, emotion, and behavior that are no longer useful and to intentionally develop new patterns that support your health and well-being. We invite you to journal your experience as you complete the exercises in this chapter and reflect upon what they mean to you. Enjoy your journey and be well. Please take some time now to complete **Reflective Exercise 10-2**.

The Concept of Self: Who Am I, and Why Am I Here?

Figure 10-1 provides a holistic model of Self that represents the meaning of Assumptions 1 and 2. It is provided to help you visualize the meaning and experience of that stillpoint within, your inner Being, or core essence. The term, self or I, is generally associated with the personal understanding of one's physical body and mental-emotional-spiritual personality. The work of Roberto Assagioli, the founder of psychosynthesis, offers another view of self based on consciousness that expands our understanding of who we are beyond a personal identity as physical beings. This view of self aligns with the unitary worldview and the concepts of being, sacred space, energetic connection, energetic presence, and other constructs that are integral to holistic nurses and nursing theorists.

Assagioli noticed a recurring theme in Eastern and Western philosophy regarding the essence of a *self* as an integrating center that *is* the essential individual. As a synonym for human growth, psychosynthesis views the self as the most elementary and distinctive part of our being—in other words, its core. This core is entirely different in nature from all elements (physical sensations, feelings, thoughts, desires, intuition, and so on) that make up our personality. Therefore, it acts as a unifying center, directing those elements and bringing them into unity and wholeness (Assagioli, 1965; Ferrucci, 1982).

The *self* or *I* is a personal center (conscious space) of pure awareness and *will*. Will is a fundamental inner power with tremendous unrealized potency, and it is considered the most direct expression of self. One can consciously experience the self as a center of pure awareness, and from this center we make the intentional choices that determine our life direction. With experience and practice, people develop their awareness and remain in this center in the face of extreme hardship. This experience is of being unshaken by changes in the body, feelings, mind, or environment and always self-aware and capable of choice. The self, then, represents our inner being and is experienced as we make choices from the point of inner stillness. Think of it as the "eye" of a hurricane—it is stable and calm amid chaos.

The *self*, lowercase, is understood to be a manifestation of a higher self, or *Self*, uppercase. The *Self* is described as an energetic source that is rarely experienced directly, is unaffected by the flow of the mind stream or by daily conditions, and can only be expressed through the personal self, which is accessible to direct experience (Assagioli, 1965). In other words, the Self is transpersonal and yet can become embodied through the personal choices an individual makes through activation of personal will. Just as there is a personal *will*, there is a transpersonal Will (also capitalized like the higher, transpersonal Self) that transcends the limitations of our personal self and unites with higher levels of consciousness to express Self more fully in the world; this can be equated with Maslow's self-actualization (Maslow, 1962).

Assagioli suggested that the purpose of life is to find forms for expressing the qualities emanating from the Self as we align our personal and transpersonal Will to express our higher potential. Awareness, acceptance, and integration of material from higher levels (energetic frequencies) of consciousness are as vital to our self-development as is processing material from the lower unconsciousness.

Finally, the Self is understood to be an individual expression of the whole—a universal being. Self is a hologram of the universal being and serves as an interface between part (individual being) and whole (universal being). Higher unconscious energies store tremendous potential for love, compassion, forgiveness, and other expressions of Self. The goal of psychosynthesis could be described as bridging spirit and matter, as creating a world at the personality level that is fully expressive of the person's spiritual being (Brown, 1983; Crampton, 1977). Psychosynthesis provides a psychoeducational approach to inner development and integration of individual energetic patterns into a harmonious whole (Schaub & Schaub, 2015). It is a synonym for human growth through self-development. It requires strengthening our awareness and will (attention and intention) to bring our personality functions into right relationship with the transpersonal Self and with one another. As we integrate and express the transpersonal qualities of Self (compassion, loving-kindness, forgiveness, etc.) into our personal way of being in the world; we discover our basic interdependence, our essential unity with one another; we expand our healing consciousness. **Figure 10-1** provides an image of the major concepts in Assagioli's system of thought (Assagioli, 1965, 1973).

Based on the view of self Assagioli presents, holistic self-development allows for integration of higher consciousness energy (compassion, loving kindness, forgiveness, etc.) into our personal way of being in the world. Dedicated practices are required to identify with our center of being and sustain our ability to act from this centered state of awareness. Thus, as we develop our understanding of self, we strengthen our capacity to act from the energetic qualities of being.

The process of identification is at the heart of all self-development. Who or what aspect of our personality we identify with either limits or challenges us to expand our capacities. Growth occurs as we disidentify from past limited perceptions of ourselves and our world and identify with new, more integrating ones. When we identify with our mind, our emotions, or our body, these thoughts, feelings, attitudes, physical sensations, and desires define who we think we are. Self-development—or learning to act from a centered state of awareness—requires that we disidentify from these limiting parts of ourselves and integrate these parts (thought patterns, images, etc.)

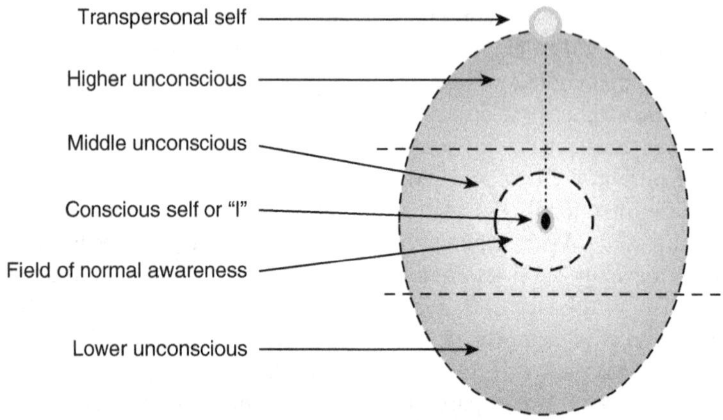

Figure 10-1 Oval diagram: Relationship between personal self and higher self.

Data from Assagoli, R. (1981). *Psychosynthesis: A manual of principles and techniques*. Middlesex, England; New York: Penguin Books.

into a larger consciousness of Self. This process of consistent identification with our center allows for the development of connection among or between parts of the whole. We develop right relationship with self, and, as Quinn suggests, right relationship to self leads to healing manifested as increased energy, coherence, and creativity in the bodymind system (Quinn, 2022). We all have the capacity for an intimate connection to the Source of all creation within ourselves. Cultivating and realizing that capacity is the ultimate purpose of our existence (Beckwith, 2013).

Reflective Exercise 10-3 is a method of letting go or disidentifying from limiting ideas of oneself and identifying with who we really are at our core, our center. Through this process, we develop the freedom of choice to be who we really are; we can more fully appreciate and use the power of our mind, body, and feelings rather than being controlled by the ever-changing nature of our thoughts and sensations (Brown, 1983). Please take some time now to complete Reflective Exercise 10-3.

Self-development, then, involves an ever-expansive awareness of and a deepening relationship with self. Reflective dialogue invites us to explore the potential meaning of the inner truths we discover and to consider patterns that support as well as hinder our growth as individuals and as holistic nurses. We connect with that sacred space of unity and stillness within—our stillpoint. How might we reach that space? We suggest that the cultivation of contemplative practice is foundational in this quest and forms the root system of the self-development process.

Self-Development and Contemplative Practices

Assumption 3: A discipline of contemplative practice is required for self-development.

Our inner being is only understood through direct experience. Contemplative practices provide direct experiential learning as we explore our inner selves; deepen awareness of our personal, aesthetic, and ethical knowledge; and intentionally develop practices that nurture our true nature (Chinn & Kramer, 2018). Centering through breath awareness, for example, allows us to move our attention inward; to pause; to become aware of and reflect upon our thoughts, emotions, and beliefs; and to choose new patterns of thinking and behavior to support our well-being. With practice, this becomes an ongoing process of well-becoming (Johns, 2021). Committing to regular contemplative practice strengthens neurological pathways that connect brain and body. Centering awareness in the stillpoint decreases sympathetic arousal associated with stress and enhances vagal (parasympathetic) balance, which calms the nervous system and connects us with right hemisphere neurocircuitry that is attuned to the

Reflective Exercise 10-3

Identification

We invite you to sit comfortably, relax your body, and allow your breathing to become slow and deep as you move into center. Read each paragraph slowly and then close your eyes and pay attention to your inner responses.

I have a body, and I value my body. I experience sensations of my body through different experiences of sickness and health, activity and rest, vigor, and tiredness. My body is my precious instrument of experience and of action, and so I treat it well and seek to keep it in good health. My body affects and expresses who I am, but it is not myself. I have a body, but I am not only a body.

I have emotions, and I value my emotions. My feelings are countless, contradictory, and changing, yet while they change, I know I always remain myself. I remain myself in times of hope or despair, in joy or pain, in a state of irritation or calm. Because I can observe and understand my emotions and then increasingly embrace and direct them, I know they are not myself. My emotions affect and express who I am, but I am not only my emotions.

I have a thinking mind, and I value my thinking mind. It is a primary tool of discovery and expression, constantly changing with new ideas, beliefs, knowledge, and experience. My mind is not the essence of my being, however, because I remain myself through all my mind's changes. My mind affects and expresses who I am but does not determine who I am. I have a thinking mind, but I am not only my thinking mind.

I have a body, emotions, and a thinking mind, and yet, I am not only these. Who am I? I am a center of consciousness and will, distinct but not separate from my body, feelings, and mind. I am *I*, capable of observing, harmonizing, and making choices about my life, my attitudes, and my actions. I am the one who is aware, the one who chooses.

Take time to honor all your experiences in this exercise. Make some notes about your experience.

present moment, to relationship, and to pattern recognition. Through regular practice, we learn to self-regulate the nervous system so that we can sustain a centered state of awareness and identify with the nonreactive, open, and nonjudgmental presence of our stillpoint. This self-regulation of the autonomic nervous system is critical to overall personal health and well-being and allows us to communicate energetically (co-regulation) to others a sense of safety and calm (Badenoch, 2023; Goleman & Davidson, 2017).

A significant body of research documents the positive impact of regular practice on health and well-being (Badenoch, 2023; Goleman & Davidson, 2017; Lomas et al., 2018; Wang et al., 2023; Wexler & Schellinger, 2023; Woods-Giscombe, 2021). Richard Davidson, director of the Center for Healthy Minds at the University of Wisconsin–Madison, has outlined four patterns of well-being that people develop through contemplative practice (Goleman & Davidson, 2017):

- Awareness—being able to pay attention, to be self-aware, and to be focused.
- Connection—cultivating emotions that underpin successful relationships with others such as kindness, gratitude, empathy, and maintaining a positive outlook.
- Insight—maintaining a healthy sense of self, the ability to deflect self-defeating narratives, and to bounce back quickly from adverse events.
- Purpose—having a clear direction and a sense that life is meaningful.

Humans are by nature relational beings, and when we develop practices that recognize our interconnectedness, we enhance our own well-being (Goleman & Davidson, 2017). Specific contemplative practices such as gratitude, loving-kindness (Metta), patience, empathy, and compassion are powerful tools for fostering well-being, resilience to stress, and generosity. When we practice gratitude and compassion, for example, we recognize the efforts that others have made on our behalf and we activate brain circuits related to loving concern for others, which helps prevent burnout, especially in caregiving professionals (Hanley, 2024).

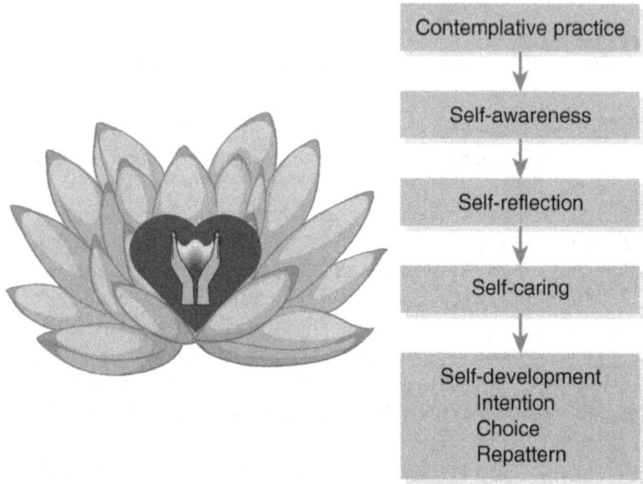

Figure 10-2 Beingcare—self-development.

Data from Shields & Stout Shaffer 2021 *Beingcare. Self-development*. Adapted from *Beingcare*. Shields. 2006.

The journey of self-development is akin to uncovering layers in our lives, revealing joy, discomfort, and insights. Contemplative practice, rooted in self-compassion and equanimity, is transformative. With deepening self-reflection, we meet ourselves where we are, listen without judgment, and develop ways to support our healing and wholeness. This shift moves us from doing self-care to self-development of our being, nurturing core resilience and embracing our imperfect selves. This is represented in **Figure 10-2** as Beingcare.

The Process of Self-Development: Pattern Recognition and Repatterning

The process of self-development emerging from contemplative practice is intentional and dynamic. It integrates personal thought patterns and behaviors leading to deeper self-awareness, and recognition of our connection with others and the environment. This deepening awareness naturally reflects the compassion and love from our heart center, cultivating personal healing and authenticity in interactions. The process is cyclical, not linear. Steps commonly used to describe the repatterning process of self-development are described below and summarized in **Table 10-1**:

1. **Centering and Grounding**: Begin by focusing attention on the stillpoint within, often using the breath as an anchor. By grounding your awareness in your body, you become attuned to internal (interoceptive) signals, like changes in stress or relaxation. This practice helps you disidentify from thoughts and emotions, allowing you to reflect on their meaning before reacting.
2. **Nonreactive (Mindful) Self-Awareness**: Mindfulness refers to the capacity to pay attention to the present moment without judgment. As you practice centering and grounding, you develop the ability to quickly re-center and observe your responses without automatically reacting.
3. **Self-Reflection and Pattern Recognition**: Nonreactive awareness allows the space for reflection and pattern recognition that helps to identify unhealthy patterns, like self-criticism, and the opportunity to consciously choose healthier responses. Through ongoing reflection, you identify and embrace patterns that are health promoting and let go of harmful patterns that do not serve growth and integration of self.

Table 10-1 Pattern Recognition and Repatterning

Key Phases	Characteristics
1. Centering and Grounding	■ Develop interoceptive awareness (body awareness; drop attention into body and focus on breath). ■ Relax and develop felt sense of being supported or connected to the earth (surface you are on; what supports you). ■ Focus, focus, focus—no judgment ■ Notice movement into the stillpoint; sense of openness to self and other. ■ Notice how it feels to be Present to Self; notice how you are more present to others.
2. Nonreactive Self-Awareness	■ Develop mindfulness over time through practice. ■ Notice the experience of observing your thoughts and feelings. ■ Practice identifying with "center" and disidentifying from negative, self-destructive thought patterns. ■ Pay particular attention to self-judgment or self-criticism that emerges and be gentle with yourself. ■ Notice how it feels, the felt sense of being connected to the heart ■ Begin to notice how others respond to you when you are centered in your heart, when you are present to self. ■ Ask the critical questions: Do I know what I do? Do I do what I know? (Chinn & Kramer, 2018)
3. Self-Reflection and Pattern Recognition	■ Pay attention to the patterns of thought and feelings that trigger negative responses when interacting with another. ■ Name the thoughts/emotions—fear, anxiety, anger—that are associated with the feelings. ■ Does this response matter; is it hurtful to self or others ? ■ What are the stories I tell myself? ■ How can I build more empowering thoughts and feelings about myself? ■ Ask how to change: What can I change, what can I accept and how do I know the difference?
4. Self-Caring and Heart Connection	■ Practice self-caring, self-forgiveness, self-compassion whenever you are aware of self-defeating thoughts, feelings, or narratives. ■ Develop the courage to authentically express your thoughts and feelings. ■ Notice when your heart feels open or closed, hurt, sad and ask yourself what you need for self-healing. ■ Develop a community of supportive peers who can support your healing.
5. Intention, Choice, and Repatterning	■ Set an intention to develop your full potential/capacity for caring. ■ Recognize you always have a choice. ■ Develop attitudes of gratitude and loving-kindness. ■ Assess where you are in developing your well-being/your ability to thrive. ■ Develop rituals that support self-care, self-reflection, and self-development. ■ What seeds are you planting and nurturing? ■ Develop practice rituals. ■ Evaluate your experiences. What is working well? What is not ?

Stout Shaffer & Shields, 2024

4. **Self-Caring and Heart Connection**: Developing a caring consciousness involves learning to love and accept yourself, including your imperfections. Awareness of self-critical thoughts signals the need for self-healing. Celebrate moments when you are gentler with yourself, as these indicate deepening self-compassion.
5. **Intention, Choice, and Repatterning**: Cultivating the ability to act with intention from a centered place is essential for creating a healing space in interactions with others (Quinn, 2022). While you may not always change a situation, you can choose how to respond in a way that empowers both yourself and others.

Holistic Caring Process: Beginning and Sustaining Your Journey

Self-development is a holistic caring process. We invite you to think of it in this poetic description "There is a song in your secret soul that cannot be silenced. It sings its existential, unceasing melody within you. Then the day comes when, through your inner work, you hear and feel the vibration of its cosmic rhythm" (Beckwith, 2013, p. 115).

Reflective Exercise 10-4 is designed to help you get started.

While there are many ways to begin, we suggest that you use the Integrative Health and Wellness Assessment (McElligott et al., 2022) in this text. This tool invites you to reflect on eight dimensions of health and wellness, consider where you are in your life, and from there, determine where you would like to be. In essence, you gently and nonjudgmentally meet yourself where you are at this moment. You can find the assessment in **Chapter 11**.

Take your time and thoughtfully complete your self-assessment. This is your dialogue with yourself, and you will notice your individual patterns. Reflect on any sensations you experience, you might feel, for example, vibrant, energized, uncomfortable, guilty, tired, steady, or anxious.

Reflective Exercise 10-4

Planting

Find a space that is comfortable and nourishing to you. Settle in and simply be for a few moments. Look around and notice what you see; listen to the space. What do you hear? Are there any aromas? Be sure to adjust yourself so that you are deeply comfortable and feel grounded. When you are ready, we invite you to do the following:

1. Take a deep breath and center your attention inward.
2. Imagine yourself holding a seed; take a moment to gaze upon it. Notice how it looks and feels, what color it is. What senses do you experience as you explore the seed?
3. As your eyes move upward, you notice a beautiful field of soil—verdant, rich, fertile. You are drawn to the earth; smell the richness of the dirt.
4. Walk to the field; in a gentle, comfortable way, lean over and scoop up a handful of soil. Let it crumble through your fingers—notice the texture, the temperature, the moisture.
5. Envision the soil as receptive—a vessel of equanimity and compassion. Sense how that knowing feels deep within you.
6. Take your seed now and nestle it into the awaiting earthen bed. Choose the depth, the position, the space of your seed.
7. Take a moment to offer nourishment to your seed: water, love, intention to grow.
8. Stay in the field as long as you should. You will know what is right for you.
9. Take a deep breath.
10. Imagine that the seed you have planted is your being, nestled in your stillpoint—safe and open—enfolded in compassion and equanimity.
11. How does this feel? Can you envision weaving contemplative practice into your life?

Your awareness is so important. Experiencing an embodied or felt sense of how these patterns affect your conscious behavior and helps you to perceive your patterns energetically. Remember that self-development invites you to accept yourself and to learn to embrace your patterns and choose actions to modify or strengthen them.

Approach your self-development with an attitude of gentle discipline. Remember that change occurs gradually; you are not likely to lose thirty pounds in 2 or 3 weeks or run a marathon without training if you have never run a block. If, however, you find that an action is not working, revise it. Always strive to notice the felt sense—the energetic response—you experience with your self-development actions.

Reassess where you are often; include both short-term (immediate feelings that reinforce your specific behavior, such as "the bubble bath was relaxing in the moment") and long-term results ("my goal of developing deeper and more restful sleep is occurring as I practice relaxation every night"). Mindful observation and reflection on your progress enhance your self-awareness; subsequently, you are more able to self-correct and discern how your self-development is progressing. As you stay the course, you become more and more observant and responsive to patterns; your embodied sense—felt sense—is shifting within you.

When we hear the word *contemplative*, we often think of meditation and prayer. We believe that contemplative practices are whatever you choose that creates the space for quiet within you. There is no right or wrong practice; each is as unique as each of you. The power of practice is your intention and your willingness to stay the course. In our busy world, it is easy to become distracted and guilty—and even to give up. Remember, contemplative practice is a gentle discipline; when you stray a bit, return with love, not self-criticism.

Table 10-2 offers some examples of contemplative practices you might consider; this is not an exhaustive list, and we encourage you to find what works for you.

It is important to choose those practices that resonate with you. Numerous chapters in this text offer ideas as you develop your plan, and we encourage you to use them. Additionally, there are numerous websites that offer tools you may find helpful in supporting your journey. Additional resources can be found on the following websites:

- American Holistic Nurses Association (AHNA) https://www.ahna.org/
- American Holistic Nurses Credentialing Corporation (AHNCC) https://www.ahncc.org/resources/self-care-response/
- The Center for Contemplative Mind in Society https://www.contemplativelife.org/body-of-practice#all

Table 10-2 Types of Contemplative Practices

Contemplative Practice Category (Examples)	Practices (Examples)
Quieting practices	Silence and breath awareness Centering and Grounding Meditation (all types) Prayer Imagery and relaxation exercises (all forms) Ritual
Creative expression	Art Writing: narrative, story, poetry, journaling Mandala Music Improvisation
Movement	Mindful walking and running Yoga, Tai Chi, Qigong, Aikido Expressive dance
Nourishment	Mindful eating Mindful drinking
Nature	Walking the labyrinth Medicine walk Sit spotting

- Center for Mindful Self-Compassion https://centerformsc.org/
- The American Nurses Foundation has produced a Gratitude Practice for Nurses Toolkit for Well-Being available online https://ggsc.berkeley.edu/gratitudefornurses
- "The Caregiver Companion," toolkit developed through support of the Samueli Foundation that has numerous exercises to support caregiver well-being https://healing-worksfoundation.org/caregiver

These websites are offered as a sampling of the work being done in contemplative practice to spark your curiosity and further exploration. Importantly, we hope that your discoveries will excite and encourage you to begin, return to, or continue contemplative practice as a foundation of your self-development. Indeed, the root system is deeply anchoring the seed of you—you, who through the journey, transforms into a beautiful flower. Please take some time now to complete **Reflective Exercise 10-5**.

Reflective Exercise 10-5

Choosing

Find a space that is comfortable and nourishing to you. Settle in and simply be for a few moments. Look around and notice what you see; listen to the space. What do you hear? Are there any aromas? Be sure to adjust yourself so that you are deeply comfortable and feel grounded. When you are ready, we invite you to do the following:

1. Take a deep breath and center your attention inward.
2. Imagine the seed you have planted earlier, your being, nestled in your stillpoint—safe and open—enfolded in compassion and equanimity.
3. Choose a contemplative practice that resonates with you.
4. See yourself engaged in that practice every day.

Notice that every day, there are more and more roots emanating from your seed—from you. They are spreading and rooting deeply into the soil of equanimity and compassion. How does that feel?

Holistic Caring Process: Continuing the Path of Self-Development

Self-development is a complex, exciting, and challenging undertaking. Sustaining the practices may seem difficult at times. While there are moments of pure joy and celebration, there can be bumps and detours along the way. Remember, this is a journey and it can take time for new patterns to become part of your lifeway; be aware, but do not criticize yourself; just keep recommitting and trust that you are evolving toward greater wholeness. We offer the following thoughts that you may find helpful as you stay the course, never giving up on you!

1. **Purpose:** Recognize that contemplative practice is foundational to self-development; it is the path to your stillpoint. Explore quieting activities and select one or two that speak to you; choose activities that are spiritually comfortable and interesting.
2. **Set time for practice.** It is helpful to carve out a bit of time on a regular schedule to practice; initially, that may be for just a few minutes daily. Try not to get caught in the linear time roadblock but rather immerse yourself in the experience. Be aware of what you are noticing: What is your felt sense? What does stillness feel like for you?
3. **Consider where you practice.** What is comfortable for you? Can you name a designated space that would support you on your path to stillness? The environment is important, but, again, try to avoid those roadblocks of needing certain props; you know where you feel best. This is the perfect place to begin your practice.
4. **Reflect on Practice**: Notice when thoughts of guilt (for taking this time when there is so much to do), need (more time, equipment, space), and even frustration (having thoughts such as, "I cannot quiet my mind," "I am never going to get this," "I am not an artist," "I cannot even draw a straight line") appear. Bear witness to your discomfort: What are you discovering about you?

5. **Breath breaks**: When it is difficult to carve out time—or even as you move through your day—begin to appreciate the stillness and immediate connection to your being that is offered with a few deep breaths. The beauty of this is that we must breathe, so this is a matter of momentarily shifting our attention to stillness to reap the benefits of the breath break.
6. **Journal**: There is much power in writing and/or drawing your practice experience. This might take the form of narrative, poetry, or some other creative expression. It is a record of *your* journey—for you. Often, rereading our journals illuminates deeper understanding and insights.
7. **Community**: Although self-development is a personal journey, your ability to stay the course may be strengthened by joining with others who share the same goal. The walker mentioned earlier may benefit from having a walking partner or from becoming part of a group activity (e.g., triweekly walks along the local bike path or at the local gym).
8. **Retreats**: These getaways are valuable if they are within your desire and ability to participate in them. There are numerous retreat venues; some are for quiet practice, others are with activities in mind, and many integrate both.
9. **Coach, guide, friend**: It is wonderful to have the support of another as you live your self-development experience. It is also important to seek professional counseling if needed; sometimes, our coaches and friends realize this is needed and guide us toward appropriate professional resources.
10. **Be attentive to your needs:** Recognize whether you may want to seek professional help if your patterns are particularly hard to break or if you are experiencing anxiety and difficulty in determining how to approach them. Please accept who you are, where you are.

Just as the journey begins with one step, our commitment to self-development will create pathways to support change in our practice and the healthcare environment. Holistic nurses understand the importance of supporting others in their self-development journey. With commitment to self-development, we integrate this knowledge and skills into our holistic nursing practice. Being present to those we serve in our practice, to colleagues, and to our earth is essential in health promotion and well-being.

Nursing Situation

Carlos M is a first-year nursing student at a small university that has been accredited by the American Holistic Nurses Credentialing Center. He enrolls in a class that focuses on the development of college success and personal well-being. He is a first-generation college student and entering the university was a little intimidating; however, Carlos is extremely strong, he works out regularly, has developed good study habits, and considers himself healthy. He works part time.

Carlos learned about the importance of taking care of oneself as an ethic of care; he learned several breath awareness centering skills and committed to practicing mindful centering 5 days a week for 10 minutes. He began to practice several other contemplative centering practices such as mindful walking in nature and journaling his thoughts and feelings. He practiced the identification guided-imagery exercise several times and began to experience what it means to mentally disconnect from the body, the mind, the emotions and connect with the felt sense of a deeper self. Gradually as he journaled, he became more aware of physical sensations, thoughts, and feelings, and this led to an awareness of a sense of loneliness, lack of connection to others, and some underlying thought patterns about not knowing how to be successful in college because of his family background. After completing his Integrative Health and Awareness Assessment, Carlos realized that he needed to develop his ability to connect with peers, support them, and be supported by them; he set this intention and began to walk that path. Carlos also actively tried to notice every negative thought pattern about non-success and change the thought to a positive affirmation of being successful. He recognized from his journal that he was developing "Pillars of a Healthy Mind": becoming more aware of his thoughts and behavior, cultivating successful relationship patterns and insight on how to change self-defeating patterns of thought. At the end of the semester, several classmates agreed to develop a long-term support network to help each other continue their self-development journey.

Implications

The practice of self-development as defined in this chapter is critically important to you, your colleagues, and the future of nursing. Given what is known about the significant impact of contemplative practices on personal well-being, the neurobiology of stress resilience and energetic renewal, and the mental capacity to remain focused and calm in chaotic situations while remaining compassionate and present to another, committing to ongoing self-development is considered an ethical imperative. Self-care has evolved from a central focus on the body and physical wellness to a deeper expression of our inner being. This is reflected in the writing of great minds from many different disciplines including nursing, neurobiology, psychoneuroimmunology, psychology, theology, and existential and esoteric philosophy.

- **Clinical Practice**: Observe your practice change over time. Nurses must appreciate the relationship between personal self-development and the provision of safe, quality nursing care. By learning to consciously slow the breath, center awareness, and regulate neurons in the body, you can intentionally change the interaction to communicate a sense of safety to client, with full presence and awareness of their needs. Notice how clients respond. As we stand in a state of "safety or calmness" at a nervous system level, this message is communicated to the client through tone of voice, the look in our eyes, and tension in our body and they feel safe (Badenoch, 2023).
- **Education**: Self-development for students must begin early in the educational program and be integrated into all courses; students need to receive course credit for self-development practice. Educators are called upon to develop experiential learning practices that develop personal, ethical, and aesthetic patterns of knowing; use of a diversity of unitary patterning processes such as meditation, visualization, imagery, therapeutic touch, motion, and the use of art, poetry writing, and storytelling will become more prominent in education, practice and research (Bartzak et al., 2023).
- **Research**: Research on self-care has not been tied to the more holistic process of self-development. Future research is needed to document this relationship and its effect on nurse well-being and perceived agency or power to participate in change. This research needs to include collection and analysis of nurses' stories. Neurobiology suggests that contemplative practices build the bodymind connections known to have a significant impact on nurse well-being and quality of care. Additional research is needed in this area.
- **Policy**: Leaders in all settings need to assume accountability for developing a culture of well-being. Although nurses are not solely responsible for creating healthy work environments, they must advocate for organizational support that address key issues such as work–life balance, collegial relationships, and whole person health (Jarden et al., 2021).
- **Global Health:** Significant data has established the relationship between personal and environmental health and health equity. Self-development sensitizes one to the felt sense, the experience, of being interrelated to everything in our environment and one begins to understand more clearly how our energetic patterns of thought affect the planet and planetary health. National and international nursing organizations need to consider advocating for self-development as a key step in evolving planetary health.

Conclusion

Self-development has evolved over the years and is now recognized as foundational to holistic practice. Self-development is a rhythm, and you are invited to find yours. There are ups and downs, and that is okay. Practices can be joyous and/or challenging, and, with an open heart, we learn from these experiences. As we move to that place of being able to let go—to not be attached to the outcomes—we live the experience.

Reflective Exercise 10-6

Developing

Find a space that is comfortable and nourishing to you. Settle in and simply be for a few moments. Look around and notice what you see; listen to the space. What do you hear? Are there any aromas? Be sure to adjust yourself so that you are deeply comfortable and feel grounded. When you are ready, we invite you to do the following:

1. Take a deep breath and center your attention inward.
2. Imagine the seed you have planted with all its roots, your being, nestled in your still point—safe and open—enfolded in compassion and equanimity.
3. Imagine completing a holistic self-assessment—notice what speaks to you. Are there any patterns being revealed?
4. Choose a holistic self-care action that resonates with you.
5. See yourself engaged in that action every day.
6. Notice that every day you are emerging higher and higher from the soil; see yourself as a flower bud, beginning to open, ever expansive.
7. See the beautiful flower that you are.
8. How does that feel?

Please take some time to complete **Reflective Exercise 10-6**. You are now the blossoming flower grown from the seed that you planted earlier in the rich soil of equanimity and compassion. Celebrate that! Congratulations on choosing you!

Flocks of geese soar
into rosygolden horizons
of the setting sun
they dance in the brilliance
unique . . . unified
reminding us . . .
the adventure is lifelong
All is . . .

References

American Holistic Nurses Association and American Nurses Association. (2019). *Holistic nursing: Scope and standards of practice* (3rd ed.). Nursesbooks.org.

Assagioli, R. (1965). *Psychosynthesis: A manual of principles and techniques*. Hobbs, Dorman.

Assagioli, R. (1973). *The act of will*. Viking Press.

Badenoch, B. (2023). *The heart of trauma: Healing the embodied brain in the context of relationships*. W.W. Norton & Co.

Bartzak, P., Butcher, H., Flanagan, J., Jones, D., Larkin, D., Malinski, V., Reed, S., & Smith, M. (2023). *Evolving Rogerian science: John R Phillips' unique contributions*. Society of Rogerian Scholars.

Beckwith, M. B. (2013). *Life visioning: A transformative process for activating your unique gifts and highest potential*. Sounds True.

Blake, N. (2022). Future of nursing 2020-2030: Supporting the health and well-being of nurses. *AACN Advanced Critical Care, 33*(1), 99–102.

Brown, M. (1983). *The unfolding self: Psychosynthesis and counseling*. Psychosynthesis Press.

Center for Contemplative Mind in Society. (n.d.). https://www.contemplativelife.org/practice/the-center-for-contemplative-mind-in-society/all/teaching-learning.

Chinn, P., & Kramer, M. K. (2018). *Integrated theory and knowledge development in nursing* (10th ed). Elsevier.

Crampton, M. (1977). *Psychosynthesis: Some key aspects of theory and practice*. Canadian Institute of Psychosynthesis.

Ferrucci, P. (1982). *What we may be: Techniques for psychological and spiritual growth*. J.P. Tarcher, Inc.

Goleman, D. & Davidson, R. (2017). *Altered traits: Science reveals how meditation changes your mind, brain, and body*. Penguin Random House LLC.

Hanley, A. (2024). A comprehensive resource for nurses' well-being. *American Nurses Journal, 19*(2), 42.

Hanley, M. A., Coppa, D., & Shields, D. (2017). A practice-based theory of healing through Therapeutic Touch: Advancing holistic nursing practice. *Journal of Holistic Nursing, 35*(4), 369–381.

Jarden, R., Jarden, A., & Gerdtz, M. F. (2021). New graduate nurse wellbeing, work wellbeing and mental health: A systematic review. *International Journal of Nursing Studies, 121*, 103997.

Johns, C. (2021). *Reflexive narrative, self inquiry, toward self-actualization and its performance*. SAGE Publications Inc.

Lomas, T., Medina, J. C., Ivtzan, I., Rupprecht, S., & Eiroa-Orosa, F. (2018). A systematic review of the impact of mindfulness on the well-being of healthcare professionals. *Journal of Clinical Psychology, 74*(3), 319–355. https://doi.org/10.1002/jclp.22515

Mariano, C. (2022). Holistic nursing: Scope and standards of practice. In B. M. Dossey, L. Keegan, (Authors) M. Blaszko Helming, D. Shields, & K. Avino, W. Rosa (Eds.), *Holistic nursing: A handbook for practice* (8th ed., pp. 25–52). Jones & Bartlett Learning.

Maslow, A. (1962). *Toward a psychology of being*. VanNostrand. https://doi.org/10.1037/10793-000

McElligott, D., Avino, K., Dossey, B., & Luck, S. (2022). Self-assessments. In B. M. Dossey, L. Keegan (Authors), M. Blaszko Helming, D. Shields, & K. Avino, W. Rosa (Eds.), *Holistic nursing: A handbook for practice* (8th ed., pp. 199–212). Jones & Bartlett Learning.

National Academies of Sciences, Engineering, and Medicine; National Academy of Medicine; Committee on the Future of Nursing 2020–2030; Flaubert, J. L., Le Menestrel, S., Williams, D. R., Wakefield, M. K., (Eds.). (2021). *The Future of Nursing 2020-2030: Charting a Path to Achieve Health Equity*. National Academies Press (US). https://pubmed.ncbi.nlm.nih.gov/34524769/

Quinn, J. F. (2022). Transpersonal human caring and healing. In B. M. Dossey, L. Keegan, (Authors) C. Barrere, M. Blaszko Helming, D. Shields, & K. Avino (Eds.), *Holistic nursing: A handbook for practice* (8th ed., pp. 97–106). Jones & Bartlett Learning.

Schaub, R., & Schaub, B. G. (2015). *Transpersonal development: Cultivating the human resources of peace, wisdom, purpose, and oneness*. Murray Court.

Wang, S. C., Hu, W. Y., Lalande, L., Chang, J. C., Tsai, S. Y., Chang, S. C., & Wen, T. K. (2023). Evaluation of guided respiration mindfulness therapy (GRMT) for reducing stress in nurses. *Journal of Holistic Nursing, 41*(2), 155–167. https://doi.org/10.1177/08980101221094973

Waters, P., & Daubenmire, M. J. (1997). Therapeutic capacity: The critical variance in nursing practice. In P. Kritek (Ed.), *Reflections on healing: A central nursing construct* (pp. 55–67). National League for Nursing.

Watson, J. (2018). *Unitary caring science*. University Press of Colorado.

Wexler, T. M., & Schellinger, J. (2023). Mindfulness-based stress reduction for nurses: An integrative review. *Journal of Holistic Nursing, 41*(1), 60–61.

Woods-Giscombe, C. L. (2021). An innovative program to promote health promotion, quality of life, and wellness for School of Nursing faculty, staff, and students: Facilitators, barriers, and opportunities for broad system-level and cultural change. *Archives of Psychiatric Nursing, 35*(2), 185–188. https://doi.org/10.1016/j.apnu.2020.10.018

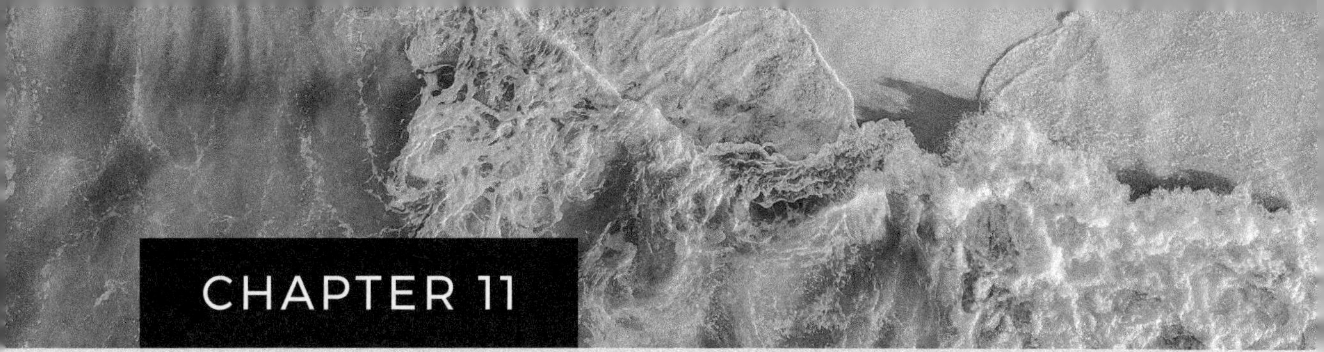

CHAPTER 11

Integrative Self-Assessment

Karen M. Avino and Deborah McElligott

NURSE HEALER OBJECTIVES

- Identify national initiatives for health and well-being and their applications for holistic nurses.
- Describe the Integrative Health and Wellness Assessment (IHWA) and its eight dimensions.
- Apply the use of the IHWA for patients who wish to self-assess and create goals to improve their health-promoting behaviors.
- Use self-assessments to guide your wellbecoming journey.

DEFINITIONS

Healing: A process of bringing into harmony and inner knowledge that leads to integration; involves an emerging pattern of relationships among elements of the whole person, leading to increased integrity, connection, and cohesion; an emergent process of the entire system that brings aspects of the self to deeper levels of inner knowing, leading to a positive, subjective process involving transformation to a new sense of wholeness, spiritual transcendence, and reinterpretation of life.

Health: A subjective sense of well-being, harmony, and unity by an individual or community supported by the experience of health beliefs and values being honored; a process of opening and widening awareness and consciousness (Office of Disease Prevention and Health Promotion [ODPHP], n.d.).

Self-efficacy: The belief that one can initiate and sustain desired behaviors with a sense of empowerment to make healthful choices that lead to enduring change.

Well-being: A static inner attitude of health and feelings of comfort and harmony in the present.

Wellbecoming: A lifelong process through which one knowingly participates in changing patterns and manifestations of wholeness and healing (Gordon & France, 2023, p. 4).

Holistic Nurses, Healthy People, and a Healthy World

It is commonly known that 21st-century conversations and initiatives focus on health promotion through healthy lifestyles, disease prevention through risk reduction, and living with chronic disease. Internationally, nurses who practice a holistic philosophy are at the forefront of this initiative, fostering change to improve the spectrum of health care, health delivery, and the lifelong health of all populations in every nation. By implementing health and wellness assessments, holistic nurses begin their self-development journey and can model that practice for others.

In 1979, the Healthy People Initiative began in the United States and continues to develop a new set of evidence-based objectives every 10 years (ODPHP, n.d.). The initiative provides a strategic framework for a national agenda and vision for holistic nurses to be pioneers on the frontier of our nation's healthcare reform, aligning with objectives and developing programs to meet the identified needs. Over the past four decades, the topic areas have increased from 15 to 42.

The Healthy People 2030 vision is to create a "society in which all people can achieve their full potential for health and well-being across the lifespan," with a mission that includes promoting, strengthening, and evaluating "the nation's efforts to improve the health and well-being of all people" (ODPHP, n.d.). The role of holistic nurse partnerships in all practice settings can support the Healthy People 2030 goals through the sharing of nursing knowledge, skills, and vision.

The National Prevention Strategy (U.S. Department of Health and Human Services, 2011) aims to improve the health and quality of life for individuals, families, and communities by shifting the nation's focus from sickness and disease to prevention and wellness. Holistic nurses are well-positioned to support national healthcare change efforts with practical strategies for lifestyle change.

Aligning with national efforts, the American Nurses Association (ANA, 2025) launched *Healthy Nurse, Healthy Nation*, designed to improve nurses' health. The aim is to engage nurses as educators and advocates for health on three levels: individual, organizational, and interpersonal. These three levels position holistic nurses to be leaders in these efforts.

The Healthy Nurse, Healthy Nation survey identified six vital areas to improve healthy behaviors: (1) physical activity, (2) rest, (3) nutrition, (4) quality of life, (5) safety, and (6) mental health. As a result, a healthy nurse population will create a healthier workforce; effective, safe, and sustainable health care; and be role models of health to others.

The World Health Organization (WHO, 2019) has included burnout of healthcare providers (ICD-11 QD85) in the 11th revision of the *International Classification of Diseases* (ICD-11) as an occupational phenomenon. Burnout is a syndrome conceptualized in ICD-11 resulting from chronic workplace stress that has not been successfully managed and is considered a factor influencing health status or contact with health services. In addition, the National Academy of Medicine's (NAM, 2019) *Action Collaborative on Clinician Well-Being and Resilience* reports that clinician well-being is essential for safe, high-quality patient care. This was followed in 2022 by the *National Plan for Health Workforce Well-Being* to restore the nation's health through collective action to strengthen health workforce well-being (NAM, 2022). In response to that paper, the American Holistic Nurses Association (AHNA) published a toolkit for organizations highlighting tools and programs to assist with healthcare workforce well-being (AHNA, 2023).

For healthcare professionals to help meet the national agenda of health promotion, the self-development, self-assessment, and self-care of healthcare providers is essential. Self-assessment is critical to individual, organizational, local, and global well-being. Many tools assess individual components and perceptions of wellness. AHNA recognizes that *Cultivating a Holistic Personal Practice* is essential and highlights various self-assessment tools to begin that process. The Integrative Health and Wellness Assessment (Dossey et al., 2015), highlighted in the kit from AHNA, is used by healthcare providers to support self-awareness and attention to improve healthy behaviors, ultimately supporting resiliency. This chapter will focus on whole-person assessment using the IHWA.

Integrative Health and Wellness Assessment

Holistic nurses recognize that integrative assessments foster awareness and choices that support healthy lifestyle behaviors, well-being, and healing. They use evidence-based nursing theories and validated tools to guide and measure the assessments in their practice.

Dossey et al. (2015) stated the IHWA long tool was developed to assess eight areas of wellness based on review of previously developed assessment tools, nursing theories, and the authors' years of clinical experience. The tool was initially developed with 139 questions and then validated by John Nelson in 2012, with a total of 132 Likert-type scale questions retained for the form.

The role of the nurse coach led to the development of a shorter form of 36 questions based on dimensions of wellness outlined by the Theory of Integrative Nurse Coaching using guidelines provided by DeVellis (2012). Pilot testing results of the short IHWA resulted in a Bartlett's test of sphericity that was significant, a Cronbach alpha overall scale of internal consistency of 0.88 (n = 36), and a Kaiser–Meyer–Olkin test that yielded a value of 0.520. This pilot indicated that the scale could be improved through additional revision (McElligott et al., 2018).

In 2022, Kenefick-Moore, Avino, and McElligott completed a factor analysis of the IHWA, and the IHWA 2.0 version was created. Using the IHWA allows clients to increase awareness of the eight dimensions of the whole person and be active participants in increasing health-promoting behaviors.

Integrative assessment is the process of going beyond the physical and mental realms. It involves partnering with the patient or self to reflect and identify patterns, concerns, and opportunities that support wholeness and meaning. This process is supported by the Grand Theory of Integrative Nurse Coaching and the IHWA long v. 2 and the IHWA short v. 2 forms.

The subscales of the IHWA involve eight dimensions: (1) life satisfaction, (2) relationships, (3) spirituality, (4) mental, (5) emotional, (6) physical (nutrition, exercise, weight), (7) environmental, and (8) health responsibility. All components of the self are interwoven and constantly interacting within the person's internal and external environment. Refer to **Figure 11-1**.

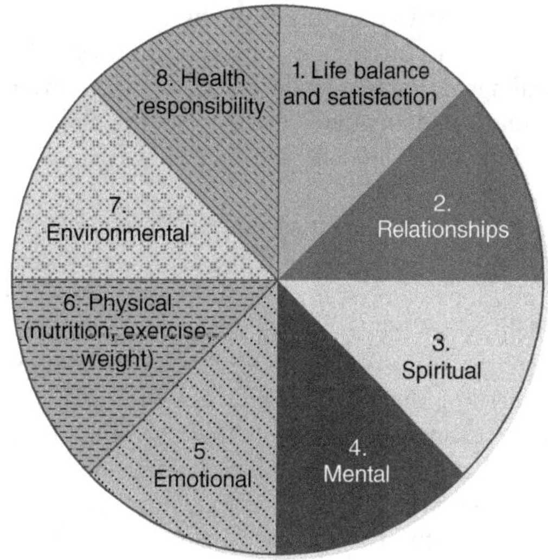

Figure 11-1 Integrative Health and Wellness Assessment (IHWA) wheel.

Used with permission: Integrative Nurse Coach Academy (2022). www.iNurseCoach.com.

The IHWA Tool assists people in becoming aware of their human potential in each category, identifying strengths and weaknesses while reflecting on their desire to create new health goals. The IHWA tool can be requested for use at IHWA.inursecoach.com.

The IHWA short form provides a brief way to begin a conversation on integrative assessment of the eight areas of wellness. The nurse's self-development parallels the patient's process, as the nurse focuses on their health and wellness from the same integral perspective. Creating the time for the nurse to practice self-development is essential. This is achieved through integrating body, mind, and spirit practices/skills; practicing integrative health knowledge; and enacting nutritional, psychological, and other integrative resources.

The IHWA short form can be provided to the patient to complete in advance of any sessions. While the tool may be scored, the score does not determine where the patient begins; this is determined by the patient regarding what is most important to them at that moment. The patient can identify barriers, discover solutions, and reach goals by starting with their own priority. The nurse skillfully creates and holds sacred space in which the patient feels trust and respect; feels listened to and not judged. In the following sections, each of the eight IHWA components is explored.

Life Satisfaction

Reflecting on life satisfaction includes identifying joys and possibilities and increasing awareness and choices that may enhance capacity, human potential, and the healing process. It attunes individuals to their healing awareness, an innate quality that everyone is born with. The healing process includes self-assessment and self-reflection to recognize feelings, attitudes, emotions, and other dimensions of wellness that are translated into our total being. Recognizing and celebrating the joys and good things in life add to experiencing life satisfaction. Life is a journey. With willingness to be present for all this life journey brings, the individual can cultivate the ability to be fully in the moment during the transformative healing process.

Assessing life satisfaction acknowledges capacity for conscious and unconscious choices. Conscious choices involve awareness and skills such as self-reflection, self-care, discipline, persistence, goal setting, priority setting, action steps, discerning the best options, and acknowledging and trusting perceptions. Both nurses and clients can be active participants in daily life, not passive observers who hope life will benefit them.

The unconscious also plays a significant role in choices. Jung (1980) conceived the unconscious as a series of layers and believed that psychic energy can become unbalanced. One of life's most significant challenges is to achieve a dynamic balance of the innate opposites and make this balancing process as conscious as possible.

Life satisfaction supports the awareness of work–life harmony, realizing that an exact balance is not always possible. Life is interconnected and part of our whole. The concepts of crossover or spillover, where others feel the effects of the workplace, and where the effects of the workplace are felt at home, are just two concepts that recognize this often-subconscious impact. Identifying these concepts by assessing work and life responsibilities and recognizing choices enable individuals to respond instead of reacting to life's challenges, enhancing satisfaction.

Relationships

Healthy people live in intricate networks of relationships and are always in search of unifying new concepts of the universe and social order. Meaningful relationships develop from understanding and nurturing those relationships, whether at work, at home, in the community, in organizations, through the ever-expanding web of electronic connection, or others worldwide.

Relationships have different levels of meaning, from the superficial to the deeply connected, and the challenges facing these relations can be multifaceted. In assessing relationships, the nurse and/or client begins with themself and explores what they hope for, what they can bring to life, and how they engage. How do they discern and decide when to exchange feelings of honesty, trust, intimacy, compassion, openness, and harmony? Assessment of relationships involves identifying both cohesiveness and disharmony and the effect of attitudes, healing awareness, and concern for self and others. Sharing life processes requires truthful and caring self-reflection and communication with others throughout the life spectrum, from the home to the workplace and to the community, whether physically or via social media. Individuals must realize that what they do locally influences the larger community—the nation and planet. Each person can take an active role in developing local networks from their relationship with self, family, and workplace teams, and these networks can have a ripple effect on local to global health concerns.

Spirituality

Throughout history, there has been a quest to understand the purpose of the human life experience. Assessing aspects of an individual's spiritual nature can be a profound learning opportunity.

Spirit comes from the individual's roots—it is a universal need to understand the human experience. It is a vital element and driving force in how people live their lives, affecting every aspect of their life satisfaction and the degree to which they develop their human potential. Usually, though not universally, spirituality involves a sense of connection with an absolute, imminent, or transcendent spiritual force, however named, and includes the conviction that ethical values, direction, meaning, and purpose are valid aspects of the individual and universe. The essence of being and relatedness permeates life and manifests in one's knowing, doing, and being. This interconnectedness with self, others, nature, and God/life force/absolute/transcendent is not necessarily synonymous with religion. Religion is the codified and ritualized beliefs and behaviors of those involved in spirituality, usually in a community of like-minded individuals (refer to **Chapter 7** on spirituality).

Spirit involves the development of our higher self, also called the "transpersonal self." A transpersonal experience (i.e., transcendence) is a feeling of oneness, inner peace, harmony, wholeness, and connection with the universe. The meaning and joy that flow from developing this aspect of human potential allow individuals to have a transpersonal view. Humans may know this transcendence through prayer, meditation, organized religion, philosophy, science, poetry, music, inspired friends, and group work.

A person's spiritual potential only develops with attention. Every day, with each of their experiences, they must acknowledge that spiritual potential is essential to developing a healthy value system. This system shapes their perception of the world and influences their experiences positively or negatively. Even through the pain and suffering of a negative experience (physical, mental, emotional, relational, or spiritual), humans can grow and transform that suffering through the healing process. The consequences of healing may involve the individual or a relationship and often include serenity, gratitude, interconnectedness, new meaning, purpose, and inner peace.

Mental

The WHO (n.d.) defines mental health as "a state of well-being in which an individual realizes his/her abilities, can cope with the normal stresses of life, can work productively, and can contribute to their community" (WHO, 2019). While one of the IHWA eight dimensions of wellness, "it is determined by a complex interplay of individual, social and structural stressors and vulnerabilities" (WHO, 2025).

Assessing mental capacity helps individuals examine their belief systems. In early life, individuals have role models who influence their beliefs, thoughts, behaviors, and values. With maturity and due to life experiences, they recognize shifts in these beliefs, thoughts, behaviors, and values and the conflicts that may arise from those shifts.

As individuals strive to perceive the world with greater clarity, they may recognize the variety of perspectives in the world. Through both logical and nonlogical mental processes, they become aware of a broad range of subjects that have the potential to enhance their full appreciation of the many great pleasures in life. Interventions such as meditation and mindfulness support being present at the moment nonjudgmentally, thus expanding mental knowing. Focus shifts from fear-based, negative thought patterns and becomes more open and receptive to life-affirming information and thought patterns. Therapies such as cognitive behavioral therapy assist individuals in assessing the feelings and behaviors attached to thoughts and reframe them more positively, supporting healing and well-being. Neuroplasticity is the brain's capacity to continue growing and evolving in response to life experiences. It highlights human abilities to change previous reactive patterns and develop new life-affirming pathways through various therapies, mindfulness, and meditative practices.

Emotional

Assessing emotional potential assists individuals in their willingness to acknowledge the presence of feelings, value them as important information, and express them. Emotional health implies that people have the choice and freedom to process and express the full spectrum of emotions, including love, joy, guilt, forgiveness, fear, and anger. Expressing these emotions provides immediate feedback about the individual's inner state, which may be crying out for a new way of being.

Emotions are responses to and are affected by the events in an individual's life as they constantly interact with their environment. These interactions may bring joy or varying degrees of chronic anxiety, depression, worry, fear, guilt, anger, denial, failure, or repression. There is no good or bad emotion; each is part of the human condition.

Emotions exist as the light and shadow of the self; thus, individuals must acknowledge all of them. People can only identify the light because they know its opposite, the shadow. When individuals recognize the value in both emotions, they can gain new insight and understanding and make more effective choices. As individuals focus on body-mind-spirit interrelationships, they can focus on the emotions that move them toward wholeness and inner understanding. Increasing emotional potential allows openness, creativity, and spontaneity to be experienced, further developing their humanness and recognizing emotions as gifts.

As the world deals with compassion fatigue, burnout in healthcare professionals, and the impact of chronic disease, a focus on the emotional stress response is vital. The global community recommends stress management and many integrative therapies focus on stress management techniques, treatments, and programs to support resilience and decrease stress. While many of these modalities have roots in ancient healing traditions, new fields of modalities are being developed and researched.

The area of emotional intelligence is receiving attention in the development of both leaders and healthcare staff. Emotional intelligence is defined as a set of core emotional abilities enabling one to interpret and respond to one's emotional states and those of others to shape thought and behavior adaptively. According to Goleman (2020), the four domains of emotional intelligence include self-awareness (recognizing the emotional state of self and others), self-regulation (using emotions to facilitate thought and behavior), social awareness (understanding how emotions shape behavior), and relationship management (regulating ones' emotional behavior). Examining these four domains enhances one's emotional wellness.

Physical

When a person's basic biological needs for food, shelter, and clothing have been met, there are many ways to seek wholeness of physical potential. Assessing physical potential includes many elements, with three significant areas being nutrition, exercise, and weight. These are frequent areas of need as individuals focus on well-being, health promotion, and healing beyond the cure factor. The physical component has received attention regarding recommendations, measurements, and interventions. However, the holistic nurse recognizes the complex interactions of the human and focuses on the whole person while attending to the physical.

Other vital areas, such as alcohol, drug use, and sleep, that are included in the long form of the IHWA can be discussed in conversations. Typically, people focus on the elements of the physical component but fail to recognize that they are not separate from—or more important than—the other components. Wellness is present when there is an integration between the components; it is more than just physical and the absence of pain and symptoms. As individuals assess biological needs, they also must consider their perceptions of these areas. Many illnesses have been documented as stress-related because consciousness plays a significant role in health and physical potential.

The body is a gift to nurture and respect. As humans nurture themselves, they increase their uniqueness in energy, sexuality, vitality, capacity for language, and connection with their other potentials. By strengthening self-image and integrating the body-mind-spirit connection, individuals create a greater sense of balance and an openness to more fully realized potentials.

Environmental

Assessing the environment increases an individual's awareness of its effect on health and well-being. The environment is the context or habitat within which all living systems participate and interact. This includes the physical body and its physical habitat; cultural, psychological, social, and historical influences; and both the external physical space and a person's internal space (physical, mental, emotional, social, and spiritual experiences). A healing environment includes everything surrounding the person and patterns not yet understood.

Florence Nightingale was an environmentalist who wrote about the effects of polluted homes and environments and the importance of avoiding anything that makes one ill or may be considered toxic. Today, this is recognized as the precautionary principle, which states that when an activity raises threats of harm to human health or the environment, precautionary measures shall be taken, even if some cause-and-effect relationships are not fully established scientifically—or it is better to be safe than sorry. If there is a suspicion about a harmful environment or substance, even though all of the evidence is unavailable, remove the person from the situation or stop using suspected harmful substances. The emphasis is on *zero*—not minimal or moderate—contamination and pollution of our environments as acceptable. The AHNA published a position statement on planetary health that calls for nurses to address planetary health through practice, research, education, and advocacy (AHNA, 2021).

Health Responsibility

Health responsibility occurs when an individual actively makes lifestyle choices to protect and improve their health. Many actions and behaviors that enhance health and well-being are explored in the IHWA. It is suggested that each person comply with all the recommended physicals, dental exams, and age-related screenings and address risk factors for individual lifestyle-related illnesses. An individual taking responsibility for their health record includes compiling all baseline personal physiologic parameters, personal history, family history, and any current symptoms. Medications and supplements, along with potential interactions, should be recognized. Allergies, hospitalizations, surgeries, and other specific medical factors should be noted.

Action toward one's health includes communicating with healthcare providers. The provider–patient relationship is vital, so one should choose a practitioner who creates a healing relationship where issues and concerns are readily discussed. Labeling a patient as noncompliant is no longer sufficient. Health care has not engaged that client in further discussion to determine the patient's health literacy and wants and to identify issues that may impact their understanding of health recommendations.

Nursing Situation

John is a robust and active 65-year-old male who anticipates retirement from his job as an economics professor at a large university in a few months. He is very anxious and unsure what to do with his free time. His wife suddenly died in her sleep 2 years ago. He is close to his two adult children (his daughter is 32, and his son is 29) and sees them weekly. His new granddaughter has brought him much joy and is his new reason for becoming healthier. He was referred to a nurse coach by a good friend at his church, where he is very active.

At the first session, John completed the IHWA and declared that he wanted to lose 30 pounds, eat healthier, begin an exercise program, and learn how to manage his anxiety. The nurse coaching process guided the sessions and supported the nurse coach–patient therapeutic relationship.

The coaching sessions explored John's strengths and prior successes in changing and maintaining new health behaviors. He demonstrated a readiness for change. He was taught various relaxation and imagery practices. He was also advised to keep a food journal to become more aware of his eating habits and to transition to mindful eating. John had six sessions with his nurse coach over 2 months and lost 15 pounds. His anxiety lessened, and he now mentors university students and volunteers at several community centers. He was thrilled to learn how to identify his strengths and not focus on his weaknesses, which gave him a new sense of joy and wellness.

Implications

- **Clinical practice**: The IHWA tool increases patients' awareness of health responsibility, which improves patient outcomes. The tool also allows for conversation about areas of health that healthcare providers do not usually approach.
- **Education**: Self-assessment of whole person potential is an effective way to teach holistic assessment to both patients and healthcare professionals. Self-care needs are identified,

and health-promoting goals and actions can be self-directed.

- **Research**: Self-assessment tools effectively evaluate changes in health behavior and perceived quality of life using IHWA's eight categories. This will inform direction for use in clinical practice and healthy lifestyles.
- **Policy**: Increased emphasis on self-assessment potential supports national efforts in health promotion and self-responsibility for health. Nurses are primarily positioned to implement the Healthy People 2030 vision to create a "society in which all people can achieve their full potential for health and well-being across the lifespan" (ODPHP, n.d.) using self-assessment tools.
- **Global health**: Each area addressed in self-assessment is intertwined with the health of an individual's family, teams, communities, and planet. The goals and action plan developed need to reflect the local-to-global perspective.

Conclusion

Self-assessment is a continuous process related to wellbecoming and whole-person healing. Assessment tools like the IHWA can engage patients, nurses, healthcare teams, and communities in self-development. Holistic nurses are challenged to expand nurse coaching knowledge and skills, assisting themselves, others, communities, institutions, and governments to develop, support, and sustain behaviors that lead to well-being for all. The IHWA may be used in two forms—the long form (for in-depth examination of specific areas of wellness) and the short form (for brief overall assessment). Individuals become healthier by changing their perceptions and beliefs and empowering themselves for effect.

References

American Holistic Nurse Association (AHNA). (2021, April). *Planetary health position paper*. https://www.ahna.org/American-Holistic-Nurses-Association/Resources/Planetary-Health

American Holistic Nurses Association (AHNA). (2023). *Promoting nurse health & well-being*. https://www.ahna.org/Portals/66/Docs/Resources/Promoting%20Nurse%20Health%20%20Wellbeing%20Toolkit%20FINAL.pdf?ver=_uPq350vOVHs1JMrBJ2JCg%3d%3d

American Nurses Association. (2025). *Healthy nurse, healthy nation*. https://www.healthynursehealthynation.org/

DeVellis, F. R. (2012). *Scale development: Theory and applications* (3rd ed.). SAGE.

Dossey, B. M., Luck, S., & Schaub, B. G. (2015). *Nurse coaching: Integrative approaches for health and wellbeing*. International Nurse Coach Association.

Goleman, D. (2020). *Emotional intelligence. 25th Anniversary edition*. Bantam Books.

Gordon, S., & France, N. (2023). *Co-creating a holistic healing environment in nursing practice*. Cognella Academic Publishing.

Jung, C. (1980). Archetypes of the collective unconscious (Vol. 9, Part 1, pp. 3–41) (R. F. C. Hull, Trans.). In *Collected works of C. G. Jung*. Princeton University Press.

Kenefick-Moore, A., Avino, K., & McElligott, D. (2022). *A factor analysis of the IHWA*. [Unpublished Manuscript].

McElligott, D., Eckardt, S. Dossey, B. M., Luck, S., & Eckardt, P. (2018). Instrument development of the Integrative Health and Wellness Assessment. *Journal of Holistic Nursing*, *36*(4), 374-384.

National Academy of Medicine. (2019). *Action collaboration on clinician well-being and resilience*. https://nam.edu/initiatives/clinician-resilience-and-well-being/

National Academy of Medicine. (2022). *National plan for health workforce well-being*. https://nap.nationalacademies.org/catalog/26744/national-plan-for-health-workforce-well-being

Office of Disease Prevention and Health Promotion (ODPHP). (n.d.). *Healthy People 2030 framework*. https://odphp.health.gov/healthypeople

U.S. Department of Health and Human Services. (2011, June). *America's plan for better health and wellness*. https://www.hhs.gov/sites/default/files/disease-prevention-wellness-report.pdf

World Health Organization. (n.d.). *Health and well-being*. https://www.who.int/data/gho/data/major-themes/health-and-well-being.

World Health Organization. (2019, May 28). *Mental health. Burn-out an occupational phenomenon: International classification of diseases*. https://www.who.int/mental_health/evidence/burn-out/en/

World Health Organization. (2025). *Social determinants of health*. Retrieved from https://www.who.int/news-room/fact-sheets/detail/social-determinants-of-health

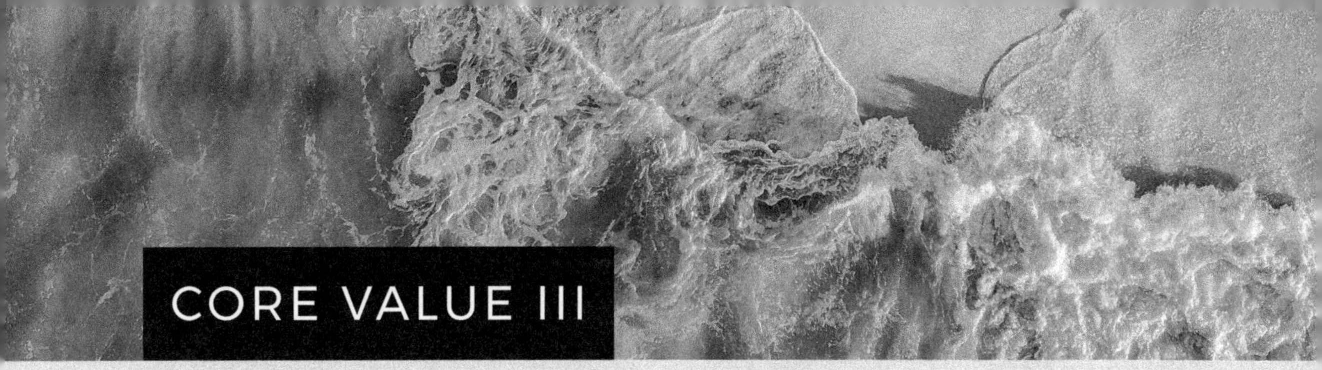

CORE VALUE III

Holistic Caring Process

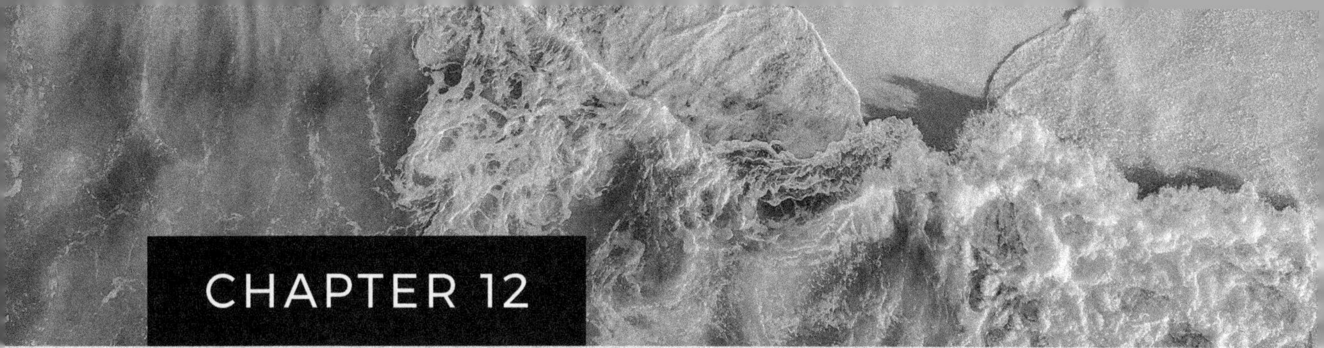

CHAPTER 12

The Holistic Caring Process

Marian Bianco Long and Margaret McGrath Brown

NURSE HEALER OBJECTIVES

- Contemplate the professional and personal value of the Holistic Caring Process during these times of significant change in health care.
- Examine the standard nursing process and enhancements of the Holistic Caring Process.
- Identify ways the Holistic Caring Process supports personal and professional nurse wellbecoming.
- Discuss applications and implications of the Holistic Caring Process in personal and professional settings, translating theory into practice.

DEFINITIONS

Health: "An individually defined state or process in which the patient (nurse, patient, family, group, or community) experiences a sense of well-being, harmony, and unity such that subjective experiences about health, health beliefs, and values are honored; a process of becoming and expanding consciousness" (American Nurses Association and American Holistic Nurses Association [ANA & AHNA], 2019, p. 116).

Holistic Caring Process: "An iterative and integrative process between a nurse(s) and people seeking care that involves six steps that may occur simultaneously: (1) assessment, (2) diagnosis or identification of health pattern(s), (3) identification of outcomes, (4) plan of care, (5) implementation of the plan of care, and (6) evaluation" (ANA & AHNA, 2019, p. 27).

Human caring: "The moral ideal of nursing, in which the nurse brings their whole self into a relationship with the whole self of the person being cared for in order to protect that person's vulnerability, preserve humanity and dignity, and reinforce the meaning and experience of oneness and unity" (ANA & AHNA, 2019, p. 118).

Human health experience: "The totality of human experience, including each person's subjective experience about health, health beliefs, illness, values, sexual orientation, and personal preferences, that encompasses health-wellness-disease-illness-death" (ANA & AHNA, 2019, p. 118).

Nursing diagnosis: A clinical judgment concerning a human response to health conditions/life processes, or a vulnerability for that response, by an individual, family, group, or community (NANDA International Knowledgebase, n.d.).

Person-centered care: "The human caring process in which the holistic nurse gives full attention and intention to the whole self of a person, not merely the current presenting symptoms, illness, crisis, or tasks to be accomplished, and that includes reinforcing the person's meaning and experience of oneness and unity; the created condition of trust in which holistic care can be given and received" (ANA & AHNA, 2019, p. 119).

Wellbecoming: An ongoing journey toward wholeness that includes all the physical, emotional, mental and spiritual aspects of well-being as well as lifelong self-discovery, transformation and transcendence (Phillips, 2015).

Well-being: "An inner attitude of feelings of comfort and harmony and acceptance of the wholeness of one's being. Integrated congruent functioning to achieve one's higher potential" (ANA & AHNA, 2019, p. 121).

Wellness: "An active process through which people become aware of, and make choices toward, a more successful existence. It is a conscious, self-directed, and evolving process of achieving full potential. Wellness is multidimensional and holistic, encompassing lifestyle, mental and spiritual well-being, and the environment. It is positive and affirming" (ANA & AHNA, 2019, p. 121).

**In this chapter, the term *patient* refers to the unit of care. However, depending on the context, *person*, *individual*, *client*, *family*, *community*, or *population* may be more appropriate.

Dear Reader,

Our message to you is We See You. You are not alone.

In this chapter, we present the concept of the Holistic Caring Process. It is based on the familiar structure of what you do every day, enhanced in depth and effectiveness by the transcendent values and the vibration of caring and love. We understand how the tasks and constraints of an overburdened system tend to crowd out what we know is the most important hallmark of nursing—loving compassionate care. And we hope that this chapter and this entire handbook speaks to your heart, renews your spirit, and sparks changes in your practice that ripple powerfully throughout your spheres of influence. Thank you for your work and your contributions to a better tomorrow. You are loved.

Introduction

People choose nursing as a profession for many reasons—a passion for caring, an interest in health, job security, competitive wages, or the appeal of a three-day workweek. Despite these motivations, some who feel drawn to nursing may now reconsider, opting for careers that are less demanding, require less training, or, unfortunately, offer greater safety. The recent decline in the nursing workforce, particularly among younger nurses, highlights the need for stronger support and retention incentives in the workplace (Auerbach et al., 2022). Furthermore, nursing education must adapt to better prepare today's learners to navigate increasingly complex healthcare environments by facilitating essential skills such as perseverance, interpersonal communication, and advanced critical thinking (Seibert, 2021).

Big changes are not new to nursing, and nurses have weathered many shifts of perception over the years. During the Crimean War, Florence Nightingale revamped well-intentioned but ineffective nursing practices, and crafted the genesis of the well-articulated, statistically sound discipline that nursing is today. Since then, nurses have gained the respect of colleagues and the public and have risen to the status of a profession. More recently, increasing numbers of advanced degree nurses have generated nursing theories that articulate the true value of nursing care. However, despite their long-standing reputation for tender care and trustworthiness, the public's perception of the healthcare system, including the profession of nursing, has suffered post-pandemic (Walker, 2024).

The healthcare landscape has changed dramatically since the last edition of this handbook. However, the vision and value of the Holistic Caring Process remains clear. In this chapter, the standard nursing process taught to all nurses as the basis for care decisions will be compared with AHNA's Holistic Caring Process, which reflects the heart of holistic nursing. Within the constraints of an overburdened healthcare system, the Holistic Caring Process promotes the vital role of caring and holistic philosophies, offering hope for the future of the nursing profession.

Nurses know that the demands of healthcare delivery require impeccable technical skills and extensive expertise. Intuitively, they understand that nursing is an art as well as a science, and the balance of both in everyday practice is sometimes an elusive but worthy effort. The Holistic Caring Process merges the *art* as well as the *science* of nursing and elevates nursing practice from the simple *doing* of tasks and interventions to a way of *being* that is truly compassionate and healing for both the nurse and those being served.

Many nurses are drawn to holistic nursing because they intuitively sense the positive impact that holism adds to their own health, personal growth, and practice. The concepts of wellness and well-being are increasingly prevalent in nursing literature today; however, their mainstream meanings can be limiting. They can imply wellness is a static state and lead to unrealistic self-imposed expectations. Phillips expanded on these definitions by introducing the term *wellbecoming* and acknowledging that wellness is not a static state, but a dynamic evolving journey (Phillips, 2015). Wellbecoming involves continual growth and transformation throughout the lifespan, which is at the heart of holistic nursing (Integrative Nurse Coach Academy, 2024).

To cultivate wellbecoming, the nurse must explore practices to increase personal capacity. Aydin et al. (2022) found that positive attitudes about work engagement increased when nurses engaged in holistic practices of self-reflection and insight. Accordingly, Riley (2024) encouraged nursing students to practice ongoing self-assessment, journaling, and meditation to improve communication in nursing as well as personal growth and professional competence. Furthermore, nurse ethicist Lazenby (2017) listed holism along with sensitivity, intimacy, vulnerability, and uniqueness as prerequisites for the healing effects of nursing presence. Truly, Jain summed up the transformative power of wellbecoming for nurses by stating, "The best way we can foster healing in others is to ensure that we are also making ourselves whole" (Jain, 2021, p. 256).

Box 12-1 Strengths of the Standard Nursing Process

- Uses a scientific approach to distinguish nursing practice from medical practice.
- Conceptualized in the 1960s to establish nursing as a unique and autonomous profession.
- Adopted into nursing curricula in the 1980s to develop critical thinking and clinical reasoning skills.
- Enables novice nurses to grasp connections between assessments, judgments, actions, and outcomes.
- Helps nurses identify nursing actions which might otherwise be unacknowledged or undervalued by reframing them as professional responses that facilitate care and healing. For example, repositioning a patient and smoothing linens enhance comfort and preserve skin integrity.
- Provides a common language and framework for nurses, administrators, and researchers to articulate and study the value of nursing thinking, interventions, and outcomes.
- Influences reimbursement, practice standards, and appreciation of nursing's unique contributions to patient care in a multidisciplinary healthcare environment.

Data from Potter, P., & Frisch, N. C. (2009). The holistic caring process. In AHNA (Ed.), *Holistic nursing: A handbook for practice* (5th ed., pp. 141–156). Sudbury, MA: Jones and Bartlett Publishers.

The Standard Nursing Process

The traditional nursing process taught in nursing schools is a linear step-by-step process that includes assessment, diagnosis, planning, implementation, and evaluation. Although this standard nursing process has many strengths (refer to **Box 12-1**), describing and guiding what nurses DO in a linear step-by-step way does not always capture the reality of human complexity and the actual experience of nurses in practice. While reductionist thinking informs how many healthcare professionals think and the way the current system is structured, it may skew nursing care into a problem-solving formula with conclusions, actions, and outcomes and can lead to judgmental perceptions of patient "non-compliance."

According to Potter and Frisch (2009), a more accurate representation of nursing practice is a circular model that recognizes a nonlinear approach. In reality, nurses often perform multiple steps at the same time or deviate from the linear order to adjust their processes based on real-time patient needs. For instance, the nurse could address several nursing diagnoses simultaneously, or adjust a planned intervention using patient input before implementing it. A nurse might assess a patient's spiritual needs while also intervening to manage pain, or begin the initial assessment by focusing on their own presence and grounding to enhance the healing process. Even sitting with a person in silence, which may appear as "doing nothing" can be an incredibly effective intervention. One could further conceptualize the Holistic Caring Process, beyond being nonlinear and circular, as multidimensional, unitary, flowing, and an ever-evolving process for supporting well becoming.

Over the years, holistic nurses and scholars have discussed and defended the vital and inherent role of *caring* within the practice of nursing. (For further study and background history, see the additional Background document in the Navigate eBook.) The next section examines how the values of holistic nursing, reflected throughout this handbook, unequivocally embrace caring as *essential* to nursing and the nursing process (ANA & AHNA, 2019).

The Holistic Caring Process

The standard nursing process emphasizes the identification and treatment of patient conditions or problems, while the Holistic Caring Process is centered around human health and wholeness and is grounded in the worldview and principles of holistic nursing. Since its inception in 1981, AHNA has provided nurses with education and resources to support this metaparadigm of healing, including the *Holistic Nursing: Scope and Standards of Practice* (ANA & AHNA, 2019), which serves as a foundational resource for nurses who choose to enhance their practice with the core values of holistic nursing:

> Holistic nursing focuses on protecting, promoting, and optimizing health and wellness; assisting healing; preventing illness and injury; alleviating suffering; supporting people to find peace, comfort, harmony, and balance through the diagnosis and treatment of human response; and advocating in the care of individuals, families, groups, communities, populations, and the planet. (ANA & AHNA, 2019, p. 1)

The Holistic Caring Process describes the practice of holistic nursing by building upon the familiar language of the first six ANA standards of care. *Holistic Nursing: Scope and Standards of Practice* identifies competencies for each ANA standard, expanding and illuminating each one through a holistic lens for both RN and advanced practice holistic nurses (ANA & AHNA, 2019). The Holistic Caring Process can be practiced in any setting and aligns with the scope and competencies of any specialty or population. Southard et al. (2021) expanded on the same ANA standards with competencies linked specifically to the practice of holistic nurse coaching. (Refer to **Chapter 26** for a discussion of nurse coaching.)

Holistic nurses view themselves as instruments of healing, fine-tuned by self-reflection and self-care practices including intentionality, mindfulness, presence, and the therapeutic use of self. By valuing the individual's broader goals, not just physical outcomes, the holistic nurse appreciates the human health experience as a complex, dynamic relationship of health/wellness, illness/disease, and wellbecoming (ANA & AHNA, 2019). Although holistic nurses are often trained and experienced in varied complementary/integrative practices such as aromatherapy, guided imagery, and energy work, they understand it is insufficient to merely insert a holistic modality into the intervention slot. Interventions are holistic when provided within a sacred space of caring, compassion, and appreciation of the inherent wholeness of human beings. Though holistic nursing may include integrative modalities in addition to standard nursing practice, it is the underlying and overarching AHNA core values that truly inform the practice as both science and art.

The Holistic Caring Process can also be applied beyond the bedside to self and colleagues as a framework to holistically assess and address personal or professional concerns. For example, a nurse may notice an internal emotional or physical response being triggered by something revealed during patient care and employ a simple practice such as deep breathing to ground and center themselves. Nurse self-reflection supports awareness of effective and ineffective coping strategies employed in response to stress and helps the nurse recognize early symptoms of burnout. A holistic nurse implements self-compassion and the power of common humanity when reaching out for stress management support. The Holistic Caring Process also supports the nursing community as a whole to advocate for psychological safety, workplace violence prevention, and workflow improvement.

CASE STUDY

Many nurses strive to practice, consciously and/or intuitively, with care, creativity, and respect for their patients, striving to forge true connections and meaningful encounters, often within the constraints of illness-oriented systems. Many nurses join AHNA from a sense of alignment with the organization's values and to network with colleagues who also embrace the principles of holistic nursing. The following paragraphs list the standards of the Holistic Caring Process (in bold), plus a few examples of the competencies for each from *Holistic Nursing: Scope and Standards of Practice* (ANA & AHNA, 2019), illustrating enhancement from a holistic caring perspective.

Standard 1. Assessment: The holistic registered nurse collects comprehensive data pertinent to the healthcare consumer's health or the situation. Nursing assessments always include quantitative physical data and the person's subjective report, updated with every interaction. In addition, the holistic nurse begins the assessment process with conscious self-preparation (centering, presence) prior to entering the energy field/environment of the person, sustaining a safe space for a co-creative mutual relationship. The person's perceived needs, understanding of their situation, and goals for care are primary sources. Significant others of the person's choosing are valued colleagues. The holistic nurse uses empirical, ethical, and aesthetic ways of knowing including awareness of family dynamics, lifestyle, and environmental factors to assess readiness and resources for change. Holistic assessments are updated with every interaction and go beyond physical findings. For example, nourishment can extend to how a person nourishes spirit as well as body; spiritual assessment explores connection, meaning, and purpose in life; deep listening, powerful questions, and intuition elicit new insights. The holistic nurse holds awareness of biofields and energetic patterns, with appreciation for the wholeness and dignity of every person.

Standard 2. Diagnosis: The holistic registered nurse analyzes assessment data to determine the actual or potential diagnosis or issues expressed as challenges/problems/needs. The holistic nurse approaches the person from a place of strength and empowerment, interpreting assessment findings as patterns/challenges/needs that can be validated by the person. Lifestyle, potential barriers, risk factors, beliefs, values, resources, and readiness are considered. Holistic nurses recognize the person's personal strengths, history, and their understanding of and response to their condition. The holistic nurse approaches the person with a beginner's mind of unknowing rather than preconceptions derived from the medical diagnosis, formulating a comprehensive holistic pattern unique to this individual and situation.

Standard 3. Outcomes Identification: The holistic registered nurse identifies expected outcomes for a plan individualized to the healthcare consumer or the situation. (The holistic nurse values the evolution and the process of healing as it unfolds. Unfolding outcomes may not be immediately evident, due to the nonlinear nature of the healing process, so both expected or anticipated and evolving or emerging outcomes are considered.) The holistic nurse appreciates the person as the expert of themselves, honoring inner wisdom and intuition. "Noncompliance" is perceived as the need to reconsider options and explore relevant barriers and insights, not as failures or disobedience. Patient goals may or may not be totally aligned with the medical plan, and the holistic nurse helps the person explore possible tweaks that individualize realistic outcomes reflecting personal values and capabilities. The holistic nurse serves as a valuable resource for physiological knowledge and evidence-informed practices, negotiating the healthcare environment, and advocating for the patient as needed. Some interventions have specific desirable outcomes, such as administering pain medication or repositioning a patient in bed, while others are facilitated with a sense of ego detachment, honoring the variances of individual healing journeys. Outcomes are formulated with intention—holding space and vision for the person's highest good and wholeness.

Standard 4. Planning: The holistic registered nurse develops a plan outlining primary strategies and suggested alternatives to attain expected outcomes. Resources for the holistic nursing plan include conventional as well as integrative modalities, providing any required information or teaching. The focus is on health promotion, recovery, and restoration, which may involve peaceful death, while enhancing personal engagement and independence. The development of the plan includes elements of the art of nursing (intuition, creativity, presence, self/personal knowing, reflection) as well as the science (data, critical thinking, evidence/research, theory). The plan is formulated in collaboration with the person or significant others as much as possible, addressing emotional, mental, spiritual, and psychosocial needs as well as physical.

Standard 5. Implementation: The holistic registered nurse implements the identified plan. (Sometimes the plan is not directed to clinical care but administrative, educational, or other foci.) Holistic implementation is a nondirective partnership. The plan may involve emotional or spiritual healing, relationship adjustments, cognitive reframing, and other psychosocial elements as well as physical factors. The person's responses inform the pace and course of implementation, and the holistic nurse provides clear information about the progress of the plan as appropriate for the person's age, level of understanding, and interest. All nursing actions are within the nurse's scope of practice, professional training, and in accordance with sound institutional guidelines and governmental regulations. As an instrument of healing, the holistic nurse recognizes that every encounter is an opportunity for caring and transcendence.

Standard 5A. Coordination of Care: The holistic registered nurse coordinates care delivery. The holistic nurse holds intention and advocates as needed throughout the process for the person's highest good; maintains collaboration with the person, significant others, and healthcare colleagues; and oversees the big picture. As the circular process continues, all steps of the process may be revisited and revised. Positive changes are noted, and even small progress is encouraged and celebrated; setbacks or barriers are addressed in an empowering way.

Standard 5B. Health Teaching and Health Promotion: The holistic registered nurse employs strategies to promote holistic health/wellness and a safe environment. Holistic nurses promote self-empowerment and are well versed in many approaches to health and healing, able to tailor teaching and suggestions to the individual's needs, abilities and desires. Recognizing true prevention as much more than screening for early detection or subsuming symptoms with pharmaceuticals, the holistic nurse encourages necessary lifestyle changes from a wellness perspective and shares methods and resources for improving stress management, nutrition, movement, sleep, play, and other self-care and health-promoting practices. Aware that humans thrive in interconnectedness, the holistic nurse assesses personal safety and available resources and support systems. Holistic nurses working in outpatient or coaching settings are especially positioned to develop ongoing relationships conducive to personal growth and wellbecoming in their patients.

Standard 6. Evaluation: The holistic registered nurse evaluates progress toward attainment of goals and health outcomes. Holistic nurses understand that healing follows a dynamic, sacred path that is distinct from the curing of symptoms or conditions, cannot be predicted or controlled, and emerges into newness rather than a return to a prior state (Quinn, 2022). Progress can be evaluated as a repatterning toward insight and wellness. Symptoms may or may not be resolved; lab values may remain persistently abnormal, and yet perceptions can be reframed and healing can occur as persons integrate or transcend their experience with self-knowledge and self-actualization. Even small changes are acknowledged and celebrated; barriers and goals of care are continuously assessed nonjudgmentally and amended as required or requested.

Implications

Practice

- The Holistic Caring Process values patient engagement, autonomy, and input, while providing the patient with a supportive and knowledgeable advocate.
- Holistic nurses value self-reflection, self-development and self-care. The wellbecoming of the nurse directly impacts patient care.
- Holistic nurses increasingly hold leadership positions as clinicians, faculty, administrators, researchers, authors, and consultants (ANA & AHNA, 2019).
- Holistic nurses practice in any setting or within any specialty, and they are in prime positions to create, train, and implement programs reflecting the public's demand for integrative care.
- Holistic nurses use ethical principles and theories to guide their decisions and actions. (Refer to **Chapter 6**, Holistic Ethics.)

Education

- Holistic nursing education emphasizes self-care and resilience, and instills principles of intentionality, presence, mindfulness, and transcendence.
- Even nurses who realize the importance of self-care may often need "permission" from self and others in order to practice self-compassion in their personal lives and workplaces (Andrews et al., 2020).
- Traits such as empathy or emotional intelligence that are often considered inherent can also be taught as skills (Stein-Parbury, 2021).
- AHNA offers continuing education to nurses and institutions online and via programs such as the Integrative Healing Arts Program and national and regional conferences.
- In *The Essentials: Core Competencies for Professional Nursing Education*, self-care is listed as a competency for personal, professional, and leadership development for both entry-level and advanced practice nursing education (American Association of Colleges of Nursing, 2021).

Research

- Holistic nursing as a specialty is dedicated to the provision of valid and reliable holistic nursing research as a foundation for education, practice, and health policy for the broader sphere of all nursing (Delaney et al., 2018).
- Holistic nursing research informs all aspects of the human lifespan and seeks to alleviate healthcare disparities among diverse and underserved populations, as well as advancing interventions tailored to the unique needs of individuals (Freysteinson et al., 2023).

> A survey of holistic nurses conducted by AHNA supported the following research priorities: (1) enhancing the wellbeing of all nurses, (2) innovating holistic nursing care practices and interventions, (3) gleaning insight into and decreasing biophysical, psychosocial, and spiritual pain across the lifespan, (4) understanding, intervening in, and reducing health inequities, and (5) exploring nature and environmental factors on the impact of health. (Freysteinson et al., 2023, p. 196)

- Holistic nursing invites research into concepts generally dismissed as nonphysical phenomena, such as the middle-range Unitary Caring Science (Smith, 2021)—a convergence of science, metaphysics, and age-old worldviews, which conceptualize humans as whole beings, fully interconnected and evolving within infinite fields of universal consciousness, energy, and unconditional love.

Policy

- Holistic nursing is proactive and visionary, acknowledging caring as a moral imperative that includes caring for self, significant others, diverse populations, and planet Earth.
- Nurses are needed in all discussions at every level regarding the state of the healthcare

delivery system and the broader profession of nursing (Wolters Kluwer, 2023).

- Hospitals and educational institutions are increasingly adopting nurse-driven initiatives using theories that honor the sacredness of human beings and compassionate care as the basis for nursing professional practice and curriculum development (Watson, n.d.).

Conclusion

While this chapter focused on the Holistic Caring Process and essential tangible nursing activities in practice, it is important to revisit the overarching worldviews that drive those actions and intentions. Holism cannot be separated from an expansive consciousness of oneness and unity, manifested in heart-centered caring, and increasingly validated by science. As nursing scholars strive to articulate a paradigm in which love is acknowledged as a high-level vibrational frequency that entrains other fields into a pattern of wholeness and healing (Smith, 2021), nurses around the world and around the clock embody caring in their practices every day. In the words of priest and paleontologist Teilhard de Chardin:

> The day will come when, after harnessing the ether, the winds, the tides, gravitation, we shall harness for God the energies of love. And on that day, for the second time in the history of the world, man will have discovered fire. (de Chardin, 1936, pp. 86–87)

References

American Association of Colleges of Nursing. (2021). *The Essentials: Core competencies for professional nursing education.* https://www.aacnnursing.org/Portals/0/PDFs/Publications/Essentials-2021.pdf

American Nurses Association and American Holistic Nurses Association. (2019). *Holistic nursing: Scope and standards of practice* (3rd ed.). ANA & AHNA.

Andrews, H., Tierney, S., & Seers, K. (2020). Needing permission: The experience of self-care and self-compassion in nursing: A constructivist grounded theory study. *International Journal of Nursing Studies 101,* 103436. https://doi.org/10.1016/j.ijnurstu.2019.103436

Auerbach, D., Buerhaus, P. I., Donelan, K., & Staiger, D. O. (2022). A worrisome drop in the number of young nurses, *Health Affairs Forefront.* https://doi.org/10.1377/forefront.20220412.311784

Aydin, A., Kaya, Y., & Erbaş, A. (2022). The effect of holistic nursing competence on work engagement, self-reflection and insight in nurses. *Journal of Holistic Nursing, 41*(3), 310–317. https://doi.org/10.1177/08980101221129716

de Chardin, T. (1936). The evolution of chastity. In *Toward the future, XI* (pp. 86–87). Harcourt.

Delaney, C., McCaffrey, R. G., Barrere, C., Moore, A. K., Dunn, D. J., Miller, R. J., Molony, S. L., Thomas, D., Twomey, T. C., & Zhu, X. (2018). Trends in contemporary holistic nursing research. *Journal of Holistic Nursing, 36*(4), 385–394. https://doi.org/10.1177/0898010117750451

Freysteinson, W. M., Enzman Hines, M., Wind Wardell, D., Friesen, M. A., Conrad, S., Zahourek, R., Gallo, A.-M., & Prather, J. G. (2023). Identifying holistic nursing research priorities for 2023–2026. *Journal of Holistic Nursing, 42*(2), 182–201. https://doi.org/10.1177/08980101231213725

Integrative Nurse Coach Academy. (2024). *Wellbeing and wellbecoming: A nurse coach's perspective on holistic growth.* https://inursecoach.com/wellbeing-wellbecoming-a-nurse-coach-perspective-on-holistic-growth/

Jain, S. (2021). *Healing ourselves: Biofield science and the future of health.* Sounds True.

Lazenby, M. (2017). *Caring matters most: The ethical significance of nursing.* Oxford University Press.

Phillips, J. R. (2015). Martha Rogers: Heretic or heroine. *Nursing Science Quarterly, 28*(1), 42–48.

Potter, P., & Frisch, N. C. (2009). The holistic caring process. In AHNA (Ed.), *Holistic nursing: A handbook for practice* (5th ed., pp. 141–156). Jones and Bartlett Publishers.

Quinn, J. F. (2022). Transpersonal human caring & healing. In M. Blaszko Helming, D. Shields, K. Avino, & W. Rosa (Eds.), *Holistic nursing: A handbook for practice* (8th ed., pp. 97–106). Jones and Bartlett Publishers.

Riley, J. B. (2024). *Communication in nursing* (10th ed.). Elsevier.

Southard, M. E., Dossey, B. M., Bark, L., & Schaub, B. G. (2021). *The art and science of nurse coaching: The provider's guide to coaching scope and competencies* (2nd ed.). Nursesbooks.org

Seibert, S. (2021). Problem-based learning: A strategy to foster generation Z's critical thinking and perseverance. *Teaching and Learning in Nursing* (*16*)1, 85–88. https://www.sciencedirect.com/science/article/pii/S1557308720301049

Smith, M. (2021). *Unitary caring*. Nursology. https://nursology.net/nurse-theories/middle-range-theory-of-unitary-caring

Stein-Parbury, J. (2021). *Patient & person: Interpersonal skills in nursing*. Elsevier.

Walker, A. (2024). *Nursing ranked as the most trusted profession for 22nd year in a row*. Nurse.org. https://nurse.org/articles/nursing-ranked-most-honest-profession/

Watson, J. (n.d.). *Watson's Caring Science and Human Caring Theory*. Watson Caring Science Institute. https://www.watsoncaringscience.org/about-wcsi/jean-bio/caring-science-theory/

Wolters Kluwer. (2023). *Why nursing needs to be included in the adverse events discussion*. https://www.wolterskluwer.com/en/expert-insights/why-nursing-needs-to-be-included-in-the-adverse-events-discussion

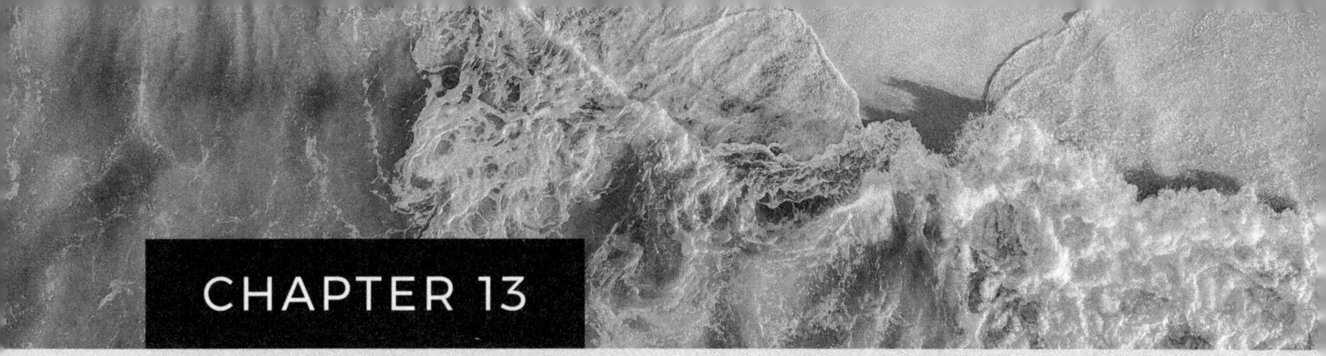

CHAPTER 13

Energetic Interconnectedness

Debra Rose Wilson

NURSE HEALER OBJECTIVES

- Describe the quantum level theory as it relates to health.
- Discuss the role of intention in nursing.
- Synthesize the knowledge of energetic interconnectedness into a better understanding of self, others, and nursing practice.

DEFINITIONS

Atom: The building block of matter consisting of a nucleus (which is made up of protons and neutrons) surrounded by a swarm of circulating electrons, each in its own orbit. There should be equal number of protons and electrons in a balanced/neutral atom. Atoms are in constant motion and emit waves of light as well as other quantum-level waves.

Antioxidants: If an atom loses an electron, it becomes unstable, and a free radical oxidant goes on a rampage, damaging the atoms around it. This translates to cell and tissue damage at the microscopic level. An antioxidant is a molecule with extra electrons that it shares with the free radical and calms it back to a neutral state.

Aura: A vague, luminous glow surrounding an object or living being. The luminous glow seems to be partly due to photons and an electromagnetic field around that contains information.

Chakra: An energy center in the subtle, or energetic, body that is described as a whirling vortex of light. Chakras are believed to be portals for energy and information flow into and out of a person and are fundamental to understanding traditional Chinese medicine.

Electromagnetic field: A field is an area where something can act on or influence something else. An electromagnetic field is a space in which there are charged objects and magnetic fields at the same time. There are numerous other quantum level waves within this field and the influence is bidirectional. The field pulls on objects, and the objects influence the field.

Electromagnetic radiation: The energy given off, radiating from an electromagnetic field.

Electron: A negatively charged tiny particle orbiting the nucleus of an atom.

Energy healing: The deliberate process of using an external energy field to induce a change in one's own or another's field for physical, mental, emotional, and spiritual healing. Energy healing may involve the presence of a caring person.

Intention: Choosing to think, act, or be a certain way; intention is deliberate.

Meridian: Microvolt electrical conduit pathways organized in an electrical mesh that permeates the body and precedes development of vessels and organs. In ancient Eastern philosophies, the meridians are said to conduct chi, qi, prana, or universal energy throughout the body and communicating to cells. Developments in quantum physics support this thinking.

Nucleus: The center of an atom, the nucleus, is composed of several structures, including the well-known protons, but also quarks, which include the delightfully named *up*, *down*, *beauty*, and *strange*. Gluons hold them together to create the nucleus of an atom. It was once thought that the atom's nucleus was the smallest piece of mass, impenetrable and unable to be broken into pieces. This was wrong.

Photon: A photon is a small packet of light; the smallest part of an electromagnetic force, considered a messenger particle. Photons give off light and carry information.

Proton: A positively charged particle found in the nucleus of an atom, made up of three quarks.

Subtle energy: Barely noticeable electrical, quantum, and magnetic fields around living organisms that we are just beginning to measure and apply to diagnosis and healing.

Introduction

Energy exists in many forms (e.g., thermal, kinetic, nuclear, chemical), but in health care, we are more attuned to electrical, electromagnetic, chemical, and other subtle energies. The concept that all matter is energy vibrating at different frequencies is basic in understanding energy physics. A fundamental assumption of energy healing is that all life is sustained by a universal life energy that moves freely. Energy fields surround the human physical body with internal and external waves signaling atoms, cells, and larger biology, waves in continuous interaction. Through this perpetual energy exchange, each field is affected and changed. In ancient Chinese medicine, illness was believed to be the result of blockages in flow or disordered patterns of the different energies in the body. Studies in the field of quantum physics support this thinking.

A Shifting Paradigm

In an attempt to provide a foundation for the energy field around living organisms, we are required to consider several different theoretical explanations. The effects of the energy fields are measurable, but the mechanism of action is not yet known. Energy fields involve numerous forces examined by physicists: magnetic fields, electrical fields, radiation, sound, electron activity, and particle/wave behavior. There are likely multiple layers of various types of energy wave networks harmoniously involved in functioning, communication between cells, and healing. This communication extends to the environment and to others. We are constantly changing and changed by the interaction.

Quantum Physics

Isaac Newton taught us that everything moves like a mechanical part, and only the solid, visible parts are relevant. Traditionally, following Newton's reductionist thinking, we have examined and studied only the solid elements and ignored the empty space between. Western medicine has focused on human biology and chemistry for the last several hundred years, and the result has been a pharmaceutical and surgical approach to disease. In the early 1900s, Berliner Max Planck described the tiny world of quantum with a mathematical formula that calculated waves of heat from a furnace. This formula changed the world, helping us understand wavelengths and their relevance. Vibrational energy could be mathematically described. Schrödinger (you may have come across his cat-in-a-box experiment) also brought the concept of quantum *entanglement* into the field of physics. It was observed that two particles that were once in contact with each other, then separated by many miles, still communicate with each other. And they communicate faster than the speed of light . . . immediately. This was at a time when everyone thought there was nothing faster than the speed of light. Einstein called this "spooky action at a distance." Particles (like electrons and photons) are usually measured for speed and position. Heisenberg noticed that the more accurate we are about one aspect, such as speed, the less we know about its position. Position changes, it is not where we expect it to be. Heisenberg's Uncertainty Principle teaches us that observing has an effect. It changes the behavior at a quantum level.

When you observe the very small quantum world, the laws of physics we know up here in the big world do not work. From a quantum perspective, biology is no longer considered the most important part of a human and their health. We now know that there are waves of energy interacting with what we once thought of as solids. Even solidity is now questioned with the wave/particle duality conversation. Sometimes, particles act like solid matter, and other times, the same particles act like light waves.

Newtonian physics does not explain the role of consciousness, thinking, attitude, and social support, other less tangible factors that are clearly involved in health. New approaches are required when thinking about health. Quantum theory is easily applied to holistic nursing practice and health. There has been a fundamental shift in our understanding of the universe and we have known about this for over 100 years. Western medicine has been slow to adapt.

Health care was viewed from a biochemical perspective and there was nowhere to address consciousness, intention, or hope and their influence on illness. Quantum physics can explain why generating hope in people with cancer is as important to recovery as the chemotherapy they are prescribed. Higher levels of hope have been shown to improve health outcomes, have greater survival among those with advanced illnesses, and improved quality of life (Corn et al., 2022).

Quantum level changes are happening long before the illness is noticed in the cells or tissue, long before symptoms are noticed. Taking antioxidants will reduce the number of unstable atoms that are missing an electron—free radicals doing damage. Currently, we use the concepts of quantum physics to diagnose and treat health issues. Quantum theory gives explanations in the field of epigenetics of how subtle waves trigger DNA changes causing cancer, or triggers genes to express that would have otherwise remained dormant, by breaking down a protective protein (Bisiani et al., 2023).

There is a well-defined range of frequencies of some of the electromagnetic radiation waves commonly tracked (**Figure 13-1**). These include extremely low frequencies, such as radio waves on a continuum up to high-frequency ultraviolet light. The human eye can see only an extremely

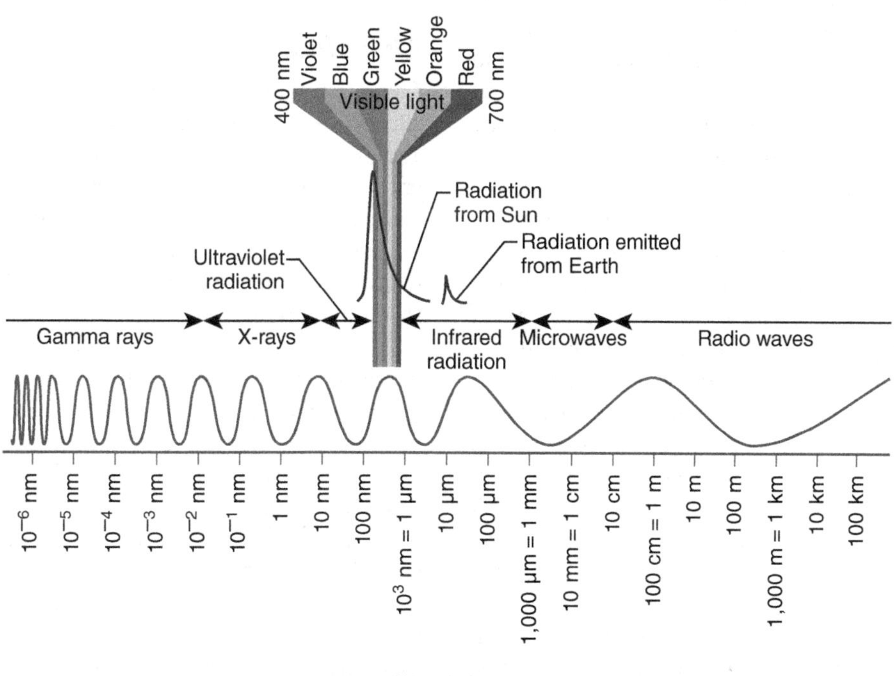

Figure 13-1 The known electromagnetic spectrum demonstrating the range visible to the eye.

narrow range of these frequencies, called the "visible spectrum." The rest of the waves still have an influence on the environment around us, even if we cannot see them.

The Biofield

All objects radiate a hierarchy of unique electrical, magnetic, and radioactive fields. Living beings are considered complex, open systems, always self-organizing, responding, and adapting to the environment to maintain homeostasis. The biofield–energy field model asserts that electromagnetic/radiation/other wave fields around living organisms are involved in homeostasis and communication of body functions. The field is always interacting with cellular health, emotions, social connections, the environment, and healing. The heart, for example, is known to give off electrical, magnetic, chemical, and thermal fields, signals that are uniquely different from all other body tissues and organs. The brain gives off electrical waves that are measured and are so important in Western medicine that decisions on whether life support should be discontinued are made based on electroencephalography (EEG). The body gives off numerous other waves, and we do not yet know how to measure or interpret them all. But they are there, and they are involved in communication between cells.

Called the "aura" in some traditions, the biofield resembles the orderly electromagnetic field you can observe when sprinkling iron filings near a magnet. Magnetic fields that were not visible to the naked eye can now be observed. One theory about what makes up an aura is that healthy human blood cells contain large amounts of iron in the hemoglobin. The electrical flow of neurons, the pulses along each cell membrane, and a vascular system that distributes iron throughout the core of the body result in electrical flow around an iron core. The result is a body that puts out an electromagnetic field. Every type of atom in the body has its own unique vibration, and gives off energy including light. There is likely an ocean of overlapping waves of energy that make up the aura around a living being, and, when we are in the presence of others, we influence each other. Historical pictures of holy figures are usually painted with an aura around them and many people report noticing auras around others.

Electricity and magnetism are different but related; they can act separately, but when combined they create an electromagnetic field that is more than either of the two. The biofield, the field around living beings, includes electromagnetic fields that are involved in organization of structure, function, communication, and health. The effects of the field on human health are not always understood. There are other waves that interact within the electromagnetic fields, including microwaves from cell towers. Concerns about 5G, a high-frequency signal, being a risk factor for disease development is an example. We would expect a cautionary, preventive approach, but epidemiological studies are needed before changes to policy will occur (Karipidis et al., 2021). UV waves from the sun break the bonds between DNA strands, changing proteins, then skin cancer begins. We are surrounded by numerous fields, always interacting.

Electrical Field

There are numerous fields influenced by electrically charged particles from molecules, cells, and organs. Atoms and molecules have different frequencies that work together harmonically and present as complex waves. Many electrical elements of a living organism's energy fields have been carefully measured, including electrocardiography (ECG) and EEG. Electricity is also used for healing. Transcutaneous electrical nerve stimulation (TENS) has been used to effectively treat chronic pain for decades and to repair tissue such as bone fractures (Johnson, 2021). Depression can be treated with electrically stimulating seizure activity or with magnetic waves (Cheng et al., 2021). Electricity can also be dangerous, even beyond electric shocks. There have been links made between the presence of high-voltage power lines and increased risk of childhood leukemia (Brabant et al., 2023). We are electrical beings, influenced by waves of electricity around us.

Magnetic Fields

Like electricity, magnetism has its uses in measurement and treatment, but also has a dangerous side. Historically, exposure to magnetic fields was not thought to be hazardous. Considerable evidence, however, has emerged on magnetic field exposure and long-term health effects including cancer, fertility issues, and numerous other health conditions. Magnetic nanoparticles are used in the diagnosis and treatment of cancer (Shivanna et al., 2022).

The magnetocardiogram (MCG) examines the heart and head's magnetic field. This device has been around more than 60 years and can measure brain waves, neuronal, and thinking activity by magnetic field changes around the head (Brisinda et al., 2023). This is a profound point. Thinking and decision making gives off a measurable field around the head, and waves are being measured from this. We can see *where* in the brain the activity is taking place with a functional MRI (*f*MRI) but we can also measure the quantum level waves that rise off of thinking or emotions. Thinking/ideas/emotional experiences are sent out as waves, and have an influence all around. There are quantum explanations of how this wave activity influences the cell membrane through a complex communication system of signals. The cell is changed.

Magnetic treatments are taking their place alongside the older electrical ones, such as electroconvulsive therapy. Repetitive transcranial magnetic stimulation (rTMS) has emerged as an alternative treatment for depression using magnetic instead of electrical stimulation of the brain. When treating those with major depression, electroconvulsive therapy is more effective than rTMS, but rTMS is better tolerated and does have measurable effectiveness (Di Iorio et al., 2022). Further, rTMS does not have the potential side effect of memory loss associated with electroconvulsive therapy. But these therapies should not be considered competing; they are both appropriate evidenced-based approaches (Di Iorio et al., 2022).

Low-Dose Radiation

The subtle energies around a living organism include a low-dose radiation given off by electrons circulating the nucleus of each atom of the body. Low doses of radiation influence cell structure and function, change ion potential of the membrane, and alter cell permeability, ion gates, and electrical potential. We clearly see this result in the radiation that comes from the sun and its effect on skin health.

Alpha, gamma, photon, and X-rays easily travel through all body tissue, passing through the body without touching any cells. At an atomic scale, the body is mostly empty space. When rays interact with human tissue, they can ionize the atoms, causing energy transfer from the rays to the atoms (usually electrons) of the tissue. We share electrons with those around us—we enter each other's subtle energy field. Low-dose radiation surrounds us and is also used as therapy (Zhou et al., 2024).

Meridian Lines

The meridians are thought to be energy flow paths marked by polarization of atomic molecules fundamental to development and perhaps preceding nervous and vascular systems. These subtle energies give off an electrical field, some of which can be measured. When energy flow is compromised, illness may result in body parts fed by that tiny energy pathway.

Acupuncture is the best-known meridian technique and involves inserting sterile needles into specific acupoints along meridian lines and points. This ancient Chinese healing technique is thought to improve the flow of qi energy through a living organism. In acupuncture, there is no anatomically defined structure compared to those in the circulatory system and Western medicine originally labeled acupuncture and traditional Chinese medicine as myth. The evidence of effectiveness of acupuncture was overwhelming, but Newtonian-thinking minds could not understand. Qi is not a biological entity, it cannot be measured, so it was dismissed and ignored. They were considering biology only, and biology is not the fundamental property. Acupressure points do not appear to correlate anatomically to body organs. Thinking in systems (respiratory system, urinary system), like we were taught in Western medicine, really does not work when considering acupuncture.

The electrical and skin conductance characteristics of acupuncture have been studied, and there is movement toward developing tools to measure skin conductance for diagnosis and treatment. However, it is unlikely that an electrical field is the only field functioning in this ancient treatment system. Energy pathways are interconnection and intercommunication systems that function at the speed of light and carry a charge of energy, influencing pH and cell function. The cell membrane is signaled from outside the cell by electro/magnetic/radiation waves, and it changes.

Research has solidified evidence for safe and effective acupuncture use and we can no longer ignore the practice because Western medicine is unable to describe how it works. There are very few risks in acupuncture beyond an occasional infection at the needle site; licensed professionals use disposable needles. This ancient approach to healing through energy systems is currently one of the better researched complementary therapies. Pain is the most common reason for acupuncture use. It has been found effective for chronic pain such as osteoarthritis, musculoskeletal back pain, and shoulder pain. Acupuncture has been found to be effective in providing relief of the symptoms of acute pain and improving outcomes post stroke such as swallowing or extremity dysfunction (Zhu et al., 2021) and chronic pain, and it does not decrease in effectiveness for up to 12 months. The World Health Organization publishes practice guidelines and recognizes acupuncture as therapeutic for more than 100 different conditions, many of which are chronic and difficult to treat with Western medicine (World Health Organization, 2021). There is strong evidence for its effective use in sleep issues, depression, infertility, GI disorders, posttraumatic stress disorder, numerous chronic diseases, various types of pain, and autoimmune diseases such as fibromyalgia or rheumatoid arthritis.

Chakras

The word *chakra*, Sanskrit for "wheel of light," describes energy centers of the body and stems from ancient understandings of energy flow within the body. These centers appear to be points where there is a continuous exchange of information between the body and the environment. There are various beliefs about the number of chakras, their location, and how they relate to the Western ideas of nerves, plexuses, neurotransmitters, neuroendocrine glands, and organs. But chakras do not translate into biology well.

Most commonly, seven major chakras are identified across Chinese, Tibetan, and Indian medicine practices. Interestingly, these chakras have been compared to Maslow's hierarchy of needs theoretically. There are energy-healing techniques developed based on the seven-chakra system. Various approaches to healing involving clearing the flow of chi (qi) through the body and many energy healing techniques center on these chakras.

Resonance

There are rhythms observed in nature that are the foundation of life. These include seasons, circadian rhythms, brain waves, planetary orbit, and the electron orbit of a nucleus. Electrons, negatively charged, circle the positively charged nucleus; they usually stay within their own ring (**Figure 13-2**).

At an atomic level, when an electron moves to a higher level of orbit, a specific quantity and

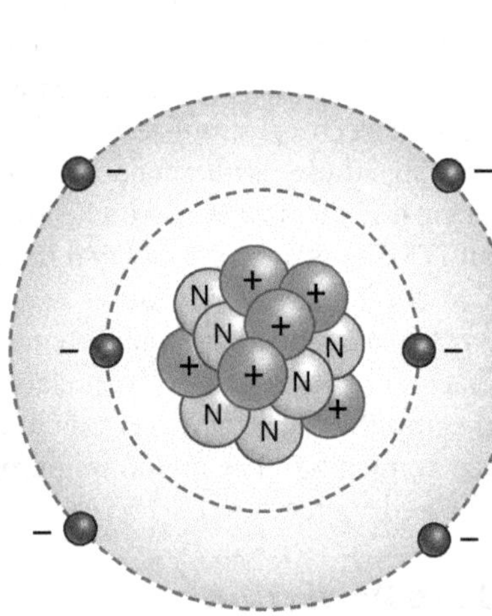

Figure 13-2 The atom, a small unit of matter. There are an equal number of electrons and protons in a stable atom.

frequency of energy is required, in much the same way that it takes more energy to speed up when passing a slower car. If an electron moves to a lower level of orbit, it radiates energy of that same frequency. In physics, this specific frequency is referred to as the *resonant frequency*. Energy is given off in the form of waves if the electron drops to a lower level and gives up energy.

Resonance is the tendency to vibrate at a specific frequency. A tuning fork creates a field of vibration around it once struck. This vibration energy moves out and influences other tuning forks of the same note. The term *resonance* is used in the field of energy psychology to describe the easy connection between two people, where it seems as if they are on the same wavelength: "I get your vibe." The experience of being close to a positive person is uplifting—it can change mood—and the connection is said to have the right vibe. Some people seem to light up the room when they enter with an upbeat, engaging energy.

Resonance in objects is best known as the effects of sound waves shattering glass, vibrating strings, or pendulum clocks beating in unison. At a specific frequency, a sound wave can shatter glass because the note matched the same resonant frequency as the glass. If you pluck a D string on a guitar, D strings on nearby guitars will vibrate and resonate. Waves are sent out, and what they touch reacts. Many energy-healing therapies, such as homeopathy, sound therapy, aromatherapy, and flower essences, use resonance as the basis for connecting in a healing and therapeutic way. The change they cause is subtle and changes are slow, but once healing occurs at an atomic level, it materializes in our macro world as measurable healing effect on cellular function and symptom reduction.

Intention and Presence

Consciousness and thinking give off waves and these transmitted signals, while subtle, can have an enormous influence on atoms, molecules, and cells. Because we all have an electromagnetic field around us (and likely several more yet to be determined fields), when we enter the biofield of another person, we change and are changed. The fields cross and interact, and electrons, energy, and information are exchanged. The mechanism of action of complementary therapies that use energy healing is thought to involve the numerous types of waves of electromagnetic radiation they emit. However, electromagnetic waves are not all we emit. Energy transferred from one to another is more than electromagnetic waves and includes a cognitive component that carries intention or caring. Emotions are not a nebulous cloud around us; they are chemicals that change cells in the body and give off waves as reactions that take place at a quantum level.

Emotions are chemicals that influence the brain neurons and thinking, and just like other chemicals, give off waves that interfere with the bonds of molecules. This can be compared to sunlight, which gives off radiation that breaks a bond between DNA strands. The cell mutates and skin cancer forms. Waves of compassion, love, and kindness cannot yet be measured, but these start out as molecules of emotion that are chemical that send out waves of information packages traveling with waves and electrons. This idea aligns with the nursing theorist Watson's identification of caring as a factor in healing.

An understanding of these principles suggests that the *presence* of a nurse brings something calming into an ocean of waves bombarding us and that the mere presence of a caring person can be healing. This concept adds to the difficulty of studying energy healing. The presence of another being—an observer, the nurse, a researcher, the practitioner—changes the experience.

Rosemarie Parse's theory of human becoming helps illustrate the importance of this concept to the practice of nursing (Parse, 1998). We are intersubjective; others influence our personal history and choices. Being in *true presence* with another reflects an experience of engaging with another at a genuine level. True presence is an intentional process, which reflects the belief that the patient knows their own way. In practice, the nurse enters the patient's perception of the world with openness and in a nonjudgmental, unconditional, and therapeutic way. The nurse's whole attention and being are with the patient, focusing on the patient's perception. This involves intentionally setting aside the nurse's own values and stepping into the patient's experience.

Intention is purposefully choosing a direction. In physics, intention has been shown to alter the activity of a particle. The particle is changed if one observes it. What is amazing is that the *intention* of observing or messing with a particle changes it.

Intention sends out a wave, and somewhere that wave influences a bond between two atoms and a molecule is changed. The nurse prepares for true presence with a quiet pause, becoming self-reflective before engaging with the patient. The nurse plans to bring some sunshine and hope to that patient behind the door. *Intention is set.* The nurse consciously allows personal worries and concerns to drift into the background while the patient's concerns are foremost. The nurse enters the room with intention, mindfully aware of the patient's words, silences, stillness, and body language. Simultaneously, the patient is aware of the nurse's genuine presence by expression of the shared feelings that exude from the nurse with facial expressions, touch, words, and energy. The nurse and patient are on the same wavelength; they are resonating.

Interconnectedness: Always Interacting

The historical exploration of energy healing invites holistic nurses to reflect on the foundations of energy as a life force in order to more deeply understand energy healing practices. Qi is the central concept of traditional Chinese medicine; it is life essence, the vital energy that is behind all physiological processes, and it flows through animals, plants, people, the earth, and the sky. Qi is distributed throughout the organism along a network of meridians that connect all parts of the organism. All life processes are based in the movement of qi. Obstructed, disordered, excess, or deficient qi flow results in problems that are unique to the person and involve disorders of the human being. In quantum physics, waves of energy are given off by all atoms, with the wave's uniqueness and strength depending on the atom.

Ayurvedic medicine is founded on the belief that there is a fundamental connection between the microcosm and the macrocosm—people are created by the universe and contain everything that composes the surrounding world. To understand people, one must understand the world and vice versa. The interdependence between individuals and society informs health and the quality of life. Energy, prana, is the basic flowing life force, the original creative power.

In modern medicine, we use fields of energy to diagnose and heal. Central to the theoretical understanding of energy in the human is the concept that energy does not stay within the realm of one's physical body. From this understanding comes the common concept originating in chaos theory: the butterfly effect. The small turbulence created when a butterfly flaps its wings can create a storm in another part of the world. One of many interpretations of this is that subtle changes do have a larger influence on bigger, more unstable systems. Released electrons, atoms, waves, and other highly subtle and difficult-to-measure factors of radiation travel to other cells in the environment. The field of radiation biology has changed significantly in the past 10 years, and the effect of low-dose radiation is no longer ignored.

We are paying more attention to these numerous, subtle energies and discovering that they also carry information packages. Einstein's famous relativity equation tells us that energy is made up of mass (can be weighed) times the speed of light (squared). $E = mc^2$ is the recipe for creating the amount of energy necessary to create mass. The very tiniest part of matter appears to be energy influenced by other energy waves in the environment. Wave/particle duality discusses how matter (hard stuff) and energy (like light) can be manipulated to change from one to another. This has been proven repeatedly, both mathematically and in a lab.

The nucleus of the atom was once thought to be the smallest building block of matter and be unbreakable. What we find when we break the atom is that it is full of energy—an atomic blast occurs. When we observe the particle very closely, it is nothing solid; rather, it appears to be waves and swirls of light and energy at the smallest level. Matter—the hard stuff—is our environment like the screen or paper you are reading this on; it is made up of waves of light and energy. Matter can no longer be thought of as the fundamental property of physics; rather, energy is. Biology can no longer be thought of as the fundamental property of health; energy is. There are oceans of waves of energy all around us, coming from us, and mingling with other waves of energy from others, from outside our body. Matter is the information packets of stuff used and organized by the energy to create the physical reality around us. This concept aligns well with Martha Rogers's nursing theory of a unitary energy system continually interacting with others and unifying with a larger universal energy.

Nursing Situation

Light is a wave of photons. Consider a patient who lives in Alaska with seasonal affective disorder using ultraviolet light therapy to improve exposure to sunlight and increased vitamin D. The sun is a wave of radiation, yet an important component of the sleep cycle is that it tones down melatonin and stimulates serotonin production. When sunlight is in short supply, biorhythms are affected, and depression is not uncommon. Yet, too much sunlight can cause skin cancer. This patient is experiencing depression and loneliness. The visits to the clinic for seasonal affective disorder light therapy provide some interaction with caring, nonjudgmental healthcare workers, and his concerns are validated. As the patient starts to feel better, he begins cooking at home again and eating better. He connects again with friends outside of work and begins meeting a friend to swim at the local pool 2 days a week. His well-being improves.

It is difficult to measure the effect of just the treatment light alone in holistic beings. Until we have ways to measure cause and effect at a quantum level, we will have difficulty showing evidence of what is happening at a quantum level. However, as nurses, we know we connect with our patients on many levels, and when our intent is examined before entering an interaction, we can enter with healing intentions, caring, and skill. Every interaction shows evidence of how we truly are interconnected.

Practice and Research

The use of energy healing has gained visibility, credibility, and use in evidence-based healthcare practice since 2000. At first met with general skepticism, research is emerging that shows efficacy beyond a placebo effect. Researching energy therapies effectively has been difficult. Recall the problem that physicists have studying photons: These tiny particles will go wherever the physicist intends, so applying this to research suggests that whatever the researcher intends will influence the outcome of an experiment. The gold-standard research approach—the experimental/control design—assumes that the people involved will not influence the results, but we now know that is not true.

Another problem with research is that most research is designed to look at cause and effect. Subtle changes in healing are difficult to measure, and we tend to use subjective measurements of the participants. We do not yet have the tools to measure changes at a quantum level, but we can measure changes when they begin to occur in the microscopic or cellular level. The technology is developing. We will one day track and interpret waves of energy that come off chemical, electrical, magnetic, gravitational, or other quantum-level reactions and better understand how that translates to health and the human condition here in the macro world.

Integration

The implications to practice are relevant since we are energetic beings; energy is involved in every health aspect of the human and in every interaction with our patients.

- In the clinical setting, there is information in the biofield around every living thing that helps the nurse understand that information is exchanged continuously.

- We are interconnected to others and the environment and this is relevant to nursing practice.
- Everything gives off waves of energy at the quantum level.
- Subtle atomic changes at the quantum level can be brought about with presence, intention, and caring.
- Subtle changes can ripple up to larger changes at the cellular and systems levels of the human being and influence health.
- Western medicine is still focused on biology, but biology is a result of what is happening at a quantum level first. Approaches to education need to change.
- There is a paradigm shift happening globally.

Conclusion

Organisms are constantly exchanging energy, electrons, and information at multiple levels, and the individual is influenced by and influencing all those around it. The mind and body cannot be separated. Fields of energy are in continuous process, and through this continuous process, the fields are in continuous change—influencing and influenced by one another.

References

Bisiani, J., Anugu, A., & Pentyala, S. (2023). It's time to go quantum in medicine. *Journal of Clinical Medicine, 12*(13), 4506. https://doi.org/10.3390/jcm12134506

Brabant, C., Geerinck, A., Beaudart, C., Tirelli, E., Geuzaine, C., & Bruyère, O. (2023). Exposure to magnetic fields and childhood leukemia: A systematic review and meta-analysis of case-control and cohort studies. *Reviews on Environmental Health, 38*(2), 229–253. https://doi.org/10.1515/reveh-2021-0112

Brisinda, D., Fenici, P., & Fenici, R. (2023). Clinical magnetocardiography: The unshielded bet-past, present, and future. *Frontiers in Cardiovascular Medicine, 10*, 1232882. https://doi.org/10.3389/fcvm.2023.1232882

Cheng, C. M., Li, C. T., & Tsai, S. J. (2021). Current updates on newer forms of Transcranial Magnetic Stimulation in major depression. *Advances in Experimental Medicine and Biology, 1305*, 333–349. https://doi.org/10.1007/978-981-33-6044-0_18

Corn, B. W., Feldman, D. B., Hull, J. G., O'Rourke, M. A., & Bakitas, M. A. (2022). Dispositional hope as a potential outcome parameter among patients with advanced malignancy: An analysis of the ENABLE database. *Cancer, 128*, 401–409. https://doi.org/10.1002/cncr.33907

Di Iorio, R., Rossi, S., & Rossini, P. M. (2022). One century of healing currents into the brain from the scalp: From electroconvulsive therapy to repetitive transcranial magnetic stimulation for neuropsychiatric disorders. *Clinical Neurophysiology, 133*, 145–151. https://doi.org/10.1016/j.clinph.2021.10.014

Johnson, M. I. (2021). Resolving long-standing uncertainty about clinical efficacy of transcutaneous electrical nerve stimulation (TENS) to relieve pain: A comprehensive review of factors influencing outcomes. *Medicina, 57*(4), 378. https://doi.org/10.3390/medicina57040378

Karipidis, K., Mate, R., Urban, D., Tinker, R., & Wood, A. (2021). 5G mobile networks and health—A state-of-the-science review of the research into low-level RF fields above 6 GHz. *Journal of Exposure Science and Environmental Epidemiology, 31*(4), 585–605. https://doi.org/10.1038/s41370-021-00297-6

Parse, R. R. (1998). *The human becoming school of thought: A perspective for nurses and other health professionals.* SAGE.

Shivanna, A. T., Dash, B. S., & Chen, J. P. (2022). Functionalized magnetic nanoparticles for alternating-magnetic field- or near-infrared light-induced cancer therapies. *Micromachines, 13*, 1279. https://doi.org/10.3390/mi13081279

World Health Organization. (2021). *WHO benchmarks for the practice of acupuncture*. https://www.who.int/publications/i/item/978-92-4-001688-0

Zhou, L., Liu, Y., Wu, Y., Yang, X., Spring Kong, F. M., Lu, Y., & Xue, J. (2024). Low-dose radiation therapy mobilizes antitumor immunity: New findings and future perspectives. *International Journal of Cancer, 154*(7), 1143–1157. https://doi.org/10.1002/ijc.34801

Zhu, J., Li, J., Yang, L. & Liu, S. (2021). Acupuncture, from ancient to current. *The Anatomical Record, 304*(11), 2365–2371. https://doi.org/10.1002/ar.24625

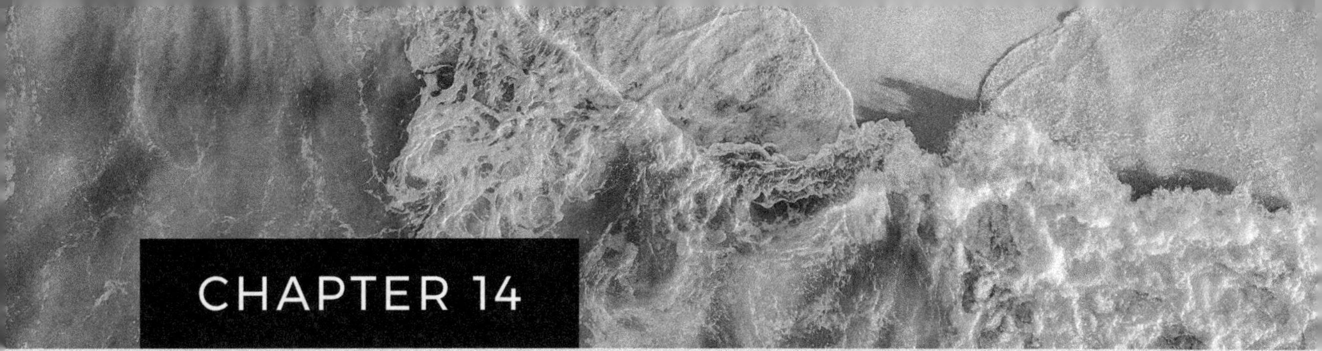

CHAPTER 14

Psychoneuroimmunology: The Science of Holistic Nursing

Debra Rose Wilson

NURSE HEALER OBJECTIVES

- Articulate the evidence behind holistic nursing interventions.
- Explain the interconnections of mind modulation and the autonomic, endocrine, immune, and neuropeptide systems.
- Recognize the totality of the human being and how all influences health, patient care, and self-care.
- Incorporate the knowledge of whole person interactions in planning nursing and self-care.

DEFINITIONS

Acute stress: The experience of reacting to something that is stressful but time limited.

Body-mind: Integration of the body and mind in an attempt to connect the duality that was lost years ago when Descartes promised the church that physicians would study the body only, not the mind or spirit. We are more than physical beings. The term *body-mind* still does not cover the whole human, but is talking about reconnecting the two when thinking about health.

Chronic stress: Stress that is of long duration, lasting weeks, months, or longer and having a far greater impact on health than acute stress. An example of chronic stress is caring for a family member with dementia in your own home.

Distant stress: Stress that may have happened a long time ago (such as from childhood sexual abuse or being in a war) but that still causes a stress response and is linked to impaired immune response and increased incidence of autoimmune disease.

Epigenetics: Part of psychoneuroimmunology, this is the study of how genes are triggered and why some stay dormant. This field examines the effect of behaviors and environment on genetic expression.

Gut microbiome: The bacteria, fungus, and other live organisms in our gut form the microbiome and, through immune function, influence our physical and mental health. Imbalance in this biome appears to be part of the trigger for many diseases.

Neuropeptides: Messenger molecules produced at various sites throughout the body to transmit body–mind patterns of communication.

Neurotransmitters: Chemicals that facilitate communication through nerves in the body. Examples are low levels of serotonin activity are associated with depressive disorder or high levels of dopamine activity associated with schizophrenia.

Psychoneuroimmunology: Often called the "science behind holistic care," psychoneuroimmunology (PNI) is a branch of research that strives to show that biology is not the only, and not even the predominant factor that determines health and illness.

Reductionism: Based on Descartes' thinking, biology was the most important part of health. Medical science reduces the human into parts, examining those physical parts they would better understand and treat the whole human.

Traumatic stress response: This response occurs due to overwhelming, unresolved, or enduring stress that changes both immune and brain function over time.

Introduction

Since the 1990s, we have developed a far better understanding of the science behind holism. The world is complex and unified. Parts complement one another and participate in the whole. Similarly, all parts of the body communicate and interact with purpose. We are starting to answer some old questions and finding ways to ask new ones.

Why is it that an attitude about illness, or the number of good friends you have, can influence on your health? How does stress make you ill? Why are there higher levels of inflammatory markers in the blood of people with depression? How is trauma linked to the development of physical disease later in life? Why do people with angry personality types develop cardiovascular disease more often? How does changing what you think and believe improve immune function? How does a psychologically toxic work environment and a sense of lack of control influence immune function? How do meditation or other stress management interventions influence health? How does prayer work to improve wound healing? The study of psychoneuroimmunology examines all these things. Psychoneuroimmunology is the eclectic science that helps us consider the human as a holistic being. Biology and chemistry are not the only "parts" relevant in healing.

The field of psychoneuroimmunology (PNI) is probably misnamed. Researchers once again tried to describe a holistic phenomenon by dividing it into systems. This is a reductionist approach, viewing a whole in parts, and maybe never seeing the whole. For decades, Western medicine has viewed the human as moving biology and chemistry. It makes sense that the response to health issues were a plethora of pharmaceuticals. But we are more than biochemistry, and the rest that isn't biology has a significant impact on health. The name has been around since the 1990s, and for now, PNI defines the science of the mind, spirit, social support, environment, genetics, biome, trauma on health, and illness. PNI is the science behind holism.

The leading causes of nonaccidental death in 2022 were cardiovascular disease (CVD), cancer, COVID-19, and stroke (CDC, 2022). The primary interventions for *prevention* of all these disease processes involve cognitive/behavioral approaches. Eating better, stress and anger management, exercise, time management, self-care, and relaxation are examples of skills that are taught to patients.

Stress suppresses immune function, which leads to increased inflammation and the development or progression of disease. CVD, cancer, and irritable bowel syndrome all begin with an inflammatory response, as do many other chronic or autoimmune diseases. Obesity is an inflammatory condition linked to cancer, asthma, CVD, and an unbalanced gut microbiome (Asthma & Allergy Foundation, 2024; Clark et al., 2024; Dai et al., 2020). Inflammation is worsened with a diet high in processed foods and saturated fats, stress, or a sedentary lifestyle. Trauma, especially in early life, can lead to autoimmune diseases by triggering inflammation. Trauma changes brain physiology over time, and the immune system changes. Depression is an inflammatory biological process influenced by the environment, diet, social support, and life satisfaction. Stress, obesity, and previous trauma are inflammatory and can trigger cancer.

PNI is innately holistic, linking systems, environment, emotions, diet, social elements, processes at a quantum level, with biology. Stress management, dietary changes, meditation, cognitive/behavioral approaches, sleep hygiene, care relating to spirituality, and social support are just a few examples of evidence-based interventions that have developed from the study of PNI. These interventions need to be used in prevention, which, from an economic and human perspective, is far less costly than treating disease.

We have to stop thinking that "biology" is the most important factor when it comes to disease. What causes disease is always more than one thing; a combination of many different factors. The study of epigenetics teaches us that even genetics does not predetermine our health.

Stress

Stress is described as a feeling of being overwhelmed, worried, or run down. Stress can affect people regardless of age, socioeconomic status, gender identity, or profession. An overabundance of stress reduces the effective function of the immune, cardiovascular, neuroendocrine, and central nervous systems. Stressors are the triggers that stress us and are a normal part of life. We are required to adapt, and when a stressor is perceived, the organism is physiologically prepared to attack or flee from the threat. When stressors are experienced, biology, emotions, social support, motivation, environment, attitude, immune function, and wellness are all relevant to how stress translates to health or disease. Stress has a profound effect on health and current levels of stress are much higher than for previous generations.

The Stress Response

There is a cascade of hormones and chemicals that begin when the brain decides there is a threat. That decision (is this a threat?) happens in milliseconds as the person reviews level of threat, access to appropriate coping mechanisms, and previous relevant experience. For example, if a teacher has a pop-quiz every single class, it is not as startling. This *fight-or-flight response* is enacted when the body moves into a sympathetic nervous system active state, preparing to expend energy and shutting down nonessential systems. Routine systems that shut down could be the production of natural killer cells that attack mutating cancer cells.

The stress response is modified by the intensity of other concurrent stressors, social support, personality, and previously learned coping skills. Perceived stressors begin in the areas of the brain that control cognition and emotions—the cerebral cortex and the limbic system. **Figure 14-1** demonstrates the physiologic stress response.

The major endocrine hormones released in the stress response are epinephrine from the adrenal medulla and glucocorticoids from the adrenal cortex. Other hormones associated with the stress response include pituitary hormones (growth hormone, prolactin, estrogen, and testosterone). The growth hormone affects the metabolism of carbohydrates, protein, and lipids. Estrogen may attenuate the stress response, changing the experience for women. Decreased testosterone levels occur in men during stressful experiences. The natural opioids (i.e., endorphins, enkephalins) are synthesized in the pituitary and other parts of the central nervous system. Opioids have a morphinelike effect with receptors throughout the body. These naturally occurring hormones produce the runner's high, increase a person's pain threshold, and explain how people can ignore their own serious injuries to save a loved one. Endorphins are secreted by immune cells during stress, leading to analgesia. Nonessential body processes are suspended. Cytokines are messenger proteins that respond to stress and trigger the body to begin inflammation. Cortisol is a steroidal hormone that produces similar effects to those of epinephrine, but the effects last from minutes to days. Cortisol stimulates increasing blood glucose levels and protein breakdown. This breakdown leads to loss of muscle, negative nitrogen balance, increased gastrointestinal secretions, more inflammation, and suppression of the immune system.

In a matter of minutes, the adrenal cortex releases glucocorticoids. Hypothalamic, pituitary, and adrenal neuropeptides interact with the immune response, completing the multidirectional circle of communication among the nervous, endocrine, and immune systems. Platelets are spilled into the blood in anticipation of injury, and glucose is released to give quick energy to react. Pupils dilate to increase peripheral vision, looking for more danger. There is increased heart and respiratory rates, tightened muscles, increased metabolic rate, and a sense of foreboding, fear, nervousness, irritability, and negative mood.

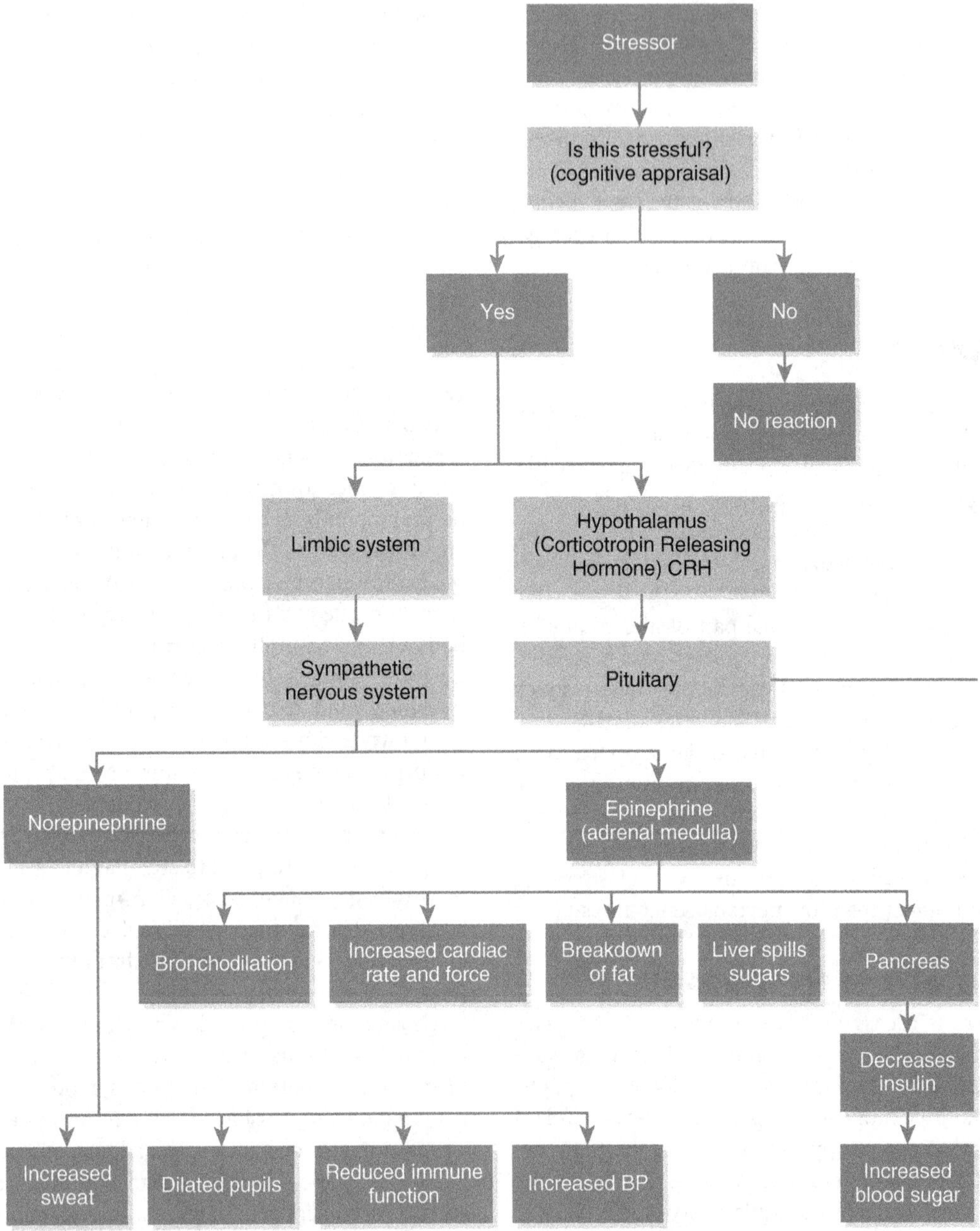

Figure 14-1 Physiologic stress response.

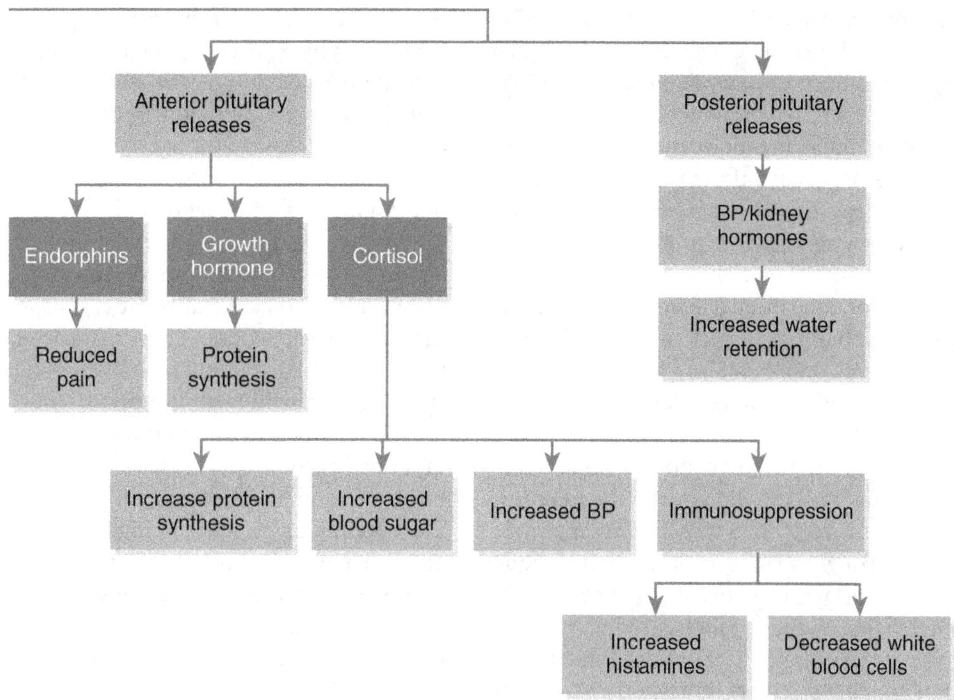

Figure 14-1 *(continued)*

Other physiologic responses include elevated blood pressure, stronger cardiac contractions, and increased levels of blood glucose, serum cholesterol, circulating free fatty acids, and triglycerides. Stress has a ripple effect on the body. The chemical response by the body affects every cell.

The stress response is designed to protect against threats. We are not supposed to be in a fight or flight response all the time. Threats may be physical, social, psychosocial, real, and/or simply part of anticipation and anxiety disorder, with no real basis in reality, and the body responds as if there was a saber-toothed tiger in the room. Thoughts and feelings alone can trigger the release cascade of chemicals described above and convey messages of distress to various systems within the body. When the stress is no longer a threat, the parasympathetic system returns the body to its normal, homeostatic state.

Types of Stressors

Duration of stress directly influences the body. *Acute stressors* are short-term and boost immune function. Taking a test or speaking in public may motivate you to pay more attention and make you feel more alive. But the longer the perceived stress, the more the body responds with the fight-or-flight response, eventually exhausting cellular immunity and triggering inflammation. *Chronic stressors* that are perceived as never-ending can have a significant impact on psychological and physical health. Family caregivers of dementia patients have been identified as one of the most stressed populations (Alzheimer's Association, 2024), and this directly affects their health. Many of us know of situations where "Aunt Betty" was caring for "Uncle Bob" until he went into the nursing home. She was financially challenged, needed respite, and was not sleeping well since he was getting up and turning on the stove. Related to this chronic stress and inflammation, she developed cancer and died before Uncle Bob. Chronic stress can occur in response to everyday stressors that are ignored, too numerous, or poorly managed. Chronic stress can occur as a response to previous traumatic events. The consequences of chronic stress are longer lasting and more serious, particularly as it contributes to inflammation and disease. Ongoing stress, such as dealing with cancer, toxic work environments, or domestic violence, has prolonged and profound effects on immune functioning over time. *Distant stressors* are traumatic experiences and include the experiences of war or childhood sexual abuse, and can also lead to posttraumatic stress disorder (PTSD). Distant stressors have the potential to continue to influence immune functioning because of the sheer length of their influence. Distant stressors are often also chronic stressors. Cortisol levels remain high for long periods after the experience.

Understanding the psychophysiologic stress response helps to clarify how many different holistic therapies work. It is possible to interrupt feelings of anxiety by using a relaxation technique to calm the self or a cognitive restructuring technique to change thought patterns. When patients learn to use relaxation, imagery, music therapy, or meditation, their sympathetic responses to stress decrease, and the calming effect of the parasympathetic system takes over, leading to holistic healing. Stress management improves immune function and reduces inflammation in patients with cancer; there is a call for stress management training to be part of the normal patient care (Antoni et al., 2023).

Trauma

Intrusive flashbacks or just thinking back on severe trauma, such as childhood abuse, war, or a near-death automobile accident, can trigger waves of the fight-or-flight responses, even when the threat is long gone. These distant stressors are unrelenting, changing immune function, coping skills, and decision making over time. Early trauma is recognized as having a significant effect on health. We can observe changes over time in brain structure, function, and circuitry in functional magnetic resonance imaging (fMRI), leaving behind a biological imprint of the trauma for those who have been traumatized (Ross et al., 2021). The amygdala is more reactive, emotions are more profound, and more chemicals are spilled (Sicorello et al., 2021). Autoimmune diseases develop; the particular disease is dependent upon genetics, physical/social/quantum environment, and lifestyle. Children who experienced trauma have higher levels of cortisol in their hair, and in a 2024 study, this translated to significantly more childhood disease compared to those who were not traumatized (Marsland et al., 2024). The earlier the trauma, the more years of profound damage to the brain and immune function. A new, severe trauma (acute trauma stress disorder) will become chronic without stress management, cognitive retraining, relaxation, self-reflection, sharing their story, and getting support.

Long-term and unremitting stress can reduce immune function and increase the inflammatory response, and the body enters an illness state. The continuous presence of high levels of cortisol and other stress chemicals triggers inflammatory processes, increasing the risk of such disorders as osteoporosis, ulcers, and Alzheimer's disease. Autoimmune diseases are also triggered.

Emotions and Cognition

The extent of the interactions that a living system can have with its environment outlines its cognitive domain. Emotions are not just an accompaniment of perception and behavior but are an inherent part of the cognitive and physical domains. For example, an anger response to a situation initiates an entire pattern of physiologic processes. Emotions are not nebulous clouds around us; rather, they each trigger unique chemical combinations that are molecules—molecules of emotion (Pert, 1999). Our emotions and feelings are sources of vital information to our physical body. Emotions are life-regulating phenomena that help maintain our health by leading adaptive changes in our body states.

Stress-related emotions can persist long after, or sometimes even without a stressful event. A substantial amount of cognitive time spent in anticipation of future stress will trigger the stress response. This cognitive state has a significant impact on the physical state as can be observed in prolonged elevated blood pressure. In some cases, the impact of rumination can increase emotion and stress, not just prolong it.

There is increasing interest in the benefits of positive emotions on the immune system, and this has been called "affective immunology," a specialty within the field of PNI. Laughter is a universal language that reduces the stress response, improves learning, increases heart rate variability, enhances cardiac output, improves endocrine function, and may be protective against metabolic syndrome (Stiwi & Rosendahl, 2022). The relationship between the immune system is bidirectional, and an unstable immune function will influence emotional response. As a result, the patient may experience an increase in pain, anxiety, unhealthy coping behaviors (such as drinking alcohol), or disturbances in interactions with others when they are ill. Studies are showing that generating happiness, hope, and other positive emotions improves immune function. This means that the healthy function of the immune system can be moderated by the conscious mind. Happiness and hope can be generated. Laughter therapy and generating hope have positive immune benefits, and programs to enhance happiness are becoming part of the evidence-based realm of patient care.

Automatic thinking elicits an emotional response. Becoming aware of automatic thinking is the first step to learning to stop negative thinking. This *cognitive restructuring* is part of the cognitive behavioral approaches to change negative patterns in thinking and emotions. Studies in forgiveness have revealed that whenever people choose to forgive, areas in the emotional limbic center of the brain are activated, health is improved, and cardiovascular stress is reduced. Numerous research studies on the relationship of forgiveness and health repeatedly show that forgiveness is good for our physical, cognitive, and emotional well-being (Mullen et al., 2023). Emotional well-being is within the realm of the nurse. Interventions to support and enhance coping offer another opportunity to promote healing and wholeness.

For those who have PTSD, writing therapy, reading, bodywork, art therapy, and even the traditional talk therapies are all ways of releasing an experience frozen in the amygdala that is capable of triggering the fight, flight, freeze, or faint response provoked by seemingly benign stimuli. Emotional healing can improve immune function and health.

Personality and Wellness

The field of PNI began in cardiovascular rehabilitation, and back in the late 1980s, it was noticed that people with cardiovascular disease tend to have controlling personalities and be quick to anger. Stress and anger management training became part of the treatment regimen in response. Personality traits are thought to be well established and difficult to change by adolescence and are both genetic and environmental. Researchers have since been finding links to personality traits and specific disease. Research is starting to ask some new questions. Can people who develop Parkinson's disease be identified as high risk before the disease begins by screening their personality characteristics (Boussac et al., 2022)? Would assessing for personality traits, such as being neurotic, help earlier diagnosis in fibromyalgia patients (Silva et al., 2022)? Personality is part of the whole human being along with genetic and environmental roots, so we cannot be surprised that wellness and disease are linked to personality and temperament.

Social Support

Another area of interest in PNI is how the environment influences health and wellness, and social networks are part of our environment. The social environment is integral to wellness. Loneliness is a risk factor for coronary heart disease (Lu et al., 2024). Women with close female friends have better breast cancer outcomes. Assessing and finding ways to enhance the social environment for our patients becomes part of the nurse's role. Nurses can refer patients to support groups and other family services with an understanding that this will improve immune function, resilience, and healing.

Stress and Disease

Metabolic syndrome is a group of risk factors that increase the likelihood of significant chronic health problems, such as diabetes, stroke, and heart disease. There are five risk factors associated with metabolic syndrome. They include a large waistline, an increased triglyceride level, low high-density lipoprotein cholesterol level, hypertension, and hyperglycemia. For an individual to be diagnosed with metabolic syndrome, they must have at least three of these risk factors (National Institute of Health, 2022). This syndrome is quite complex, but an underlying factor is low-grade inflammation. Prevention of metabolic syndrome will protect the individual from these major life-threatening diseases. Lifestyle changes, weight and stress management, lowering cholesterol with diet and medication, increasing activity, and self-care are all recommended for those at risk.

Being stressed or chronically ill can be depressing in itself. Depression must be considered holistically and has many different possible contributors. These probably include genetics, resiliency, current internal and external resources, brain neurotransmitters, hormones, diet, environment, and stress. Stressful events are known to be triggers for depression. Stress also leads to overactivity of the body's stress-response system. The failure of the body to stop the rush of hormones related to stress is also known to influence depression. If sleep is poor, the immune system does not get to repair and replenish itself in deep sleep. When people are stressed or depressed, they neglect self-care, diet, and exercise and engage in lifestyle practices (like smoking and using drugs or alcohol) that further contribute to depression. Depression causes even further stress and life crisis. High levels of inflammation markers are found in those who are depressed.

One of the new ways of thinking about depression also includes the immune system in the equation. When an injury or infection happens, the immune system directs inflammatory agents to rush through the blood to the wound. Cytokines (interleukins) signal for help and trigger sickness behaviors (fatigue, appetite changes, reduced motivation, fever). White blood cells arrive to kill any invading bacteria. Red blood cells bring extra oxygen for the healing tissue. Clotting factors arrive in case there is bleeding. The result is swelling and redness that is uncomfortable enough that one has to rest a little so the body can heal, further contributing to the sickness behavior. Depression is accompanied by this same inflammatory response; we tend to observe higher levels of cytokines in the blood. Stress hormones (such as cortisol) tend to be higher in people with depression. Stress leaves behind a biological footprint. For example, babies of women who experienced high levels of stress or trauma during pregnancy have higher levels of cortisol in their hair, and the stress reaction often continues in the infant after birth (Strahm et al., 2020).

Depression is disproportionately higher in people with inflammatory chronic diseases. There is a strong link between inflammation and the development of depression (and other psychiatric illnesses). People who have a history of depression are more likely to develop cancer and atherosclerosis, which are also inflammatory. Depression is an inflammatory condition that worsens autoimmune diseases.

Autoimmune diseases are a group of inflammatory (often chronic) diseases in which the immune system is attacking the self. Stress has an instrumental role in autoimmune disease genesis. In rheumatoid arthritis, for example, the immune system believes the cells of the tissue around joints are foreign invaders and attacks them. Inflammation, pain, and eventually disability result. Cancer is another example of an autoimmune disease. Stress management, self-care, meditation, guided imagery, yoga, music, and exercise are found to release endorphins as the sympathetic system is calmed. The immune system steps out of the emergency mode and back into maintenance of function and symptoms of autoimmune diseases are reduced. This is a concept worth reflecting on.

Sleep

Relevant to the connection between thoughts, behaviors, and health is sleep. Immune function maintenance and repair occur during deep and prolonged stages of sleep. Less than 4 hours of sleep results in higher blood pressure and reduced function of the entire cardiovascular system. Inflammatory markers increase in the blood, amplifying any chronic pain or inflammatory diseases. Cells begin showing insulin-resistant behaviors that are known to lead to diabetes (Sleep Foundation, 2024). Chronic inadequate sleep increases appetite and activity decreases, predisposing the individual to obesity. Those who are sleep deprived develop less immunity from vaccines, implying impaired immune function. Sleep apnea, teeth grinding, and other sleep disorders have been directly linked to increased perceived stress and subsequent health issues. Sleep apnea significantly increases inflammation in the body and has been shown to lead to cardiovascular disease. Sleep deprivation increases symptoms of mental health disorders and decreases perceived coping ability. Inadequate sleep is strongly linked to an increased risk of dying. Those who have experienced trauma tend to feel overstimulated and have difficulty falling asleep and staying asleep. Nightmares and flashbacks are the antithesis of relaxed sleep, flooding the body with the hormones and neurotransmitters of alertness and fear. In the other direction, sleep deprivation has been shown to be associated with increased responsiveness to stress and sensitivity to stress-related disorders.

Sleep hygiene training should include assessment of sleep patterns, identification of barriers to good sleep, and tips for quality sleep. The field of behavioral sleep medicine is expanding. More studies are needed on effective treatment approaches, and focus needs to turn to prevention of sleep disorders. An early focus on healthy sleep and dissemination of sleep hygiene education can be expected to reduce the incidence of chronic, expensive, and debilitating disease.

Epigenetics

Our genes are not fixed; we are not simply genetically determined. Choices and behaviors trigger a gene, otherwise it remains dormant, wrapped in a protective protein. Our genes are modulated by our inner environment—the emotional, chemical, mental, energetic, and spiritual landscape—as well as our outer environment—the social, physical, quantum, and ecological systems in which we reside. Genes may be activated or deactivated by the meaning we assign to an experience, the emotions experienced, or the trauma felt.

The process by which a gene produces a result in the body is well established. Signals pass through the cell membrane to the nucleus, enter the chromosome, and activate a specific strand of DNA. Each strand of DNA is protected by a protein. The protein serves as a barrier between the information in the DNA and the rest of the intracellular environment. As long as the DNA is wrapped by the protein, the DNA lies dormant. When the right signal arrives, the protein around the DNA unwraps, and, with the assistance of RNA, the DNA molecule replicates a protein molecule. A gene is expressed. At this point, the targeted gene moves into active expression where it constructs, assembles, or alters products. What was dormant potential is moved into active expression by a signal that comes from outside the cell, not from the DNA.

Key neuronal genes are modified by early life experience and govern learning and memory throughout life. Enriched early childhood experience enhances spatial learning, whereas chronic early life stress may result in persistent deficits in the structure and function of hippocampal neurons. Epigenetics allows people who have a strong genetic history of bowel cancer (for example) to avoid triggering that gene with proper nutrition, fiber, stress management, or exercise. A lifetime of stress accelerates the processes of epigenetic aging, and cells are changed. Environmental pollution, allergens, and even maternal stress during pregnancy can activate the genes, and the disease begins. Epigenetics is a new field of study, and we are beginning to understand that our genes do not define us; rather, we can influence them positively and negatively.

Microbiome

The bacteria and other live organisms in our gut microbiome can influence our mental health and appear to be part of the trigger for diabetes and other inflammatory diseases (Clark et al., 2024). There is also increasing evidence that we can use probiotics to help persons suffering from a variety of illnesses. These include not only bowel disease

Nursing Situation

A person with asthma that increasingly interferes with their activities may remember that their mother's asthma also became more severe as she aged. They may begin to become resigned to what they see as an inevitable decline in their health. However, sadness and depression associated with those thoughts release stress hormones. The body responds with chemicals of stress, cytokines tell the body there is danger and that inflammation is needed, and responses to allergens worsen. One day, they learn that they do not have to be a slave to their genetics. They decide they do not want to be as miserable as their mother was, and they begin to educate themself. Subsequently, they learn how to monitor their asthma. They begin to see a pattern to their attacks, identify potential triggers, and use both traditional and holistic interventions to gain more control. They change their environment, reduce triggers and stress, and begin using meditation as a way to reduce inflammation in their body. They choose to forgive those who have given them worry or injury and improve their social support network. The asthma attacks decrease in severity and frequency.

such as Crohn's, but also depression and diabetes. One of the functions of the gut microbiome is to produce neurotransmitters (i.e., serotonin, GABA). Deficiency in the neurotransmitters and serotonin and gamma aminobutyric acid (GABA) are found with depression. A probiotic cocktail of *Lactobacillus helveticus* and *Bifidobacterium longum* was found to reduce cortisol (stress) levels. We have to consider the negative effects of overused antibiotics on the helpful bacteria in our gut, when rest and fluids would have been sufficient. Humans are in symbiotic relationship with these microorganisms.

Quantum Physics

The field of quantum physics in health examines the continuous, tiny atomic levels of interaction between the self and the environment. There are chemical, electrical, and subatomic waves that are able to change bonds within molecules, changing cell structure. Thoughts induce emotions, emotions are chemicals that give off waves as they react, chains of protein have bonds broken, and the protein twirls and changes into something else. The cell changed. A better understanding of quantum physics in health will help us demonstrate the importance of intention, kindness, self-talk, hope, and true presence in healing, providing more insight into how we each make a ripple of change.

Integration

- In clinical practice, diseases previously regarded as psychological (depression) or physical (cancer) can no longer be categorized.
- In patient education, teaching patients about relevant and *doable* options they can employ can reduce feelings of helplessness and generate hope.
- Nursing research can continue to examine the impact of cognitive or behavioral interventions on health.
- Recognizing that biology is not as important as once thought, when it comes to health or disease, is a paradigm shift happening globally.

Implications

Stress management training and life coaching are part of the nurse's role in promoting wellness. Being aware of how personality, environment, social support, and other factors influence the holistic being will help the nurse assess and enhance those factors. The field of psychoneuroimmunology is demonstrating that holism is a solid, measurable science that calls for change on how nurses view and provide care to their patients.

Conclusion

We are increasingly faced with challenges of complexity. People with heart disease, a major and costly public health concern with high hospitalization and mortality rates, also experience disproportionately high rates of depression. We are just beginning to understand the neurohormonal and cytokine activation link to these comorbid disorders. Simple cause-and-effect explanations are no longer sufficient. The exploration of the extensive interactions among psychological and behavioral factors, the nervous system, the immune system, the endocrine system, and the environment should help us understand the mechanisms underlying health, wellness, and diseases. Existing evidence already supports the relationship between unmanaged stress, depression, and inflammation with disorders such as cardiovascular disease, skin diseases, obesity, diabetes, arthritis, and Alzheimer's disease.

Patients are increasingly knowledgeable about complementary interventions and incorporate them with positive results. Effective interventions can educate and empower the patient and generate hope. The meaning of the illness, the method of giving the diagnosis, the tone of voice, the touch of the nurse, and the relationships to family and friends are all part of the experience for the patient.

Consider, for a moment, the metaphorical implications of autoimmune disease where the self is attacking the self. Negative self-talk and low self-esteem create a similar tangible self-attacking-self analogy. Changing beliefs about self, learning to recognize and stop toxic self-talk empowering self, learning life skills for success, embracing the power of self-care, and stress management also reduce inflammation and help balance immune function, and ultimately promote wellness. We are holistic beings.

References

Alzheimer's Association. (2024, March). *Alzheimer's disease caregivers.* https://www.alz.org/news/2024/facts-figures-report-dementia-caregiver-stress

Antoni, M. H., Moreno, P. I., & Penedo, F. J. (2023). Stress management interventions to facilitate psychological and physiological adaptation and optimal health outcomes in cancer patients and survivors. *Annual Review of Psychology, 74*, 423–255.

Asthma and Allergy Foundation of America. (2024). *Asthma: Emotions, stress, and depression.* https://aafa.org/asthma/asthma-triggers-causes/emotions-stress-depression/

Boussac, M., Arbus, C., Colin, O., Laurencin, C., Eusebio, A., Hainque, E., Corvol, J. C., Versace, N., Rascol, O., Rousseau, V., Harroch, E., Ory-Magne, F., Fabbri, M., Moreau, C., Rolland, A. S., Jarraya, B., Maltête, D., Drapier, S., Marques, A. R., Auzou, N., … PREDISTIM study group. (2022). Personality assessment with temperament and character inventory in Parkinson's disease. *Parkinsonism Related Disorders, 103*, 34–41. https://doi.org/10.1016/j.parkreldis.2022.08.004

Centers for Disease Control and Prevention (CDC). (2022). *Deaths and mortality.* https://www.cdc.gov/nchs/fastats/deaths.htm

Clark, T., Butler, K., & Wilson, D. R. (2024). The gut biome and health. *American Nurse,19*(4). https://www.myamericannurse.com/gut-microbiome-and-health

Dai, S., Mo., Y., Wang, Y., Xiang, B., Liao, Q., Zhou, M., Li, X., Li, Y., Xiong, W., Li, G., Guo, C., & Zeng, Z. (2020). Chronic stress promotes cancer development. *Frontiers in Oncology, 10*, 1492. https://doi.org/10.3389/fonc.2020.01492

Lu, Y., Wang, R., Norman, J., & Yu, P. (2024). Loneliness status transitions and risk of cardiovascular disease among middle-aged and older adults, *Nutrition, Metabolism and Cardiovascular Diseases, 34*(3), 718–725.

Marsland, A. L., Jones, E., Reed, R. G., Walsh, C. P., Natale, B. N., Lindsay, E. K., & Ewing, L. J. (2024). Childhood trauma and hair cortisol response over the year following onset of a chronic life event stressor. *Psychoneuroendocrinology, 165,* 107039. https://doi.org/10.1016/j.psyneuen.2024.107039.

Mullen, L. M., Bistany, B. R., Kim, J. J., Joseph, R. A., Akers, S. W., Harvey, J. R., & Houghton, A. (2023). Facilitation of forgiveness: Impact on health and well-being. *Holistic Nursing Practice, 37*(1), 15–23. https://doi.org/10.1097/HNP.0000000000000559

National Institute of Health. (2022). *Metabolic syndrome.* https://www.nhlbi.nih.gov/health-topics /metabolic-syndrome

Pert, C. B. (1999). *Molecules of emotion: The science behind mind–body medicine.* Simon & Schuster.

Ross, M. C., Heilicher, M., & Cisler, J. M. (2021). Functional imaging correlates of childhood trauma: A qualitative review of past research and emerging trends. *Pharmacology Biochemistry and Behavior, 211,* 173297. https://doi.org/10.1016/j.pbb.2021.173297

Sicorello, M., Thome, J., Herzog, J., & Schmahl, C. (2021). Differential effects of early adversity and posttraumatic stress disorder on amygdala reactivity: The role of developmental timing. *Biological Psychiatry: Cognitive Neuroscience and Neuroimaging, 6*(11), 1044–1051. https://doi.org/10.1016/j.bpsc.2020.10.009.

Silva, M. P. S., Carvalho, J. F., & Rodrigues, C. E. M. (2022). Evaluation of big five personality factors in women with fibromyalgia: A cross-sectional study. *Rheumatology International, 42*, 503–510. https://doi.org/10.1007/s00296-021-04936-x

Sleep Foundation. (2024). *Effects of sleep deprivation.* https://www.sleepfoundation.org/sleep-deprivation/effects-of-sleep-deprivation

Stiwi, K., & Rosendahl, J. (2022). Efficacy of laughter-inducing interventions in patients with somatic or mental health problems: A systematic review and meta-analysis of randomized-controlled trials. *Complementary Therapies in Clinical Practice, 47*(101552).

Strahm, A. M., Bagne, A. G., Rued, H. A., Larson, K. J., Roemmich, J. N., & Hilmert, C. J. (2020). Prenatal traumatic stress and offspring hair cortisol concentration: A nine year follow up to the Red River flood pregnancy study. *Psychoneuroendocrinology, 113*(104579). https://doi.org/10.1016/j.psyneuen.2019.104579

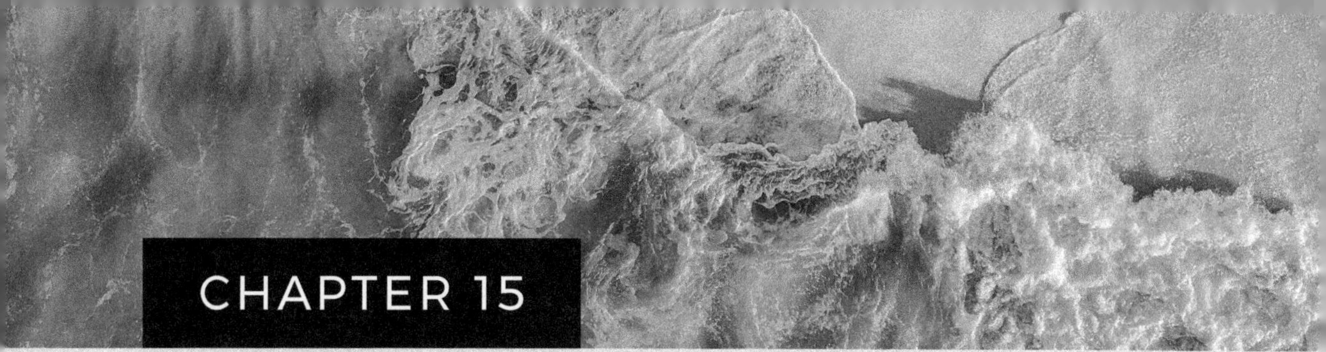

CHAPTER 15

Integrative and Complementary Health Approaches

Jennifer S. Browning and Marci Resnicoff

Introduction

Holistic nurses provide whole-person care, recognizing the interconnectedness of all and the totality of the human experience. Holistic nurses, in partnership with the person and significant others, create a plan of care that focuses on well-being in health promotion, recovery, restoration, or peaceful dying, honoring each person's unique journey and meeting them where they are. In the provision of whole-person care, holistic nurses may utilize complementary health approaches and therapies along with conventional medical care. Although using complementary health approaches on their own does not designate the nurse "holistic," holistic nurses know the importance and value of an integrative approach to health care, enabling the person to benefit from the best of all treatments available.

According to the National Center for Complementary and Integrative Health's National Health Interview Survey (NHIS), more than 30 percent of adults and about 12 percent of children use healthcare approaches that are not typically part of conventional medical care or that may have origins outside of traditional Western healthcare practice (NCCIH, 2024). Most complementary health approaches fall into one of two subgroups—natural products or mind and body practices. *Natural products* include a variety of natural remedies, such as herbs (also known as "botanicals"), vitamins and minerals, and probiotics. *Mind and body practices* include a large and diverse group of procedures or techniques.

For example, in 2017, the NHIS Survey revealed that the number of American adults and children using yoga and meditation had significantly increased over previous years, while the use of chiropractic and osteopathic manipulation had increased as well. Other complementary health approaches reported by investigators included those that did not fit into either of the two groups, for example, Ayurveda, Traditional Chinese Medicine, homeopathy, naturopathy, and energy healing. A more comprehensive list of additional therapies may be found in *Holistic nursing: Scope and standards of Practice*, 3rd ed. (American Nurses Association & American Holistic Nurses Association, 2019).

The purpose of this chapter is to introduce a number of complementary therapies that you could integrate into your holistic nursing practice such as mindfulness, meditation, clinical imagery, touch and hand-mediated therapies, energy-based practices, and aromatherapy. The contributors are holistic nurses, all experts in their chosen therapy. While the chapter is not intended to teach the practices in their entirety, we hope that your interest is piqued. Perhaps you will discover a practice that you can use right away, or maybe you will choose to delve more deeply into one of these and undertake studies to deepen your knowledge, skills, and expertise. Enjoy the journey!

References

American Nurses Association & American Holistic Nurses Association. (2019). *Holistic nursing: Scope and standards of practice* (3rd ed.). Nursesbooks.org

National Center for Complementary and Integrative Health (NCCIH). (2024, December). *Complementary, alternative, or integrative health: What's in a name?* https://www.nccih.nih.gov/health/complementary-alternative-or-integrative-health-whats-in-a-name

Mindfulness and Meditation

Toyoko Yasui with credit to the former work of Jeanne Anselmo

NURSE HEALER OBJECTIVES

- Define mindfulness and meditation.
- Explore ways that a chosen meditation/mindfulness practice supports self-care, well-being, and the ability to connect deeply with oneself, others, community, and beyond, helping create a healing environment and supportive organizational culture.

DEFINITIONS

Meditation: Originally based in spiritual traditions, now recognized in both religious and secular forms of a variety of practices including insight, open awareness, cultivating compassion, and concentration. Through dedication, meditation practice evolves over time and is known to provide self-regulation health benefits and is a pathway for personal and spiritual transformation.

Mindfulness/mindful awareness: Awareness arising through nonjudgmental, present purposeful attention in the service of self-understanding and wisdom. One can practice mindfulness during everyday activities like walking, eating, breathing; mindfulness is enhanced by meditation practice but is not contingent on it.

Oneness: A united state, wholeness, not separate; identity in harmony with beings and/or nature.

Introduction: Cultivating Awareness for Personal and Collective Nursing Practice

Jean Watson (2005) describes "Caring" (p. 6) as a sacred art in which the transpersonal caring field and the relationship between the nurse and the patient create new possibilities for how to be in the moment through a unitary field of consciousness and energy that transcend time, space, and physicality. Margaret Newman (1994) also informs us of the great importance of being fully present in the moment and knowing that whatever the experience, it is a manifestation of the process of evolving to higher consciousness (p. 68). Our "presence" with the patient, holding time and space, allows us, nurses, to witness how resilient patients grow through challenges, their turning points while expanding their consciousness with every challenge. Mindfulness and meditation are keys to actualizing in care what Watson and Newman thus theorize regarding presence, intention, mutuality, and transformation. They cultivate both individual and organizational consciousness/awareness, helping manifest a healing moment and environment. While being there with patients, mindful awareness allows the nurse to witness the patient's strength and vulnerability on their journey; in our "presence," we attend and live with challenges patients face even when the circumstance appears to be in crisis or disharmony. It is not only a beauty but a privilege for us nurses to witness patients' transformation by finding meaning in the experience.

Mindfulness: Cultivating Conscious Mindful Awareness

Often described as paying more attention and bringing more awareness, mindfulness refers to conscious awareness of the self, others, and the time and space/environment in which the self is placed. Mindfulness practice, therefore, brings your awareness to your whole being in the now with your mind and heart. In other words, your heart and mind are here and now with and/or in your physical being, as expressed in 念, the Japanese Kanji/Chinese character that presents mindfulness with its elements "heart" and "now."

Focus on your breaths or activity, and then you will notice your body being placed in a certain environment (exteroception, proprioception). Observe what you see and/or hear and feel and/or sense in your body (exteroception, proprioception), then also become aware of and explore what impressions and/or emotions you recognize inside your heart (interoception) in that moment and the space you occupy. Now, you are fully present (centered and grounded). "There are only two days in the year that nothing can be done," expresses the Dalai Lama. "One is called yesterday, and the other is called tomorrow, so today is the right day to love, believe, do and mostly live" (Wise Blue Sky, 2025). Bring your awareness to today and to the moment, whatever you are doing, to make a conscious effort to be fully present in the moment in daily life.

Mindfulness practice cultivates compassion. Practicing alone or together will create and enable you to feel connectedness and oneness in the group, community, nature, space, and time beyond, nurturing compassion toward loving and kindness. Any activity can qualify for such mindfulness practice (Thich Nhat Hanh, 1991). In walking, for example, you just slow down and pay more attention to each step and each breath, which can be a form of meditation. By being mindful of what you do, you come to appreciate small things that you normally may not pay attention to, such as chewing food slowly and washing dishes. Mind or consciousness expands through mindfulness practice with each moment acquiring more depth with new insights and sensations. With increased gratitude, connectedness and oneness grow with and within one's environment and nature while fostering within the self-appreciation of and kindness to oneself and other beings.

Mindfulness in Practice: For Centering and Presence in Creating the Healing Environment

Any state of being and nursing activity or event offers a moment for mindfulness as you make a conscious choice to Pause, Center, Ground, Reflect, and Be or Engage. Simple awareness practices help the nurse become fully present in the moment with an inner awareness of both the self and the patient (refer to **Box 15-1**). Mindful presence, cognizant of one's own consciousness and energy in the moment and space, fosters a healing environment while empowering both the nurse and patient together in a cultivated mutual relationship. Our interconnected being is the most significant contributor to the environment; we are the environment (Quinn, 1992). The first step to mindful presence is being aware of and in touch with our own interior and exterior selves through

Box 15-1 Awareness Practices to Pause, Center, Ground, and Reflect

- Mindful handwashing before and after seeing the patient (required for infection control at the hospital) as a moment to pause, breathe, calm, and center
- Reciting a mindful intention affirmation: "May I offer my care and presence unconditionally, knowing it may be received with gratitude, indifference, anger, or anguish" during walking meditation between your patient visits
- Simple deep breathing; offering a personal meditation or prayer
- Blessing food and water with good intention
- Self-reflective journaling as a mindfulness practice to reflect on yourself or events
- Visualizing; embodying yoga poses, such as a superperson or warrior asana pose
- Smiling to yourself and others: practicing yoga with your face
- Doing what you love, such as gardening, singing, dancing, and drumming, to learn to be fully in the moment and be with whatever is unfolding
- Finding something or someone to appreciate in every moment, such as a sunset or a patient's or colleague's smile

Awareness practice, allowing pausing between activities or events, enables nurses to center and ground and to learn to be fully present in the moment, thus being with whatever they are engaged in. Integrating awareness practice improves both patients' and nurses' satisfaction rates (Alkhawaldeh et al., 2024; Dil & Çam, 2024).

reflective practices such as meditation, prayer, mindfulness, spiritual practice, journaling, dialogue, and art.

Integrating Mindfulness in Hospital Programs, the Community, Society, and Globally

In-hospital programs (refer to **Box 15-2**) may effectively incorporate mindfulness practices, cultivating and transforming both individual and organizational consciousness/awareness through practices of presence, intention, mutuality, and transformation to create a healing environment. Such mindfulness integration has a far-reaching potential for a supportive culture and healing environments to be expanded to community, society, and globally.

Any moment, space, activity, or event can offer nurses a cue to breathe in and out and become aware, which is a reminder of our ability to make a conscious choice. Sharing mindful intentions takes the participants on a spiritual journey together in oneness, transformed into community awareness of our interconnectedness. Mindfulness, thus practiced together and successfully integrated into organizational programs, can further transform organizational and leadership emotional intelligence, a constituent of mindfulness, assisting the organization in building a supportive organizational culture.

Meditation

Originating in Sanskrit, the word *meditation* means wisdom. With many health benefits substantiated through research studies and as a path to spiritual transformation in many spiritual traditions, meditation provides wisdom of life, health, and well-being. Now presented in both spiritual/religious and secular forms, meditation offers various ways to practice. Two significant practices are Concentrative Meditation and Mindfulness Meditation. Transcendental Meditation, introduced by Herbert Benson to promote relaxation response, is an example of the former. Jon Kabat-Zinn was the first to bring Mindfulness Meditation to the clinical and research for stress reduction. Whereas Transcendental Meditation focuses on specific words, mantras, sounds, or objects when meditating, Mindfulness Meditation instructs one

Box 15-2 Integrating Mindfulness in Hospital Programs

- **Transition to practice/nursing orientation for new nurses**: Offer holistic self-care tools for stress management, including awareness practices such as mindful dialogue and deep listening.
- **Care Code©** and **Nurses Week for mindful healing moments**: Provide nurses and employees an opportunity to experience and practice mindfulness through healing sessions, breathing, movement, and sound. Care Code© at the author's hospital responds to staff crises, offering a healing moment on demand and regularly.
- **Healing modality class**: A class, such as on energy healing, can cultivate mindful presence while promoting nurses' self-care and well-being and fostering patient-centered quality care.
- **Bell project**: A new parent offers a bell when leaving the labor and delivery room. Hearing its sound, all staff take a breath with an intention for the highest good for the newborn baby and their family. Using this cue as a time and space for one's conscious choice for all to be in the moment with deep breathing fosters mindful awareness in nurses, employees, and patients. Applications of this mindful act can also be used at other vulnerable times such as when hearing a patient code and/or a patient passes; one may choose to pause, be present, and send the highest intention to the patient, their family, and staff involved in care.
- **Ikebana as mindfulness meditation** as both an in-hospital and an outreach program: The philosophy of this Japanese flower arrangement is to learn impermanence, mindfulness, and oneness with the universe. Ikebana is a fun way to learn meditation: becoming more aware of the inner self, the present moment, and the surroundings and nature, one transforms their whole being and environment.

to notice or be aware of breaths and incoming thoughts and feelings while breathing but without judgment.

Meditation requires focused attention, discipline, and practice from a few minutes to an hour to clear your mind. Imagine, for example, a snow globe shaken with snowflakes swirling and glittering all over the place. First, you find your mind to be filled with stuff, a chatter mind, in other words. With each mindful breath, you quiet your mind, snowflakes come down, and your mind becomes clearer. Daily meditation for up to 10–30 minutes can lead one to physical and mental well-being (Fincham et al., 2023; Schmidt & Pilat, 2023). Regular meditation practice helps one find peace in any moment of life with answers, solutions, and inspirations.

In practice and discipline, one can develop new insights into self and others, bring about inner calmness, increase energy levels, and find new ways of perceiving and reaching out to the world. Yoga and Qigong are also forms of meditation, namely moving meditation in which breathing practice moves, balances, and enhances chi/ki/prana (energy).

Mindfulness Meditation takes various forms, to be done either in a sitting position or walking while focusing on breathing and with or without phrases or sentences. One simple way to engage in Mindfulness Meditation is to recite, either in mind or in voice, "Breathe in peace, breathe out tension, and I smile."

Loving Kindness Meditation, also called Cultivating the Heart of Compassion Meditation, consisting of three parts, is another form of Mindfulness Meditation. First, plant a healing seed within your heart: "May I be safe, May I be peaceful...." while following your breath and focusing on your intention to cultivate compassion. Secondly, visualize someone you care about while centering your thoughts on offering compassion: "May you be safe, May you be peaceful...." Thirdly, you visualize all beings on Earth, the universe, and beyond time and space to offer compassion: "May all beings on Earth be safe, May all beings on Earth be peaceful...." The author uses a modified meditation of this Loving Kindness Meditation when seeing patients in transition to support them, their family members, and the staff in charge, pausing for a moment and promoting a peaceful transition.

The precautions and contraindications for meditation practice need to be explored prior to recommending meditation and its apps, especially for patients with a history of mental health challenges, such as posttraumatic stress disorder (PTSD) and acute psychosis. Meditation may trigger painful past experiences, and overwhelming emotions may arise. If this occurs, try not to panic and remember your intention to help and support. Breathe and stay centered and ground yourself, then, reassure and ground your patient.

Mindfulness and Meditation as Self-Care for Nurses and Nursing Leaders

Awareness of one's own being as a whole (body-mind-spirit) is fundamental to patient care and self-care. Mindfulness and meditation are awareness practices and paths to connect with who we really are. As nurses, cultivating ourselves becomes vital to being a good conduit/nurse in our care and presence with intention. Cultivating awareness is also a significant part of self-care. Acknowledging, allowing, appreciating, and accepting both strengths and weaknesses cultivate self-awareness.

Awareness practice and reflective practice are essential for nurses to build resilience to manage life stresses and challenges. As Dr. Krieger (2006) taught, "TT [Therapeutic Touch] is you," your being, including energy and consciousness, affects your care, patients, colleagues, family, and those around you. Mindfulness of self, awareness of one's own being as whole (body-mind-spirit), being in the moment, quieting your mind, and reflecting on events and/or yourself helps you align, connect, and balance your own energy, assisting you on your spiritual journey. With compassion cultivated toward others and care for the self through the practices, we understand and relate and connect better with the experiences of people from different backgrounds and cultures.

Ever since the COVID-19 pandemic, which has foregrounded a necessity of self-care for healthcare workers, mindfulness and meditation practices have played ever more significant roles in self-care, not only for nursing individuals but for healthcare leadership and organizations. Awareness and effective utilization of emotional intelligence, as an example of organizational and leadership mindfulness, help nurture patients and staff in wholeness, whereas the leadership equipped with high emotional intelligence can raise their competence and performance, de-stressing themselves and clearing their minds while engaging with staff and colleagues.

Mindfulness as emotional intelligence underscores feedback with active listening and uplifting responses and encouragement (Daniel et al., 2022). Such hospital programs as Care Code© and Nurses Week in Box 15-2 illustrate integrating mindfulness/meditation practice at the institutional level in collaboration with nursing councils that represent the voice of staff nurses. Mindfulness, which encompasses organizational and leadership's emotional intelligence, practiced by both nursing individuals and the leadership, will significantly impact healthcare organizations, creating a collaborative organizational culture for a healing environment, thereby providing patient-centered quality care.

Mindfulness and Meditation AI and Apps

Artificial intelligence (AI) is becoming an inseparable part of our daily lives, including in health care. AI-guided mindfulness meditation, despite privacy concerns and lack of human touch, has been readily accessible, offering flexible, personalized programs with quick feedback. Although it is uncertain if AI-assisted applications (apps) help improve connectedness with oneself, others, and the universe, its clearer communication and fast connection may render apps useful in teaching and promoting mindfulness practices, thus improving individual lives. These apps can also be an excellent supplement to teaching and learning mindfulness and meditation as they support personal at-home practice, patient care, and nurses' self-care. Many apps are free and/or have

Nursing Situation

Nurses, on their busy work shifts, find themselves multitasking, often encountering unexpected challenges or demands. Every nursing practice presents an opportunity for mindfulness practice in patients' care and nurses' self-care. Nurses who wish to be more present with their patients, to practice own self-care, and to awaken to the simple sacredness of every nursing practice may want to incorporate simple mindfulness breathing into their daily practice, to center and ground before, during, and between their routine nursing tasks. Begin with your breaths to become mindful in each moment, aware of your inner and external environments without judgment. Be it hanging an intravenous bag, administering medications, documenting nursing notes, eating, or walking down a hall, every nursing task provides an occasion to be mindful, which nurtures self-compassion while serving as self-care. In practicing simple mindful breathing, as in the scripts in **Box 15-3**, a nursing moment becomes a cue to breathe in and out, to be aware, and to be present with intention, creating a healing environment for oneself and others.

Box 15-3 Mindful Breathing Exercises/Practices for Patient Care and Self-care

Script I: Breathing in, I am aware of breathing in.
Breathing out, I am aware of breathing out.
Breathing in, I am aware of introducing this healing medication through this intravenous line.
Breathing out, I send my healing intentions along with the medication to help support this patient's healing.

Script II (Walking Meditation): Breathing in, I am walking down this hall
Breathing out, I smile, enjoying my steps.
Breathing in, I am fresh.
Breathing out, I celebrate my aliveness.

Script III: Practice sitting or resting comfortably. You may use this script in nursing practice for your patient or yourself.
Breathing in, I am aware of breathing in.
Breathing out, I am aware of breathing out.
In.
Out.
Breathing in, I am calm.
Breathing out, I smile. (Thich Nhat Hanh, 1993, p. 17)

Data from Thich Nhat Hanh. (1993). *The blooming a lotus: Guided meditation exercises for healing and transformation* (p. 17). Beacon Press.

paid subscription options. Some of the frequently used include Headspace, Calm, Insight Timer, the Plum Village app, and The Mindfulness App. As the ease of use for some patients is a concern, when supplementing teaching and supporting at-home practice with apps, the nurse needs to be familiar with and able to instruct patients on how best to use apps.

When preparing medication, for example, ***Script I or III*** helps the nurse to be present in the moment, centered and grounded, and focused on the task, which may contribute to fewer medication errors (Ekkens & Gordon, 2021; Łoś et al., 2022). The nurse may utilize ***Script I*** or ***III*** to guide patients when administering pain or other medications, thereby helping promote relaxation while potentially easing patients' anxiety (Maddock & Blair, 2023), stress (Fisher et al., 2023), and pain (O'Connor et al., 2022; Pérez-Fernández et al., 2022). Once learned, patients can use mindful deep breathing independently to address the anxiety and stress that frequently accompany pain. Such multimodal pain management maximizes the benefits of conventional treatments for the patient. Mindfulness and meditation techniques can also help nurses reduce their stress and anxiety (Knudsen et al., 2023; Kriakous et al., 2021), connecting with who they really are, to be more self-compassionate (Alkhawaldeh et al., 2024), ultimately building resiliency. If we act in each moment with compassion and mindfulness, with these simple techniques illuminating our caring intention, each moment of our nursing intervention can be a work of art.

Individually practiced and/or organizationally integrated into hospital programs as self-care resources, mindfulness and meditation techniques, including mindful listening/dialogue, can effectively be applied to a crisis and a trauma, assisting in equipping nurses and their team with mindfulness to better cope with challenges while building resiliency. If not organizationally incorporated, interdisciplinary teams and holistic nurses can serve as resources for nurses, patients, the organization, and the community to learn and practice mindfulness as self-care and stress management.

Mindfulness and meditation practices may not change the reality, but they enable us nurses to be present in the very moment and place, to feel/share the pain together, and to uplift the involved in care, helping nurture resilience and create a supportive environment for diverse individual and team needs. Mindfulness requires practice and discipline. Practicing mindfulness and meditation over time may change the perception of stresses and stressful situations (Toniolo-Barrios & ten Brummelhuis, 2023) to better cope with threatening situations (Bartlett et al., 2021). Once acquired, requiring no cost, nurses can utilize mindfulness techniques anytime, anywhere, and in any situation. To know that we nurses have control over our minds and challenges is empowering.

Integration

Clinical Practice

- Mindfulness and meditation practices have been demonstrated to reduce stress, anxiety, and pain and to promote mental, emotional, and physical health and well-being.
- While reality may not be changed, the practices may ease the perception of challenges that patients, their families, and the community face, assisting them in coping with their illnesses, conditions, and/or crises.
- Mindfulness (and its practices) incorporated into the organization and its leadership as emotional intelligence can transform awareness of the organization and its greater community and beyond, creating a supportive culture and a healing environment.

Education

- Education on mindfulness practice and meditation for individual patients and their family members, nursing staff, healthcare organizations, patient support groups, and/or schools in the community has greater implications and outcomes for wholeness, health, and well-being. In-person or virtual classes are available for anyone interested in the practice.
- Recent AI technology advancements render various AI-assisted apps accessible for patients' individual needs and utilization to provide personalized education and fast feedback in mindfulness and meditation.
- The goal is to help individuals and their community obtain resources and develop skills to address and improve their concerns, concentration, emotional regulation, self-care, and compassion.

Research

- Research has substantiated many physical and mental health benefits of mindfulness and meditation. Further research with specific populations, such as children with gun violence, toxic stress, trauma, or physical illnesses, can be explored due to current studies often being limited to healthy pediatric populations. Age-appropriate contents, frequencies, and duration of the practice can also be explored.
- With our society now facing more aging populations with nearly 7 million people living with Alzheimer's in the United States (Alzheimer's Association, 2024), mindfulness and meditation can support older populations in delaying cognitive instability or dementia as the practice helps improve coping skills with stress and attention. Further research with a significant number of participants, optimum contents, duration, frequencies, and other lifestyle factors needs to be explored.

Policy

- Many schools across the country are now including mindfulness practices to increase physical and mental well-being, enhance social-emotional learning, and improve school culture. For example, since fall 2023, all public schools (pre-kindergarten to grade 12) in New York City require two to five minutes of mindful breathing practices every day in school. Such mindfulness practice helps encourage physical and mental health in both students and educators.

Global Health

- Gun violence has been the leading cause of death in children in recent years in the United States (Johns Hopkins, 2024), while wars have increased their presence and considerable impact on the world scene. Violence, toxic stress, and childhood trauma can exert an immeasurable impact on children's emotions and coping skills.
- Holistic nurses can help individuals and the community, teaching mindfulness and meditation through our presence and intention to promote peace and healing in those, especially children, with psychological and physical trauma from gun violence (Francis, 2024).
- Promoting mental and emotional well-being in children is crucial for global health and our shared future. "The energy of mindfulness is a real energy, and whenever energy is applied there is a change"—Thich Nhat Hanh (Flippin, 2025).

Conclusion

Awareness practices of mindfulness and meditation are even more relevant and needed now in a world divided and surrounded by much violence. Our work and home environments have become so busy, and we are often easily distracted and disconnected by the media and events. Cultivating conscious, mindful awareness through the practice of mindfulness and meditation can lead to creating resilience and compassion in individual nurses while promoting self-care. Through fostering mindfulness as emotional intelligence, administrative leadership can help transform and build a healing environment and supportive culture for all involved in care while supporting themselves and other staff in the organization.

We, nurses, can disseminate and engage in mindfulness awareness practice and reflective practice to bring a moment of peace at work and everywhere we go, to be fully present in the moment in our wholeness, with intention and for mutual relationships for insights and new possibilities while witnessing our consciousness expand. It all begins with us finding who we really are, our lineage of hope, compassion, and healing that began with Nightingale and was expanded by Watson, Newman, and others. AI-assisted apps assist in promoting mindfulness and meditation education, facilitating individual and community access to much-needed resources with tailored practice and feedback, fostering a better community and society. Sharing mindful intentions can take us together on a spiritual journey in oneness, nurturing community awareness of our interconnectedness created within a healing moment and space. With mindful intention, a simple act, being still in the moment with nature or taking a breath, can promote caring, thereby creating a healing, compassionate environment for all. Especially in times of community crisis and loss, these mindfulness and mediation practices offer a simple yet profound experience for all individuals and the community globally.

References

Alkhawaldeh, J. M., Khawaldeh, M. A., Mrayyan, M. T., Yehia, D., Shudifat, R. M., Anshasi, H. A., Al-Shdayfat, N. M., Alzoubi, M. M., & Aqel, A. (2024). The efficacy of mindfulness-based programs in reducing anxiety among nurses in hospital settings: A systematic review. *Worldviews on Evidence-Based Nursing, 21*, 395–406. https://doi.org/10.1111/wvn.12722

Alzheimer's Association. (2024). *Alzheimer's disease facts and figures*. https://www.alz.org/alzheimers-dementia/facts-figures

Bartlett, L., Buscot, M., Bindoff, A., Chambers, R., & Hassed, C. (2021). Mindfulness is associated with lower stress and higher work engagement in a large sample of MOOC participants. *Frontiers in Psychology, 12*. https://doi.org/10.3389/fpsyg.2021.724126

Daniel, C., Daniel, P. A., & Smyth, H. (2022). The role of mindfulness in the management of projects: Potential opportunities in research and practice. *International Journal of Project Management, 40*(7), 849–864. https://doi.org/10.1016/j.ijproman.2022.07.003

Dil, S., & Çam, M. (2024). The mediator role of mindfulness in the relationship between the listening skills and anger management skills of emergency health care professionals. *International Emergency Nursing, 75*. https://doi.org/10.1016/j.ienj.2024.101475.

Ekkens, C. L., & Gordon, P. A. (2021). The mindful path to nursing accuracy: A quasi-experimental study on minimizing medication administration errors. *Holistic Nursing Practice, 35*(3), 115–122. https://doi.org/10.1097/HNP.00000000000004

Fincham, G. W., Mavor, K., & Dritschel, B. (2023). Effects of mindfulness meditation duration and type on well-being: An online dose-ranging randomized controlled trial. *Mindfulness, 14*(5), 1171–1182. https://doi.org/10.1007/s12671-023-02119-2

Fisher, V., Li, W. W., & Malabu, U. (2023). The effectiveness of mindfulness-based stress reduction (MBSR) on the mental health, HbA1C, and mindfulness of diabetes patients: A systematic review and meta-analysis of randomized controlled trials. *Applied Psychology: Health and Well-Being, 15*(4), 1733–1749.https://doi.org/10.1111/aphw.12441

Flippin, P. (2025). *The energy of mindfulness, meditation, and prayer*. Still Water: Mindfulness Practice Center. https://www.stillwatermpc.org/dharma-topics/the-energy-of-mindfulness-meditation-and-prayer/

Francis, M. (2024). Holistic approach to gun violence. *Journal of Holistic Nursing, 42*(3), 291–299. https//:doi.org/10.1177/08980101231207697

Johns Hopkins. (2024, September 12). *New report highlights U.S. 2022 Gun-related deaths: Firearms remain leading cause of death for children and teens, and disproportionately affect people of color.* https://publichealth.jhu.edu/2024/guns-remain-leading-cause-of-death-for-children-and-teens

Knudsen, R. K., Ammentorp, J., Storkholm, M. H., Skovbjerg, S., Tousig, C. G., & Timmermann, C. (2023). The influence of mindfulness-based stress reduction on the work life of healthcare professionals: A qualitative study. *Complementary Therapies in Clinical Practice, 53*. https://doi.org/10.1016/j.ctcp.2023.101805.

Kriakous, S. A., Elliott, K. A., Lamers, C., & Owen, R. (2021). The effectiveness of mindfulness-based stress reduction on the psychological functioning of healthcare professionals: A systematic review. *Mindfulness, 12*(1), 1–28. https://doi.org/10.1007/s12671-020-01500-9

Krieger, D. (2006). *TT is you*. Advanced therapeutic touch class at Pumpkin Hollow Retreat Center, Craryville, New York.

Łoś, K., Łuczyński, W., & Waszkiewicz, N. (2022). Can the practice of mindfulness reduce medical errors? *Postepy Psychiatrii Neurologii, 31*(3), 121–127. https://doi.org/10.5114/ppn.2022.120158

Maddock, A., & Blair, C. (2023). How do mindfulness-based programmes improve anxiety, depression and psychological distress? A systematic review. *Current Psychology*, 42, 10200–10222. https://doi.org/10.1007/s12144-021-02082-y

Newman, M. A. (1994). *Health as expanding consciousness*. Jones and Bartlett Publishers.

O'Connor, S., Mayne, A., & Hood, B. (2022). Virtual reality-based mindfulness for chronic pain management: A scoping review. *Pain Management Nursing, 23*(3), 359–369. https://doi.org/10.1016/j.pmn.2022.03.013.

Pérez-Fernández, J. I., Salaberria, K., & Ruiz de Ocenda, Á. (2022). Mindfulness-based pain management (MBPM) for chronic pain: A randomized clinical trial. *Mindfulness, 13*, 3153–3165. https://doi.org/10.1007/s12671-022-02023-1

Quinn, J. (1992). Holding sacred space: The nurse as healing environment. *Holistic Nursing Practice, 6*(4), 26-35.

Schmidt, H., & Pilat, C. (2023). Effects of meditation on pain intensity, physical function, quality of life and depression in adults with low back pain: A systematic review with meta-analysis. *Complementary Therapies in Medicine, 72*. https://doi.org/10.1016/j.ctim.2023.102924

Thich Nhat Hanh. (1991). *Peace is every step: The path of mindfulness in everyday life*. Bantam Books.

Thich Nhat Hanh. (1993). *The blooming a lotus: Guided meditation exercises for healing and transformation.* Beacon Press.

Toniolo-Barrios, M., & ten Brummelhuis, L. L. (2023). How does mindfulness reduce stress at work? A two-study examination using a stress appraisal perspective, *Personality and Individual Differences, 215*. https://doi.org/10.1016/j.paid.2023.112392

Watson, J. (2005). *Caring science as sacred science*. E. A. Davis Company.

Wise Blue Sky. (2025). *Dalai Lama positive thinking quotes*. https://wisebluesky.com/quotations/quotes-from-dalai-lama/?_page=4

Clinical Imagery

Bonney Gulino Schaub

NURSE HEALER OBJECTIVES

- Learn how to incorporate imagery interventions into clinical practice.
- Understand how to use the power of the imagination to activate physiological, psychological, or spirituality-related healing.
- Learn how to use imagery techniques to rehearse new behaviors or prepare for activities or procedures.

Introduction

Imagery is an essential aspect of holistic nursing practice because it brings the natural powers of the mind into the process of health and healing. Distinct from thinking, imagery as a technique interacts with the image-making function of the brain, which, in turn, acts on the subtle energies of our entire physiology. This aspect of subtle energy brings the value of imagery as an asset when used in conjunction with therapeutic touch, meditation, biofeedback, Reiki, reflexology, massage, and other holistic practices. Martha Rogers was the visionary nurse who opened nursing up to the holistic model. She viewed people and their surroundings as "unitary, indivisible wholes." She fully embraced the importance of energy fields and the environment in "wellbecoming" (Malinsky, 2022).

Imagery

The research definition of imagery is the perception of a stimulus in the absence of that stimulus (Richarson, 1969). For example, if a person imagines a lemon and begins to taste the lemon juice, they are having a perception (tasting the juice) of a stimulus (lemon) that is not present. Commonly, in addition to tasting the lemon, the person begins to salivate, demonstrating a rapid physiologic alteration in response to the imagery suggestion. Magnetic resonance imaging (MRI) investigations of the brain's recording of tactile information demonstrate that imaged tactile stimulation and actual tactile stimulation are registered in partially overlapping areas of the brain. Investigators also used functional MRI to examine brain activity in healthy volunteers who mentally imagined walking along a curved path. The outcome suggested a close neurophysiologic relationship between locomotion and mental imagery.

In another study, researchers found that individuals gazing at water, such as in a pool, a creek, or a small lake, experienced a relaxation effect. This was evidenced by a reduced average heart rate or lower blood pressure (systolic/diastolic ratio) (Coss & Keller, 2022). If the nurse has discovered that patients love going to the beach, or swimming or some other water setting, it offers an opportunity to have them close their eyes, connect with the breath, and imagine themself in that setting. The nurse has now taught the patient a self-care practice that can be used in any setting.

Current Trend

The Placebo/Nocebo Effect and Imagery

The absence-of-stimulus definition is relevant to the crucial issue of the placebo effect, a phenomenon where the patient thinks (imagines) they are receiving a potent medication and experiences its anticipated effects, both positive (placebo) and negative (nocebo). In recent times, there were significant controversies related to the COVID-19 vaccine. In a study that took place at Beth Israel Deaconess Medical Center, investigators reported that a third of the trial participants who received a placebo injection containing no vaccine reported adverse effects from the treatment such as headache and fatigue (Haas et al., 2002).

Utilizing the Power of the Imagination in Health Care

This information challenges the holistic nurse to understand and work with the power of the patient's imagination when providing care. Clinical imagery is the conscious use of the power of the imagination with the intention of activating physiological, psychological, and higher unconscious awareness. The essential word here is *conscious*.

People imagining negative futures and employing their intelligence and energy to be consumed with worry are creating obstacles to well-being and healing. Regarding understanding the power of imagination when working with patients, the imagination is not just present as visible images. That is the limitation in the use of the word *imagery*.

A patient may convey, "I can't work with imagery because when a person took me through a guided imagery, I didn't see anything." Individuals have different ways of experiencing their imagination. Some don't have a visual sense, but they experience words, an inner voice. This may be clear to the person, but they may feel self-conscious sharing that they experienced hearing a voice. Others may experience a physical or emotional response instead of visual images (Roebuck & Lupyan, 2020).

When working with imagery, as with other integrative approaches, nurses need to have their own experience with the techniques. This will build confidence in using this technique/tool clinically with their patient.

There are common concerns when beginning to use these skills such as what if nothing happens, too much happens, or "I don't do it the right way"? The answer is that everyone has their unique way of connecting with their imagination. Some individuals have intense visual imagery, while others may experience multisensory inner experiences. These variations also reflect differences in cognitive styles. With greater experience, nurses can be serene and present in a way that creates calmness and trust in the patient as well as feeling open and interested in the diversity and how imagery work can be adapted for integration into patient care (Takahashi et al., 2023).

Transpersonal Imagery

Cultures throughout the world have used prayer, imagery, physical training, contemplation and study, rituals, art, music, and chanting as methods to experience states of consciousness beyond their personality (i.e., transpersonal). People seek these states because they tend to provide a subtler understanding of the universal patterns of reality and a more peaceful perspective of the "little self" living in the immensity of creation. Nurses frequently cite their own transpersonal experiences and perspectives as one of the reasons they have been drawn to bringing holistic skills and practices into their work.

The role of imagery in evoking transpersonal experiences is a crucial one. This connection can be interpreted as a connection with God, with all of humanity, with higher power, with the wonder of the universe and nature, or with the mysterious nonverbal communication that occurs between people at the level of intuitive knowing and caring. The nurse's openness to the individual's process results in these skills being effective for cross-cultural work; this may take the form of a patient imagining a scene of praying with their rosary beads and someone else visualizing a small shrine in their home or other creative practices that are sources of peace, inner joy, and healing (Schaub & Schaub, 2003).

Integration

Clinical Practice

- Individuals generally have a particular sensory (visual, auditory, kinesthetic, emotional, sensorial) way that they experience their imagery and imagination.
- The nurse can invite the patient to reflect on the imagery suggestions and be open to whatever form feels most natural to them.

Nursing Situation

Here is an example of a clinical application of imagery. Felicia, a 40-year-old woman with two children, was referred to a nurse working in an outpatient setting. She was referred by her gynecologist because she had cancelled her hysterectomy surgery at the last minute two times. She had large uterine fibroids and had been experiencing extremely heavy menstrual periods that were occurring frequently. She was also getting painful urinary tract infections (UTIs). Her doctor suggested that she meet with a nurse to help her process what she was feeling.

In the first meeting, Felicia didn't fully understand her intense anxiety and fear. She informed her doctor that she didn't want any more children and was reassured that the surgery was not going to be severely disabling. The nurse suggested that they work with some basic stress management skills. They started with breath awareness. Felicia really needed to learn how to relax, and she appreciated the experience. The nurse then returned Felicia to the relaxed state and guided her through a process of body awareness.

After spending a few moments with this process, Felicia started to cry. She shared that what came to her was a vivid memory of her mother going to the hospital when she was a little girl. Her mother never returned; she had died there. Felicia judged herself because she hadn't connected her personal fear of the hospital with this early memory.

The nurse then processed this experience with Felicia and asked her what she thought she needed at this point. Felicia expressed, "I need to say goodbye to her." The nurse then shared that it was important, and whenever she was ready, Felicia could go back into her relaxation state and reconnect with the image in whatever way felt best for her.

This clinical example reflects how guiding someone into a quiet inner space and connecting with the imagination can be deeply therapeutic. Felicia was relieved that she could experience saying goodbye to her mom. She was relieved to understand why she had been so fearful about entering a hospital. Felicia was then able to practice the breath work on her own, and the nurse suggested that it might be helpful for her to take some notes about her experience when she returned home. This experience resulted in a dramatic shift in Felicia's outlook, and she was able to have her surgery. She also wanted to continue working with her imagination for her own well-being after she was discharged.

Education

- The diversity of possible experiences that patients can have when working with their imagination as a healing tool.
- The importance of nurses experiencing their own imagery and inner knowing as a way of resonating with the imagery suggestions they are bringing into their clinical practice.

Research

- Understanding the scholarly evidence on the direct effect of imagery and consciousness on the body.
- Understanding the value of positive imagery and consciousness states for health and well-being.

Policy

- Imagery and consciousness practices can be offered in diverse clinical settings.
- Imagery is a safe and effective practice.

Global Health

- Transpersonal imagery is a skill adaptable to any tradition because the patient creates healing images that are personally meaningful.
- The treatment can be provided in any care setting.

References

Coss, R. G., & Keller, C. M. (2022). Transient decreases in blood pressure and heart rate with increased subjective level of relaxation while viewing water compared with adjacent ground. *Journal of Environmental Psychology*, *81*(101794).

Haas J. W., Bender, F. L., Ballou, S., Kelley, J. M., Wilheim, M., Miller, F. G., Reif, W., & Kapchuk, T. J. (2002). Frequency of adverse events in the placebo arms of COVID-19 vaccine trials: A systematic review and meta-analysis. *JAMA Network Open, 5*(1), e2143955. https://doi.org/10.1001/jamanetworkopen.2021.43955

Malinsky, V. M. (2022). Unitary human-environment field mutual process: Knowing participation in patterning the environment. *Nursing Science Quarterly*, *35*(2). https://doi.org/10.1177/08943184211070603

Richarson, A. (1969). *Mental imagery*. Routledge & Kegan Paul.

Roebuck, H., & Lupyan, G. (2020). The Internal Representations Questionnaire: Measuring modes of thinking. *Behavioral Research Methods, 52*(5), 2053–2070. https://doi.org/10.3758/s13428-020-01354-y

Schaub, B. G., & Schaub, R. (2003). Imagery and spiritual development. In A. A. Sheikh (Ed.), *Healing images: The role of imagination in health* (pp. 489–498). Baywood.

Takahashi, J., Saito, G., Omura, K., Yasunaga, D., Sugimura, S., Sakamoto, S., Horikawa, T., & Gyoba, T. (2023). Diversity of aphantasia revealed by multiple assessments of visual imagery, multisensory imagery, and cognitive style. *Frontiers in Psychology*, *14*, 1174873. https://doi.org/10.3389/fpsyg.2023.117483.

Touch and Hand-Mediated Therapies

Jennifer Browning and Marci Resnicoff

NURSE HEALER OBJECTIVES

- Reflect on ways nurses may use the art of touch and hand-mediated therapies for self-care and in the care of others.

Introduction

To introduce the section on touch, we invite you to find a quiet space in which you are able to reflect for a moment. Consider lowering your gaze or closing your eyes and spend the next few moments imagining a world without human touch in health care. This is a world in which a programmed robot places the IV, hangs the medications, and even gives the patient a bed bath complete with a back rub at a preprogramed strong, medium, or light touch setting (Arcega et al., 2020). Would the robot understand how to comfort the patient with phobia of needles or adjust the strength of the touch during the backrub? How would the robot respond if the patient began to cry because the last person to give him a backrub was his deceased spouse?

Now lift up or open your eyes and reflect on the reality that touch in nursing has become diminished as technological skills have become more important. Couple that with social movements to expose the misuse of touch that have led to the fear of touch, especially by male nurses, being misinterpreted, thus decreasing its use as a natural gesture of caring (Burgess et al., 2023). The COVID-19 pandemic expanded on that fear. Fear of contagion by the quickly spreading virus encouraged "touchless" care whenever possible. Care was completed in gloved hands, masks, and eye shields and conversations were held from doorways. Backrubs were not offered and bed baths were only completed as a necessity. Post-pandemic, nurses realized that their long "To-Do" list is made slightly shorter by foregoing stroking a patient's head as a form of comforting or moisturizing their feet when they have trouble reaching.

What is the importance of touch? Does touch still play a part in caring for patients? Research has shown skin-to-skin "kangaroo care" between new mothers and preterm babies lowers the cortisol level in the babies (Cristóbal Cañadas et al., 2022). It helps calm them both so they feel safe enough to bond (Cristóbal Cañadas et al., 2022; Kerr et al., 2019). The preterm babies who experienced kangaroo care often gain a healthy amount of weight and flourish, whereas those babies and children not receiving adequate nourishment from touch could experience delays in reaching developmental milestones (Kerr et al., 2019).

Appropriate touch benefits nurses and other healthcare workers in a caregiving role. It may offer a deeper connection to those they are caring for, bringing meaning and a deeper purpose to their work (Burgess et al., 2023; Mühlenpfordt et al., 2020).

Once again, return to that quiet reflective space. This time, visualize a nurse at the bedside of an anxious patient—just being present and holding the person's hand. Notice that it is a nurse, not a robot, giving the widower the backrub. It is a nurse who takes a moment to gently place a hand on the widower's shoulder as he shares a story of his late wife. In this chapter, we will explore the ways in which touch, without the need of a prescription, can be used in a safe and appropriate way to care for and support our patients and ourselves.

Self-Soothing Touch

Research in the field indicates more and more that caring for oneself in body, mind, spirit, and emotions is imperative if the nurse is to give competent, heart-centered care without experiencing burnout. However, Udoudo et al. (2023) pointed out that most nurses cite lacking time to engage in self-care activities that also help them reduce or manage their stress level. As per the American Nurses Association Code of Ethics, Provision 5 (2025), learning how to incorporate brief, simple, and effective tools that help engage the parasympathetic nervous system, thereby activating the relaxation response, into work routines is an important part of being a nurse.

Supportive gestures are various motions often used unconsciously to self-soothe the nervous system and reduce cortisol levels, in order to elicit calm and notify the brain that you are safe (Dreisoerner et al., 2021; Franco & Christie, 2021; Franco & Gregory, 2023). One such gesture is for the individual to place their open palms on their chest at their heart, while taking a couple of deep slow breaths. Another gesture, while engaging in deep slow breaths, is to rest your palms on your shoulders and let your arms, with elbows bent, gently hang. A third is for the person to give themself a supportive hug, arms crossed and the opposite hands resting on the upper arms as the person either gently strokes their upper arms or just gives a squeeze (Franco & Gregory, 2023; Franco & Christie, 2021). These, and others, are gestures that a nurse could do to self-calm in less than two minutes during a hectic shift at work.

Finger Tracing with Mindful Breath

Another self-calming modality is the different forms of finger tracing with the incorporation of mindful breathing. Fingers have many nerve endings to assist us in distinguishing what we are touching and sending signals to the brain. By consciously slowing down the breath while connecting to some of these neurovascular points, the brain becomes very present and calm.

A popular version of finger tracing while mindfully breathing is to trace the fingers as if you were drawing a sketch of your hand. This comes from the program Greater Good in Education (2025; McKeering & Hwang, 2019). With the palm of your dominant hand facing you and those fingers spread wide, place the pointer finger of the other hand at the base of the thumb. As you slowly inhale, trace your finger up the outside of the thumb to the top. As you slowly exhale, bring the finger down the other side of the thumb into the crevice between the thumb and the pointer finger. Continue up the side of the pointer finger to the top on the inhale and down the other side on the exhale. This is continued until you end at the outer base of the pinky finger. Repeat on the other hand if you have time. This mindful sensory modality is effective, self-soothing, and can be completed in less than 5 minutes, which may help a nurse having a stressful moment to reset.

Therapeutic Massage

The category of somatic and musculoskeletal therapies encompasses the generic work known as *therapeutic massage*. As a nursing intervention, therapeutic massage is effective in stimulating circulation of blood and lymph, dispersing nutrients, removing metabolic wastes, and enhancing relaxation. Although they may be called by different names (e.g., Swedish massage, deep tissue massage), many of the techniques of therapeutic massage are similar.

Nurses have routinely performed therapeutic massage primarily on the backs, hands, and feet of their patients. Back care is not new; for decades, it has been incorporated into the standard bathing and evening care routine of most hospitals. Technology, task-oriented care, and time constraints have affected nurses providing therapeutic back, feet, and hand massages.

Patients receiving hemodialysis often experience fatigue. In a randomized controlled trial, patients receiving hemodialysis received either hand massage, foot massage, or no massage three times per week over four weeks. The hand and foot massage groups' mean fatigue score decreased after massage compared to the control group (Çeçen & Lafcı, 2021).

Foot and hand massage were studied for their benefit of providing pain relief for mothers who had cesarean sections. Twenty-minute hand and foot massages were given to the mothers, resulting in statistically significant reductions in incisional pain compared to the control group receiving routine hospital care (Sharma & Kumari, 2019).

Reflexology

Reflexology is a complementary therapy that nurses can incorporate into their practice. Reflexology involves applying manual pressure to specific points of the feet, hands, and ears. The reflex points correspond to different internal organs. Applying manual pressure to the reflex points can stimulate body zones and promote the self-healing powers of the organs. Congestion or tension in any area affects the entire zone running laterally throughout the body.

Research supporting the effectiveness of reflexology for physical and psychological symptoms is growing. In a randomized controlled trial, the effects of foot reflexology on burn patients for the alleviation of pain and anxiety was examined (Davodabady et al., 2021). Treatments were provided to the intervention group prior to dressing changes for six days. The control group received routine care. Patients receiving foot reflexology had improved pain and anxiety scores on days 4–6 of treatment. By learning foot reflexology as an intervention, nurses can provide more support and comfort for patients experiencing pain and anxiety

Acupressure

Acupressure is a complementary therapy based on principles of Traditional Chinese Medicine. Pressure is applied to specific points on the body, known as *acupoints*, and works on the concept of energy pathways or meridians that flow through the body. Gentle, but firm, pressure using the fingers, knuckles, or palms is applied to acupoints and may be held for several seconds to a few minutes. This pressure stimulates the body's natural healing processes.

Nurses can receive training and certification in acupressure and, in turn, empower patients by teaching acupressure techniques. In a randomized controlled trial with patients with colon and pancreatic cancer receiving chemotherapy, the effects of self-applied acupressure for decreasing pain and anxiety and improving sleep quality were examined (Bahçecioğlu Turan et al., 2023). Self-acupressure was found to be effective in reducing pain, anxiety, and sleep disorder scores in the intervention group compared to the control group. In nursing practice, the use of acupressure can be an effective integrative modality.

Nursing Situation

The busy night-shift nurse noticed the call bell had been activated for the patient A.G.'s room. The 72-year-old female patient had received a stage 3 colon cancer diagnosis and was recovering from surgery (post-op day 3). Her adult-aged son lived a 4-hour plane ride away. He had been present for the surgery but then had to return home. Feeling very alone, anxious, and unable to sleep, A.G. pressed the call bell.

The nurse paused outside of A.G.'s room to center herself by placing her feet flat on the floor and her hand on her heart while taking a deep, slow breath. She then entered the room and found that A.G. was sitting up in the bed, fiddling with her blanket. As soon as A.G. noticed the nurse, she began to ask questions about her upcoming radiation treatment.

The nurse sat at the bedside with A.G., quietly taking her hand. Before answering A.G.'s questions, the nurse slowed her breathing, encouraging A.G. to do the same. As A.G. became visibly more relaxed, the nurse explained the treatment protocol including what she may expect to experience from the treatment.

Since A.G. was having trouble sleeping, the nurse asked her if she would like to experience an acupressure point activation to help her feel calmer and encourage sleep. A.G. agreed, and the nurse introduced her to the Heart-7 (Shen Men) acupressure point on her wrist. The nurse pressed the point and held it for one minute on each wrist while encouraging A.G. to take slow breaths. At the end of the two minutes, A.G. noticed she was feeling more relaxed.

Before she left the room, the nurse taught A.G. how to activate the Heart-7 acupressure point herself, and A.G. was able to demonstrate the technique successfully. The nurse encouraged A.G. to press the point while taking slow breaths whenever she began to feel anxious or was unable to sleep. She also let A.G. know she would check on her again soon to evaluate how she was doing but also encouraged her to use the call bell anytime she needed help.

A.G. thanked the nurse and shared that for the first time since her diagnosis, she felt like there was something she could do to help herself as opposed to just feeling dependent on everyone. The nurse gently took A.G.'s hand, and they shared one more slow breath. Then, A.G. settled down in bed to sleep.

Integration

- **Clinical Practice:** Nurses can implement touch and hand-mediated techniques into clinical practice as a stand-alone therapy or in conjunction with other modalities. Cultural differences are vital for nurses to understand when deciding which therapies are best suited for various health concerns and populations.
- **Education:** Nurses can educate parents and caregivers on how to provide touch and hand-mediated therapies to loved ones and those they are caring for, providing comfort and a satisfying experience for all. Nursing schools can be the frontline in effectively teaching nursing students the importance of touch for their patients.
- **Research:** Nurses can take part in research endeavors and strengthen the evidence base for practicing touch and hand-mediated therapies, including the development of reliable evaluation tools and demonstrating the effectiveness of these practices in patient care.
- **Policy:** Nurses can develop procedure and policy in their areas of practice to promote patients receiving holistic care.
- **Global Health:** Nurses practicing touch therapies can impact global health by addressing physical and emotional well-being, providing holistic care and fostering human connection across cultures.

Conclusion

The simple, yet profound, use of touch can enhance the quality of life across the age span, especially during times of both acute and chronic health challenges. Many techniques are simple to learn and implement, and they can provide positive outcomes for the practitioner as well as the receiver. Nurses can be instrumental in furthering the use of touch modalities that promote healing and well-being for themselves and their patients.

References

American Nurses Association. (2025, January 6). Code of Ethics, Provision 5. https://www.nursingworld.org/globalassets/covid19/provision-5_-self-care--covid19-final.pdf

Arcega, J., Autman, I., De Guzman, B., Isidienu, L., Olivar, J., O'Neal, M., & Surdilla, B. (2020). The human touch. *Critical Care Nursing Quarterly, 43*(3), 294–302. https://doi.org/10.1097/CNQ.0000000000000314

Bahçecioğlu Turan, G., Özer, Z., Yanmış, S., & Aksoy, A. (2023). The effects of self-acupressure on pain, fatigue, and sleep quality in colon and pancreatic cancer patients receiving chemotherapy. *Cancer Nursing, 46*(6), 457–466. https://doi:10.1097/NCC.0000000000001193

Burgess, J. E., Gorton, K. L., Lasiter, S., & Patel, S. E. (2023). The nurses' perception of expressive touch: An integrative review. *Journal of Caring Sciences, 12*(1), 4–13. https://doi.org/10.34172/jcs.2023.31903

Çeçen, S., & Lafcı, D. (2021). The effect of hand and foot massage on fatigue in hemodialysis patients: A randomized controlled trial. *Complementary Therapies in Clinical Practice, 43*, 101344. https://doi.org/10.1016/j.ctcp.2021.101344

Cristóbal Cañadas, D., Parrón Carreño, T., Sánchez Borja, C., & Bonillo Perales, A. (2022). Benefits of kangaroo mother care on the physiological stress parameters of preterm infants and mothers in neonatal intensive care. *International Journal of Environmental Research and Public Health, 19*(12), 7183. https://doi.org/10.3390/ijerph19127183

Davodabady, F., Naseri-Salahshour, V., Sajadi, M., Mohtarami, A., & Rafiei, F. (2021). Randomized controlled trial of the foot reflexology on pain and anxiety severity during dressing change in burn patients. *Burns, 47*(1), 215–221. https://doi.org/10.1016/j.burns.2020.06.035

Dreisoerner, A., Junker, N. M., Schlotz, W., Heimrich, J., Bloemeke, S., Ditzen, B., & van Dick, R. (2021). Self-soothing touch and being hugged reduce cortisol responses to stress: A randomized controlled trial on stress, physical touch, and social identity. *Comprehensive Psychoneuroendocrinology, 8,* 100091. https://doi.org/10.1016/j.cpnec.2021.100091

Franco, P., & Gregory, L. (2023). *Resiliency training facilitator guide.* The Center for Resiliency.

Franco, P. L., & Christie, L. M. (2021). Effectiveness of a one-day self-compassion training for pediatric nurses' resilience. *Journal of Pediatric Nursing, 61,* 109–114. https://doi.org/10.1016/j.pedn.2021.03.020

Greater Good in Education. (2025, January 3). Finger tracing: Mindful breathing for students. *Greater Good Science Center Magazine.* https://ggie.berkeley.edu/practice/finger-tracing-mindful-breathing-for-students/#tab__3

Kerr, F., Wiechula, R., Feo, R., Schultz, T., & Kitson, A. (2019). Neurophysiology of human touch and eye gaze in therapeutic relationships and healing: A scoping review. *JBI Database of Systematic Reviews and Implementation Reports, 17*(2), 209–247. https://doi.org/10.11124/JBISRIR-2017-003549

McKeering, P., & Hwang, Y.-S. (2019). A systematic review of mindfulness-based school interventions with early adolescents. *Mindfulness, 10,* 593–610. https://doi.org/10.1007/s12671-018-0998-9

Mühlenpfordt, I., Stritter, W., Bertram, M., Ben-Arye, E., & Seifert, G. (2020). The power of touch: External applications from whole medical systems in the care of cancer patients (literature review). *Supportive Care in Cancer, 28*(2), 461–471. https://doi.org/10.1007/s00520-019-05172-7

Sharma, K., & Kumari, R. (2019). Study to assess the effectiveness of foot and hand massage on reducing pain among post-natal mothers who had undergone caesarean section. *International Journal of Nursing Education*, 11(1), 79–84. https://doi:10.5958/0974-9357.2019.00017.5

Udoudo, D. A., Agu, C. F., Lawrence, E. S. Woolcock, A. M. M., Emanuel-Frith, M., & Kahwa, E. (2023). Factors influencing nurses' self care practices. *Journal of Holistic Nursing, 41*(3), 285–293. https://doi.org/10.1177/08980101221119776

Energy Healing

Mary Anne Hanley, Marjorie S. Anderson, Deborah A. Shields

NURSE HEALER OBJECTIVE

- Examine the integration of energy healing into holistic nursing practice.

DEFINITIONS

Energy healing: The deliberate process of using an external energy field to induce a change in one's own or another's human energy field for the purpose of supporting their physical, mental, emotional, and spiritual healing.

Entrainment: The phenomenon of rhythmic processes synchronizing with one another.

Healing: "An inner experience, a human potential and function, expressed as a shift in consciousness in which the practitioner and healing partner experience transformation or change" (Hanley et al., 2017, p. 374).

Healing partner: The recipient of biofield practices is a partner in the healing process. The holistic nurse and patient or client are partners in healing (Hanley et al., 2017; Krieger, 2021).

Human energy field: "A luminous field of energy that comprises a person, extends beyond the physical body, and is in a continuous mutual process with the environmental energy field. It is a vital energy that is a continuous whole and is recognized by its unique pattern; it is dynamic, creative, nonlinear, unpredictable, and flows in lower and higher frequencies. The balanced HEF is characterized by flow, rhythm, symmetry, and gentle vibration" (Shields et al., 2017, p. 352).

Intention: Choosing to think, act, or be a certain way.

Subtle energy: Barely noticeable energy fields of living organisms that may be related to internal electrical and magnetic activity.

Introduction

The National Center for Complementary and Integrative Health divides complementary health approaches into two general areas: nutritional approaches and psychological and/or physical approaches, which include mind–body practice (National Center for Complementary and Integrative Health, 2018). Mind–body practices include meditation, tai chi, guided imagery, hypnosis, yoga, and energy healing (National Center for Complementary and Integrative Health, 2018). There are many energy healing (biofield) practices. Therapeutic Touch®, Reiki, and Healing Touch are widely known in the interprofessional healthcare community (Guarneri & King, 2015). In an interview, Richard Gerber described these practices as vibrational therapies as well as sound, light, color, aromatherapy, flower essences, and homeopathy (Brown, 1999). He proposed that biofield or vibrational therapies are used to assess and help a person's energetic system to restore a balanced vibration and resonance, providing an environment to support the person's potential to self-heal (Brown, 1999). These practices are used for personal well-being and in a variety of healthcare settings.

Practice of Energy Healing in Holistic Nursing

The holistic nurse weaves together historical, philosophical, theoretical, and research knowledge to create a foundational framework for the practice of energy healing. Holistic nurses apply a synthesis of knowledge about energy therapies as they enter into helping relationships with healing partners with the intention to promote their healing partners' highest good and potential for healing. The nurse is aware that healer and healing partner are changed through this helping relationship (Hanley et al., 2017).

Overview of the Practice of Energy Healing

Krieger (1979) and Kunz (1995) theorized that healing is a human potential, and humans possess an innate capacity to access inner wisdom and guidance. A fundamental assumption of energy healing is that all life is sustained by universal life energy that moves freely within and without sentient beings. In health, we are in harmonic resonance within ourselves and with our environment; illness is generally associated with lower frequency and unbalanced vibrations. Perhaps this is why, when our bodies, minds, and/or spirits hurt, we feel drained (Shields et al., 2017).

Energy healing practices intentionally influence the flow of subtle energy within the human energy field (Krieger, 1987) to support people moving toward greater balance, coherence (Ross, 2019), and equilibrium.

Rogers (1992) asserted that energy is the fundamental building block of the universe and human beings. The human and environmental energy fields are in continuous process. Rogers's Principles of Homeodynamics explain change, its nature, mutuality, and direction. These principles inform how the nurse and healing partner cocreate healing, a human potential (Kunz & Krieger, 2004).

Within a holistic perspective, human biofield energy patterns explain the intricacies and complexities of a human energy system that is designed to gather process, store, and transmit information. Beginning within the body and closely surrounding it, the aura reflects our history and current energy patterns; moving inward, our chakras receive and process universal energetic information quickly; finally, meridians spread the word slowly and completely, transmitting and interpreting information, interpenetrating and connecting throughout the energy field. These interconnecting systems help us understand how energy therapies work.

Energy Healing Interactions

All healing interactions—or interactions of any sort—are energetic. Energy practitioners agree on five basic assumptions (Krieger, 2002; Levin, 2011):

1. Energy moves within and through living beings.
2. Energy is part of a universal field.
3. The human energy field is dynamic.
4. The human energy field can be perceived by another.
5. Imbalances and disorders in human energy flow are associated with illness and stress.

The relationship between the energy practitioner and the healing partner is integral and interconnected within the universal field, yet practitioners respect energetic boundaries. Energy healing is a highly intimate process, and as such, these practices are rooted in ethical knowing, authenticity, and compassion. Energy healing practitioners know that "the outcome of the patient is not in [our] . . . hands" (Kunz, 1995).

Energy Healing Process

Hands-on energy healing practices often begin with the practitioner quieting their mind, often referred to as *centering*. Practitioners use a variety of approaches to purposely shift their awareness inward to a stillpoint, which facilitates responding to another's need for help or healing (Krieger, 2015), and to focus on the energetic cues revealed during the assessment. This process creates a space for presence and deep listening. It may also alter the practitioner's electromagnetic field (Slater, 2013). Within this sustained centered state of consciousness, energy healing practitioners and healing partners experience a sense of well-being (Hanley et al., 2017, 2018).

The second step that practitioners use in the energy healing process is assessment. At this point, the practitioner uses their hands and intuitive knowing to search for cues about the healing partner's energy patterns. A healthy energy field is characterized by a sense of balance, flow, rhythm, symmetry, and gentle vibration. An unbalanced field is disordered in some way (Shields et al., 2017). The practitioner discerns these imbalances and intervenes to support balance in the healing partner's energy field and potential for healing.

Nursing Situation

Patsy was a pediatric nurse. She had been in a car accident and suffered a fractured sternum and deep brain injury. During her recovery, she experienced pain described as 7 on a scale of 0–10 and was unable to return to work. She felt that her energy centers (chakras) were out of alignment, which made her feel disoriented and unbalanced. She requested a series of energy healing sessions to ameliorate her pain and disorientation.

During the first session, Patsy demonstrated signs of physical tension and emotional anxiety. As we centered together, Patsy was asked to take a few cleansing breaths. I attuned to the characteristics of her unique energy field. Using my hands as a focus, I sensed energetic tightness and congestion around her neck and along her spine, while the area of her chest was cool, indicating a lack of energy flow. Focusing on releasing the congestion, I shifted my awareness and intention to promote flow and balance throughout her energy field and energy centers. As the congestion lessened, I modulated the flow of energy, bringing fresh energy into her field. I sustained a centered state throughout session, simultaneously assessing and modulating Patsy's energy field. When the cues indicated her energy was flowing uninterrupted throughout her energy field, I concluded the session, thanking Patsy as she continued to integrate the new energy. She reported that her pain reduced to a 4 on a scale of 0–10.

Patsy identified the ways her energy field changed, opening and balancing, during and following each session. She identified this process as healing, feeling as if she were embodying loving energy, making her more sensitive to people and her environment. Patsy continued to participate in energy healing sessions throughout her recovery and as she returned to her nursing practice.

The third step in the process is to identify from a variety of approaches those most useful to foster balance and flow within the energy field. Practitioners use intention to facilitate the flow of human energy that is integrated by the healing partner as needed. The healing partner's autonomous potential for healing is supported rather than controlled by the practitioner.

Reassessment and intuitive knowing guide the practitioner in determining when the session is complete. Energetic cues such as deeper breathing, facial flushing, or muscular relaxation reflect changes toward balance within the healing partner's field. These shifts in energy patterns inform the practitioner to allow the healing partner to rest and integrate the energy; the practitioner takes time to reflect on the interaction. The practitioner and healing partner discuss the treatment and plan further sessions. This process exemplifies the cocreation of healing relationships.

Various intentional actions used during energy healing are taught in a stepwise, linear process. The relationship between the healer and healing partner unfolds improvisationally and is informed through continual assessment and rebalancing actions or intentions (Hanley, 1991). The holistic caring process is a beautiful circular process.

Energy Healing Practitioner

Krieger (1979) and others found that energy healing practices can be learned. Energy healing practitioners deepen and advance their practice through self-development, study, and practice (Levin, 2011). Krieger reminds us that practitioners must be willing to do the inner work necessary to be present in healing interactions (Krieger, 2002). Perhaps this inner journey reveals the depth of and our capacity for compassion—a quality important to the healing process and the motivator for healing.

Authentic presence, an intentional process, calls the practitioner to meet people where they are with clear focus, attention, a willingness to walk with another, bearing witness, and trusting. Our self-compassion and inner wisdom allow us to appreciate another's healing journey. Healing is an individual experience, and the outcome is not in our hands (Krieger, 2013).

Evidence-Informed Energy Therapies

Energy healing approaches are evidence-informed, noninvasive, gentle, caring, and affordable. Often requested by patients and clients, these practices have gained visibility and credibility and are widely integrated into health and wellness care (Jain et al., 2015). We may consider all nursing interactions with patients, including bed baths and sitting with a patient as energetic in nature. Regardless of what we are doing, it is our way of being with another that makes a difference.

Holistic nurses are familiar with several energy healing therapies. According to Guarneri and King (2015), Therapeutic Touch was the first biofield therapy introduced and researched by nurses. Developed by Dolores Krieger and Dora Kunz in 1972, Therapeutic Touch is an evidence-informed therapy that incorporates the intentional and compassionate use of universal energy to promote balance and well-being; it is a contemporary interpretation of ancient healing traditions (Kunz & Krieger, 2004). Traditional East Asian practices involving energetic applications of the hands in healing include qigong (originating in China) and Reiki (originating in Japan). Nurses also incorporate energy-based therapies developed in Western contexts, including Healing Touch, Hands of Light, Touch for Health, Polarity Therapy, and Quantum Touch. The reader is invited to visit the websites of the professional associations representing these therapies and peruse the research reported by the practitioners/researchers.

Mounting evidence supports the positive impact of these energy healing practices on health and well-being. Numerous reviews of biofield research have been conducted to better understand the usefulness of biofield therapies (Garrett & Riou, 2021; Jain et al., 2015; Rao et al., 2016). These inquiries illuminate the many factors revealing the complexity of energy healing and elucidate the effectiveness, commonalities, and differences associated with energy therapies, including Therapeutic Touch, Healing Touch, and Reiki, with a variety of conditions such as cancer, pain, and cardiovascular disease. Jain et al. (2015), among others, examined the use of these biofield therapies with those experiencing health challenges, such as managing symptoms experienced by people at the end of life (Henneghan & Schnyer, 2015), people living with HIV (Bremner et al., 2015), and pain management during labor (Wang et al., 2024). The evidence from these reviews supports the use of biofield therapies in relieving pain, reducing stress, and improving well-being and quality of life.

Gronowicz et al. (2015) pointed out that preclinical trials investigating biofields could potentially increase our understanding of how/why biofield therapies are effective, leading to increased integration of these into healthcare practices.

Researching energy therapies effectively has been difficult. Warber and colleagues asserted that it is important to integrate multiple approaches into biofield research (Hannemann, 2014). Jain et al. (2015) identified methodological issues with three aspects of energy/biofield therapy research: (1) treatments—dosing, type, and delivery; (2) moderators, mediators, and mechanism of action; and (3) outcomes—biomarkers, qualitative data, whole-person effects. In randomized controlled trials, researchers assume the people involved will not influence the results, but we know this is not true. The inclusion of a sham provider is likely to have a healing effect. People, as open fields of energy in continuous process, are not neutral and always have some intention; both process and intention must be considered within the context of any inquiry or protocol.

This brief view of work being done in biofield research is intended to encourage you to dig deeper into areas of inquiry about energy healing. Further exploration of energy therapies is essential as we deepen our understanding of these therapies within the context of holistic nursing.

Integration

Education–Academic or Continuing Education Online and/or in Person

1. Introduce human energy field concepts early in healthcare education.
2. Expand interprofessional collaboration to develop standardized education, and credentialing of energy therapy practitioners as posited by Guarneri and King (2015).

3. Develop Continuing Education workshops that include energy healing approaches within clinical settings.
4. Increased education and understanding will lead to a greater pool of funders.

Clinical and Finance Policy

1. Work within institutions and engage voices of consumers to develop policies that incorporate the inclusion of energy healing therapies within clinical practice.
2. Although funding remains limited and outside of the dominant biomedical paradigm (Warber et al., 2015), participation in governmental and nongovernmental financing sources is critical.
3. Call for investments in education and inquiry about energy healing therapies.

Research

1. Design novel approaches that provide an entirely new model for researching human-to-human energy field interactions and measuring immediate and long-term results of treatments.
2. Moving forward, it is critical to be mindful of questionable methodological designs and be proactive in addressing them.

Global Health

1. Energy healing therapies emerged from contemporary interpretations of ancient healing approaches from across the globe. Through the application of these therapies, holistic nursing is aligned with global understandings of health and well-being.

Conclusion: The Tapestry Revealed

This is a new world, a new time alive with endless possibilities! Holistic nurses can choose to be trailblazers—to design educational curriculum, policies, and research studies that contribute to the body of nursing knowledge and contribute to the art and science of holistic nursing. As holistic nurses and energy therapy practitioners, we speak the truth, listen, and stay the course.

All we are asked is to remember what matters—and what matters is the healing partner. Energy therapies are used by practitioners and healing partners who are convinced that these approaches not only work but may be more appropriate, and perhaps more successful in some cases, than biological medicine.

As we bring closure to our exploration of energy healing, we ask: How does energy healing work? Weaving together patterns of knowing, we are offered a beginning idea. Drawing on life experiences and healing encounters, empiric, intuitive, and personal ways of knowing inform practitioners and healing partners as they cocreate the potential for healing (Krieger, 2021). The relationship between the practitioner and healing partner is grounded in compassion, respect, and trust.

Centering, coming to a stillpoint, is a compassionate ethical practice, which enables practitioners to appreciate the energetic boundaries. Ego is not a part of the healing interaction; rather, humility and gratitude are manifest. Aesthetically, energy healing practitioners are compassionately present, engaging, and willing to cocreate healing relationships with healing partners. It is beautiful.

References

Bremner, M., Blake, B., & Stiles, C. (2015). The experiences of persons living with HIV who participate in mind-body energy therapies: A systematic review protocol of qualitative evidence. *JBI Database System Review Implement Report, 13*(10), 41–49. https://doi.org/10.011124/jbisrir-2015-2321

Brown, E. (1999, April). *New choices for healing ourselves: Interview with Richard Gerber*. http://share-international.org/archives/health-healing /hh_ebnewch.html

Garrett, B., & Riou, M. (2021). A rapid assessment of recent Therapeutic Touch research. *Nursing Open, 8*(5), 2318–2330. http://doi.org/10.1002/nop2.841

Gronowicz, G., Bengston, W., & Yount, G. (2015). Challenges for preclinical investigations of human biofield modalities. *Global Advances in Health and Medicine*, 4(Suppl.), 52–57. https://doi.org/10.7453/gahmj.2015.013.suppl

Guarneri, E., & King, R. P. (2015). Challenges and opportunities faced by biofield practitioners in global health and medicine: A white paper. *Global Advances in Health and Medicine,* 4(Suppl.), 89–96. https://doi.org/10.7453/gahmj.2015.024.suppl

Hanley, M. A. (1991). Therapeutic Touch: The art of improvisation. *Journal of Holistic Nursing*, 9(3), 26–31.

Hanley, M. A., Coppa, D., & Shields, D. (2017). A practice-based theory of healing through Therapeutic Touch: Advancing holistic nursing practice. *Journal of Holistic Nursing, 35*, 369–381. https://dx.doi.org/10.1177/0898010117721827

Hanley, M. A., Shields, D., & Anderson, M. (2018). Living the experience of Therapeutic Touch. *Beginnings, 35*, 369–381. https://dx.doi.org/10.1177 /0898010117721827

Hannemann, D. (2014). *Biofield science & healing: A new chapter*. https://tiih.org/who/blog/biofield -science-healing-new -chapter/JOURNAL

Jain, S., Hammerschlag, R., Mills, P., Cohen, L., Krieger, R., Vieten, C., & Lutgendorf, S. (2015). Clinical studies of biofield therapies: Summary, methodological challenges, and recommendations. *Global Advances in Health and Medicine*, 4(Suppl.), 58–66. https://doi.org/10.7453/gahmj.2015.014.suppl

Krieger, D. (1979). *The Therapeutic Touch: How to use your hands to help or heal*. Prentice Hall.

Krieger, D. (1987). *Living the Therapeutic Touch: Healing as a lifestyle*. Dodd-Mead.

Krieger, D. (2002). *Therapeutic Touch as transpersonal healing*. Lantern Books.

Krieger, D. (2013). *Experiential knowledge of destiny during healing*. Lecture at Therapeutic Touch Dialogues, Whitefish, Montana.

Krieger, D. (2015). *Seeking ISSIE'S "native tongue."* Lecture at Therapeutic Touch Dialogues, Whitefish, Montana.

Krieger, D. (2021). *A healer's journey to intuitive knowing*. Bear & Co.

Kunz, D. (1995). *Spiritual healing: Doctors examine Therapeutic Touch and other holistic treatments*. Quest Books.

Kunz, D., & Krieger, D. (2004). *The spiritual dimensions of Therapeutic Touch*. Bear & Co.

Levin, J. (2011). Energy healers: Who they are and what they do. *Explore: The Journal of Science and Healing*, 7(11), 13–26.

National Center for Complementary and Integrative Health. (2018, July). *What's in a name?* https://www.nccih.nih.gov/health/complementary-alternative-or-integrative-health-whats-in-a-name

Rao, A., Hickman, L., Sibbritt, D., Newton, P., & Phillips, J. (2016). Is energy healing an effective non-pharmacological therapy for improving symptom management of chronic illnesses? A systematic review. *Complementary Therapies in Clinical Practice*, *25*, 26–41. https://doi.org/10.1016/j.ctcp.2016.07.003

Rogers, M. E. (1992). Nursing science and the space age. *Nursing Science Quarterly*, *5*, 27–34.

Ross, C. L. (2019). Energy medicine: Current status and future perspectives. *Global Advances in Health and Medicine, 8*, 1–10.

Shields, D., Fuller, A., Resnicoff, M., Butcher, H. K., & Frisch, N. (2017). Human energy field: A concept analysis. *Journal of Holistic Nursing, 35*, 352–368. http://dx.doi.org/10.1177/0898010116678709 https://doi.org/10.1177/2164956119831221journals.sagepub.com/home/gam

Slater, V. (2013). Energy healing. In B. Dossey, L. Keegan, C. Barrere, & M. A. Helming (Eds.), *Holistic nursing: A handbook for practice* (6th ed., pp. 751–773). Jones & Bartlett Learning.

Wang, R., Lu, J., & Chow, K. M. (2024). Effectiveness of mind-body interventions in labour pain management during normal delivery: A systematic review and meta-analysis. *International Journal of Nursing Studies, 158*, 104858. https://doi.org/10.1016/ijnurstu.2024.104858

Warber, S., Bruyere, R., Weintrub, K., & Dieppe, P. (2015). A consideration of the perspectives of healing practitioners on research into energy healing. *Global Advances in Health and Medicine*, 4(Suppl.), 72–78. https://doi.org/10.7453/gahmj.2015.014.suppl

Aromatherapy

Denise J. Joswiak

NURSE HEALER OBJECTIVES

- Identify elements of a safe, effective clinical aromatherapy program.
- Articulate the gap that prompted international support to promote evidence-informed essential oil use.

DEFINITIONS

Essential oils: Concentrated volatile aromatic compounds produced by plants and used in the process of aromatherapy.

Chemical components: Individual compounds that make up complex essential oils. An essential oil may have over 300 different components (Example: linalool in lavender). Also known as *constituents*.

Latin binomial: Genus and species of a plant, part of the taxonomic hierarchy, written after the common name in italics within parentheses (Example: Lavender [*Lavandula angustifolia*]).

Introduction

Plant medicine has been used for millennia with knowledge handed down as oral tradition and in the written word. Among the seminal resources is the *Ebers Papyrus*, a comprehensive document that dates to about 1550 BCE and lists approximately 800 medicinal and aromatic plants. An important revelation occurred in France in 1910 when Rene-Maurice Gattefossé severely burned his head and hands in a laboratory explosion. When the customary treatment was not helping and his wounds started to give off a gangrenous odor, he remembered that lavender growers informed him that burns could be healed with lavender essential oil. Using the oil, his infection cleared and the wounds healed without scarring.

For René-Maurice, this experience confirmed the hypothesis that lavender essential oil had antiseptic and healing properties. Profoundly changed by this experience, René-Maurice worked with military and civilian hospitals to demonstrate that essential oils constituted a new way of treating and healing. He coined the term *aromatherapie* in 1937 and published *Aromathérapie: Les Huiles Essentielles Hormones Végétales*. This text explored the antimicrobial properties of essential oils using medical case studies. René-Maurice authored over 30 technical books and scientific articles (Fondation-Gattefossé, 2025b).

True aromatherapy utilizes the essential oils of plants to effect therapeutic changes in body, mind, emotions, and spirit and bring healing to the places that need it. Aromatherapy is an effective, low-cost, therapeutic modality that can be easily integrated into a holistic self-care routine or patient care plan. Essential oils can provide a comforting, invigorating, and sometimes fun aromatic option for self-care. Clinical aromatherapy is the controlled and therapeutic use of essential oils in the clinical setting for specific, measurable outcomes.

True aromatherapy utilizes essential oils, while some products labeled as aromatherapy contain synthetic fragrance. Many plants have similar common names, so essential oils are referred to by the Latin binomial for accurate identification. For instance, some plants in the Asteraceae family appear similar and have the common name Chamomile. German Chamomile *(Matricaria recutita)* and Roman Chamomile *(Chamaemelum nobile)* are both commonly used in aromatherapy but have different chemistry and therefore different therapeutic properties. Essential oils are obtained from plants in one of two ways: steam distillation or expression. Although most aromatherapists believe plant extracts are considered essential oils only if they are obtained by steam distillation or expression, various types of solvent-extracted aromatics are also used in therapeutic applications.

Chemistry

Chemistry helps us understand potential healing properties, safety considerations, and shelf life of individual essential oils. Knowing the chemistry of an essential oil prior to purchase is important, as many variables can change the chemistry including country of origin, altitude, seasonal temperature, and rainfall. Research has been conducted on some essential oils and on many chemical components found within essential oils. Knowing the primary components of an oil aids in predicting which therapeutic effects the essential oil will likely have. If chemical components are significantly different, the therapeutic effect of the oil will likely be quite different too.

Gas chromatography/mass spectrometry (GC/MS) testing combines two analytic techniques to determine percentages of chemical components and detect adulterants. Essential oils used in the healthcare setting must have batch-specific GC/MS testing. Reputable companies provide GC/MS reports for each essential oil they sell.

Therapeutic Properties and Methods of Application of Essential Oils

Research suggests that essential oils may have therapeutic properties including the following: analgesic, anesthetic, antibacterial, antifungal, anti-inflammatory, antimicrobial, antioxidant, antiseptic, antispasmodic, antiviral, anxiolytic, cicatrisant, hypotensive, insecticidal, mucolytic, repellent, and sedative. Knowing the therapeutic properties of essential oils supports evidence-informed practice.

Essential oils are commonly used via inhalation, a highly effective method of application. Topical application is also used in clinical aromatherapy and allows essential oil blends to be absorbed into the skin to promote skin healing or to provide targeted pain relief to muscles and joints. Essential oils used topically should be diluted in carrier oils in almost every situation. Topical dilution of 1–3 percent is recommended for most preparations. Higher dilutions, or full-strength essential oils, may be used under the recommendation of a certified aromatherapist or qualified aromatherapy practitioner, especially for short-term, acute situations. Internal use of essential oils is not recommended except under the supervision of a certified aromatherapist or qualified aromatherapy practitioner who has received additional training on internal methods of application.

Trends and Resources for Gaps in Knowledge, Practice, and Research

Knowledge Gap

Millions of people around the world currently use essential oils, yet many utilize essential oils with little knowledge about safety and therapeutic indications. Adverse reaction databases document irritation and damage to the skin, digestive tract, and respiratory system from the improper use of essential oils. Education is key. The basic level of professional aromatherapy is a minimum of a 200-hour training program, commonly known as an *aromatherapy certification program*. Those interested in learning about essential oils can seek education provided by a qualified aromatherapist, and students are encouraged to enroll in one that is approved by a professional aromatherapy organization and endorsed by the American Holistic Nurses Association.

Practice Gap and Resources

Many healthcare facilities utilize essential oils without having formally trained staff or patient education, policies, protocols or guidelines, documentation, and evaluation protocols in place. Maddocks stated, "It remains critical that when aromatherapy is offered to patients as part of holistic care, there are clear guidelines for use and policies around handling and storage of oils" (Maddocks, 2023, p. 82). Documentation is key for monitoring efficacious utilization and future publication of findings.

Sustainability of essential oil plants is an important consideration that is just starting to be acknowledged within the aromatherapy community. The Convention on International Trade in Endangered Species of Wild Fauna and Flora (CITES) and Airmid Institute are excellent resources on such topics for those using plant medicine.

Research Gap and New Resources

"The increase in both quality and quantity of research is evident since 2005, supporting the growth of expertise in conducting research in this area" (Maddocks, 2023, p. 82). Although the amount of research is growing, more studies of improved quality are needed. Sometimes, entire articles must be disregarded due to insufficient information regarding the essential oils, chemistry, or protocols.

New initiatives support adding to the body of credible aromatherapy research. During the past five years, both the Gattefossé Foundation (GF) and the Aromatic Research Quality Appraisal Taskforce (ARQAT) wrote white papers outlining the need for more and better research, and both organizations made advances in these areas. The ARQAT, comprised of aromatherapy professionals with varied expert backgrounds, created the "open access" Transparent Reporting for Essential Oil & Aroma Therapeutic Studies (TREATS) checklist to evaluate reporting of nonpharmacologic aromatic research (Reven et al., 2024).

GF aims to strengthen the role of aromatherapy within integrative health and supports the development of a more sustainable and human-centered integrative healthcare model. The GF created two international awards to support evidence-based clinical aromatherapy programs that collect and intend to publish their data and gave a grant to the Alliance of International Aromatherapists (AIA) Research Academy (2025) to create an Aromatherapy Research Academy (Fondation-Gattefossé, 2025a).

AIA is an international professional aromatherapy member organization offering benefits for clinical aromatherapists and aromatherapy business owners. The AIA Research Academy launched in 2024 and offers mentoring and free educational webinars. The Research Academy started with basic presentations about research and continues to focus on publishing case studies, creating research posters, and elements needed to conduct and publish research (AIA, 2025).

Case studies are another important way for aromatherapists to share their work. Nurse aromatherapists are encouraged to share such information through the Aromatherapy Case Study Collaborative (CSC) and publish in an aromatherapy, holistic, integrative, or population-specific journal.

Why Integrate Aromatherapy into Holistic Nursing Practice?

Clinical Aromatherapy

Patients and clients request aromatherapy, and those receiving aromatherapy in a clinical setting often describe greater satisfaction with their care. Aromatherapy is an empowering, simple, and effective nonpharmacological option. In one study, a hospital-based, nurse-delivered aromatherapy program reported results from 10,372 aromatherapy sessions showing decreases in patient anxiety, nausea, and pain with average pain reduction of 3.31 units. Measurement was based on a numeric scale with 0 indicating no pain and 10 indicating the worst possible pain (Johnson et al., 2016). As the United States Department of Veterans Affairs leads the way with a person-centered Whole Health focus, many nurses are becoming certified in aromatherapy and implementing aromatherapy programs for their patients and clients.

Self Care

Holistic nurse self-care remains a core value. Many hospitals have added restoration rooms that include aromatherapy. Several facilities give aromatherapy inhalers or patches as a gift during Nurses' Week with essential oils that have been shown to decrease anxiety and depression and support resilience. Aromatherapy has the potential to support nurses during a stressful workday or personal situation.

Patient Consults

Advanced Practice Nurses and Nurse Coaches increasingly offer aromatherapy to their clients. In some facilities, specific nurses who are Certified Aromatherapists provide individual consultations and create specific blends to address their patient's or client's unique needs.

Integration

- **Clinical Practice:** Research and give rationale for essential oil choices. Create a clinical aromatherapy program or improve an existing program that includes policies, procedures and guidelines, staff and patient education, documentation, and evaluation protocols.
- **Education:** Utilize essential oils from a reputable vendor or seek appropriate education. A minimum of a 200-hour aromatherapy certification program is the minimum level of education to work as an aromatherapist in a clinical setting.

- **Research:** Utilize research, set aromatherapy programs up to capture data, and if possible, publish case studies or other research investigations. Credible research is foundational and supports dissemination of information about therapeutic efficacy.
- **Policy:** Be certain that aromatherapy falls within your scope of practice. In the United States, Nurse State Practice Acts might define whether integrative therapies fall within the nursing scope of practice.
- **Global Health:** The World Health Organization promotes safe and effective use of traditional medicine, like the utilization of essential oils, and encourages research to support its application in health care. Several international organizations such as AIA, ARQAT, and the GF are working to encourage quality research, promoting safe and effective clinical essential oil use with the goal of improving global health. Similarly, the National Center for Complementary and Integrative Health recognizes aromatherapy as a complementary and integrative modality and offers information through their "Resources for Researchers" portal.

Conclusion

There is clear evidence that aromatherapy benefits patients. Nurse-driven aromatherapy programs continue to gain momentum. Research is essential to support evidence-informed aromatherapy practice.

Nursing Situation

Nancy, a night nurse, realized her patient, Mrs. Smith, was not sleeping. This was due to pain and anxiety about a procedure she was having the following day. Mrs. Smith did not want a sleeping pill. Alliance Hospital, where Nancy worked, had just provided education for all of their nursing staff about their aromatherapy program, which included lavender (*Lavandula angustifolia*) to assist with anxiety, pain, and sleep. Lavender was available via inhalation in an aromastick (also called a personal inhaler) and as a 2-percent blend in lotion to be used topically. Nancy educated Mrs. Smith about lavender's therapeutic properties, the methods of application, and that this species of lavender has a high degree of safety. The patient was willing to try a hand massage, so Nancy retrieved the single-patient bottle of lotion from the supply cart.

Nancy asked the patient to smell the aroma of the lotion before beginning the hand massage. The patient liked it. Nancy documented the aromatherapy intervention, including Mrs. Smith's level of pain and anxiety on the hospital's Pain, Comfort and Well-being flowsheet. Nancy asked Mrs. Smith to inhale the lotion for five slow, deep breaths and suggested Mrs. Smith imagine her body relaxing more and more each time she exhaled. Nancy then sat and quietly massaged each of Mrs. Smith's hands. Within about seven minutes, Mrs. Smith thanked Nancy and reported that she felt relaxed. Nancy left and checked on Mrs. Smith again about 30 minutes later, finding Mrs. Smith asleep. Nancy opened the aromatherapy intervention on the flowsheet and added "sleeping" as an outcome.

References

Alliance of International Aromatherapists Research Academy. (2025). https://aoia.mclms.net/en/researchacademy

Fondation-Gattefossé. (2025a). *Call for applications.* https://www.fondation-gattefosse.org/en/our-actions/rene-maurice-gattefosse-prize/

Fondation-Gattefossé. (2025b). *The foundation; René-Maurice Gattefossé.* https://www.fondation-gattefosse.org/en/rene-maurice-gattefosse/

Henneghan, A. M., & Schnyer, R. N. (2015). Biofield therapies for symptom management in palliative and end-of-life care. American Journal of Hospice & Palliative Care, 32(1), 90–100. https://doi.org/10.1177/1049909113509400

Johnson, J. R., Rivard, R. L., Griffin, K. H., Kolste, A. K., Joswiak, D., Kinney, M. E., & Dusek, J. A. (2016). The effectiveness of nurse-delivered aromatherapy in an acute care setting. *Complementary Therapies in Medicine*, 25, 164–169. https://doi.org/10.1016/j.ctim.2016.03.006

Maddocks W. (2023). Aromatherapy in nursing and midwifery practice: A scoping review of published studies since 2005. *Journal of Holistic Nursing*, *41*(1), 62–89. https://doi.org/10.1177/08980101221078736

Reven, M. E., Bowles, E. J., Audia, D. D., Cohen, M. M., Joswiak, D. J., Kurkas Lee, B. A., May-Fitzgerald, A. C., Peppers-Citizen, M., Resnick, J. A., Tomaino, J. M., & Unger, B. J. (2024). Quality appraisal of research reporting for aromatherapy and essential oil studies in humans: Proposed checklist for "Transparent Reporting for Essential Oil and Aroma Therapeutic Studies". *Journal of Integrative and Complementary Medicine*, *30*(5), 469–477. https://doi.org/10.1089/jicm.2023.0006

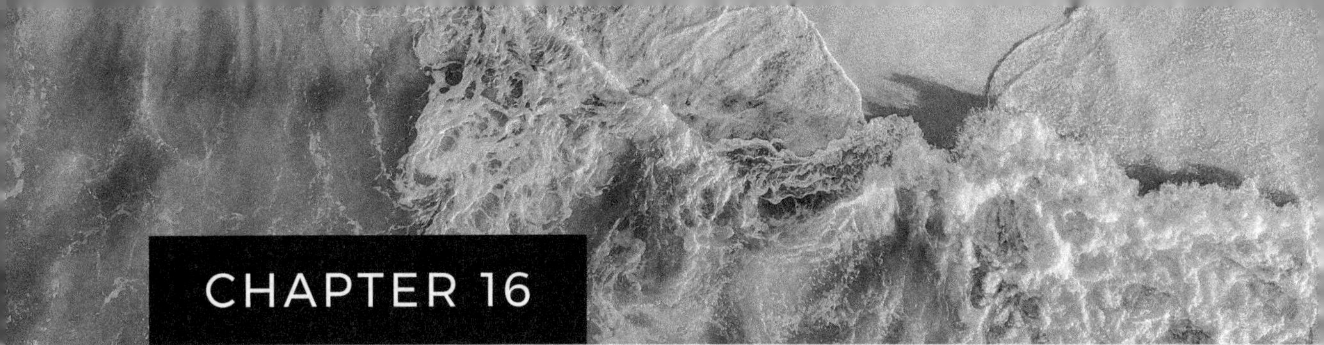

CHAPTER 16

Aesthetics and Self-Reflection in Holistic Nursing

Jennifer L. Reich, Mary Anne Hanley, Deborah A. Shields, and Lorrine Hall

NURSE HEALER OBJECTIVES

- Examine aesthetics as a way of knowing in nursing.
- Explore strategies to incorporate aesthetics into holistic nursing practice.
- Describe the benefits of reflection within the healing environment.

DEFINITIONS (AS AESTHETIC INTERPRETATION OF THE CHAPTER CONTENT)

Aesthetics:
An expression of our higher self
As we move about this Earth
Inspirations and creations
Allowing hope to birth-
Our presence with each other
A beauty we are feeling
Creating meaning in our lives
As a catalyst for healing-

Reflection:
Beyond any description
It takes us deep inside
To a space where our awareness lies
And our spirit may confide-

Introduction

Aesthetic practices are those that bring a sense of awe, wonder, and harmony and contribute to healing by facilitating an expanded expression of self that is unique and meaningful to the person. Bringing beauty into what we do and how we do it facilitates mind-body-spirit shifts in awareness and healthy biochemistry, mediating the chaos and confusion of a health crisis into meaningful form and substance. With the growth of neuroscience and psychoneuroimmunology, we can trace the neuropathways that give us this sense of safety, well-being, and relaxation. Aesthetic practices can be integrated into our personal healing journeys, as well as with the individuals, families, and communities for whom we care.

Aesthetics, as a way/pattern of knowing in nursing, was introduced in 1978 by Dr. Barbara Carper (Carper, 1978). Her seminal work sought to move nursing from a reductionist, autocratic model of practice and education to one that was holistic and individualized (Benner, 1982). She proposed four essential ways/patterns of knowing; empirics, ethics, personal, and aesthetics. Since then, other nursing scholars have expanded the original four patterns and proposed others (Benner, 1982, 1983; Chinn et al., 2022; Munhall, 1993).

Aesthetic knowing is the art of nursing. This way of knowing is a complex set of creative, imaginative, and self-reflective practices that nurses interweave into their work. Chinn et al. (2022, as cited in Lindell & Chinn, 2022) have described how aesthetic knowing is expressed in nursing practice as "...transformative acts that reveal the meaning and the significance of the experience" (para. 4).

Aesthetics in holistic nursing requires a solid foundation in the science of holism as well as in the evidence that supports artistic expression. Frequently, art leads us to new healthcare and self-care practices before theory or evidence does.

Art allows us to find ways to express our world and our relationship with our world through nonverbal means. Having made that journey, we can begin to express meaning and create new patterns of being. It is that *aha* moment.

Self-Reflection

Self-reflection, one of the essential tools of holistic nursing, is also essential to our work as nurses. Self-reflection allows us this opening of spirit, to knowing self (Levin & Reich, 2013).

As nurse healers, it is helpful to become familiar with a self-reflection practice through personal experience before introducing it to a patient/client. As you explore the self-reflection strategies offered throughout this chapter, tune in to what resonates with your body-mind-spirit. In addition, be gentle and respectful of the inner guidance you receive through your sensations, thoughts, feelings, and intuition. From there, you can envision how these might resonate with the person with whom you are working. Each patient/client is unique, and each moment of their healing journey is as well. Taking time to assess each person's preferences and interests as you bring aesthetic ways of knowing, being, and doing into your healing practice is essential.

Smith and Parker (2020) discussed how reflection on the experience of nursing is connected to an understanding of aesthetic knowing. "Through such reflection, the nurse understands that nursing practice has in fact been created, that each instance of nursing is unique, and that outcomes of nursing cannot be precisely predicted" (Smith & Parker, 2020, p. 27).

As you read and reflect through the tapestry of aesthetic practices in this chapter, imagine yourself as the artist who attends to beauty, harmony, and wholeness through art, movement, sound, nature, and reflective writing strategies. Allow . . . be spontaneous . . . trust . . . and enjoy.

The chapter also includes self-reflection moments for you to pause for self-reflection and contemplation. The purpose of these pause moments is to create a space for you to move more deeply into your own creativity and personal inquiry. These moments mirror how we engage in our lives, consciously taking time to pause and reflect on meaning, direction, and how we are bringing ourselves to the world.

As you visit the self-reflection moments, we invite you to consider the following questions in addition to those within each section:

1. What arises for you when you consider this aesthetic practice? Consider excitement, resistances, and/or fears.
2. How might you integrate this aesthetic practice in your holistic nursing work? What barriers do you anticipate? How might you address these?

Self-Reflection Moment: Art

Reflection: *As you begin your exploration of art, we invite you to take a virtual tour of the Notre Dame Cathedral. Pause and take a few deep breaths, and when you feel centered activate this link https://www.youtube.com/watch?v=uJ0f_HzODfM* (AFP News Agency, 2024).

Immerse yourself in the experience, noticing the stonework, sculptures, paintings, and stained glass. Listen to the music that accompanies you on your tour. Just dwell on that for a moment. How do you feel? Was there anything particularly beautiful and exciting? Were you unsettled by anything? When you feel ready, leave the experience without judging, be kind to yourself, and allow yourself to move on.

As an aesthetic expression art is transcendent, touching our heart, mind, and soul and transporting us to realms beyond the ordinary. Art engages the senses and intellect, invoking an emotional response that ranges from beauty and awe to discomfort. It is a medium through which individuals and cultures can convey their interpretations of their world and the meaning it holds for them (FAH, 2025; Mensink, 2023; World Health Organization [WHO], 2025).

To glimpse at the history of art and health is to visit the yesteryear. Art, religion, and healing developed synchronously, in the same social space. Archaeological evidence includes a variety of art forms that reveal insight into people's daily lives, ceremonies, rituals, and transitions. From paintings on cave walls and bodies to ancestral stories, we better understand the significance of art across cultures and throughout human evolution.

Art can be active (e.g., creating art) or something you receive. Both creating and receiving engage our inner being. Creating art takes many forms, including drawing, painting, writing, poetry, sculpting, fabric work, photography, singing, and dancing. We appreciate receiving art from many sources, such as art galleries, concerts, street art, reading, theaters, and special items that we use in our personal and professional life.

Holistic nurses utilize their intuitive knowing of art to create caring spaces designed to support the healing of self and others. This begins with presence, meeting people where they are with kindness and respect. When attending to the environment—lighting, color, air quality, scents, sounds, and general ambiance, we are tuning into the sense of aesthetics as part of the healing milieu. Integrating opportunities for yourself and your patient/client to create and receive art are important touchstones in the healing journey.

A scan of the healthcare landscape reveals an increasing presence of art both in system designs and in services offered as part of healthcare interventions. The World Health Organization (WHO) has long drawn the ability of art to help us communicate and understand concepts by drawing on all our senses and capacity for empathy. This has been a foundation for health promotion. In 2019, the WHO issued a report of a scoping review of the literature that addressed the question, "What is the evidence on the role of the arts in improving health and well-being." Over 900 publications were reviewed and the findings demonstrated that the arts can potentially impact both mental and physical health. The researchers clustered the results of the review under two broad themes: prevention and promotion, and management and treatment (Fancourt & Finn, 2019). The WHO began testing art interventions to advance specific health goals, including universal health coverage, mental health, suicide prevention, and collaboration with global media companies to provide local language programming on health issues. The work of the WHO demonstrates the global impact of art and the extraordinary potential to combine the arts with modern science and health practices.

The Foundation for Art & Healing (FAH) was founded in 2003 to explore the relationship of art and creativity with science and health. It includes a diverse membership of individuals who, in collaboration with community groups, are dedicated to bringing art and health together to enhance well-being. Some projects the foundation has initiated include providing art therapists and creative expression toolkits to the community after Hurricane Sandy, the Sandy Hook Shootings, and the Boston Marathon bombings. The Black Health & the Arts Initiative was created to address systemic racism as a public health crisis and, in 2016, The UnLonely Project was created to address the widespread issue of loneliness and use film as a vehicle to promote connection (FAH, 2025).

Social isolation and loneliness are global epidemics posing serious threats to our health (Centers for Disease Control and Prevention [CDC], 2024; WHO, 2025). It is estimated that about 1 in 4 U.S. adults report not having social and emotional support (CDC, 2024). Lack of social connection is common when a person does not have relationships or contact with others and has little to no social support. Loneliness is feeling alone or disconnected from others, like you do not have meaningful or close relationships or a sense of belonging—even a person with a lot of friends can feel lonely. Both loneliness and social isolation have far-reaching effects on our health and well-being. They are associated with an increased risk of cardiovascular disease and stroke, anxiety and depressive disorders, dementia, self-harm, experiencing suicidal ideation, and early death (CDC, 2024). Art programs designed to support social connection and community building are one approach being used to combat the loneliness widespread issue and can be done live or virtually. The arts offer a powerful lens to better understand ourselves, each other, and the world. Art draws us inward, allowing us a chance to improve personal health through individual reflection, expression, and action. Creativity also acts as a catalyst to promote interpersonal engagement that strengthens community connections and well-being. Creative arts help people develop a shared sense of belonging and togetherness, and to form stronger bonds with others and with themselves (FAH, 2025; Mensink, 2023).

Research has demonstrated the potential health benefits of art in various populations, including its role in reducing stress, helping with focus, processing emotions, and imagining a more hopeful future. There is increasing awareness of the mind-body-spirit effects of art. The pleasure associated with creating or gazing upon aesthetically pleasing art can stimulate endorphin release. A stress response may be modulated, as engaging in art seems to increase natural killer and T cells and decrease cortisol levels (Mensink, 2023). Art helps with whole-brain integration, bringing together the emotional, intuitive, nonverbal right side with the logical, problem-solving left side of the brain. Indeed, through art, the brain reveals its plasticity.

In the 1990s, Semir Zeki coined the term *neuroaesthetics* to describe a field of study that seeks to understand the neurological basis of beauty, art, and the aesthetic experience; to explore how our brains process and respond to aesthetic stimuli (LeGrand, 2024). Neuroaesthetics may help us better understand the intersection of art and science and the promotion of well-being. You are encouraged to read more about this fascinating field of study and some of the ethical implications of attempting to measure objectively the subjective experience of engagement with the arts. As neuroaesthetics continues to grow, it promises to unlock new understandings of what it means to be human, enriching our relationship with beauty, creativity, and each other (LeGrand, 2024; University of Pennsylvania, 2025).

Art can be a powerful expression of self-reflection, moving us to depths not yet discovered but alive with wisdom. In this state of unknowing, we become open to possibilities and new ways to articulate our understanding of our experiences (Levin et al., 2020). Michael Meade (2024) reminds us that creative practices can help us stay centered and grow "a greater sense of self and soul." He suggests that through meaningful practice, we can gain emotional stability, as well as creative ways to express our true selves. The two paths of practice are the inward path of contemplation, meditation, and self-reflection and the expressive path of creative arts. Both pathways can help us develop core strength and become more resilient and able to rebound no matter what happens (Meade, 2024).

We may be reluctant to undertake art projects because we believe that we are not artistic or that we lack in some way the abilities needed to create art. As a self-reflective expression, we are invited to consider that the healing journey is about process, not outcome. Who are we when we gaze upon a work that we find beautiful or when we create a piece that represents something deep within our hearts? There are no rules, no requirements, as we pick up the paintbrush or sing the song. It is our chance to express, to feel the joy of liberation! So... let your inner artist manifest in all its beauty!

Art Exemplar: Mandala Art

The most profound aspects of any art form, traditional or spontaneous, will be felt and recognized as universal; a mandala is one of these. Rooted in Sanskrit, the word *mandala* is translated to mean *circle*. The circle represents a sacred container that most traditions have used as a meditative and/or symbol relating to spirituality for thousands of years. Crafting a mandala is an ancient practice used for insight, healing, self-reflection, and self-expression. The mandala is said to be the bridge between the higher and lower realms and represents wholeness, unity, and the interconnectedness of all things (Thakker, 2023). How might we create our own mandala journey?

The mandala process is a merging of art, science, and ancient wisdom for reconnection to meaning and purpose within the sacred circle. It is an opportunity to dwell within ourselves and, through the process of drawing within the circle, for our authentic selves to be revealed. The mandala process may serve as a(n):

1. self-care reflective process of awareness and stress management;
2. healing tool for someone wishing to experience a nonverbal expression and release of emotions related to relationships, transitions, or health challenges; and/or
3. opportunity to connect with one's spirituality and inner wisdom.

The basic tools required include an unlined sheet of white or black paper with a circle; black, white, or colored pencils; and a simple pencil sharpener. If you wish to make a collage mandala, with pictures and symbolic images, you will need scissors and paste. No artistic ability is necessary—only the intention to dwell within and express what emerges into the circle.

Self-Reflection Moment

Create your mandala. Gather your equipment, and create a space that is comfortable, safe, and feels right. Pause...breathe... and move inward to your stillpoint. Set your intention for this mandala. You may ask yourself, "What would be most helpful to know about ____ right now? What would be healthy to release from my worries? What does my worry, anger, fear, joy, healing practice look like?" There is no right way to draw, let go of prejudging, and release expectations. Let your mandala evolve from the inside out. Recall that the center, the bindu, represents your origin (Purple & Pure, 2022). When you feel complete, rest, be. Gaze upon your creation. What do you feel as you observe it? Are any insights unfolding for you? If not, it is okay—do not get caught in the analysis trap. Over time, new insights may emerge and reveal the unconscious messages expressed within the mandala.

Aesthetics of Sound

Sound, vibration, and rhythm are universal energetic pulsations. Awakening through our awareness of and being present to sound and vibration around us affects us in unique and varying ways. Our world is abundant with sound and its vibrational patterns.

Seward posited, "Quantum physics established the theory that everything is energy, hence, the effect of vibrations on anything can be powerful" (Seward, 2005, p. 171). Every cell is vibrating at a particular resonance; each organ and tissue is pulsing in continuous motion. Energy (qi/chi) pulses throughout us along meridian lines. Vibrating atoms create our energy field, these vibrating patterns communicate information and extend outward from our body to interact with the environmental energy field (Wilson & Pappas, 2024).

Rechtschaffen (1996) discussed how living beings become entrained or synchronized with the rhythms around them. The aesthetic use of sound emerges through the purposeful use of vibration and rhythm through voice, song, and music with our healing partners to support and promote well-being.

Rhythm is a given: if you have a heartbeat, you have rhythm; if you are breathing, you have rhythm. The pattern manifestations of rhythms inherent in our lives derive from the synchronous attunement of the heartbeat and breath. It is inherently this rhythm from within where we may find a connectedness with the self; energetically, the soul's heartbeat is a constant. The energy center or chakra of the heart holds the vibrational quality for each individual's own unique rhythm—as unique as a fingerprint or the iris.

We experience many variations of sound and rhythm throughout our lives. The earliest experience of sound is primordial, infrasound heard and felt below the perception of hearing and is associated with spiritual traditions and scientific discoveries (PopTech, 2011). A variety of traditions relating to spirituality consider *om*, from

Hinduism (pronounced *aum*), as a primordial sound. The Tibetan sacred word *Hum*, Follower of Islamic faith *Amin*, and Egyptian, Greek, Roman, and Follower of Christianity *amen* are all considered to be primordial sounds (AWGP, 2005). We use these primordial sounds to shift or raise our awareness of ourselves and our connection with the universe.

In his exploration of voice, Tomatis helps us understand that the voice can only reproduce what the ear can hear (Campbell, 1997). He found that "the mother's voice serves as a sonic umbilical cord for her developing baby and a primal source of nurturing" (Campbell, 1997, pp. 17–19). We begin hearing low-frequency sounds at close to 4.5 months of fetal life; we experience the vibration of our mother's breath moving in and out, her heartbeat, and her stomach rumbling (in hunger and satisfaction). Through this entrainment to the mother, we are moved to seek places and spaces filled with peaceful nurturing sounds and vibrations, and even silence, that provide relief from the background noise that is constant in our daily lives.

The throat is a physical and symbolic bridge between the head and the heart. Producing and engaging with sound vibrations are empowering approaches to self-reflection and healing. Since ancient times, mantras, chanting, toning, and, more commonly in our culture, humming (a quiet form of toning) are ways to enliven the vocal cords that actually create a healing vibration throughout our body-mind-spirit. Singing connects the mind with the emotions. Gaynor (1999) noted that for the Sufis, singing as breath is one of the most powerful ways of healing.

Humming occurs consciously or unconsciously in our daily lives is humming. Humming, with the mouth closed creates a resonance within one's energy field that has been found to express happiness or satisfaction. This vibrational pattern releases neurochemicals that enhance the body's comfort and pleasure, contributing to a sense of well-being and peace (Trivedi et al., 2023).

Rhythm, a dominant vibrational feature of the universe—indeed, ubiquitous in nature—emanates through all musical genres. Music is present throughout life and is used by people from before birth to transition to entertain or to comfort individuals experiencing physical and emotional discomfort (Ergin & Yucel, 2019; Sung et al., 2010).

To use the aesthetic forms of music for healing means to transform the environmental field into a state of *holos* or becoming whole. "Defining wholeness in musical terms means we must go beyond the contemporary model of the body and think of it as an orchestra receiving and producing a symphony of sounds, chemicals, electrical charges, colors and images" (Campbell, 1997, p. 62). Music helps the body rebalance, allowing the music of one's own heart song to strengthen and regain a sense of peace, healing, and wholeness, whether into life or death.

As partners in healing, through the thoughtful and intentional use of the aesthetics of sound, voice, rhythm, vibration, through music, song, or humming, holistic nurses support whole person's synchrony and harmony.

Nursing Situation: Anna's Story

Anna was a brilliant woman and nurse who for the past several years experienced progressive signs and symptoms of dementia with full knowledge of the course of her illness and its impact on her life. She was not happy with her changing cognitive abilities. Each day she lost connections with the larger world, retreating into her home and into herself. She described herself as being alone even though she lived with others. Finding ways to help her gain a sense of peace or joy, even momentarily, was a challenge. At times when she felt confused or disoriented in the current moment, her past life experiences provided the best clues for ways to access those moments of joy in the present and help her to reorder her thinking and ability to relate in the moment.

As a youthful woman, Anna was a pianist and organist who was unable to play following a serious back injury. Yet music and dance always brought her pleasure. Her favorite artists were Harry Belafonte and Hugh Masekela. Alvin Ailey and Judith Jameson's Dance Theatre was her favorite dance troupe. Throughout her adult life she attended performances by these artists. A particular favorite was Alvin Ailey's production of *Revelations* that she attended every year during the holidays.

Anna traveled the world. In her later days she conveyed, "I have no regrets, I did everything on my 'bucket list' when I was young enough to enjoy them." During one trip to the Netherlands, we visited Keukenhof Gardens. Walking among the beautiful colors of the tulips, the deep green of the lawns, and sounds of nature created a vibrant and enduring memory for Anna.

As Anna's illness progressed, she felt increasingly isolated and sad. She could not imagine what she could do to improve her life situation or improve her mood. I would remind her how she enjoyed her trips and how her favorite music gave her pleasure. I proposed that by drawing on her memories she could access feelings of joy embedded in those special experiences. Through this process she might experience a sense of clarity and connection with herself and reduce her sense of isolation, confusion, or disorientation. One of the approaches we used was to play music by artists she enjoyed. Later, we found YouTube videos of these artists and tours of the Keukenhof Gardens.

On days Anna felt disconnected and that her world was shrinking, I would play a video of spring in Keukenhof Gardens, and we would literally share our walk through the nature trails and the tulips again, amazed as if for the first time at tulips' beauty. During the tours she would comment on the brilliant colors, changing flowers and trees, recalling our last trip to the Netherlands.

At other times, when Anna was isolated or disoriented, or confused, I would ask if she wanted to listen to music. We searched YouTube for Harry or Hugh, or Alvin Ailey Dance Theatre to create concerts, sometimes for 30 minutes and sometimes 2–3 hours. During the concert she tapped her feet and played her invisible piano, singing along with Hugh and Harry, and the dancers.

Dementia separated Anna from the woman she knew herself to be and the life she lived. Watching the videos provided audio and visual connections that enabled Anna to recall and relive distant memories and make them a part of her present reality. Following our excursions into her past experiences, she shared memories, relationships, travels, and expressed a deep contentment with her life. The concerts and trips we took from her living room expanded her sense of connection with the life she knew, bringing her joy and peace. The concerts and journeys via music and travel videos gave me a sense of contributing to Anna's reality and helping us to connect with each other in the present moment, reflecting on our shared experiences.

Self-Reflection Moment–Humming

As you move through your day, take a moment to hum. Place your tongue behind your upper teeth, open your lips slightly, and breath through the space you created. Do this for a moment as you breathe in and out. Notice how your body vibrates with the humming. You can use the hum as a way of centering before entering a patient's room or home. Notice any change in your awareness. Consider, how did you feel before you hummed? Were there any changes in your mood or stress?

What more can you do in your work with patients/clients to bring the aesthetics of sound to support calm, joy, and healing? Perhaps inquire how their music preferences make them feel and if they would want to listen to music to aid in their healing and well-being.

Aesthetics Through Writing

Writing for self-reflection is another aesthetic form and practice to explore one's conscious and unconscious experiences. Some individuals feel drawn to the creative forms of poetry and story writing, and some journal daily to track ongoing thoughts, brainstorm creative ideas, and record insights.

Journaling

Journaling can be a powerful tool for self-reflection and critical thinking. Numerous studies have been conducted on the use of journaling with nursing students. A 2022 systematic review found journaling to be an effective tool for promoting reflection, as well as for developing clinical judgment and emotional competency (Greenleaf Brown et al., 2022).

Nurses at any stage of their career may find journaling a beneficial strategy for themselves or their patients/clients. Whether using traditional pen and paper or technology such as a journaling app, reflecting through journaling may reveal to us our unique inner world while also connecting us to our shared human experience. Through the inner experience of reflection, journaling can be viewed as a form of storytelling—sharing the story of your experiences with yourself. You can read your journal out loud, noticing how it sounds in a space of nonjudgment.

Poetry

Poetry is an aesthetic form of reflective practice that facilitates exploration of nursing issues (Jack, 2016). Through exploration of our feelings and emotions, poetry expresses what prose language cannot, connecting us to the art of nursing.

Poetry has been studied as one way to foster empathy in nursing students. Jack and Illingworth (2023) suggest poetry as a safe space for students to rehearse and foster empathy and self-awareness. Through strategies incorporating poetry, learners may explore empathy with patients, self, and others (Jack & Illingworth, 2023).

Some nurses, including some of the authors of this chapter, write poetry and use poetry as both a self-reflective and a reflective practice with nursing and healthcare students. However, for others, poetry may feel intimidating in this realm of aesthetic expression. For example, perhaps they had an experience in childhood where they felt that they were not good at poetry, or they were taught it had to fit a certain meter or rhythm. In these situations, offering nonjudgmental support and encouragement may foster a new perspective on creating poetry.

Exemplar: Poetry and Reflection

In a July 2024 AHNA webinar for nurses, participants engaged in an exercise to create a self-caring poem. After learning about reflection and ideas to begin a reflective writing practice, prompts were provided for crafting this personal poem. Some of the prompts included "What do I love about myself?" "What brings me joy?" "What is going well for me now?" After writing and spending time in quiet reflection, participants had the opportunity to share their experience with the writing process.

Self-Reflection Moment: Journaling and Poetry

How can you bring these forms of reflective writing into your personal self-care practice and that of those you care for? Consider the following suggestions and adapt them to the environment you are in and the presences you have and the preferences of your patient/client. Remember, when working with another person, first explore their preferences for an aesthetic practice by inquiring if they have ever journaled, written poetry, or any other forms of reflective writing. Describe how these aesthetic practices may support self-understanding and insight into the health challenges they are facing.

For journaling, gather a notebook and pen, and set a timer for 10 minutes. Sit in quiet meditation for a few moments and take this time to consider an issue of importance or even notice something in the environment you or the patient/client wants to reflect on. Then begin to write. Allow whatever wants to be expressed to take form on the page. Write until the buzzer goes off, or beyond, *without* editing. The writing may take any number of forms. Use this writing as a guide for reflection throughout the day.

To explore poetry, attend a poetry reading, or choose a poem that speaks to you from a book or poetry blog or website. After listening to or reading the poem, reflect on the experience. Can you relate to the experience shared in the poem? How did reading the poem make you feel?

Next, find a quiet space to sit. Close your eyes and take three slow breaths, expanding the belly as you breathe in and fully emptying the belly before your next breath. Gently open your eyes. Now, try writing a poem about a personal experience, allowing the words to flow without expectation or judgment.

Reflections on the Journey

As holistic nurses, we participate in the unfolding and enfolding of the environmental fields to support greater consciousness and healing processes for ourselves and those we work with. The use of aesthetic practices of sound, movement, nature, art, and reflective writing adds meaning, depth, texture, substance, and nuance to the dynamic and pandimensional human healing journey experience.

As we integrate aesthetic expressions into our lives, we learn to model the lived experience of the art of nursing and our holistic nursing philosophy more fully through thoughts, words, and actions.

Take a moment now to reflect on ways in which your personal well-being and your holistic nursing practice are enriched by your explorations and self-inquiry into the aesthetics of nursing.

Implications

As you progressed through this chapter, you experienced many ways to bring aesthetic practices into your own well-being with added suggestions on how to integrate aesthetic ways of being and knowing into the work you do with others. Consider, as well, the following implications for education, research, and policy.

Academic, Staff, or Continuing Education Online and/or in Person

1. Incorporate aesthetics and reflective practice into class topics and experiences.
2. Use performance to facilitate understanding of aesthetic knowing. For example, engaging in interdisciplinary collaboration to present topics of importance of nursing in health care.
3. Develop Continuing Education workshops that include aesthetics and opportunities for reflection.

Policy

1. Work within institutions, through grants or public policy venues, to call for investments in aesthetics for healthcare professionals.
2. Participate in local arts campaigns and bring attention to the importance of the arts for the well-being of communities.

Research

1. How does the use of aesthetics enhance the holistic nurses' understanding of the patient/client?
2. Explore the lived experience of nurses and patients/clients who incorporate aesthetic strategies in their personal and professional lives.
3. What contributions does the use of music, film, or videos make in promoting healing relationships with your clients or patients?

Conclusion

Through our aesthetics journey, we have taken time out to explore the interface of our experiences and the meaning these have for our personal lives and holistic nursing pract0ice. Consider these as initial guides that contribute to your personal life and holistic nursing practice.

- Holistic care may be enhanced when nurses and patients engage with aesthetically creative expressions that allow mindful self-reflection.
- Consider aesthetic strategies you currently practice and others you might try in the future for your own and your patients'/clients' inner growth.
- Bring yourself into attunement with your patient/client and the environment simultaneously; identify an aesthetic strategy you can draw on to enhance your patient/client healing relationship with themselves and the environmental field.

Our ongoing personal and professional development flourishes as we purposefully and intentionally ponder and invite ourselves to imagine the unknown through reflection.

References

AFP News Agency. (2024, December 4). *A look inside the restored Notre Dame Cathedral* [VIDEO]. YouTube. https://www.00youtube.com/watch?v=uJ0f_HzODfM

AWGP. (2005, September–October). (Om)—The primordial sound, the eternal syllable. *Akhandjyoti Magazine*. https://www.awgp.org/en/literature/akhandjyoti/2005/Sep_Oct/v1.OmEternalSyllable

Benner, P. (1982, March). From novice to expert. *American Journal of Nursing, 82*, 402–407.

Benner, P. (1983). Uncovering the knowledge embedded in clinical practice. *Image: The Journal of Nursing Scholarship, 15*(2), 36–41.

Campbell, D. (1997). *The Mozart effect*. Avon Books.

Carper, B. A. (1978). Fundamental patterns of knowing in nursing. *ANS Advances in Nursing Science, 1*(1), 13–23.

Centers for Disease Control and Prevention. (2024, May 15). *Health effects of social isolation. and loneliness*. https://www.cdc.gov/social-connectedness/risk-factors/index.html

Chinn, P. L., Kramer, M. K., & Sitzman, K. (2022). *Knowledge development in nursing theory and process* (11th ed.). Elsevier.

Ergin, E., & Yucel, S. C. (2019). The effect of music on the comfort and anxiety of older adults living in a nursing home in Turkey. *Journal of Religion and Health, 58*(4), 1401–1414.

Fancourt, D., & Finn, S. (2019). *What is the evidence on the role of the arts in improving health and well-being? A scoping review [Internet]*. WHO Regional Office for Europe. (Health Evidence Network synthesis report, No. 67). SUMMARY. https://www.ncbi.nlm.nih.gov/books/NBK553775/

The Foundation for Art and Healing (FAH). (2025). Art and Healing. https://www.artandhealing.org

Gaynor, M. (1999). *Sounds of healing*. Broadway Books.

Greenleaf Brown, L., Briscoe, G. S., & Grabowsky, A. (2022). The influence of journaling on nursing students: a systematic review. *Journal of Nursing Education, 61*(1), 29–35. https://doi.org/10.3928/01484834-20211203-01

Jack, K. (2016, May 19). Using poetry writing to help students explore empathy. *Nursing Times*. https://www.nursingtimes.net/careengland/using-poetry-writing-to-help-students-explore-empathy/7004923.article

Jack, K., & Illingworth, S. (2023). Rehearsing empathy: Exploring the role of poetry in supporting learning. *Arts & Health, 16*(3), 303–316. https://doi.org/10.1080/17533015.2023.2256361

LeGrand, E. (2024, January). *What is neuroaesthetics? Science origins. Science*. https://neuroaesthetics.med.upenn.edu/

Levin, J., Reich, J., Hanley, M., Shields, D., & Murname, S. (2020). Aesthetics in holistic nursing. In M. A. B. Helming, D. A. Shields, K. M. Avino, & W. E. Rosa (Eds.). *Dossey & Keegan's holistic nursing: A handbook for practice* (8th ed.). Jones & Bartlett Learning.

Levin, J. D., & Reich, J. L. (2013). Self-reflection. In B. M. Dossey & L. Keegan (Eds.), *Holistic nursing: A handbook for practice* (6th ed., pp. 247–260). Jones & Bartlett Learning.

Lindell, D., & Chinn, P. (2022, October 27). Aesthetic knowing. *Nursology*. https://nursology.net/patterns-of-knowing-in-nursing/aesthetic-knowing/

Meade, M. (2024). *Arts and practices. Antidote to overwhelm. Sources of resiliency*. Webinar. Presented November 21, 2023, by The Mosaic Multicultural Foundation. https://www.mosaicvoices.org/arts-and-practices

Mensink, S. (2023, October). *The intersection of art and health: How art can help promote well-being*. Living Well. Mayo Clinic Press Editors. https://mcpress.mayoclinic.org/living-well/the-intersection-of-art-and-health-how-art-can-help-promote-well-being

Munhall, P. L. (1993). Unknowing: Toward another pattern of knowing in nursing. *Nursing Outlook, 41*, 125–128.

PopTech. (2011). *Milton Garcés: Primordial sounds* [VIDEO]. YouTube https://www.youtube.com/watch?v=sFqU8tNJ3PY

Purple and Pure. (2022). *The beauty and meaning of mandala art: A guide to creating and appreciating*. https://purpleandpure.com/blogs/blogs/the-beauty-and-meaning-of-mandala-art-a-guide-to-creating-and-appreciating-1?srsltid=AfmBOorb7-QbLxyRuqg_A3dyTpPzSKs6cc_KpyUN-JrhoWP6_dTFCuUz

Rechtschaffen, S. (1996). *Timeshifting: Creating more time to enjoy your life*. Doubleday.

Seward, L. (2005). *Achieving the mind-body-spirit connection*. Jones and Bartlett Publishers.

Smith, M. C., & Parker, M. E. (2020). Choosing, evaluating, & implementing nursing theories for practice. In M. C. Smith (Ed.), *Nursing theories and nursing practice* (5th ed.). F. A. Davis Company.

Sung, H. C., Chang, A. M., & Lee, W. L. (2010). A preferred music listening intervention to reduce anxiety in older adults with dementia in nursing homes. *Journal of Clinical Nursing, 19*(7-8), 1056–1064.

Thakker, A. (2023, July 26). *The deep and sacred symbolism behind the mandala*. shunspirit. https://shunspirit.com/article/mandala-symbol-meaning

Trivedi, G., Sharma, K., Saboo, B., Kathirvel, S., Konat, A., Zapadia, V., Prajapati, P. J., Benani, U., Patel, K., & Shah, S. (2023). Humming (Simple Bhramari Pranayama) as a stress buster: A Holter-based study to analyze heart rate variability (HRV) parameters during Bhramari, physical activity, emotional stress, and sleep. *Cureus, 15*(4).

University of Pennsylvania. (2025, January). *Penn Center for Neuroaesthetics*. https://neuroaesthetics.med.upenn.edu/

Wilson, D. R., & Pappas, J. (2024). Sound waves and holistic healing. *Beginnings, 44*(3), 14–16.

World Health Organization. (2025). *Arts and health*. https://www.who.int/initiatives/arts-and-health

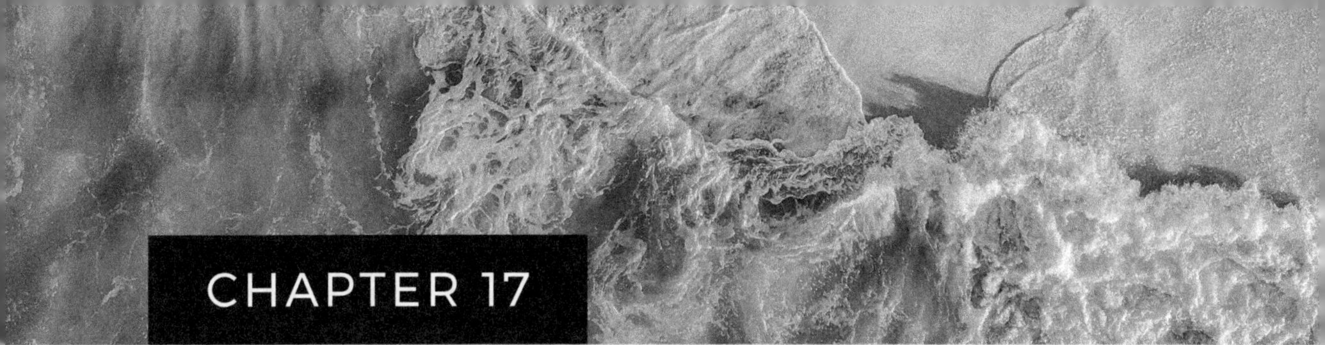

CHAPTER 17

Peaceful Transitions at the End of Life

Lynn Keegan and Janet Booth

NURSE HEALER OBJECTIVES

- Apply theories of grief, self-transcendence, and culture to assist the dying in peaceful and meaningful death.
- Contribute to the dying person's peace of mind through the nurse's Presence and natural approaches.
- Support the natural closing down of the body as it prepares for the final exhale.
- Utilize trends in end-of-life care to maximize the dying person's holistic caring process.

DEFINITIONS

Death: Moment in time when the spirit transitions out of the body.

Dying: Final stage of physical life that fits into a broader awareness, giving meaning to both life and death.

Nearing death awareness: A dying person's knowledge of death and attempts to describe this experience to healthcare providers, family, and friends.

Self-transcendence: A spiritual concept referring to moving oneself into a larger sense of consciousness that is more than the physical mind and understanding.

Introduction

To die well is to die peacefully, with the knowledge that life has had meaning and that one is connected through time and space to others, to the universe, and, for some, to one or several higher powers. Supporting people to die well requires knowledge and skill, as well as a willingness to be intensely involved in the most intimate phases of another's life. Care for the caregiver, both professional and personal, is a necessity and an often-overlooked part of caring for the dying. The dying and their families are the units of care. Additionally, although some nurses will work specifically at end of life, nurses in any practice setting can impact how people navigate serious illness and how they die. Open conversations about goals of care and what matters most, taking place throughout the trajectory of illness, are one way to support patients and families to make thoughtful decisions about their care—long before they are dying. This conscious preparation for the last stage of life is part of upstreaming and normalizing advance care planning conversations (Prince-Paul & DiFranco, 2017). In fact, the American Nurses Association (2016) position statement on Nurses Roles and Responsibilities for Providing Care and Support at the End of Life stated that decision making for the end of a patient's life should occur over years rather than just in the minutes or days before death, and nurses are ideally positioned to contribute to those conversations.

Theoretical Frameworks

Developing theoretical frameworks to guide end-of-life care is based on standards of care including scope and standards of practices, state laws, and national laws. Theories related to grief and loss, self-transcendence, and nearing death awareness are particularly useful in developing holistic caring process plans for care for the dying. In addition, like other aspects of patient care, nurses will want to recognize, acknowledge, and modify care based on the varying practices of different cultures.

Watson's Theory of Human Caring

One holistic overarching approach to easing the burden for those who are caring for people at the end of life is based on Jean Watson's Theory of Human Caring, which focuses on the relationship between the whole self of the nurse and the whole self of the patient/family as it protects and preserves the humanity and dignity of the patient (Watson, 2021). In this important partnership or relationship between the caregiver and the dying person and their family, the burden becomes shared; each can ease the other's burden. Caring science and the concept of conscious dying work together as an emerging metaparadigm to deepen the nurse's awareness of both the sacred nature of the dying process as well as the nurse's own spiritual and emotional relationship with death (Rosa et al., 2019).

Conscious Dying

From classic books like *Who Dies?* (Levine & Levine, 1982) and *The Tibetan Book of Living and Dying* (Rinpoche, 1992) to more recent integrative trends in nursing literature (Rosa et al., 2019), the concept of conscious dying has become more examined in popular culture. Rosa et al. (2019) described conscious dying as the process of imagining the end of life as an opportunity to become more present and loving, to experience profound healing and spiritual awakening, and to look at suffering from a whole-person lens. During the pivotal time of dying, the energetic, spiritual, and existential aspects of the patient are also in transition.

Kübler-Ross

Spiritual development is also related to the phases of grief originally identified by Elisabeth Kübler-Ross (1969). Nursing care during each of the phases takes into account the spiritual maturity of the griever, whether it is the dying person or those who love that person. A person who is in the early stages of spiritual development, whether a child or an adult, needs external help, information, and experience to strongly develop the ability to trust. Learning to accept a loss through integration and transcendence seems to occur alongside spiritual growth and development. People with well-developed spiritual practice may use rituals, rites, symbols, and other comforting activities when planning their own funerals.

Nursing care requires a careful assessment of a dying person's spiritual resources to assist with a peaceful death. In one survey of registered nurses caring for the actively dying in an academic medical center, it was found that nurses' self-perceived professional capability and comfort levels in caring for dying patients is positively influenced by older age, greater clinical experience, and extensive continuing education (Toh et al., 2021). This suggests that it is important to recruit experienced nurses to care for the dying and their families and to mentor inexperienced nurses to increase their comfort in working with the dying.

Evolution of Grief Theories

Kübler-Ross' classic model for understanding grief was pivotal in shifting the focus to the experience of the dying person, and her work in the 1960s and 1970s brought in a new cultural paradigm of more open and honest conversations about death and dying. She normalized the variety of stages a dying person might experience and emphasized the value of empathy and deep listening. Subsequent thought leaders have continued to expand our understanding of the purpose and value of grief after loss. As summarized by Tyrrell et al. (2023), J. William Worden encouraged grieving people to more actively engage with grief in his four-phase task model—accepting the reality of the loss, experiencing the pain of grief, adjusting to an environment without the deceased, and redirecting emotional energy to engaging with new activities. Tyrell et al. also described how Alan Wolfelt shifted the attention from a more clinical approach of grief therapy to a model of accompanying, where anyone can serve as a witness and companion to another as they walk their grief journey. This companioning approach views grief as a natural extension of our ability to give and receive love; not something to avoid but instead meant to be fully experienced and embraced in the path to healing.

Weller (2015) offered another model of grief experience called "The Five Gates of Grief," which invites people into a more soulful approach to the losses they experience as human beings. The first gate is the loss of all that is loved, which is the most common context for experiencing loss. He added four other gates into grief that include what might be considered both personal and cultural losses: the places that have not known love, the sorrows of the world, what was expected but not received, and ancestral grief. This expanded perspective of loss might increase the nurse's awareness of what Weller called "unmetabolized grief" in both themselves and their patients and impact their ability to be compassionately present for those who are experiencing emotional distress.

Lastly, the concept of collective grief brings another dimension to the isolated grief that many people experience. *Participatory grieving* is the act of involving families and communities in the dying process and after-death care. Community death care is a movement to reclaim practices and rituals to enhance family engagement in care of the dying and community presence to support those who are grieving (Hope et al., 2023).

Self-Transcendence

Many people have studied self-transcendence, the sense of a temporal integration of self, the feeling that past and future enhance the present, and the drive to benefit others beyond self (Kang, 2019). In studying survivors of concentration camps, Frankl (1963) discovered that those who survived seemed to transcend beyond self either toward other people or toward meaning. Self-transcendence gives people a greater sense of well-being and ability to cope with grief. Those with a sense of transcendence live in the present and are able to see death as part of the impermanence of physical life. Encouraging people to seek meaning and connections, either in the present or through the ages, helps people move toward self-transcendence and thereby achieve peace.

For some people, finding meaning through sharing their stories is part of leaving a legacy. Research with older adults (Neller et al., 2023) shows that when they share their stories and values with others, they are better prepared to live out the remainder of their lives. Story-telling or narrative therapy helps people change the language of their own experience and how they view themselves within and outside of their disease (Saxena, 2019). Narrative approaches have helped patients and their families create new meaning and become empowered to own the circumstances of their environment and disease, leaving them feeling more peaceful and hopeful with an enriched sense of self at the most vulnerable period in their lives. Additionally, narrative therapy can support patients and their families in their spiritual development (Saxena, 2019). By constructing a life-limiting diagnosis in a different way, patients and their families—individually or together—can create new meaning of the terminal illness and the end-of-life experience.

Hwang et al. (2019) found that among long-term care workers, those who experience greater self-transcendence also report higher subjective well-being—and that this is partly because self-transcendence fosters caring behaviors. Nurses can better advocate for the self-transcendence and well-being of their patients when they use holistic end-of-life assessment tools. Multiple studies have looked at the relationship between spiritual assessment tools and patient care and have found positive effects (Henry & Gilley, 2024). The tools help the provider to understand the context in which patients are making medical decisions, guide the team in encouraging the patient's use of their own spiritual resources, and help to identify both the patient's hopes and their fears. (Refer to Chapter 7, *Spirituality and Health.*)

Another aspect of self-transcendence can be found in the emerging field of entheogen or plant-based psychedelics that are being studied for their medicinal and spiritual properties. For example, compelling research from Johns Hopkins University and New York University has shown significant reduction in end-of-life anxiety for people with life-threatening cancer after taking a single dose of psilocybin (Ross et al., 2022). Patients reported improvements in quality of life, feelings of peacefulness, and spiritual insight that lasted for many months. Nurses are being encouraged to collaborate and advance knowledge about psychedelic-assisted therapies in palliative care and beyond (Rosa et al., 2019; Ross et al., 2022).

Nearing Death Awareness

Nearing death awareness begins with a person's realization that the inevitable is happening to them and that there is a definite ending of days. Most dying persons have a generalized understanding of human mortality and their increasing nearness to the end of their life. Interestingly, in a meta-analysis of advanced/terminal cancer patients, fewer than half understood their prognosis (Lee et al., 2020). As the person gets closer to death, health changes and progressive deterioration become more apparent, and the reality of impending death becomes more real. This is often in the last few hours or days of life. At this point, the dying person may attempt to describe what they are experiencing while dying, and they may request something that they need for a peaceful death. This awareness is not to be confused with near-death experiences that happen as a result of cardiac arrest, drowning, or trauma in which a person feels the self suddenly leave this life but quickly return.

The phenomenon of nearing death awareness, also called "end-of-life experiences," includes end-of-life dreams and visions (ELDVs). Depner et al. (2020) researched ELDVs with hospice patients and reported that the most prevalent ELDVs were those in which dying patients describe seeing deceased family, friends, or religious figures. These visions can occur months, weeks, days, or hours before death and typically decrease the fear of dying, making transition from life to death easier for those experiencing them. Rabitti et al. (2024) conducted a qualitative study of ELDVs in hospice settings, and their evidence showed that about 50 to 60 percent of hospice patients report a "visitation" by someone who is not there while dreaming or awake. The researchers recommended that healthcare professionals and families be educated about ELDVs and learn how to support patients in sharing these emotional and identity-related experiences for meaning-making at end of life. Grant et al.'s (2020) research with ELDVs focused on the emotional transformation they observed in families when patients experience such visions. Interestingly, favorable attitudes toward dreams and positive ELDV perceptions are correlated with better bereavement outcomes. Lastly, recent research by the Shared Crossing Research Initiative (2021) has used anecdotal evidence to suggest that some loved ones and caregivers of dying patients experience a type of end-of-life phenomenon known as a "shared death experience," in which one feels that they have participated in a dying person's transition to an after-death existence. Their analysis revealed three major domains of shared death experience effects: changes in belief, the reconciliation of grief, and the perception of ongoing relational bonds with the person who died. A common theme across this research is the importance of nurses and healthcare providers supporting open, validating conversations about end-of-life experiences, and exploring how these experiences can enhance psychological, spiritual, and bereavement care.

Nurses and caregivers should respond to the dying person's wishes and needs while listening to what dying is like for them during this in-between or liminal time. These responsibilities can be challenging for caregivers, and nurses must help both the dying person and their loved ones to cultivate a peaceful death amidst the fully human and unknowable phenomenon of death. Upstream conversations before imminent death can have an impact on how people come into this time of dying. The concept of dying well is shaped by each individual's values, beliefs, and priorities. As healthcare providers, holistic nurses can meet dying individuals and their loved ones wherever they are (emotionally, spiritually, and clinically) while also recognizing the value of early preparation and clear goals in creating well-being throughout the dying process (Drick et al., 2022). Individuals who are tired of living, or are not ready to die, describe the dying process differently from those who are prepared to depart. The dying person ready for death has clarity of spoken words, softness in their eyes, and gentleness in their touch. Their Presence comes shining through in all its radiance, and they are at peace.

Assisting Peaceful Death

It could be said that the two most important aspects of holistic nursing care at the end of life are the nurse's Presence and the natural approaches that are brought to the bedside to assist in the transition. The nurse's Presence creates the atmosphere of safety, caring, and compassion while the natural approaches assist and support that atmosphere. This atmosphere is supportive of not only the dying person but also their family, friends, and anyone who enters the room.

Presence

Presence is foundational to all holistic nursing (American Nurses Association & American Holistic Nurses Association, 2019). Nowhere is Presence seen more exquisitely then with the dying person and their loved ones. Presence is so much more than taking a few breaths before entering the patient's room; it is a nurse's deepening way of life—an expanded pathway for living, unbound by the influences of the past or the fears of the future. Presence is not to be taken lightly or for granted. Just like the breath and heartbeat, presence can only be experienced now. Stepping into Presence and remaining in this expanded consciousness, the nurse can be open and receptive to how this moment unfolds and respond with intention.

Natural Approaches

First and foremost, pain is one factor, if not the primary factor, that can complicate a peaceful death. The mind's fear of pain is often more intense than the physical pain. Acute pain has the qualities of suddenness and surprise that can evoke anxiety, fear, and even dread. With sudden pain, encouraging the dying person to breathe rhythmically often softens the pain, thereby decreasing the resistance to the experience. With chronic pain, the nurse or caregiver can still encourage the dying person to rely on their oldest and closest friend—the breath. Chronic pain becomes exhausting for the dying person, but paying attention to the rhythm of their breath can keep their mind occupied. Remember, the mind cannot hold two thoughts at the same time. With practice, this simple technique can dramatically decrease the pain sensation they are feeling. The rhythm of the breath is remarkably powerful and can lull the dying person into a place of deeper peace and tranquility.

Current clinical approaches support effective symptom management, but there is growing interest in the benefits of cannabis-based medicine for those living with serious illnesses. While some individuals report that cannabis products are effective in alleviating their neurological pain, cancer-related pain, and anxiety, current research presents mixed findings regarding their benefits (Doppen et al., 2022; Herbert & Hardy, 2021; Modesto-Lowe et al., 2018). Despite ongoing uncertainty regarding the effectiveness of cannabis-based medicine, many palliative and hospice care clinicians support its use for symptom management (Maximillian & Stevenson, 2023).

In addition, other natural approaches are also available to assist in reducing or eliminating emotional and/or physical pain. A systematic review of complementary and alternative medicine in hospice and palliative care showed short-term benefit for patients with symptom burden with the following therapies: acupressure, acupuncture, aromatherapy, massage, breathing, hypnotherapy, massage, meditation, music therapy, reflexology, and reiki (Dingley et al., 2021). Among these available techniques, two are especially relevant to the end of life—meditative techniques and aromatherapy.

Meditative Approaches at the End of Life

All types of meditative approaches are readily available including mindful meditation, visualization, guided imagery, and prayer or even a mix of approaches. The key is for the nurse or caregiver to find what speaks to the individual in need and then allow it to flow through themselves in the moment.

There is no set time or place to meditate. Even in a busy or noisy place, the attention can be focused within. The approach can be as simple and short as "Take a few easy breaths" or "Let's breathe together" or "Focus on your breath gently in and out, allowing the exhale to get longer and longer." The key is for the individual to be present and let themself be guided.

Even the simple release of the breath and the ah-h-h-h sound is an ancient ritual for dying in peace. Often called "co-meditation," this approach is based on the principle that breathing brings one into the present moment and is a direct link to the nervous system. *Note*: Nurses often get caught up in the procedure rather than allowing the natural process to flow through them. Beginners may need more guidelines to assist others until the words begin to flow naturally. Spontaneous communication is more powerful as it is fresh, alive, and specifically for this moment in time.

Prayer as a meditative approach has a broad and rich background in all religions. The essence is quieting the mind and turning inward often through the breath, mantras, or moving into spontaneous communication with a higher power. Whether the prayer is directed, nondirected, or centering, every faith group has prayers that provide both comfort and joy during the dying process.

Aromatherapy at the End of Life

Perhaps the most important goal of nursing care at the end of life is assisting the dying person to die well, based on what matters most to them. The real challenge is to minimize end-of-life symptoms while improving quality of life during the final hours. Aromatherapy can do both. This natural approach can decrease both terminal agitation and fear while increasing quality of life with familiar smells and gentle touch. Farrar and Farrar (2020) noted that aromatic scents and oils used in clinical aromatherapy can be beneficial for symptom management such as pain, nausea, vomiting, anxiety, depression, stress, insomnia, agitation with dementia, cancer pain, and end-of-life symptoms. Another study of palliative care patients showed therapeutic benefit from the use of lemon oil pads for nausea and vomiting (Kreye et al, 2022). (Refer to Chapter 15, *Integrative and Complementary Health Approaches*, which includes aromatherapy.)

The Body Shutting Down: What Is Natural and What to Expect

The moment of death comes with the last exhale and when the heart stops beating. Before that moment, the body orchestrates the most exquisite symphony of shutting down systematically and logically as all the energy is withdrawn from the periphery and moved to the internal organs. Then each system in turn shuts down gently.

Closing down of the body is simple, logical, and sequential. Once understood, the experience of death can become less demanding and problematic for the patient and loved ones. Death comes when all the bodily systems cease to function. This normal sequential, unromantic process is *not* a medical emergency that requires intervention; rather, this is the time for the family, caregivers, and nurses to give love, compassion, and comfort measures.

As the bodily functions gradually cease, the limbs become cold, and circulation is withdrawn.

The skin becomes mottled and discolored. When food is refused, thirst often becomes the last craving and eventually even it is refused. Terminal dehydration then occurs where the body naturally and painlessly dehydrates, which assists the process by providing chemical changes that reduce pain and anxiety. Most dying persons become mouth breathers to assist in respirations, yet this results in the mouth and lips becoming dried and cracked. Even though they are asleep or unconscious, their eyes remain open as the eyelid muscles relax. Most dying individuals can hear until the moment of death.

Imminent death can be within hours or minutes. It is often difficult to judge. Signs of imminent death include the following:

- Speech lessens
- Movement ceases
- Pulse weakens so it can be difficult to feel
- Blood pressure continues to drop
- Respirations change (Cheyne–Stokes pattern slowing/pausing of breaths 5–60 seconds)
- Secretions may accumulate ("Death rattle" gurgling, breathing sound)
- Pupils become dilated and fixed

Remember, there is no pain; this is a normal natural process of closing down all body functions.

The moment of death comes unbidden without notice. To each it has to be entered alone. Loved ones and health professionals can only go to the edge. Death is simply a moment in time. The body knows how to create itself from the moment of creation; at the moment of death, the body immediately begins to rapidly decompose or uncreate itself. The picture of death, the final closing down of all the body functions, typically unfolds as follows:

- The heart stops pumping
- Breathing comes to an end
- All muscles relax—urine/stool may be released
- The jaw usually opens slightly
- The eyes remain fixed and dilated

In the final days of life, all systems of the body are systematically closing down. None is exempted. This process is natural, exquisite in its grand design, and experienced by everyone. Once the process is understood, death can begin to take its rightful place in physical life. It is the major event in everyone's life, second only to physical birth. Without death, life itself would have no conclusion, no culmination. To live forever would become a dreaded curse. But death itself is not a disease to be treated and fought; rather, death is a normal, natural process holistic nurses can respond to with love, compassion, comfort measures, and dignity.

It is for the nurse to meet the dying where they are and support this natural process. It is for the nurse to protect the dying during the dying process and to prevent anything from deterring or prolonging the process. It is for the nurse to assist the loved ones in understanding and then accepting this process. It is for the nurse to be deep in Presence and to meet the dying where the river meets the sea and then bid them a gentle farewell.

Trends in End-of-Life Care

Home surpassed the hospital as the most common place of death in the United States in 2017, for the first time since the early 20th century (Cross & Warraich, 2019), although only about half of Americans die while receiving hospice services. Current statistics from the National Hospice and Palliative Care Organization (2024) show Alzheimer's/nervous system disorders/organic psychosis as the top category of diagnosis for hospice beneficiaries (25%), followed by cancer and circulatory diseases. These three diagnosis groups account for almost three-fourths of all hospice diagnoses. In 2022, the average hospice length of stay for Medicare decedents was 95.3 days—an increase from 2021, which had declined following a significant rise in 2020. The median length of stay was 18 days, which has stayed consistent for several decades. From 2021 to 2022, the number of Medicare-certified hospices increased by over 500, reaching a total of 5,899 in 2022 based on submitted claims. A significant change is that three-fourths of hospices in the United States are now for-profit, many of which are affiliated with regional and national chains (Teno, 2023). A 2023 study found that family caregivers reported poorer care experiences in for-profit hospices. The researchers also noted that perceptions of care quality varied across both for-profit and not-for-profit providers (Anhang Price et al., 2023). In 2021, hospice was a $23 billion industry that made up roughly 20 percent of the overall U.S. home-based care market (Vossel, 2022).

In the Lancet Commission's report on the "Value of Death," Sallnow et al. (2022) emphasized that the public's relationship with death and dying has become unbalanced, and many people (including medical professionals) are no longer familiar with dying as a natural, human event. At the heart of this rebalancing are relationships and partnerships among people who are dying, families, communities, health and care systems, and the wider society. This system's approach is considered essential for an emerging transformation in global care at the end of life. Five underlying principles will likely be familiar to holistic nurses, and include:

- tackling the social determinants of death, dying, and grieving;
- understanding dying to be a relational and spiritual process rather than solely a physiological event;
- community networks of care leading support for people dying, caring, and grieving;
- conversations and stories about everyday death, dying, and grief becoming commonplace;
- death being recognized as having value.

Some of the changes and transformation seen in end-of-life care in the United States reflect the imperative value of these principles.

Caregiving Patterns

Palliative Care

Palliative care commences with supportive care beginning with a serious, complex, or life-limiting diagnosis when new goals and direction are determined. Rather than invasive, oftentimes painful care that strives to keep patients alive, palliative care goals prioritize quality of life rather than quantity of life. The Center to Advance Palliative Care (2022) reported that since 2000, the percentage of hospitals (with 50 or more beds) with a palliative care program has more than tripled. As of 2020, more than 83 percent of these hospitals had a palliative care team. Despite this growth, millions of Americans with serious illness do not have access to palliative care due to understaffed programs and geographical limitations. Ideally, the next phase of growth will bring more palliative care into the community via nursing homes, office practices, and patients' homes.

Innovative models of care have been developed to provide high-quality and home-based care to persons living with serious, life-limiting illness, such as advanced cancer. These include inpatient and outpatient palliative care, telehealth and home-based palliative care, home and inpatient hospice, and palliative care provided through integrated mobile technologies (Grudzen et al., 2022). Comfort care homes or Omega homes are innovative models of nonmedical care in a community setting that offer a comfort-based, person-centered home-away-from-home for people in the last months and days of life. Varying in size, appearance, and individual policies, they share a common foundation and philosophy. Currently, there are over 100 open or developing Omega homes located in multiple U.S. states (Omega Home Network, 2023).

Hospice

Although not new, hospice centers and inpatient care are proliferating both in the United States and other parts of the world. Hospice aims to create a compassionate environment where a professional team works with family and/or friends to manage symptoms and end-of-life issues either at home, in the hospital, or in a freestanding center. This methodology has grown in acceptance and use over the past several decades. Although hospice programs have been around since the 1970s, it is discouraging to note that the median length of stay for someone in a hospice program is still only 18 days (National Hospice and Palliative Care Organization, 2023)—a short amount of time for a dying person and their loved ones to benefit from the holistic, interdisciplinary care and expertise of a hospice care team.

In-Home, Community-Based Services

Home health agencies have historically rendered in-home care. There has been an awakening of community-based national and local conglomerates offering more structured and focused services. These services may have a cost associated with them depending on the person's insurance and personal finances.

Within the context of home and community is the presence of internet information, where numerous blogs, websites, workshops, and consultants offer advice, information, and a plethora of services to the consumer. Technology has become part of home health services, including end-of-life advice and resources.

Shared Decision Making

There is a growing emphasis on shared decision making in transitioning dying patients from hospital settings to home-based care. In shared decision making, care decisions are done in collaboration with the patient, the patient's family, and a healthcare professional or an interdisciplinary team. This patient-centered care enables patient autonomy—a cornerstone of palliative care. In the past, nurses were less involved in shared decision making for palliative care patients. The focus was mainly on specific medical interventions, rather than the holistic nurse-driven palliative care model. Today, nurses who work in inpatient hospital settings can advocate and facilitate the decision-making process during day-to-day clinical activities. In the palliative decision-making phase, the nurse's role is especially significant—offering the option to refrain from life-prolonging treatment (if not communicated by the physician) and supporting patients to explore their attitudes and feelings about their end-of-life care (Bos-van den Hoek et al., 2021).

Death Doulas (or End-of-Life Doulas)

Death doulas assist people at the end of life in a variety of ways that are still emerging as the role develops and becomes better known. The essence of doula care is to provide nonmedical, holistic, nonjudgmental support and guidance to individuals and families before and during the end of life. These professionals can offer advance care planning, vigil support, legacy work, grief companioning, end-of-life coaching, or community end-of-life education. Over the past few decades, there has been a new wave of options for innovative end-of-life care and education. As a result, different doula roles have evolved—comfort doulas, delirium doulas, hospice doulas, end-of-life doulas, death doulas, and palliative care doulas (Lentz, 2023). There are educational training and certificate programs, but at this point, standardization of education and/or certification has not been consistent. Many doulas are volunteers, and others are paid for their services.

Death doulas represent an emerging model of personalized, person-directed care. They may serve as a complementary addition to existing services—or, depending on perspective, as an unregulated form of care provision. Given that most people experience a gradual decline over months or years, many medical professionals are uncomfortable initiating conversations about goals of care, end-of-life wishes, or hospice involvement. This has created a gap in support—one that death doulas increasingly seek to fill by providing guidance to individuals living with serious illness and their families.

Death Positive Movement

Death doulas are part of a growing phenomenon of what some people call the "death positive movement" (Leland, 2018). A coined phrase by mortician Caitlin Dougherty, *death positivity* encourages open dialogue about death, dying, and grief. It reflects a movement away from the concepts of the medicalization of death and "death as failure." This movement represents the reclaiming of death as a natural, purposeful part of life, and represents a shift from death and grieving in isolation towards a more community-oriented approach. Many emerging trends and ideas fall under the umbrella of death positivity and a more conscious approach to dying: death cafes, podcasts and TED talks about death, green burials, home funerals, water cremation, doula and conscious dying training programs, comfort care homes, research with psilocybin and death anxiety, grief ceremonies, and options for hastening death through "voluntarily stopping eating and drinking" and "medical aid in dying". Many small, interwoven movements around community death care have begun to gain traction over the past 10 or so years. Community death care is a grassroots movement that educates and supports families to care for their dying loved ones, and guides communities in caregiving skills that many have forgotten (Hope et al., 2023). Holistic nurses would benefit from doing a community assessment to identify which of these newer trends and initiatives exist in their own communities and consider how they might bring their own depth of experience to community end-of-life care.

Allow Natural Death

The discussion between the Allow Natural Death (AND) and Do Not Resuscitate (DNR) directives began in the late 1990s and continues today. Both the AND and the DNR have comparable clinical outcomes emphasizing comfort and pain management. That is where the resemblance ends. The AND and the DNR infer dissimilar messages. While the DNR speaks to taking away possible care, the AND emphasizes allowing a natural, gentler death. The AND reflects a positive, growing care philosophy in providing comfort care, rather than the DNR's model of death as treatment failure (Fan et al, 2018). The AND can feel less threatening to patients and families, thereby opening the door for families to potentially communicate earlier and realize that being comfortable (palliative care) is the most supportive of the natural closing down of the body. In this way, the AND can be seen by the dying person as a positive choice rather than a last resort.

Newer forms of advance directives are the Medical Orders for Life-Sustaining Treatment or Physician Orders for Life-Sustaining Treatment (POLST) forms. The forms are completed by a physician, summarize a person's end-of-life wishes, and give medical orders for emergency healthcare professionals to follow. They go into

CASE STUDY

This case study represents nursing actions based on the holistic caring process, which includes the elements of holistic assessment, identification of patterns/challenges/needs, outcome identification, development of a therapeutic care plan and interventions, and evaluation.

Patient: Sarah is a 45-year old woman with two children (ages 9 and 11) and a partner (Jonathan). She has been living with metastatic breast cancer for three years, but her condition has significantly worsened over the past six months. While Sarah is in physical pain, she is most concerned about her emotional and psychological well-being, especially regarding her family's response to her illness and impending death.

Setting: Sarah's home, with partner Jonathan present.

Patterns/Challenges/Needs

1. Moderate pain related to a diagnosis of cancer
2. Family anticipatory grieving support
3. Spiritual well-being and effective individual coping related to the patient's desire to die in alignment with their values

Sarah has asked for a conversation with her holistic palliative care nurse to create a plan for more community support for herself and her family. Having always been spiritually inclined, she hopes to make the most of the time she has left by creating an environment of love, peace, and intention. She wishes to die in a way that honors her values and beliefs while easing the burden on her young family. To do this, she is requesting the integration of holistic care practices, including a death doula and hospice support, and would like to form a care circle from her friends to provide ongoing support for her family in the time ahead.

The most important outcome of the conversation between Sarah, Jonathan, and the nurse was clarity about the different kinds of support they are asking for—hospice care for the interdisciplinary team support 24/7 to manage symptoms and create a safe home environment; a death doula to help with care coordination, the creation of legacy projects and meaningful rituals with her family, the development of a vigil plan for her last days; and the integration of holistic practices like music therapy, energy work, and aromatherapy that have been important to her throughout her healing journey.

This case highlights the importance of integrating holistic nursing care with a multidisciplinary approach, including collaboration with death doulas, palliative care/hospice teams, and healing professionals. For Sarah, this holistic and intentional approach to her end-of-life care allows her to experience a dignified, conscious death, addressing her physical, emotional, and spiritual needs while ensuring her family is supported throughout the process.

the person's medical record and are portable, so the patient's wishes can be accessed wherever they are in a healthcare system. However, not all states have these forms available. (For more information on advance directives, refer to Chapter 6, *Holistic Ethics*.)

Implications

Clinical Practice

During a patient's transition period between active life and end of life, nurses will want to know the what, why, and wherefore of applying end-of-life caregiving skills. They do this to ease pain and allow for patient preferences and values in addition to including family and friends.

Education

End-of-life caregiving requires an additional skill set to provide effective care in this special setting. New trends and opportunities to improve one's ability in this area are available, and specialty end-of-life care certifications are now available. (Refer to Resources). Ongoing personal development and becoming peaceful with impermanence are highly recommended.

Research

End-of-life care is a burgeoning area of practice; hence the research is proliferating. To keep their knowledge base current, nurses will want to seek, read, and generate their own research and library around end of life.

Policy

It is critical to stay informed of end-of-life policies. They differ widely from state to state and are rapidly changing. Federal organizations such as the Coalition to Transform Advanced Care (refer to Resources) are critical to monitor and even join to be apprised of legislation and advances in end-of-life care. Nurses are in a key position to help create policy changes that will enhance and facilitate these precious life experiences.

Conclusion

In today's society, the last phase of life more often consists of a series of medical emergencies for which medical care can only give fleeting and brief relief. This route is unpredictable, with the pauses between emergencies always being variable. Unfortunately, or fortunately, after a certain point, the direction of this route becomes clear. The question then becomes, "Treatment for what purpose?" Increasingly, many are beginning to accept and take what time they have, and some are even comprehending that the finitude of one's time could be a gift. It is a gift to redefine one's life identity into something new. A dying person might not be able to control their circumstances, but they can become the author of what their life means *and* remain in control of what they do with their lives.

Dying is the one thing that each and every one of us will go through in our lives. Nurses will experience it with themselves, their families, and their patients. Therefore, it behooves every nurse to spend the time now to understand their own personal feelings about death. The more nurses accept and find peace with the idea of impermanence and the transition from this mortal plane into another, the more capable they will be in assisting others on their incredible final journey through life.

Resources

Certified Hospice and Palliative Nurse (CHPN): https://www.advancingexpertcare.org/hpcc/credentials/chpn/

Advanced Certified Hospice and Palliative Nurse: https://www.advancingexpertcare.org/hpcc/credentials/achpn/

Coalition to Transform Advanced Care: https://thectac.org/

References

American Nurses Association. (2016). *Position statement: Nurses' roles and responsibilities in providing care and support at the end of life*. https://www.nursingworld.org/~4af078/globalassets/docs/ana/ethics/endoflife-positionstatement.pdf

American Nurses Association & American Holistic Nurses Association. (2019). *Holistic Nursing: Scope and Standards of Practice* (3rd ed.). ANA & AHNA.

Anhang Price, R., Parast, L., Elliott, M. N., Tolpadi, A., Bradley, M., Schlang, D., & Teno, J. (2023). Association of hospice profit status with family caregivers' reported care experiences. *JAMA Internal Medicine, 183*(4), 311–318. https://doi.org/10.1001/jamainternmed.2022.7076

Bos-van den Hoek, D. W., Thodé, M., Jongerden, I.P., Van Laarhoven, H. W. M, Smets. E. M. A., Tange, D., Henselmans, I., & Pasman, H. R. (2021). The role of hospital nurses in shared decision-making about life-prolonging treatment: A qualitative interview study. *Journal of Advanced Nursing, 77*(1), 296-307. https://doi.org/10.1111/jan.14549

Center to Advance Palliative Care. (2022). *Growth of palliative care in U.S. hospitals: Snapshot*. https://capc.org/documents/download/1031/

Cross, S. H., & Warraich, S. J. (2019). Changes in the place of death in the United States. *New England Journal of Medicine, 381*(24), 2369–2370. https://doi.org/10.1056/NEJMc1911892

Depner, R., Grant, P., Byrwa, D., LaFever, S., Kerr, C., Tenzek, K., LaValley, S., Luckiewicz, D., Wright, S., & Levy, K. (2020). Expanding the understanding of content of end-of-life dreams and visions: A consensual qualitative research analysis. *Palliative Medicine Reports, 1*(1), 103–110.

Dingley, C., Ruckdeschel, A., & Lekhak, N. (2021). Implementation and outcomes of complementary therapies in hospice care: An integrative review. *Journal of Hospice & Palliative Nursing, 15*. https://doi.org/10.1177/26323524211051753

Doppen, M., Kung, S., Maijers, I., John, M., Dunphy, H., Townsley, H., Eathorne, A., Semprini, A., & Braithwaite, I. (2022). Cannabis in palliative care: A systematic review of current evidence. *Journal of Pain and Symptom Management, 64*(5), e260–e284. https://doi.org/10.1016/j.jpainsymman.2022.06.002

Drick, C., Keegan, L., & Sanders, P. (2022). *The last journey: A road map for ending of days*. Sacred Life Publishers.

Fan, S., Want, Y., & Lin, I. (2018). Allow natural death versus do-not-resuscitate: Titles, information contents, outcomes, and the considerations related to do-not-resuscitate decision. *BMC Palliative Care, 17*, 114. https://doi.org/10.1186/s12904-018-0367-4

Farrar, A. J., & Farrar, F. C. (2020). Clinical aromatherapy. *Nursing Clinics of North America, 55*(4), 489–504. https://doi.org/10.1016/j.cnur.2020.06.015

Frankl, V. (1963). *Man's search for meaning* (3rd ed.). Simon & Schuster.

Grant, P., Levy, K., Lattimer, T., Depner, R., & Kerr, C. (2020). Attitudes and perceptions of end-of-life dreams and visions and their implications for the bereaved family caregiver experience. *American Journal of Hospice and Palliative Medicine, 38*, 104990912095231. https://doi.org/10.1177/1049909120952318

Grudzen, C. R., Barker, P. C., Bischof, J. J., Cuthel, A. M., Isaacs, E. D., Southerland, L. T., & Yamarik, R. L. (2022). Palliative care models for patients living with advanced cancer: A narrative review for the emergency department clinician. *Emergency Cancer Care, 1*(1), Article 10. https://doi.org/10.1186/s44201-022-00010-9

Henry, N. L., & Gilley N. (2024). Spiritual assessment. In *StatPearls*. StatPearls Publishing. https://www.ncbi.nlm.nih.gov/books/NBK599554

Herbert, A., & Hardy, J. (2021). Medicinal cannabis use in palliative care. *Australian Journal of General Practice, 50*(6).

Hope, S., Booth, J., & Rosa, W. (2023). Chapter 12. Bearing witness to suffering at end of life. In W. E. Rosa & B. R. Ferrell (Eds.), *The nature of suffering and the goals of nursing* (2nd ed., pp 156 157). Oxford University Press.

Hwang, H. L., Tu, C. T., & Chan, H. S. (2019). Self-transcendence, caring, and their associations with well-being. *Journal of Advanced Nursing, 75*(7), 1473–1483.

Kang, Y. (2019). Examining interpersonal self-transcendence as a potential mechanism linking meditation and social outcomes. *Current Opinions in Psychology, 28*, 115–119.

Kreye, G., Wasl, M., Dietz, A., Klaffel, D., Groselji-Strele, A., Eberhard, K., & Glechner, A. (2022). Aromatherapy in palliative care: A single-institute retrospective analysis evaluating the effect of lemon oil pads against nausea and vomiting in advanced cancer patients. *Cancers (Basel), 14*(9), 2131. https://doi.org/10.3390/cancers14092131

Kübler-Ross, E. (1969). *On death and dying*. Macmillan.

Lee, H., Ko, H. J., Kim, A. S., Kim, S. M., Moon, H., & Choi, H. I. (2020). Effect of prognosis awareness on the survival and quality of life of terminally ill cancer patients: A prospective cohort study. *Korean Journal of Family Medicine, 41*(2), 91–97. https://doi.org/10.4082/kjfm.18.0113

Leland, J. (2018, June 22). The positive death movement comes to life. *The New York Times*. https://www.nytimes.com

Lentz, J. (2023). The doula model in American health care in the 21st century: A narrative literature review. *Journal of Hospice and Palliative Nursing, 25*(1), 18–23. https://doi.org/10.1097/NJH.0000000000000913

Levine, S., & Levine, O. (1982). *Who dies? An investigation of conscious living and conscious dying*. Anchor Books.

Maximillian, H., & Stevenson, L. S. (2023). Symptom control in palliative care settings: The role of cannabis-based medicines. In V. Preedy, V. Patel, & C. Martin (Eds.), *Medicinal usage of cannabis and cannabinoids* (pp. 401-413). Academic Press. https://doi.org/10.1016/B978-0-323-90036-2.00025-9

Modesto-Lowe, V., Bojka, R., & Alvarado, C. (2018). Cannabis for peripheral neuropathy: The good, the bad, and the unknown. *Cleveland Clinic Journal of Medicine, 85*(12), 943–949. https://10.3949/ccjm.85a.17115

National Hospice and Palliative Care Organization. (2023). *NHPCO facts and figures: 2023 edition*. https://allianceforcareathome.org/wp-content/uploads/NHPCO-Facts-Figures-2023.pdf

National Hospice and Palliative Care Organization. (2024). *NHPCO facts and figures: 2024 edition*. https://allianceforcareathome.org/wp-content/uploads/2024/09/Facts-Figures-2024_FINAL.pdf

Neller, S. A., Cloyes, K. G., Edelman, L. S., Wong, B., Baines, B., & Towsley, G. L. (2023). Preparing for the future while living in the present: Older adults' experiences creating a legacy of values. *Gerontologist, 63*(9), 1488–1496. https://doi.org/10.1093/geront/gnad019

Omega Home Network. (2023). About. In *Omega Home Network*. https://www.omegahomenetwork.org/about/

Prince-Paul, M., & DiFranco, E. (2017). Upstreaming and normalizing advance care planning conversations: A public health approach. *Behavioral Sciences, 7*(2), 18. https://doi.org/10.3390/bs7020018

Rabitti, E., Cavuto, S., Díaz Crescitelli, M. E., Bassi, M. C., & Ghirotto, L. (2024). Hospice patients' end-of-life dreams and visions: A systematic review of qualitative studies. *American Journal of Hospice and Palliative Care, 41*(1), 99–112. https://doi.org/10.1177/10499091231163571

Rinpoche, S. (1992). *The Tibetan book of living and dying*. Harper.

Rosa, W., Estes, T., Hope, S., & Watson, J. (2019). Conscious dying: Human caring amid pain and suffering. In W. Rosa, S. Horton-Deutsch, & J. Watson (Eds.), *Handbook for caring science: Expanding the paradigm* (pp. 156–157). Springer Publishing.

Ross, S., Agrawal, M., Griffiths, R. R., Grob, C., Berger, A., & Henningfield, J. E. (2022). Psychedelic-assisted psychotherapy to treat psychiatric and existential distress in life-threatening medical illnesses and palliative care. *Neuropharmacology, 216*, 109174. https://doi.org/10.1016/j.neuropharm.2022.109174

Sallnow, L., Smith, R., Ahmedzai, S. H., Bhadelia, A., Chamberlain, C., Cong, Y., Doble, B., Dullie, L., Durie, R., Finkelstein, E. A., Guglani, S., Hodson, M., Husebø, B. S., Kellehear, A., Kitzinger, C., Knaul, F. M., Murray, S. A., Neuberger, J., O'Mahony, S., … Wyatt, K. (2022). Report of the Lancet Commission on the value of death: Bringing death back into life. *The Lancet, 399*(10327), 837–884. https://doi.org/10.1016/S0140-6736(21)02314-X

Saxena, R. (2019). Pain, palliative care, and end-of-life SIG: The impact of narrative therapy in shaping end-of-life perceptions among terminal cancer patients. *Palliative & Supportive Care, 17*(3), 257–264. https://doi.org/10.1017/S147895151800088X

Shared Crossing Research Initiative (SCRI). (2021). Shared death experiences: A little-known type of end-of-life phenomena reported by caregivers and loved ones. *American Journal of Hospital Palliative Care, 38*(12), 1479–1487. https://doi.org/10.1177/10499091211000045

Teno, J. M. (2023). Hospice—The time is now for additional integrity oversight. *JAMA Health Forum, 4*(5), e232045. https://doi.org/10.1001/jamahealthforum.2023.2045

Toh, S. W., Hollen, V. T., Ang, E., Lee, Y. M., & Devi, M. K. (2021). Nurses' communication difficulties when providing end-of-life care in the oncology setting: A cross-sectional study. *Support Care Cancer, 29*(5), 2787–2794. https://doi.org/10.1007/s00520-020-05787-1

Tyrrell, P., Harberger, S., Schoo, C., & Siddiqui, W. (2023). Kubler-Ross stages of dying and subsequent models of grief. In *StatPearls*. StatPearls Publishing. https://www.ncbi.nlm.nih.gov/books/NBK507885/

Vossel, H. (2022). Hospice market to nearly double by 2030: Palliative care to see large gains. *Hospice News*. https://www.hospicenews.com

Watson, J. (2021). *Caring science as sacred science, New revised edition*. Lotus Library.

Weller, F. (2015). *The wild edge of sorrow: Rituals of renewal and the sacred work of grief*. North Atlantic Books.

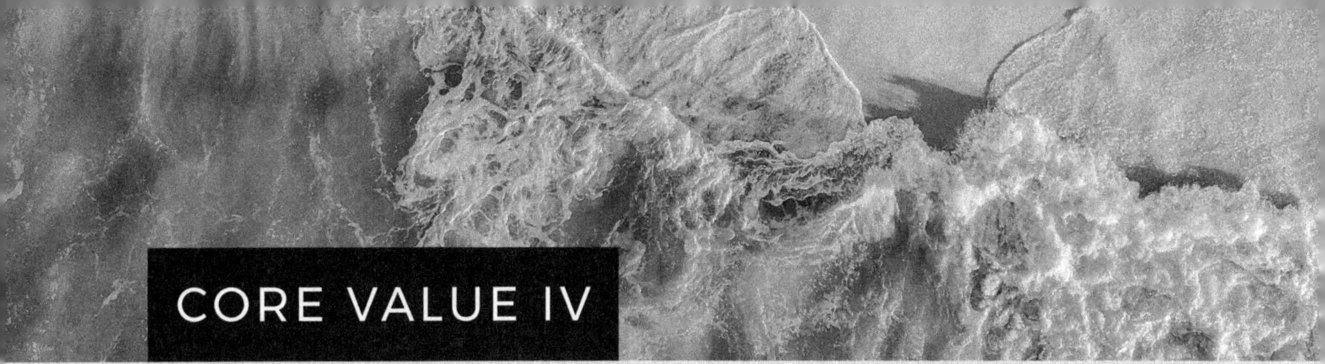

CORE VALUE IV

Holistic Communication, Therapeutic Relationship, Healing Environments, and Cultural Care

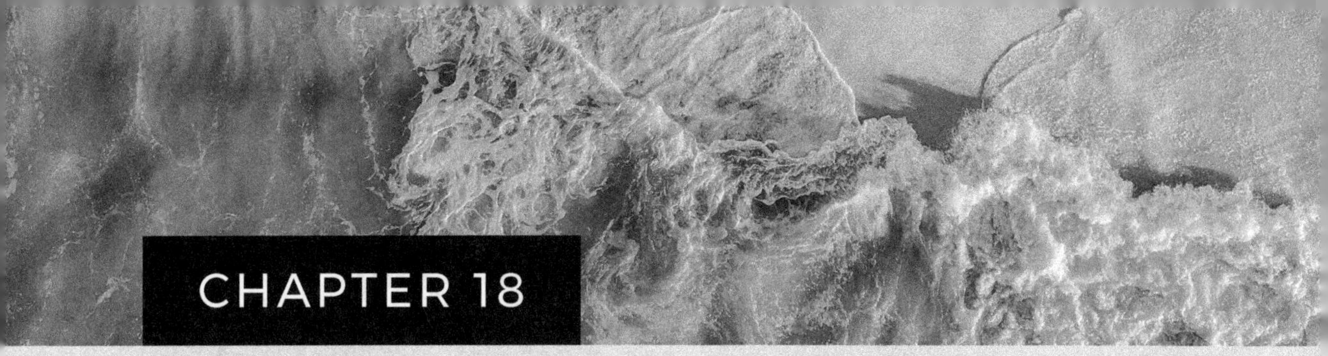

CHAPTER 18

Holistic Communication for Caring–Healing Relationships

Mary A. Blaszko Helming, Carla Mariano, and Lucia M. Thornton

NURSE HEALER OBJECTIVES

- Identify and describe the concepts that distinguish holistic communication.
- Identify practices that enhance holistic communication.
- Identify holistic nursing competencies in relationships.
- Gain insight into relationships and how to manage them effectively.

DEFINITIONS

Boundaries: Artificial separations between people that define relationship parameters.

Defense patterns: Protective mechanisms used to justify individual actions that may interfere with good relationships.

Holistic communication: A caring, healing process that calls forth the full use of self in interacting with another. It incorporates the constructs and processes of therapeutic communication within a framework that acknowledges the infinite, spiritual, and energetic nature of Being; the centrality of being heart-centered; and the importance of intention, self-knowledge, transcendent presence, and intuition in our interactions (Thornton & Mariano, 2022, p. 363).

Therapeutic communication: A goal-directed form of communication used to achieve goals that promote patient/client health and well-being. Empathy, unconditional regard, genuineness, respect, concern, caring, and compassion are conveyed through active listening, active observing, focusing, restating, reflecting, and interpreting (Thornton & Mariano, 2022, p. 363).

Introduction

Communication is the cornerstone of all relationships. Communication arising from respect, trust, compassion, and sincerity fosters positive and healthy relationships. Therapeutic and holistic nurse–patient communication results in positive physical, mental, and emotional outcomes for both the patient and the nurse. However, when faced with illness, disease, and possible death, therapeutic and holistic communication can be extremely challenging. This chapter will illuminate ways that nurses can develop caring–healing relationships with their patients in the face of distress and illness. Moving from therapeutic to holistic communication adds a healing dimension to the nurse–patient relationship. This chapter will explore dimensions inherent to holistic communication and ways the nurse can cultivate a caring–healing presence. Further, holistic nursing competencies in the nurse–patient relationship will be explored along with insights into problematic relationships and how to manage them more effectively. Defense mechanisms, relationships disorders, and boundary issues are highlighted.

Therapeutic Communication Skills: A Prerequisite for Holistic Communication

Traditional models of therapeutic communication do the following: define and prescribe various stages or phases, delineate various roles for the nurse or therapist, identify verbal and nonverbal communication skills, and identify therapist characteristics that are essential to creating a therapeutic milieu.

It is important for nurses to be familiar with the various stages of relationship formation and to develop and refine communication skills. It is also important for nurses to understand and integrate the qualities and attributes that are important in creating a therapeutic exchange. Empathy, unconditional regard, genuineness, respect, concern, caring, and compassion are vital and essential attributes for therapeutic communication. Developing and refining communication skills, including active listening, active observing, focusing, restating, reflecting, and interpreting, is also important in facilitating the therapeutic process. The aforementioned knowledge, skills, techniques, and attributes are foundational to the therapeutic communication process and are prerequisites to engaging in the caring–healing exchange that characterizes holistic communication. Acquiring these skills takes time and is enhanced by experience. Mastering these skills is a lifelong process that is facilitated by reflective practices, guidance, sage mentoring, and a commitment to self-knowledge and awareness.

The next step is to identify the distinguishing characteristics of holistic communication and how we can integrate these to create caring–healing relationships.

Distinguishing Characteristics of Holistic Communication

Pre-Access Phase: Heart-Centering and Intention Setting

The holistic communication process involves being centered and creating an intention before engaging in a caring–healing interaction with another. These two processes, being centered and creating intention, constitute the pre-access phase involved in holistic communication. This phase lays the foundation for caring–healing communication and occurs before any person-to-person interaction takes place.

Heart-centering is one of the first processes the nurse engages in prior to any interaction. This process involves the nurse focusing their attention on the heart, setting aside concerns and thoughts, and connecting with feelings of love and compassion.

Maintaining this heart-centeredness throughout interactions has many positive effects for the nurse. Seminal research conducted at the HeartMath Institute showed that the resultant feelings of caring and appreciation from heart-centering creates coherence in the electromagnetic energy field; balances heart rhythms; increases IgA (immunoglobulin A) levels and natural killer cell levels; increases mental clarity and problem-solving; and reduces sleeplessness, body aches, fatigue, anger, sadness, hypertension, and other chronic problems (McCraty & Reese, 2009).

Heart coherence, also referred to as *resonance*, is a functional mode measured by heart rate variability analysis, wherein a person's heart rhythm pattern becomes ordered (McCraty & Childre, 2010). In addition to the positive mental, psychological, and physiologic effects, coherence may help to connect people with their intuitive inner guidance. Research suggests that the heart's energy field (energetic heart) is coupled to a field of information that is not bound by the classic limits of time and space. This evidence comes from a rigorous experimental study that investigated the proposition that the body receives and processes information about a future event before the event actually happens (McCraty et al., 2004). McCraty and Childre explained that the intuitive heart or heart intelligence is coupled to a deeper part of oneself, what some may call their *higher power* or their *higher capacities*. When we are heart-centered and coherent, we have a tighter coupling and closer alignment with our deeper source of intuitive intelligence (McCraty & Childre, 2010, p. 15–16).

Research also shows that the positive mental and physiologic effects from heart-centering can be transmitted to the patient. When a person maintains a coherent electromagnetic field through the process of centering, that person's energy field positively affects those in the surrounding environment. It is believed that information about a person's emotional state is encoded in the heart's electromagnetic field and is communicated into the external environment (McCraty & Childre, 2010, p. 20). When the nurse becomes heart-centered, a caring–healing field is created, and in it, the person feels safe, nurtured, and loved; this is in an optimal environment for healing communication to occur.

Setting an intention involves identifying and internalizing what you would like to happen in your communication and interaction with the patient. Setting an intention is considered to be the first part of the healing process as it sets into motion the healing dynamic. Examine the following intention: "I am here for the greater good of this person. I set aside my own concerns and worries and am fully present to the person here and now." With this intention, the nurse is consciously setting aside their own concerns and focusing on the patient, thus putting into motion the dynamic that this interaction will be for the greater good of this person. The nurse is also making a conscious decision to be fully present. Through this intention, the nurse creates an environment that promotes and sustains a caring–healing relationship.

Acknowledgment of the Infinite and Sacred Nature of Being

Holistic nursing acknowledges that people are infinite, sacred, and spiritual beings. Florence Nightingale spoke of human beings as a reflection of the Divine with physical, metaphysical, and intellectual attributes. Jean Watson teaches that we are sacred beings, and Martha Rogers speaks of unitary human beings as energy fields that are infinite in nature. Thus, from the perspective of holistic nursing theorists, people are infinite and sacred in nature. This orientation makes a difference in how we approach one another. It shifts how we speak, listen, relate, and interact. When we perceive human beings as infinite and sacred, our words, actions, and behaviors are significantly affected.

This alters our relationship to illness, disease, and death. Communication may be oriented to the soul's purpose in addition to symptom relief. This creates a potential to explore and derive meaning from life's challenges and create a healing environment even in the face of death and terminal illness.

When one understands that this physical life is a small part of the infinite journey, the stigma of death becomes obsolete. It allows the nurse to be fully present and communicate with compassion and empathy to persons with terminal illnesses and facing imminent death.

Grounding

Grounding is the process of connecting to Earth and Earth's energy field to calm the mind and focus one's inner flow of energy as a means to enhance healing endeavors.

Often, communication can bring up many feelings and thoughts that are emotionally charged and difficult for the nurse to deal with. Grounding provides the nurse with a steady physical, psychological, and energetic platform on which to anchor the communication process. In physical terms, grounding provides a connection between an electric circuit and the earth. In psychological terms, grounding helps establish a feeling of self-awareness and provides a connection to the consciousness of one's own self.

Energetically, grounding establishes an awareness of the unity of body, mind, and spirit, as stated by McCartney:

> The practice of grounding connects you with your spiritual intelligence. To heighten this experience, visualize your spiritual intelligence as energy or light. To ground your spiritual intelligence into your body, visualize this light in the center of your head expanding straight down your body and anchoring into the earth. In this way you are affirming [that] I am a spirit grounded in my body and anchored to the earth. (F. McCartney, personal communication, July 13, 2024)

Caring, Healing, Transcendent Presence

Presence has been defined as a way of being, a way of relating, a way of being with, and a way of being there. These perspectives each speak to different facets of the quality and characteristics of the attention that one person gives to another in a relationship.

What distinguishes holistic communication from other types of communication is the depth and profound quality of presence. When the nurse becomes heart-centered, they have the capacity to resonate with the person at a heart-and-soul level. At this level, the nurse connects with the person at a deep psychosocial, heartfelt, and spiritual level. This is a difficult concept to describe and remains more of a felt experience. The nurse must be able to access and rest in the depth of their own beingness before bringing this caring, healing, transcendent presence into a relationship.

Being able to communicate from more profound levels of presence is the result of experience and engaging in processes of deep reflection and inquiry. Various self-reflective practices such as journaling, meditation, relaxation, contemplation, dream analysis, narrative, and storytelling in one's personal daily practice can help cultivate a deeper relationship with the essence of one's existence that can then be brought into a relationship with another. The nurse must be able to connect with their own heart, soul, and transcendent nature before establishing that connection with others.

Intuition

Intuition is a foundational element in the holistic communication process. It is defined in the *Merriam-Webster*. dictionary (Intuition, n.d.) as "the power or faculty of attaining to direct knowledge or cognition without evident rational thought and inference." The usefulness of intuition in the nursing process is well-researched and documented. Intuition allows the nurse to access the subtle energies and the conscious and unconscious fields that are not readily perceived. Although intuitive knowing is something that occurs more readily with the experienced nurse, it can be consciously cultivated through various practices. Ways to cultivate intuition are listening to music, engaging in relaxation and mindfulness practices, reflective journal writing, and meditation.

Ways and Practices to Enhance Holistic Communication

Increasing Self-Knowledge

Awareness and understanding of one's self, one's values, beliefs, motivations, goals, feelings, and actions are imperative to relating in a caring–healing manner. When we understand who we are and know the basis for our own attitudes, preconceptions, and reactions, we are in a much better position to empathize, appreciate other people's differences and uniqueness, and encourage their self-revelations. To nurture caring–healing communication and relationships, we need to conduct assessments of ourselves as individuals, as well as our communications, spirituality, and cultural beliefs and traditions. All these factors influence behavior and, without a thoughtful reflection and understanding of them, we deny the very people we care for the opportunity to understand themselves.

Meditation

Meditation is a quiet turning inward—the practice of focusing one's attention internally to achieve clearer consciousness and inner stillness. Meditation is perhaps the single most useful reflective practice to help gain self-awareness and self-knowledge, increase intuition, and enhance development relating to spirituality. Because self-awareness, self-knowledge, and intuition are foundational to creating caring–healing relationships, meditating regularly is an important practice in which to engage. (Refer to Chapter 15, *Integrative and Complementary Health Approaches*, for more information about meditation.)

Engaging Your Observer

Engaging your observer is a process that is useful when confronting a situation or communication that is particularly difficult and emotionally charged. It also helps the nurse be present to a person or situation with clarity and without bias. This practice has its roots in Buddhist psychology.

The nonjudgmental aspect of yourself is called the *Observer* or *Witness*. Some perceive this aspect as our High Self. It can be likened to a wise grandparent who looks lovingly on the thoughts and reactions of our childlike minds. The Witness is our ability to observe life without engaging our past patterns of reacting and becoming emotionally charged. The Observer acts as a third party who allows the nurse to separate from difficult emotions and feelings so that communication occurs from a space of clarity and wisdom. Utilizing this technique enhances self-knowledge and self-awareness because it provides constant feedback related to one's responses and reactions to situations. The Observer can transcend the ego while embracing the whole of the moment so that one responds with wisdom rather than reacting from conditioned response.

Engaging the Observer involves centering, being aware of internal reactions, gratefully acknowledging these reactions, and responding from the High Self. This is a technique that allows one to access the High Self and move from that place of higher consciousness in interactions with another. This entire process takes about 15 seconds and allows the nurse to set aside thoughts and feelings that interfere with a caring–healing interaction.

This is central to the transpersonal caring process and communicating from a holistic perspective (**Box 18-1**).

Box 18-1 Engaging Your Observer in a Difficult Situation

Situation: You just realized that you gave your patient the wrong medication.

- **Center yourself and create an intention:** Take a breath and bring your consciousness or attention to the area around your heart; connect with a feeling of love and compassion. You might imagine holding a newborn baby, hugging a loved one, or cuddling your pet.
- **Observer relates your internal reactions—emotionally, mentally, and physically:** This makes you feel horrible. You are upset that you made this mistake. You are concerned about your patient, what your supervisor will think, and filling out an incident report. Your stomach is churning, and you feel like crying.
- **Acknowledge your reactions:** "I feel horrible when I make mistakes and I am concerned about my patient, my supervisor's response, and having to fill out an incident report. My stomach hurts and I feel like crying."
- **Respond from a place of wisdom and compassion:** Take another deep breath, bring your attention to the area around your heart, connect with a feeling of love and compassion, and respond silently to yourself with a self-compassionate remark: "Making mistakes is part of being human. Don't be so hard on yourself. This is a valuable opportunity to learn and grow and become a better nurse."

Data from Thornton, L. (2013). *Whole person caring: An interprofessional model for healing and wellness* (p. 104). Sigma Theta Tau International. (Copyrighted 2013 by L. Thornton); Thornton, L. *Whole person caring: Healing ourselves, healing our patients*. Forthcoming.

Clear Communication: An Acronym for Holistic Communication

Nurses use this acronym, CLEAR, to help remember some of the processes involved in holistic communication. Being CLEAR in communication means we Center, Listen, Empathize, pay Attention, and Respect (**Box 18-2**):

Box 18-2 Holistic Communication: Be CLEAR

Center Yourself

- Pause for a moment.
- Breathe deeply.
- Connect with a feeling of love and compassion.
- Create a silent intention that your thoughts, words, and actions will be for the greater good.

Listen Wholeheartedly

- Set aside your own thoughts, emotions, and feelings.
- Focus on understanding the person's perspective.
- Pay close attention to verbal and nonverbal clues.
- Do not judge or analyze.
- Open your heart to what is being communicated.

Empathize

- Come from a place of genuine concern.
- Ask yourself: How does this person perceive the situation? What does the world look like through this person's eyes? What are they feeling?
- Empathy involves an understanding that comes from sensing into the being of another.

Attention: Be Fully Present

- Be aware of what you are feeling and sensing. Stay present to yourself.
- Bring the fullness of yourself to every moment: emotionally, mentally, physically, and spiritually.

Respect

- Respect all that is.
- Respect yourself. Set boundaries if needed.
- Respect the person. Honor cultural, social, ontological, and ideological differences.
- Welcome diversity.

Reproduced from Thornton, L. (2013). *Whole person caring: An interprofessional model for healing and wellness*. (Copyrighted 2013, L. Thornton); Thornton, L. *Whole person caring: Healing ourselves, healing our patients* Forthcoming.

Drawing Out the Person's Story

A cornerstone of holistic communication is assisting individuals to find meaning in their experience as well as deeper meanings related to the person's purpose in life.

One of the best ways to understand what the person is most concerned about and the meaning something has for that person is by using narrative and story. Patient/client narratives, whether they arise from individuals, families, or communities, provide the context of the experiences and are used as an important focus in understanding the person's situation. The nurse first ascertains what the individual thinks or believes is happening to them and then assists the person to identify what will help the situation. The assessment begins from where the individual is. Space and time are allowed for exploration. Each person's health encounter is seen as truly unique. This requires a perspective that the nurse is not the expert regarding another's health/illness experience. Thoughtfully asking, "What do you think is going on with you (or is happening to you)?" and "What do you think would help?" allows patients time to share their story and give their perspective. The same principle applies to cultural competence. Asking, "What do I need to know about you culturally (or your culture) to care for you?" provides much more individualized and useful information about various cultures, their health beliefs and practices, and needs. The nurse then discusses options, including the person's choices, across a continuum, with the possible effects and implications of each.

Listening to the patient's story provides a holistic perspective and allows the nurse to get an overall sense of what the person is experiencing. This is more than using therapeutic techniques such as responding, reflecting, and summarizing. This is deep listening or, as some say, "listening with the heart and not just the ears." It is done with conscious intention and without preconceptions, busyness, distractions, or analysis. Using active listening responses, such as "Uh huh . . . uh huh," "Oh," "I see," and "Can you tell me more?" indicate that the nurse is listening, gives the person permission to continue, and keeps the patient focused on the story. It takes place in the now within an atmosphere of shared humanness—that is, human being to human being. Through presence or being with in the moment, nurses provide each person with an interpersonal encounter that is experienced as a connection with one who is giving undivided attention to the needs and concerns of the individual. Using unconditional positive regard, nurses convey to the individual receiving care the belief in their worth and value as a human being, not solely as the recipient of medical and nursing interventions (Mariano, 2020).

Creating Caring–Healing Relationships

Caring–healing relationships are developed by incorporating holistic communication. The term *caring–healing relationship* refers to special connections between two or more individuals, which may be brief, intermittent, or long-lasting. Patient-centered care and a solid nurse–patient relationship are key to achieving a caring–healing relationship. Relationships and interconnectedness exist between human beings, a Higher Power, animals, and Earth's environment. As social beings, humans are not suited to living alone.

Interrelationships

The term *interrelationship* implies the existence of a subtle web of life that connects all human beings, their environment, and spirituality. Each person's actions are capable of directly and indirectly affecting others that can create healing energy or toxic responses. For holistic nurses, the concept of relationship transcends individual patient care to include everyone and everything in the patients' environment—families, significant others, coworkers, and interdisciplinary staff.

Relationships in Holistic Nursing

The nurse–patient relationship plays a potentially immense role in healing. Advanced practice nurses in primary care, and psychiatric care especially, form beneficial, longer lasting, therapeutic relationships with their patients. Emotional intelligence skills enhance a nurse's empathy, holistic communication, and ability to reduce patient stress (Faubion, 2024). Recognizing nonverbal body language is an essential communication skill as well.

The American Nurses Association (ANA) Nursing Resources Hub (2023) states that trust is foundational to the nurse–patient relationship. This relationship enhances patient satisfaction and cooperation, potentially leading to better health outcomes. Without feeling judgment, patients are more inclined to reveal helpful, sensitive information (ANA Nursing Resources Hub, 2023). Oppositely, discontent with healthcare providers may cause patients to avoid treatment and misunderstand vital information.

Relationship to Other Living Beings and Nature

Relationships with animals can be equally vital. Unconditional love, bonding, and comfort can be provided with pets and other animal-assisted therapies, especially with dogs. Animal-assisted therapy includes emotional support animals, service animals trained to perform tasks for people with disabilities, and therapy animals owned by organizations. Typical benefits include anxiety, stress, depression, and PTSD; helping people with hearing and vision impairment; assisting special needs populations, including children and adults with dementia; as well as providing safety and security (Therapist.com Team, 2024).

Relationship to nature is exemplified by activities such as peacefully walking on a woodland path, inhaling sea air at the ocean, and nurturing gardens. Activities involving nature demonstrate relationships to living waters, plants, and ecosystems. The American Horticultural Therapy Association describes therapeutic gardens, often located within hospitals, long-term care, and hospice grounds, as plant environments designed for nature-healing while involving the senses (American Horticultural Therapy Association, 2024).

Spirituality and Relationship to a Higher Power

Physician–researcher Dr. Herbert Benson, author of the classic, *Timeless Healing: The Power and Biology of Belief* (1996), emphasized that human beings are "wired for God" and many have agreed. This implies the importance of relationship with a Higher Power, however the individual conceives that to be.

Through practices such as prayer, solitude, contemplation, meditation, music, scripture reading, and being in nature, people can increasingly seek a relationship with their Higher Power. As with any other caring–healing relationship, complete honesty, trust, and time are essential. Helming (2011) described the lived experience of being healed through prayer when 20 participants attributed their healing to prayer, even if they had used allopathic and integrative modalities.

Qualities that Enhance Caring–Healing Relationships

Qualities for healthy relationships include trust, forgiveness, and appropriate boundary setting.

Trust

Trust is an essential element of both the caring–healing relationship and the therapeutic relationship. A belief in the essential goodness of humankind assists people to trust rather than distrust.

Forgiveness

A key aspect of the healing relationship is forgiveness, a deliberate decision to release resentment. Forgiveness allows for peace of mind and freedom from bitter anger. Forgiveness improves mental health, may improve physical health such as reduced blood pressure and heart rate, and sustains connectedness (Greater Good Magazine, 2024).

Boundary Setting

Boundaries serve as healthy emotional or physical spaces between two or more people, but problematic boundary issues can occur. Rigid boundaries are found in more formal relationships, while family and friend relationships may have relaxed boundaries. Select boundary issues are presented in **Table 18-1**.

Nurses often encounter boundary issues observing patients' personal and family struggles. The nurse–patient relationship is asymmetrical since the nurse holds more power; while emotion can be expressed by holistic nurses, significant personal information should not be revealed in order to maintain healthy boundaries and safety.

Disorders in Relationships

Selected psychological issues that create unhealthy relationships are described in this section. These include psychological defense mechanisms, anger, power, and control issues.

Defense Mechanisms

Defense mechanisms are Freudian-based unconscious strategies to protect people from the anxiety of unacceptable emotions (McLeod, 2024). **Table 18-2** summarizes several common defense mechanisms with examples.

Anger

Anger is a transient but forceful emotion arising from threats, and it can be simple annoyance to major rage often expressed as aggression (American Psychological Association, 2023). Three means of manifesting anger include expressing it assertively, not aggressively, as the healthiest option. Secondly, suppressed anger may be

Table 18-1 Selected Boundary Issues and Symptoms

Boundary Issues	Symptoms
Martyr or victim	People who feel the world is against them and unfortunate things always happen to them.
Smothering	Parents may continue to try to control an adult child's life. Partners may try to constantly know where the significant other is or what they are involved in.
Over-enmeshment	Boundaries become entangled between two people so that individual aspects of personalities are blurred. Fears of abandonment and rejection may be significant.
Disassociation	Stress causes blanking out and forgetting what has happened. The person is out of touch with their feelings.
Codependency	One person in the relationship puts the other's needs ahead of their own, allowing the other to take no responsibility. There is often a need to fix or rescue the other person.
Chip on the shoulder	A person who carries a grudge against others and is easily angered into confrontations.

Source: Mary Helming

Table 18-2 Selected Common Defense Mechanisms

Defense Mechanism	Description	Example
Denial	Inability to acknowledge a real fact, to avoid anxiety.	Denial of addiction or violent crime, blocking memories.
Repression	Unconsciously blocking unpleasant feelings.	Adult woman has blocked her past sexual victimization but has trouble forming normal relationships now.
Regression	Reverting back to earlier stage of development due to anxiety.	Child regresses back to earlier developmental stage when sibling is born.
Projection	Unconsciously ascribing one's feelings to another to avoid taking responsibility.	Unfaithful partner accuses the significant other of infidelity.
Rationalization	Unconscious justification of behaviors or thoughts, differentiated from lying.	Explaining one did not get required work done because of being "too busy."
Acting out	Primitive mechanism uses self-injury, tantrums, or violent actions because of inability to express feelings.	Adolescent throwing a tantrum when denied permission to go on a date.

Source: Mary Helming

channeled into positive actions or instead turned internally, causing cardiac issues and depression, as examples. Third, if anger is not expressed, it can funnel into hostility or passive-aggressive behaviors, causing more subtle revenge such as gossiping behind another's back.

Resentment may persist long-term and overlap with anger and hostility. As a complex layering of emotions, resentment can occur when people feel wronged, mistreated, ignored, and undermined (Cleveland Clinic, 2024). Common anger defense mechanisms include withdrawal, isolation, rage, insults, and aggression. All nurses, including advanced practice nurses, frequently encounter patients angry at their illnesses, themselves, others, and life. Helping patients deal with overt or repressed anger and move toward forgiveness is an essential aspect of the healing relationship.

Power and Control Issues

Controlling people may exert power over others and cause resentment. The underlying issue may be anxiety if the person fears a loss of control (Tiwari, 2022). These people may also experience *obsessive-compulsive personality disorder,* focused on extreme control of self and others, perfectionism, and stubbornness. This is differentiated from *obsessive-compulsive disorder*, with obsessions and ritualistic behaviors such as handwashing and counting (Zimmerman, 2023).

Integration

Clinical Practice

- Incorporate heart-centering and intention setting before patient interactions.
- Utilize the Observer technique in difficult and challenging patient communications.
- Identify problematic defense mechanisms, personality patterns, and boundary issues in patients, self, and colleagues.
- Promote therapeutic and caring–healing relationships.

Nursing Situation

Being Wanted Saved My Life by Carla Mariano

For a couple of months, I had several falling episodes, but the last one left me with a severe concussion. I knew I had some serious decisions to make about my future. After spending a week in Bellevue Hospital's Trauma Center, I transferred to a nursing home for Physical and Occupational Therapy. I could not stand or walk.

During my first PT visit at the nursing home and after working with me for a little bit, the physical therapist said, "We can't work with you because you can't even stand up." I thought to myself, "Why am I spending money on this nursing home if I can't even get the treatment that I need to stand up?" I was going into this extremely dark place, and I didn't know what to do. I was beginning to feel like I didn't care if I lived or died. It just didn't matter anymore. I was extremely numb about the whole thing. If I lived fine, if I died fine.

My brother contacted an assisted living center and Randy, their admission advisor, came to visit me. I wasn't particularly interested in seeing them. Little did I know that this woman would change my life! What she said exemplified the essence and power of a caring–healing interaction. She said to me:

> Carla, we want you at the Village. We want you there. We can Hoyer lift you wherever you need to be or to go. We can work with you as slow or as fast as you are able. We can work with all your abilities and disabilities. We really want you to come to the Village because we think we can help you; we know we can help you.

After Randy said that, it was like a miracle burst forth inside of me. I knew, "I can do this—they're going to help me. And somebody wants me and will work with me." Randy saved my life just by letting me know that I was wanted.

When I arrived at the assisted living facility, I weighed 105 lbs. They worked with me incredibly slowly. I had to use a Hoyer lift for quite a while. I had pneumonia a couple of times. But the will to live was there. If I had stayed in that nursing home and if Randy had not visited me, I would have died. I know I would have died—I didn't care. I just didn't care. The moral of the story is "To be wanted and to know that you're wanted is a life saver."

Education

- Include concepts of holistic communication in undergraduate education.
- Basic and advanced holistic nurse education should include study of relationships, defense mechanisms, boundaries, and relationship disorders.
- Simulation scenarios can assist learning to practice therapeutic and healing relationships.

Research

- Identify means to integrate civility into healthcare workplaces.
- Research the effects of utilizing holistic communication techniques on patient outcomes.

Policy

- Create hospital policy on holistic and therapeutic communication that addresses nurse–patient and coworker interactions.
- Include components of holistic and therapeutic communication in employee evaluation criteria.

Global Health

- Apply principles of holistic communication to global partnerships.
- Apply principles of healing and therapeutic relationships to global partnerships.

Conclusion

Holistic communication calls forth the full use of self in interacting with another. It incorporates the constructs of therapeutic communication while acknowledging the infinite, spiritual, and energetic nature of Being; the centrality of being heart-centered; and the importance of intention, self-knowledge, transcendent presence, and intuition in our interactions. This creates the basis for caring–healing relationships. Basic and advanced holistic nurses improve patient care by utilizing principles of therapeutic and caring–healing relationships. A quality nurse–patient relationship provides improved physical and emotional healing. The holistic nurse brings a sense of therapeutic presence to the encounter and allows patients to share their stories. Relationships go beyond dealing with patients to dealing with coworkers, friends, family, animals, the environment, and a Higher Power. Skill in holistic nursing competencies provides healing care with the use of presence, intentionality, and therapeutic use of self.

Still, there are many ways for relationships to become destructive. Nurses must be informed about defense mechanisms, boundary setting, and issues of anger, control, trust, and forgiveness.

References

American Horticultural Therapy Association. (2024). *Horticultural therapy.* https://www.ahta.org/horticultural-therapy

American Nurses Association Nursing Resources Hub. (2023, September 13). *Nurse-patient relationship.* https://www.nursingworld.org/content-hub/resources/becoming-a-nurse/nurse-patient-relationship-trust/

American Psychological Association. (2023, November 3). *Control anger before it controls you.* https://www.apa.org/topics/anger/control

Benson, H. (1996). *Timeless healing: The power and biology of belief.* Simon & Schuster.

Cleveland Clinic. (2024, May 15). *Resentment: How it can creep in and take hold.* https://health.clevelandclinic.org/what-is-resentment

Faubion, D. (2024). *12 simple tips to IMPROVE emotional intelligence in nursing.* https://www.nursingprocess.org/emotional-intelligence-nursing.html

Greater Good Magazine. (2024). *What is forgiveness?* https://greatergood.berkeley.edu/topic/forgiveness/definition#what-is-forgiveness

Helming, M. A. (2011). The lived experience of healing through prayer: A qualitative study. *Holistic Nursing Practice, 25*(1), 33–44.

Intuition. (n.d.). In *Merriam-Webster.com dictionary.* https://https://www.merriam-webster.com/dictionary/intuition

McLeod, S. (2024, January 25). *Defense mechanisms in psychiatry explained.* https://www.simplypsychology.org/defense-mechanisms.html

Mariano, C. (2020). Holistic nursing: Scope and standards of practice. In M. Helming, D. Shields, K. Avino, & W. Rosa (Eds.), *Dossey & Keegan's holistic nursing: A handbook for practice* (8th ed., pp. 25–52). Jones & Bartlett Learning.

McCraty, R., Atkinson, M., & Bradley, R. T. (2004). Electrophysiological evidence of intuition: The surprising role of the heart. *Journal of Alternative and Complementary Medicine, 10*(1), 133–143.

McCraty, R., & Reese, R. (2009). *The central role of the heart in generating and sustaining positive emotions* (Institute of HeartMath, Publication no. 06-022). HeartMath Research Center.

McCraty, R., & Childre, D. (2010). Coherence: Bridging personal, social, and global health. *Alternative Therapies, 16*(4), 10–24.

Tiwari, D. (2022). Control issues: Signs, causes, & ways to overcome. ChoosingTherapy.com https://www.choosingtherapy.com/control-issues/

Therapist.com Team. (2024, May 16). *Animal-assisted therapy (AAT) and emotional support animals.* https://therapist.com/types-of-therapy/animal-assisted-therapy/

Thornton, L. (2013). *Whole person caring: An interprofessional model for healing and wellness.* Sigma Theta Tau International.

Thornton, L. *Whole person caring: Healing ourselves, healing our patients.* Forthcoming.

Thornton, L., & Mariano, C. (2022). Evolving from therapeutic to holistic communication. In D. Tiwari (Ed.), *Control issues: Signs, causes and ways to overcome.* https://www.choosingtherapy.com/control-issues/

Zimmerman, M. (2023). *Obsessive compulsive personality disorder.* https://www.merckmanuals.com/professional/psychiatric-disorders/personality-disorders/obsessive-compulsivepersonality-disorder-ocpd

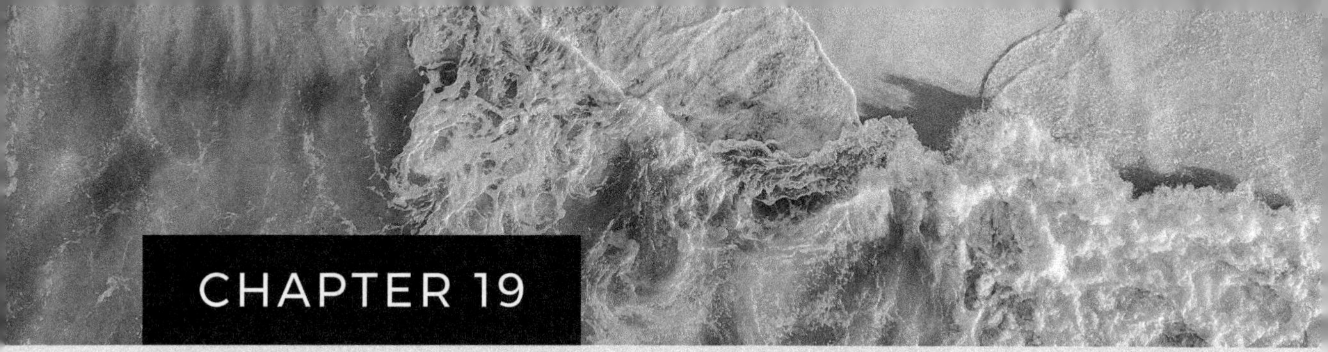

CHAPTER 19

Transcultural Engagement

Shu-Fen Wung, Chiyoung Lee, Joan C. Engebretson, and Hyochol Ahn

NURSE HEALER OBJECTIVES

- Define culture.
- Discuss cultural influences on health and illness.
- Cultural safety continuum.
- Describe the components and principles of cultural competence.
- Cultural humility and transcultural engagement.

DEFINITIONS

Acculturation: This is a process through which an immigrant or immigrant group adapts to a new culture. It also refers to the changes in values, beliefs, language, and behaviors resulting from interactions with culturally diverse people and social influences.

Cultural safety in healthcare: It involves a heightened awareness and accountability among healthcare professionals and organizations. It necessitates a commitment to continuous self-reflection and self-awareness to ensure the provision of culturally safe care, as defined by the client. The effectiveness of such care is assessed through measurable progress toward health equity.

Culturally competent health care: This involves providing care with an understanding of and sensitivity to the cultural factors that influence the health and illness behaviors of individual clients, families, or communities.

Culture: The values, beliefs, customs, social structures, and patterns of human activity, along with the symbolic structures that provide meaning and significance to human behavior.

Ethnocentrism: A worldview significantly influenced by the socialization experiences of individuals within their own culture. It fosters the belief that all others perceive and interpret the world in a manner consistent with one's own cultural perspective.

Transcultural engagement: An interactive process aimed at fostering understanding and connection with individuals from different cultural backgrounds, promoting such without seeking to change or judge them. It involves creating structures that support ongoing cultural exchange, resulting in transformative learning and deep changes in individual and group identities.

Culture

Culture constitutes a complex combination of values, beliefs, languages, customs, traditions, practices, skills, and artistic expressions that are collectively shared among a group, distinguishing it from an individual perspective. It is frequently associated with race, ethnicity, and nationality; however, cultural or subgroup affiliations can also arise from various other factors, including religion, socioeconomic status, age, shared beliefs, lifestyle, sexual orientation, educational background, and professional domains such as healthcare disciplines. Members of a cultural group inherently share values, beliefs, and behavioral patterns that foster a collective identity, resulting in a profound influence on individual behavior, often operating at a subconscious level.

Ethnicity and Race-Based Culture

Ethnicity refers to the shared culture, including language, food, music, dress, values, and beliefs, that stems from common ancestry and history (American Psychological Association, 2023). Generally, *ethnicity* pertains to nationality, denoting a collective that shares a common social and cultural heritage. While ethnicity serves as the most common criterion for cultural classification, variations within an ethnic group may prove to be more significant than those differentiating between various ethnicities, particularly in a culturally pluralistic society. *Race* is the social construction and categorization based on perceived shared physical appearance, which is resolved in the preservation of a sociopolitical hierarchy (American Psychological Association, 2023). Genetic diversity is greater within self-identified racial groups than between them (Bonham, 2025). Genomic scientists are studying the connection between self-identified race and genetic heritage. Nonetheless, in some literature, the term *race* has been erroneously used to delineate differences among individuals that lack any biological foundation. Demographic data are commonly gathered without distinguishing between ethnicity and race.

Gender and Sexuality Identity-Based Cultures

All cultures develop socially sanctioned roles for different genders. Over the past century, the role of women has progressed from a traditional emphasis on childbearing and rearing to encompass active participation in both the workplace and the marketplace. The feminist movement has advocated for this expanded role and has heightened awareness of opportunities aligned with the American values of individualism, equality, and political freedom. Recently, the lesbian, gay, bisexual, transgender, queer/questioning, intersexual, asexual, and more (LGBTQIA+) community has illuminated the diversity inherent within sexuality and gender identity–based cultures. The "+" in the acronym LGBTQIA+ signifies the extensive spectrum of sexual orientation and gender identities recognized by society.

Culture is acquired from birth through language acquisition and socialization, and it represents the process by which individuals adapt to an organized way of life of their groups. This process ensures the transmission of cultural knowledge from one generation to the next. Culture is largely implicit, as it is not typically articulated or discussed at a conscious level. Consequently, most culturally driven actions derive from subtle cues rather than formalized written or spoken rules. Additionally, culture is dynamic and continually evolving as individuals encounter and adapt to various cultural influences. *Acculturation* refers to the transformation of values, beliefs, language, and behaviors that ensue from the integration of culturally distinct individuals, groups, and social influences.

Cultural Influences on Health and Illness

The concepts of health and healing are fundamentally rooted in cultural beliefs. Activities conducted to promote, maintain, or restore health are performed within a specific cultural framework. Culture exerts a significant influence on individual health and illness behaviors as well as shapes responses to illness and health care. The term *disease* generally refers to the diagnostic labels or classifications of disorders addressed by medicine, whereas *illness* incorporates the personal, social, and cultural dimensions of the experience. This includes the timing, context, and social interactions influencing an individual's decisions regarding the pursuit of help or treatment. Cultural beliefs and practices significantly determine which health issues are prioritized and the strategies employed to address them. Furthermore, these cultural beliefs, values, and practices are particularly important in events surrounding birth and death. Religious affiliation and practices also constitute important aspects of culture and cultural health behavior.

There exist important correlations among race, ethnicity, and culture in relation to health conditions, as biological differences can predispose certain demographic groups to specific diseases. Certain illnesses often result from a combination of genetic predisposition and lifestyle choices, including nutritional patterns and other behaviors that may be more prevalent in specific populations. For instance, both Indigenous American and Hispanic communities demonstrate a disproportionately high prevalence of diabetes. Moreover, certain diseases associated with lifestyle risks—such as substance use disorder and human immunodeficiency virus (HIV) infection—are linked to particular social behaviors. The field of pharmacogenomics has emerged from growing literature that examines variations in pharmaceutical responses among different ethnic and racial groups (Jordan et al., 2023; Marazziti et al., 2021).

Despite the genetic similarity of 99.9 percent among humans at the DNA level, notable differences in illness prevalence persist across various populations. These discrepancies can be explained by a multitude of factors, including genetic differences, dietary and cultural practices, environmental conditions, and socioeconomic status (Emeny et al., 2021; Pérez-Stable & Webb Hooper, 2023). According to a recent report by the Centers for Disease Control and Prevention, key social determinants of health encompass education, income, housing quality, air quality, and health insurance coverage (Department of Health and Human Services). Healthy People 2030 establishes data-driven national objectives within five principal areas of social determinants of health: healthcare access and quality, education access and quality, social and community context, economic stability, and neighborhood and built environment. Socioeconomic status serves as a foundational element impacting three major determinants of health: access to healthcare, environmental exposure to health-related agents, and health behaviors (Adler & Newman, 2002).

Health disparities in the United States impact various health outcomes, and one prominent example is the persistent racial disparities in infant mortality rates (Venkatesan et al., 2023). While the average infant mortality rate has declined from 33.71 deaths per 1,000 preterm births annually between 1995 and 1997 to 23.32 by the years 2018 to 2020, Black infants remain at a higher risk of mortality from preterm birth compared to non-Hispanic White infants, with respective rates of 31.09 and 21.81 deaths per 1,000 preterm births (Venkatesan et al., 2023). Furthermore, longstanding disparities in cardiovascular disease (CVD) mortality rates exist between Black and White adults. From 2010 to 2020, age-standardized CVD mortality rates were consistently higher among Black adults than among their White counterparts (Woodruff et al., 2024). In particular, Black adults exhibited the highest CVD mortality rates when compared to other ethnic groups, particularly in rural areas (Chaturvedi et al., 2024; GBD US Health Disparities Collaborators, 2022). Additionally, non-Hispanic Black adults experience higher rates of hypertension relative to non-Hispanic White and Hispanic adults (Ostchega et al., 2020). They also display higher systolic blood pressure levels and lower rates of blood pressure control among those receiving antihypertensive treatment, a trend that has persisted for several decades (Hardy et al., 2021).

The nursing profession has a unique culture that emphasizes the importance of applied science, efficacy, and cost-effectiveness. It also includes a biomedical–social understanding of health, along with recognition of power structures within healthcare systems. Nurses and other healthcare providers undergo a rigorous educational process and accumulate substantial working experience, allowing them to become acculturated to the healthcare environment. In contrast, patients engage with the healthcare system through the lens of their own cultural perspectives, which are shaped by factors such as ethnicity, social groups, geographic location, religion, education, personal beliefs, and experiences. For many individuals, the initial experience within the healthcare setting may resemble an entry into an unfamiliar culture.

Cultural factors heavily influence the dynamics of communication and the nature of relationships between clients and healthcare providers. Given the cultural diversity within the United States, nurses and other healthcare providers frequently encounter individuals and groups whose health maintenance behaviors, responses to illness, and healthcare utilization patterns diverge from their own experiences. Acknowledgment of and sensitivity to the cultural dimensions of health and illness behaviors are essential for the promotion of health and well-being. This understanding facilitates the integration of professional knowledge with an awareness of clients' cultural backgrounds. Consequently, comprehending clients' perceptions and the contextual factors influencing their lives is necessary for delivering optimal care. Culturally competent care entails the provision of health services with skill, knowledge, and sensitivity to the relevant cultural factors. In light of the increasing cultural pluralism in North America, it is essential for nurses to develop cultural competency to provide comprehensive and holistic care.

Cross-cultural health belief paradigms, which represent broader philosophical worldviews, provide various frameworks for understanding and explaining health and illness across cultures. According to Andrews and Boyle, there are three major types of cross-cultural health belief paradigms: magico-religious, holistic, and scientific/biomedical (Andrews & Boyle, 2002). Within the magico-religious paradigm, health and illness are attributed to supernatural forces and forces relating to spirituality. The holistic paradigm asserts that optimal health is achieved through an interconnected balance of physical, mental, and spiritual well-being. Conversely, the scientific/biomedical paradigm attributes illness to biological factors such as bacteria or genetics and relies on scientific, evidence-based interventions. While many cultures may blend elements from all three paradigms, one is more prominent. To facilitate effective communication, healthcare providers must recognize the health belief paradigm or paradigms that influence their patients.

Cultural Safety Continuum

There is a growing recognition of the importance of cultural competency and cultural safety at both the individual healthcare practitioner and organizational levels to achieve equitable health care. Although definitions and understandings of cultural competency and related concepts—such as cultural sensitivity, cultural humility, and cultural safety—can vary, a shift toward a broader concept of cultural safety is recommended (**Figure 19-1**). This approach aims to ensure that the healthcare system provides appropriate and equitable care (Curtis et al., 2019).

This healthcare cultural safety model illustrates the progression of an individual practitioner from cultural awareness and cultural sensitivity to cultural competence and ultimately to cultural humility. It emphasizes that both the practitioner and the healthcare organization/system must engage in critical self-reflection to understand power dynamics, privilege, and biases. This understanding is essential for delivering culturally safe care, moving beyond mere cultural knowledge.

Cultural awareness is the ability of healthcare practitioners to recognize, understand, and respect the cultural backgrounds, beliefs, values, and behaviors of clients from diverse populations. This essential first step begins with an insight into the practitioner's own cultural beliefs, values, and attitudes, which may include ethnocentric, biased, or prejudiced views toward others.

Cultural sensitivity goes beyond merely being aware of cultural differences. It involves accepting and respecting these differences and being willing to adapt one's behavior and communication style when interacting with people from various cultures. Foronda (2008) analyzed cultural sensitivity and identified key attributes, including knowledge, consideration, understanding, respect, and the ability to tailor interactions to meet individual needs. The antecedents of cultural sensitivity include diversity, awareness, and personal encounters with different cultures. Its outcomes involve effective communication, successful interventions, and overall client satisfaction. The benefits of nurses becoming culturally competent include providing more attentive and positive emotional responses to clients, demonstrating higher self-esteem, and enhancing their capacity for empathy (Sharifi et al., 2019). Recent scoping reviews indicate that both undergraduate nursing programs and postgraduate education are increasing focused on promoting cultural sensitivity

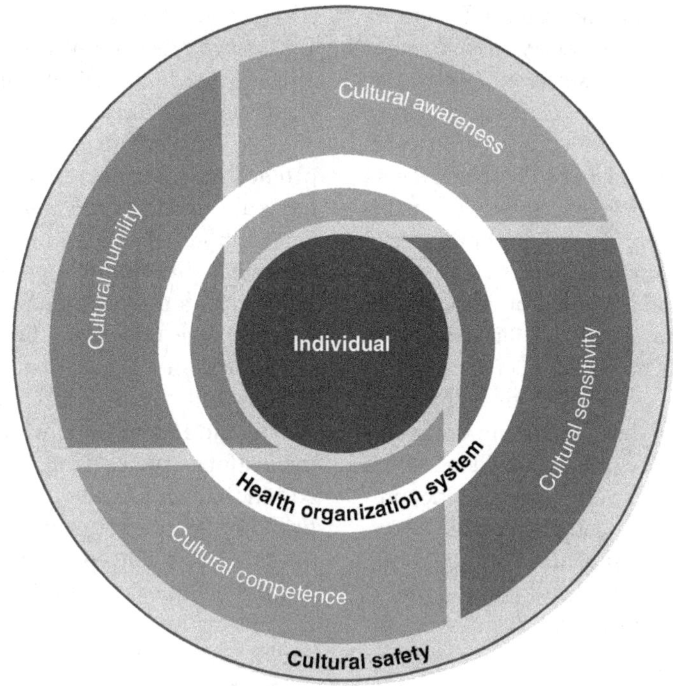

Figure 19-1 Healthcare cultural safety model

This healthcare cultural safety model © is co-created by Shu-Fen Wung and Chang-Chun Chen.

through effective teaching strategies (Gradellini et al., 2021). Active engagement in culturally competent practices for healthcare providers includes using culturally appropriate communication methods, respecting clients' cultural preferences in treatment plans, and committing to ongoing education about various cultural practices and beliefs. This may also involve adapting healthcare interventions to better align with clients' cultural values and expectations.

Culturally competent care is defined as healthcare delivered with a deep understanding of and sensitivity to the cultural factors that influence a client's health and illness behaviors, whether at the individual, family, or community level. Cultural competence is frequently discussed in literature as a continuous process whereby healthcare providers strive to work effectively within the cultural context of their clients. For healthcare providers, being culturally competent necessitates a thorough understanding of their own cultural background and biases, as well as a conscious effort to comprehend their client's cultural context. This involves acknowledging the client's cultural identity and understanding how it influences their health behaviors and attitudes toward illness and treatment. Cultural competence is widely promoted as essential for healthcare providers to effectively serve diverse populations, ultimately aiming to reduce health disparities.

Alizadeh and Chavan (2016) highlighted in a systematic review that the key elements of most cultural competence frameworks are awareness, knowledge, and cultural skills/behaviors. *Cultural knowledge* refers to the ongoing acquisition of information about different cultures. *Cultural skills* or *behaviors* involve the ability to communicate and interact effectively with individuals from diverse backgrounds. *Cultural desire* encompasses an individual's motivation to engage with and learn about cultural diversity. *Desired outcomes* include improved patient quality of life, satisfaction, and treatment adherence.

The National Center for Cultural Competency at Georgetown University developed a widely cited conceptual framework illustrating a continuum from cultural destructiveness to cultural competency (Cross et al., 1989). This framework positions cultural destructiveness at the lowest level, progressing through four intermediary steps to reach cultural proficiency at the top. The continuum, along with parallel values in biomedicine and a recent emphasis on evidence-based practice, is illustrated in **Figure 19-2** (Engebretson et al., 2008).

Practicing in a culturally competent manner should include three key components of evidence-based practice: the best evidence from valid and clinically relevant research, the provider's clinical expertise, and the client's values, unique preferences, and situations (Sackett, et al., 2005). Emphasizing the client's values, preferences, and situations moves evidence-based practice toward cultural competence and proficiency. Unfortunately, much of the literature on cultural competency tends to focus on studies from specific ethnic groups. It is important to recognize that applying information relevant to a particular ethnic group is at best a level of pre-competence. To achieve true competency, practice must be individualized and client-centered during each client–provider interaction.

The concept of developing cultural competence has been increasingly discussed in the literature, and the term *competency* has been challenged more recently; however, it is essential to remember that cultural competence is a process rather than a destination (Young & Guo, 2020). In 2000, the Office of Minority Health developed the National Standards for Culturally and Linguistically Appropriate Services (CLAS) in Health and Health Care, which included recommendations applicable at both the institutional and individual provider levels. This marked the first time a federal agency operationalized and advanced this concept (Lee, 2021). These standards were enhanced in 2013 to provide guidance for national leadership in promoting CLAS and health equity, supporting language assistance in healthcare institutions, and outlining processes for quality improvement, community engagement, and evaluation (U.S. Department of Health & Human Services, 2025). Additionally,

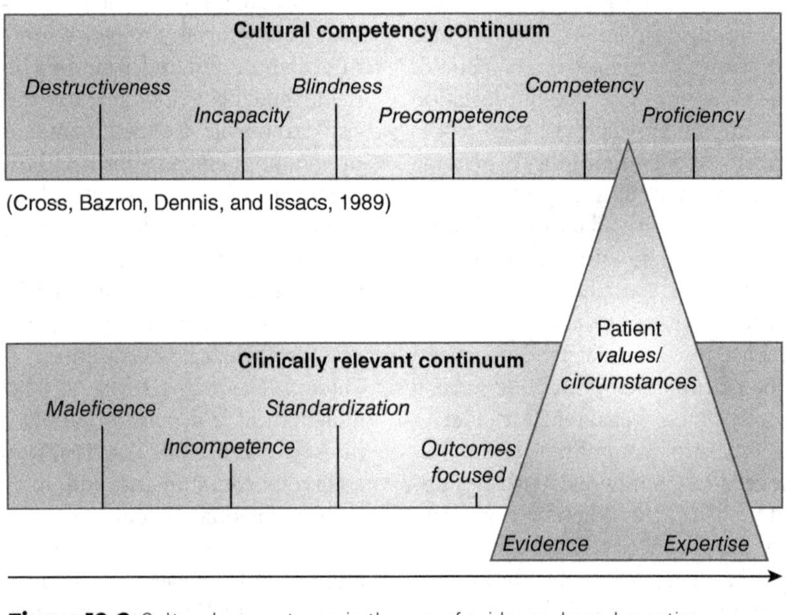

Figure 19-2 Cultural competence in the era of evidence-based practice

Reprinted from the *Journal of Professional Nursing*, volume 24, issue 3, by J. Engebretson, J. Mahoney, and E. Carlson, titled "Cultural Competence in the Era of Evidence-Based Practice," pages 172–178, Copyright 2008, used with permission from Elsevier.

a guide/toolkit for implementing the CLAS standards was developed in 2016. This toolkit can be applied across various healthcare contexts and addresses all populations, with special sections dedicated to minorities, individuals with low health literacy, racial and ethnic minorities, as well as sexual and gender minorities (Barksdale et al., 2017).

Cultural Humility and Transcultural Engagement

While *competency* refers to the achievement of a specific skill set or mastery, *cultural humility* is an intrapersonal and interpersonal approach that encourages person-centered care Minkler (2012). There is a growing recommendation for training that promotes cultural humility. Tervalon and Murray-García (1998) described *cultural humility* as a lifelong commitment to self-evaluation and self-critique, aimed at addressing imbalances in the patient-provider dynamic and developing mutually beneficial, non-paternalistic clinical and advocacy partnerships with patients and communities. This concept is particularly relevant in nursing care.

Foronda et al. (2016) conducted a concept analysis of cultural humility to identify its antecedents, attributes, and consequences, emphasizing that it is a lifelong process. This framework can be beneficial in contexts involving individuals with ethnic or racial differences, as well as variations in sexual orientation, social status, interprofessional roles, and provider–patient relationships. Achieving cultural humility leads to mutual empowerment, respect, partnerships, optimal care, and lifelong learning (Foronda et al., 2016).

In a multicultural world marked by power imbalances, cultural humility encourages the *attributes* of openness, self-awareness, egolessness, supportive interactions, and self-reflection and critique. *Openness* represents an initial willingness to explore new ideas, crucial for healthcare providers working with diverse patient populations. *Self-awareness* involves understanding one's strengths, limitations, values, beliefs, behaviors, and how one is perceived by others, which is vital for interpreting others' behaviors accurately. *Supportive interaction* is the positive exchange that occurs when individuals engage, interact, and shape one another's experiences. *Self-reflection and critique* entail thinking critically about one's actions and questioning oneself.

The *antecedents* of cultural humility include diversity and power imbalance. *Diversity* encompasses a wide range of factors such as multiculturalism, various belief systems, social group memberships, social power, social class, oppression, health disparities, and differing concepts of sickness and health. It also includes healthcare demands, language differences, varying attitudes, material privilege, customs, lifestyles, taboos, and ethnic or religious affiliations. *Power imbalances* intersect with diversity and relate to social injustice, manifesting in various social contexts characterized by inequality, oppression, group membership, injustice, power, cultural imposition, stigma, stereotyping, biases, entitlement, and differing levels of power.

Consequences of cultural humility include mutual empowerment, partnerships, respect, optimal care, and lifelong learning. *Respect, mutual empowerment, and partnerships* are essential components that reflect in our connections, trust, patient-clinical dynamics, and the development of honest and trustworthy relationships. Advocacy also plays a significant role. Providing *optimal care* involves effective treatments, informed decision-making, and improved communication, all of which contribute to enhanced patient outcomes. This process often leads to *lifelong learning*, which is evident through self-reflection, constructive critique, and ongoing learning.

In contrast, the *antonyms* of cultural humility include prejudice, oppression, intolerance, discrimination, stereotyping, exclusion, stigma, inequity, marginalization, misconceptions, labeling, mistrust, hostility, misunderstanding, cultural imposition, judgment, undermining, and bullying.

To foster mutual understanding and improve human interactions, Foronda proposed a grand theory to guide nurses and other professionals in appreciating diversity and applying cultural humility (Foronda, 2020). This theory emphasizes recognizing diversity, addressing power imbalances, considering contextual factors, understanding perspectives, managing conflicts, and maintaining flexibility, all while promoting ongoing self-reflection to cultivate positive intercultural interactions. The application of this theory in nursing practice is expected to enhance patient outcomes, yielding benefits such as improved communication, increased satisfaction, empowerment, stronger partnerships, mutual respect, optimal care, better health, and overall wellness.

Hughes et al. emphasized that fostering cultural humility in nursing begins with training future faculty to advocate for this approach (Hughes et al., 2020). This initiative helps create a pipeline of nurses who embody respect and empathy toward their patients. Equipping future generations of nurses with the practice of cultural humility is essential for advancing the profession and improving outcomes for students, clinicians, and patients alike. Enhanced training in cultural humility, which includes both intrapersonal and interpersonal aspects, promotes deeper introspection and critical thinking among students and clinicians. This ultimately leads to better interactions within interdisciplinary teams and between patients and healthcare providers.

Transcultural engagement goes a step further by actively involving both healthcare providers and clients in a collaborative process aimed at bridging cultural gaps. This ensures that care is not only culturally aware but also mutually enriching and empowering. Transcultural engagement emphasizes a proactive and intentional effort to understand and integrate diverse cultural perspectives into healthcare practices, fostering a more inclusive and effective healthcare environment.

The term *think like a native*, coined by anthropologists who studied cultures through extensive fieldwork, highlights the importance of understanding the behaviors and beliefs of different cultures. With increased travel and electronic communication, we encounter diverse cultures more frequently. This exposure can present challenges for healthcare providers as they meet patients with differing health-related beliefs and behaviors. Conversely, exposure to various cultures can influence the practices and perspectives of the providers themselves.

Transcultural engagement is distinct from cross-cultural, intercultural, and multicultural engagement, which can be illustrated using a fruit metaphor (Winschiers-Theophilus et al., 2019). Cross-cultural engagement is akin to a set of distinct adjacent fruits, where each entity is identifiable based on clear differences. Intercultural engagement resembles processed fruits arranged to represent something else, reflecting how interactions create varied expectations and expressions. This approach acknowledges that marginalized and Native communities, which were previously silenced, can now express their voices and develop counternarratives. Multicultural engagement is best depicted as a fruit salad, where fruits are mixed but remain distinguishable. This approach focuses on building bridges for peaceful coexistence with mutual benefits. In contrast, transcultural engagement can be likened to a smoothie, where the fruits contribute their flavor, but individual distinctions become less significant. "Transculture is a new sphere of cultural development that transcends the borders of traditional cultures (ethnic, national, racial, religious, gender, sexual, and professional). Transcultural overcomes the isolation of their symbolic systems and value determinations and broadens the field of 'supra-cultural' creativity" (Epstein, 2009).

Transcultural engagement is centered on meeting others with the intention of sharing, understanding, and forming authentic connections, rather than aiming to change or judge them (Walsh, 2006). This type of interaction fosters the creation of frameworks that support continuous engagement. By approaching others in this way, we promote a deeper and more meaningful connection. Those who participate in transcultural engagement embark on a journey that explores different cultures, embraces change, and fosters transformative learning. When the interaction is sincere, it has the potential to alter the fundamental aspects of both individual and group identities, reshaping our perspectives on the world and ourselves.

Common Myths and Errors

Errors stemming from stereotyping are prevalent among individuals who perceive the world through rigid constructs of ethnicity or race. It is also misleading to presume that all members of a culture adhere to a single pattern, ignoring individual characteristics and the diversity within cultural groups. For example, some may believe that all African Americans enjoy "soul food" or that all Hispanic individuals are Catholic. This oversight can lead to the stereotyping of cultures, as values within a particular group can vary over time and across different locations, contradicting current individuals' thoughts or behaviors. Stereotyping can manifest in subtle ways, such as when a nurse manager assigns all Hispanic clients to a Mexican American nurse. This approach fails to acknowledge the differences among individuals within the Hispanic community and presumes that all individuals within this group have the same characteristics.

Ethnocentrism, often an unconscious tendency, leads individuals to regard their own values as the only objective reality, viewing others through the lens of their cultural norms and customs. This can result in "cultural blindness," where people ignore real diversity and overlook cultural differences as if they do not exist. Ethnocentric views often stem from a lack of understanding of other cultures, along with the mistaken belief that one's behavior is unaffected by culture. Many individuals from dominant cultures may falsely assume they possess no cultural practices or beliefs. This narrow worldview can lead to the perception of different cultures and beliefs as inferior. An extreme and more deliberate form of ethnocentrism is *xenophobia*, which is an inherent fear of cultural differences. This fear can drive people to reinforce their own values by disparaging the beliefs and traditions of others. Such attitudes frequently manifest as prejudice or racism.

Cultural imposition refers to the belief that successful adaptation to a culture requires individuals to change their beliefs and practices to align with those of the dominant group, regardless of their own cultural backgrounds. This perspective suggests that the dominant culture is superior and that its values should be imposed on others. Such impositions can have serious implications for marginalized groups, such as LGBTQIA+ individuals, who may express different sexual behaviors.

Technology and Culture

Technology is advancing rapidly in the Information Age, significantly influencing values, religion, politics, economics, and the arts and sciences. In particular, medical technology has seen remarkable progress, resulting in the development of sophisticated instruments that enable complex procedures such as computer-based imaging, microsurgery, gene mapping, targeted therapies, and pharmacogenomics. The introduction of these technologies brings forth new ethical and cultural questions regarding their human and social implications. Often, the deployment of technology challenges established cultural values. Once technology is introduced, it frequently sparks ethical debates on topics such as resource allocation, fetal tissue transplantation, genetic testing, the right to life, and the right to privacy.

Moreover, technology exerts a profound influence on culture, especially in the realm of communication. It not only shapes how information is conveyed but also determines what types of knowledge are valued (Giger & Haddad, 2021). In today's electronic culture—dependent on cell phones, radio, television, tablets, and computers—its impact on contemporary beliefs, values, and behaviors is immense. In the healthcare sector, clients now have access to a wealth of health-related information from multiple sources. This abundance of information presents new challenges for healthcare providers, who must assist clients in interpreting these data and making informed choices.

Ethnic Groups in North America

Culturally diverse groups in the United States have grown significantly, now representing a substantial portion of the population. According to the United States Census Bureau, the probability that two randomly selected individuals will belong to different racial or ethnic groups increased from 54.9 percent in 2010 to 61.1 percent in 2020 (Jensen et al., 2021). In their practice, nurses often encounter individuals from various ethnic backgrounds. While general descriptions of these ethnic groups can provide valuable insights, it is essential to recognize the considerable diversity that exists within each ethnicity. Cultural beliefs are also dynamic, influenced by globalization and exposure to other cultures. Therefore, it is crucial for nurses to avoid stereotyping. Engaging in reading, discussions, and activities with members of these cultural groups can help to prevent stereotypic interpretations and enhance cultural competency.

Additionally, the delivery of cross-cultural care faces challenges such as personal struggles, cultural conflicts, diverse expressions of pain and suffering, and the need to navigate both personal and organizational constraints (Shahzad et al., 2021). To effectively address these challenges, nurses should engage in self-reflection, embrace cultural differences, cultivate strong interpersonal and psychological skills, and work collaboratively with colleagues and patients' families.

Nursing Applications

Six phenomena are common across all cultural groups and have variations relevant to providing culturally competent nursing assessments and care (Giger & Haddad, 2021). A comprehensive understanding of these variations enhances clinical practice.

1. *Communication.* Cultural differences can significantly influence the expression of emotions, the use of touch, body contact, as well as verbal and nonverbal communication. Language not only shapes individual experiences but also influences perceptions and actions. Elements such as warmth and humor are interpreted differently across cultures. For example, individuals from many Asian-descent cultures may refrain from overt emotional expression due to concerns about "losing face."
2. *Personal space.* Personal space refers to the comfort level associated with the area surrounding an individual's body. Spatial territoriality indicates the necessity to possess and control this personal space. Acceptable proximity varies across cultures. For example, Western culture typically categorizes personal space into three distinct zones: the intimate zone (less than 18 inches), the personal zone (18 inches to 3 feet), and the social zone (3 to 6 feet). Furthermore, cultural backgrounds influence perceptions regarding orderliness, cleanliness, and the structural boundaries associated with furniture and architecture.
3. *Time.* Cultural orientations toward time exhibit notable differences, encompassing both social time and clock time. *Social time* relates to patterns and orientations that shape social interactions, while *clock time* conveys an objective, linear perception of time that implies causality. Certain cultures adhere to cyclical approaches, linking time to recurring natural events such as seasons or migration patterns. For example, in mystical contexts, magic or rituals may provoke a reversal of temporal causality associated with specific events. All cultures recognize the past, present, and future, although one orientation is typically dominant.
4. *Social organization.* Social organizations include families, religious groups, kinship networks, workplace collectives, and special interest associates. The structure, dynamics, and roles within families may vary significantly across cultural contexts. Additionally, the geographical distribution of family members has sociocultural implications. Religious organizations not only provide social connections but also offer a framework for individuals to understand their relationships with the world and the cosmos.
5. *Environmental control.* Cultural perspectives concerning an individual's ability to exert control over nature, the environment, and personal relationships are diverse. The locus of control may be ascribed to external factors (such as luck or fate), internal attributes (dependent on one's behaviors or characteristics), or an alignment with natural harmony,

as is often observed in certain Asian descent cultures. In traditional medicine practices, events are categorized as natural or unnatural, with natural occurrences representing an existence aligned with divine intention, while unnatural occurrences disrupt this balance.

6. *Biological variations.* In pluralistic societies, it is essential to distinguish between factors that are strictly biological (e.g., genetic) and those related to ethnic adaptations resulting from environmental conditions (e.g., food availability) or specific social circumstances (e.g., socioeconomic status, lifestyle). Biological considerations include variations in body size and structure, encompassing differences in teeth, facial features, and skin color, as well as metabolic variations impacting medication reactions, interactions, and sensitivities. Additionally, an awareness of nutritional issues, including food preferences, dietary habits, and conditions such as lactose intolerance, carries significant medical implications.

This overview serves as a foundational guide for understanding cultural variations in nursing practice. Nevertheless, comprehensive individual assessments remain imperative, as intracultural variation often exceeds intercultural differences.

Holistic Caring Process

The interactions between healthcare providers and clients are influenced by the communication between the two, reflecting their respective cultural backgrounds. Both the provider and the client bring their personal beliefs, values, and cultural perspectives to these interactions. These elements significantly impact the transfer of information, decision-making, adherence to treatment, and overall healing outcomes. The professional dynamic of the encounter also incorporates the culture of the healthcare system, even when meetings occur in the client's home or within a community setting. A comprehensive understanding of both the client's cultural context and the healthcare system's culture enables the provider to deliver culturally competent care. In many cases, nurses act as cultural brokers, facilitating communication between the client and the biomedical culture. In today's world, a vast amount of health information is accessible through various media outlets. Patients engage with different media and possess varying levels of formal education regarding health matters. Both the nurse and the patient contribute their personal or intuitive knowledge to the encounter.

Central to this interaction is the nursing process, a fundamental approach to problem-solving. Holistic nurses have long advocated a process that fosters active engagement between the patient and the clinician. This model empowers the patient with greater agency, or influence, in the relationship, contrasting with the traditional nursing process where the clinician typically holds the majority of the authority and the patient merely complies. In this new model, agency is fluid; for example, if a patient is too ill to exert much influence, the nurse and medical team take on a more assertive role. Conversely, in situations focused on promoting health or managing chronic conditions, the expectation is that the patient will assume greater responsibility. This perspective is reflected in the reconfiguration of the steps in the nursing process (refer to **Exhibit 19-1**).

Integration

Clinical Practice

- Formulate protocols that facilitate the integration of cultural beliefs and practices into individualized care plans, thereby enhancing patient outcomes.
- Implement transcultural engagement practices that actively involve patients and their families in the healthcare process, ensuring that their cultural beliefs and values are respected and incorporated into care plans.
- Promote ongoing cultural competence training for healthcare providers to improve com munication and foster positive relationships with clients.
- Establish multidisciplinary teams, inclusive of cultural liaisons, to effectively navigate cultural differences within clinical settings.

Exhibit 19-1 Nursing Process

Traditional Nursing Process Model	Negotiated Holistic Model of the Nursing Process
1. Nursing Assessment	■ A collaborative exchange of expert knowledge between the client and the nurse
2. Nursing Diagnosis	■ An analysis and interpretation of information gathered from both the client and the nurse
3. Planning	■ A collaborative decision-making process involving both the client and the nurse
4. Intervention	■ The implementation of mutually developed action plans that include specific, agreed-upon tasks for both the nurse and the client
5. Evaluation	■ Evaluation of the outcomes related to goals and processes is a collaborative endeavor

Nursing Situation

A 72-year-old man of Asian descent presented to the clinic with knee pain due to osteoarthritis. His nurse, Emily, asked him to rate his current pain on a scale from 0 (no pain) to 10 (worst pain imaginable), but he hesitated to respond. Recalling an article on cultural differences in pain perception, Emily recognized the importance of healthcare professionals understanding how their own cultural backgrounds can shape their attitudes toward pain. She observed that patients from Asian American/Pacific Islander cultures often exhibit stoicism when experiencing pain, which reflects their strong cultural values regarding self-discipline. Therefore, Emily chose to proactively assess multiple dimensions of his knee pain. Upon examining his radiographs, she identified severe sclerosis and evident bony deformities in both knees. In this case, Emily demonstrated cultural competence, emphasizing the significance of healthcare providers' ability to work effectively within their clients' cultural context.

- Continuously monitor and evaluate patient satisfaction and health outcomes to ensure the effectiveness of culturally competent care practices.

Education

- Integrate cultural competence modules into nursing curricula to equip students for engagement in diverse clinical environments.
- Employ case studies and simulations that reflect a range of cultural scenarios to enhance students' practical skills in cultural competence.
- Provide continuous professional development opportunities that focus on cultural humility and competence for nursing educators.
- Develop assessment tools designed to measure students' cultural competence and track their progression throughout their educational experience.
- Promote student engagement with diverse communities through service-learning projects and clinical rotations in multicultural settings.

Research

- Investigate patterns of utilization of healing modalities across various cultural backgrounds.
- Develop efficient and effective methodologies for assessing the degree of acculturation among clients from diverse cultural contexts.
- Analyze effective models for interaction between biomedical and traditional healthcare systems.
- Evaluate the extent to which healthcare goals are achieved when nurses deliver culturally competent care.
- Analyze various instructional methods for focusing on teaching nursing students and staff how to provide culturally competent care.

Policy

- Advocate for the establishment of policies that mandate cultural competence training for all healthcare professionals as a requirement for licensure.
- Establish guidelines that facilitate the incorporation of culturally competent practices into every dimension of patient care.
- Promote policies that necessitate healthcare institutions to offer language assistance services and culturally appropriate educational materials.
- Encourage the integration of cultural competence metrics in healthcare quality assessments and accreditation standards.
- Foster transcultural engagement by creating policies that promote ongoing cultural exchange and transformative learning within healthcare settings.

Global Health

- Develop global health initiatives that emphasize the importance of cultural competence in international healthcare contexts.
- Foster cross-cultural exchanges and collaborations to disseminate best practices and enhance global cultural competence.
- Address global health disparities through the promotion of culturally tailored interventions aimed at underserved and diverse populations.
- Support international research initiatives that examine the impact of cultural competence on health outcomes on a global scale.
- Advocate for global health policies that acknowledge and incorporate cultural diversity into healthcare planning and delivery.

Conclusion

Culture encompasses the shared values, beliefs, and norms that shape human behavior. It often represents the "taken-for-granted" aspects of our lives, influencing our interpretations and understandings of various experiences. Culture plays a crucial role in health care, where each setting—be it hospitals, clinics, or specific units—has its own distinct culture. Healthcare providers adapt to these environments through education and experience, often becoming so accustomed to these cultural norms that they overlook the process of acclimatization. In contrast, patients frequently navigate this "foreign culture" while seeking and receiving care.

As global travel and communication expand, healthcare professionals increasingly interact with individuals from diverse cultures and subgroups, whose contexts may differ widely from their own. This underscores the importance of cultivating cultural humility among providers, enabling them to understand their biases and deliver culturally safe care to their clients. Transcultural engagement enhances this process by fostering an ongoing and interactive exchange of cultural knowledge and practices, ultimately contributing to improved health outcomes and more equitable healthcare delivery.

References

Adler, N. E., & Newman, K. (2002). Socioeconomic disparities in health: Pathways and policies. *Health Affairs (Millwood)*, *21*, 60–76. https://doi.org/10.1377/hlthaff.21.2.60

Alizadeh, S., & Chavan, M. (2016). Cultural competence dimensions and outcomes: A systematic review of the literature. *Health and Social Care Community*, *24*, e117–e130. https://doi.org/10.1111/hsc.12293

American Psychological Association. (2023). *Race and ethnicity*. https://www.apa.org/topics/race-ethnicity

Andrews, M. M., & Boyle, J. S. (2002). Transcultural concepts in nursing care. *Journal of Transcultural Nursing, 13*, 178–180. https://doi.org/10.1177/10459602013003002

Barksdale, C. L., Rodick, W. H., 3rd, Hopson, R., Kenyon, J., Green, K., & Jacobs, C. G. (2017). Literature review of the National CLAS Standards: Policy and practical implications in reducing health disparities. *Journal of Racial Ethnic Health Disparities*, *4*, 632–647. https://doi.org/10.1007/s40615-016-0267-3

Bonham, V. (2025). *Race.* National Human Genome Research Institute. https://www.genome.gov/genetics-glossary/Race#:~:text=Race%20was%20constructed%20as%20a,social%20factors%20and%20cultural%20backgrounds

Chaturvedi, A., Zhu, A., Gadela, N. V., Prabhakaran, D., & Jafar, T. H. (2024). Social determinants of health and disparities in hypertension and cardiovascular diseases. *Hypertension*, *81*, 387–399. https://doi.org/10.1161/hypertensionaha.123.21354

Cross, T. L., Bazron, B. J., Dennis, K. W., & Isaacs, M. R. (1989). *Towards a culturally competent system of care: A monograph on effective services for minority children who are severely emotionally disturbed.* Georgetown University Child Development Center.

Curtis, E., Jones, R., Tipene-Leach, D., Walker, C., Loring, B., Paine, S. J., & Reid, P. (2019). Why cultural safety rather than cultural competency is required to achieve health equity: A literature review and recommended definition. *International Journal of Equity Health*, *18*, 174. https://doi.org/10.1186/s12939-019-1082-3

Department of Health and Human Services. *Healthy People 2030: Social Determinants of Health.* https://odphp.health.gov/healthypeople/objectives-and-data/social-determinants-health

Emeny, R. T., Carpenter, D. O., & Lawrence, D. A. (2021). Health disparities: Intracellular consequences of social determinants of health. *Toxicology and Applied Pharmacology*, *416*, 115444. https://doi.org/10.1016/j.taap.2021.115444

Engebretson, J., Mahoney, J., & Carlson, E. D. (2008). Cultural competence in the era of evidence-based practice. *Journal of Professional Nursing*, 24, 172–178. https://doi.org/10.1016/j.profnurs.2007.10.012

Epstein, M. (2009). 12. Transculture: A broad way between globalism and multiculturalism. *The American Journal of Economics and Sociology*, 68, 327–351.

Foronda, C. (2020). A theory of cultural humility. *Journal of Transcultural Nursing*, *31*, 7–12. https://doi.org/10.1177/1043659619875184

Foronda, C. L. (2008). A concept analysis of cultural sensitivity. *Journal of Transcultural Nursing*, *19*, 207–212. https://doi.org/10.1177/1043659608317093

Foronda, C., Baptiste, D. L., Reinholdt, M. M., & Ousman, K. (2016). Cultural humility: A concept analysis. *Journal of Transcultural Nursing*, *27*, 210–217. https://doi.org/10.1177/1043659615592677

GBD US Health Disparities Collaborators. (2022). Life expectancy by county, race, and ethnicity in the USA, 2000-19: A systematic analysis of health disparities. *Lancet*, *400*, 25–38. https://doi.org/10.1016/s0140-6736(22)00876-5

Giger, J. N., & Haddad, L. G. (2021). *Transcultural nursing: Assessment and intervention* (9th ed.). Elsevier.

Gradellini, C., Gómez-Cantarino, S., Dominguez-Isabel, P., Molina-Gallego, B., Mecugni, D., & Ugarte-Gurrutxaga, M. I. (2021). Cultural competence and cultural sensitivity education in university nursing courses. A scoping review. *Frontiers in Psychology*, *12*, 682920. https://doi.org/10.3389/fpsyg.2021.682920

Hardy, S. T., Chen, L., Cherrington, A. L., Moise, N., Jaeger, B. C., Foti, K., Sakhuja, S., Wozniak, G., Abdalla, M., & Muntner, P. (2021). Racial and ethnic differences in blood pressure among US adults, 1999-2018. *Hypertension*, *78*, 1730–1741. https://doi.org/10.1161/hypertensionaha.121.18086

Hughes, V., Delva, S., Nkimbeng, M., Spaulding, E., Turkson-Ocran, R. A., Cudjoe, J., Ford, A., Rushton, C., D'Aoust, R., & Han, H .R. (2020). Not missing the opportunity: Strategies to promote cultural humility among future nursing faculty. *Journal of Professional Nursing*, *36*, 28–33. https://doi.org/10.1016/j.profnurs.2019.06.005

Jensen, E. J. N., Rabe, M., Pratt, B., Medina, L., Orozco, K., & Spell, L. (2021). *The chance that two people chosen at random are of different race or ethnicity groups has increased since 2010.* Bureau UC.

Jordan, I. K., Sharma, S., & Mariño-Ramírez, L. (2023). Population pharmacogenomics for health equity. *Genes (Basel)*, *14*. https://doi.org/10.3390/genes14101840

Lee, S. (2021). Evaluation of the National CLAS Standards: Tips and resources, by Malcolm V. Williams, Laurie T. Martin, Lois M. Davis, Linnea Warren May and Alice Kim, The U.S. Department of Health and Human Services (HHS) Office of Minority Health (OMH), 2018. *Journal of Gerontological Social Work*, 64, 442–445. https://doi.org/10.1080/01634372.2021.1882638

Marazziti, D., Mucci, F., Avella, M. T., Palagini, L., Simoncini, M., & Dell'Osso, L. (2021). The increasing challenge of the possible impact of ethnicity on psychopharmacology. *CNS Spectrums*, *26*, 222–231. https://doi.org/10.1017/s1092852920000073

Minkler, M. (2012). Community Organizing and Community Building for Health and Welfare. 3rd ed.: Rutgers University Press.

Ostchega, Y., Fryar, C. D., Nwankwo, T., & Nguyen, D. T. (2020). Hypertension prevalence among adults aged 18 and over: United States, 2017-2018. *NCHS Data Brief*, 1–8.

Pérez-Stable, E. J., & Webb Hooper, M. (2023). The pillars of health disparities science-race, ethnicity, and socioeconomic status. *JAMA Health Forum*, 4, e234463. https://doi.org/10.1001/jamahealthforum.2023.4463

Sackett, D. L., Strauss, S. E., Richardson, W. S., Rosenberg, W., Haynes, R. B. (2005). Evidence-Based Medicine: How to Practice and Teach EBM. 2nd ed.: Churchill Livingstone.

Shahzad, S., Ali, N., Younas, A., & Tayaben, J. L. (2021). Challenges and approaches to transcultural care: An integrative review of nurses' and nursing students' experiences. *Journal of Professional Nursing*, 37, 1119–1131. https://doi.org/10.1016/j.profnurs.2021.10.001

Sharifi, N., Adib-Hajbaghery, M., & Najafi, M. (2019). Cultural competence in nursing: A concept analysis. *International Journal of Nursing Studies*, *99*, 103386. https://doi.org/10.1016/j.ijnurstu.2019.103386

Straus, S. E., Glasziou, P., Richardson, W. S., & Haynes, R. B. (2018). *Evidence-based medicine: How to practice and teach EBM*. Elsevier.

Tervalon, M., & Murray-García, J. (1998). Cultural humility versus cultural competence: A critical distinction in defining physician training outcomes in multicultural education. *Journal of Health Care for the Poor and Underserved*, *9*, 117–125. https://doi.org/10.1353/hpu.2010.0233

U.S. Department of Health & Human Services. (2025). *National Culturally and Linguistically Appropriate Services Standards*. https://thinkculturalhealth.hhs.gov/clas/standards

Venkatesan, T., Rees, P., Gardiner, J., Battersby, C., Purkayastha, M., Gale, C., & Sutcliffe, A. G. (2023). National trends in preterm infant mortality in the united states by race and socioeconomic status, 1995-2020. *JAMA Pediatrics*, *177*, 1085–1095. https://doi.org/10.1001/jamapediatrics.2023.3487

Walsh, T. (2006). Changing culture. In B. Treacy, A. V. Martin, & T. Walsh (Eds.), *No longer strangers: Cultural integration in church and society in Ireland*. Dominican Publications.

Winschiers-Theophilus, H., Zaman, T., & Stanley, C. (2019). A classification of cultural engagements in community technology design: Introducing a transcultural approach. *AI Society*, *34*, 419–435. https://doi.org/10.1007/s00146-017-0739-y

Woodruff, R. C., Tong, X., Wadhera, R. K., Loustalot, F., Jackson, S. L., & Vaughan, A. S. (2024). Cardiovascular disease mortality disparities in black and white adults, 2010–2022. *American Journal of Preventive Medicine*, *66*, 914–916. https://doi.org/10.1016/j.amepre.2023.12.007

Young, S., & Guo, K. L. (2020). Cultural diversity training: The necessity of cultural competence for health care providers and in nursing practice. *Health Care Management (Frederick)*, *39*, 100–108. https://doi.org/10.1097/hcm.0000000000000294

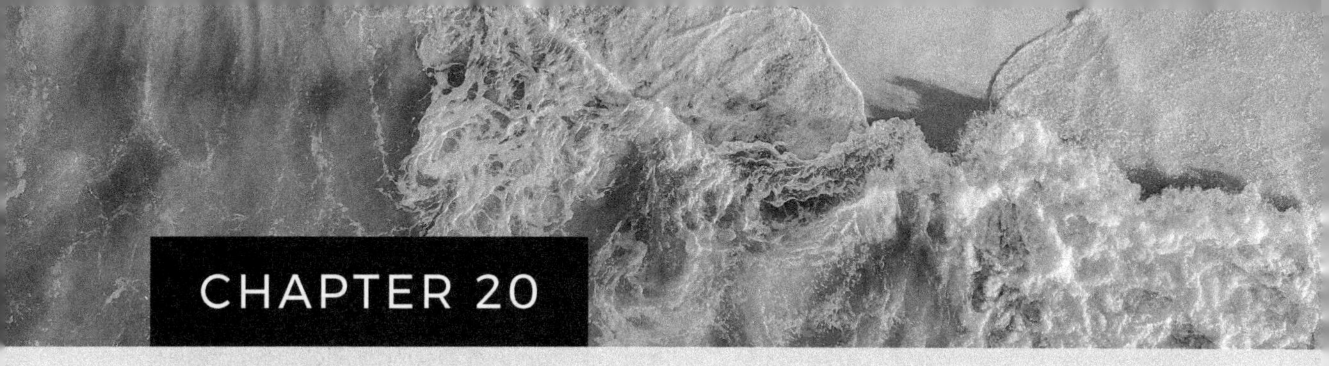

CHAPTER 20

Planetary and Environmental Health

Heidi Honegger Rogers, Mitzie Rains Meyers, Jennifer Rasmussen, and Katherine E. Zychowski

NURSE HEALER OBJECTIVES

- Introduce the framework for planetary health as a lens to inform the education and practice of holistic nursing.
- Review the environmental and ecological determinants of health and how they impact human health and well-being.
- Discuss the concept of interconnection within nature as the paradigm shift needed in modern healthcare systems and services.
- Explore the role of systems thinking and complexity in the daily practice of holistic nursing for planetary and environmental health.
- Apply the holistic nursing values for social justice and equity to nursing advocacy and actions with patients and communities.
- Connect holistic nurses to the resources they need to apply principles of planetary and environmental health with their patients, families, systems, and communities.
- Describe how holistic nurses can integrate the values and ethics of holistic nursing for planetary and environmental health.
- Review how holistic nurses can use the Planetary Health Education Framework to advance planetary health by integrating its principles into their practice, leadership, education, advocacy, scholarship and personal and community engagement efforts.

DEFINITIONS

Anthropocene: The period of time in which human activity has become the dominant influence on Earth's climate, ecosystems, and geological processes. It recognizes that human decisions—particularly related to industrialization, consumption, and land use—are reshaping planetary systems in unprecedented and potentially irreversible ways.

Biodiversity: The variety of life forms in a particular ecosystem or on the planet as a whole. Greater biodiversity supports resilient ecosystems and is essential for maintaining food webs, medicine development, and climate stability.

Complexity theory: A way of understanding how interconnected systems—like communities, environments, and health—operate in unpredictable and adaptive ways. It helps explain why interventions in one area can have ripple effects elsewhere.

Decarbonization: Reducing carbon dioxide emissions—primarily from fossil fuel use—to slow climate change. This involves shifting toward renewable energy sources and more sustainable practices across industries and communities.

Ecosystem: A complex, dynamic system made up of interdependent components—biological, social, environmental, or technological—that influence and sustain one another. These systems can range from natural environments (like forests or oceans) to human systems (like healthcare, education, or community networks).

Epigenetics: The study of how environmental factors (like stress, nutrition, or toxins) can influence gene expression without changing the DNA sequence itself. These changes can affect health outcomes and may be passed on to future generations.

Genomics: The study of all an organism's genes, including how they interact with each other and the environment. It helps researchers understand disease patterns and how genetics and exposures combine to affect health over time.

Microbiome: The community of microorganisms (such as bacteria, viruses, and fungi) that live on and inside the human body. These microbes play key roles in digestion, immune function, and even mental health, and are influenced by environmental exposures.

Systems thinking: A holistic approach to problem-solving that emphasizes the relationships and interdependence among parts of a system.

Introduction

Holistic nursing centers the importance of healing environments to support the health, well-being, and flourishing of patients and communities. Inherent in this paradigm is the understanding that human health is intricately interconnected with the health and well-being of all ecosystems, which include cellular (genetics, epigenetics and microbiome), individual (behavioral), social, spiritual, geopolitical, informatic, and environmental as well as planetary-scale ecological systems. At this unprecedented moment in time, these ecosystems—from the microbiome to the planet—are sick from air, land, and water pollution, global climate change, biodiversity loss, degradation of arable land and fresh water, land use and land cover decisions, scarcity, conflict and neglect, as well as disregard for sustainable and peaceful collaborative living. Human waste and pollution are exceeding the planet's ability to sustain the nine critical processes that compose the planetary-scale ecosystems (Stockholm Resilience Centre, n.d.), contributing to compounding health crises locally and globally. Holistic nurses are paying attention to the environmental destruction and "Planetary Vital Signs" (Ripple et al., 2023) and the status of Mother Earth's health. Holistic nurses are responding to these complex problems by using planetary health sensibilities to inform their nursing practice, leadership, education, advocacy, scholarship, and research, as well as through their personal and community engagement. Holistic nurses are recognizing that the damage humans have caused to each other, the environment, and the planet as a whole are immoral and unsustainable. Holistic nurses can show up for this work, and bring their unique perspectives, experiences, and intuitive senses to imagine and cocreate solutions for a collective ecological, social, physical, and emotional well-being. They can inform the already emerging systems and sensibilities of the "Great Transition" that are called for by the World Health Organization (WHO, 2024a); United Nations (UN, 2024), and the Sao Paulo Declaration on Planetary Health (Planetary Health Alliance, 2021), which reminds nurses that:

> Every dimension of human health and well-being is now affected by global environmental change. The planetary health science is clear: we can no longer safeguard human health unless we change course. We need a fundamental shift in how we live on Earth, what we are calling the Great Transition. (Myers et al., 2021, p. 1)

Planetary Health

Planetary health is a transdisciplinary field, a framework, and a movement. Planetary health helps people understand the connections of human-caused damage and disregard on their cellular, individual, societal, and planetary-scale ecosystems. It provides a lens to examine how these disruptions influence the health and well-being of current and future generations. Planetary health recognizes that health is not solely based on individual/behavioral and social determinants, but also on the interconnectedness of human health, environmental health, planetary-scale ecosystems, and the well-being of nature (Whitmee et al., 2015).

In holistic nursing, this framework is particularly relevant as it aligns with the core principles of recognizing the whole person—body, mind, spirit, and emotion—adding all the environments and ecosystems within which humans live and recognizing the profound interconnection of the health of the natural world and the environment on individual and community well-being. Holistic nurses can follow the work and advocacy of the Planetary Health Alliance to learn more.

The Planetary Health Education Framework

The Planetary Health Alliance (n.d.) has developed the Planetary Health Education Framework, freely available through their website as a strategy for building common knowledge sets and a shared language and sensibility across all disciplines within planetary health.

Interconnection Within Nature

Interconnection Within Nature is the central domain in the Planetary Health Education Framework that reminds humanity that health and well-being are intricately interconnected with the health and well-being of all others, human and more than human, and that people are part of nature, not separate. Holistic nurses can play several important roles in fostering an understanding and appreciation of the interconnections within nature, contributing to planetary health, and promoting sustainable practices. Nurse healers recognize that the paradigm for health is not separate and entirely self-determined, but connected and interdependent on the health of all ecosystems—social, structural, environmental, and planetary. They should recognize that this idea is not new; it is a central paradigm in many Indigenous wisdom traditions. Holistic nurses can follow the guidance that is given to them from their local Indigenous communities, when available. There are several books, as well as national and international organizations of Indigenous scholars and wisdom keepers that are helping to direct this work. Interconnection within nature involves integration of the cognitive, affective, and behavioral domains within this paradigm, and includes respecting the ways of knowing and the many Indigenous wisdoms around the world. Using this experiential knowledge, individuals and communities can bring about transformational change (Guzmán et al., 2021).

Anthropocene and Health

Anthropocene and Health recognizes that the Earth has adapted over millions of years to geological changes. In the period called the "Holocene," the Earth was stable and predictable. As within any system, there is cause and effect; in the Anthropocene, human degradation has caused imbalances within the Earth system (Guzmán et al., 2021). *Anthropocene and Health* is the sensibility that brings together the narrative of how humans are causing damage to environments and how these activities impact health and well-being. It incorporates the science and current understanding of how climate change, biodiversity loss, global air, land and water pollution, novel entities (like chemicals and plastics), land use decisions, nutrient cycling, marine degradation, and resource scarcity impact communicable and noncommunicable diseases, nutrient deficiencies, mental health, reproductive health, and injuries.

Equity and Social Justice

Equity and Social Justice is a core domain with important concepts of the Planetary Health Education Framework. It is essential for holistic nurses to recognize that certain populations bear a disproportionate burden of illness due to environmental and planetary disruption. In terms of climate change, some communities are living on the front lines of wildfires, extreme weather, heat, drought, and flooding. Communities that lack public health and organized infrastructure for water, electricity, transportation, food production, and delivery as well as social, economic, and basic safety infrastructure are at increased risk in the face of climate change and other planetary-scale problems (Guzmán et al., 2021).

Systems Thinking and Complexity

Systems Thinking and Complexity discusses how systems are organic, dynamic, and fluid. Systems are about relationships interacting and working together to ensure survival of the whole. The planet Earth, the human body, social, structural, and healthcare systems can all be viewed through systems thinking. Universally, a variety of elements within ecosystems interact as part of complex systems. Holistic nurses can use complexity theory and a systems-thinking approach to understand the dynamic forces within planetary health to join transdisciplinary partnerships to address these complex problems and transform the whole (Albert et al., 2022; Guzmán et al., 2021).

Movement Building and Systems Change

Movement Building and Systems Change is the work that humanity must attend to. The scale of these problems requires people to imagine new systems and ways of being. People must design the future from the understanding that humans are nature, and that all life is intricately interconnected. Movement building and systems change are the outcomes and solutions that the Planetary Health Education Framework and the work that planetary health is requiring. It is not just understanding the science of how health is impacted, but redesigning how people all live together, based on the values of health for all life, fairness and equity, sustainability, and stewardship. Holistic nurses can work from these sensibilities to imagine a future where humans and nature can flourish together (Macy & Johnstone, 2022).

Sustainable Development Goals and Planetary Health

In 2015, the UN developed the Sustainable Development Goals as a 2030 agenda for sustainable development, with the overall goal of peace and prosperity for all people and the planet through a global partnership (UN, n.d.). The Sustainable Development Goals provide specific guidance and recommendations to move toward a future of mutual flourishing. These goals can guide holistic nurses in their own work in all domains of nursing. While the guidance represents a clear vision and a broad collaboration across the United Nations, the global community remains off track from achieving these goals by 2030, with only 17 percent of targets progressing to expectation (refer to **Box 20-1** for details) (UN, 2024; UN General Assembly Economic and Social Council, 2024).

Box 20-1 **SDGs at Risk: Key Goals Off Track for 2030**

- Goal #6 Clean Water: None of the targets are on track to be met. According to 2020 data, 2.2 billion people did not have access to safe drinking water; droughts affected 1.4 billion people, and half of the world's population experienced water scarcity.
- Goal #7 Clean Energy: There is insufficient investment in clean energy in many countries.
- Goal #12 Responsible Consumption and Production: Material consumption and carbon footprint continue to increase, contributing to climate change, pollution, and biodiversity loss. It is estimated that one billion meals worth of edible food are wasted every day globally.
- Goal #13 Climate Change: 2023 was the warmest year on record, breaking every single climate indicator.
- Goal #14 Life Below Water: Trends indicate declining fish stocks from overfishing, water pollution, ocean acidification, bleached coral reefs, increased water temperatures, and habitat destruction.
- Goal #15 Life on Land: Species extinction risk continues to worsen, and forests continue to decline.

Data from United Nations. (2024). *The Sustainable Development Goals Report 2024*. Retrieved from https://unstats.un.org/sdgs/report/2024/The-Sustainable-Development-Goals-Report-2024.pdf
United Nations General Assembly Economic and Social Council. (2024). *Progress toward the sustainable development goals*. https://unstats.un.org/sdgs/files/report/2024/SG-SDG-Progress-Report-2024-advanced-unedited-version.pdf

Nurses have a responsibility to promote and work toward these goals, and the holistic nursing community can be a driving force in this work.

Planetary-Scale Ecological Determinants of Health and Holistic Nursing Considerations

To understand the core concepts of planetary health, nurses can become familiar with how human activities threaten the Earth's ecosystems. The Stockholm Resilience Centre (n.d.), which tracks and studies the planetary boundaries, provides useful educational resources to help holistic nurses understand this science. In addition, the Planetary Health Alliance (n.d.) provides excellent summaries on how current and future human health and well-being is determined by these ecosystems. The planetary-scale ecological determinants of health are air, land, and water pollution, chemical pollution and other novel entities, biodiversity loss, land use and land cover changes, climate change, nutrient overloading, ocean/marine degradation, and resource scarcity.

Air, Soil, and Water Pollution

Air, soil, and water pollution are impacting local communities and are contributing to widespread acute and chronic health conditions. These pollutants impact the health of human bodies and all animal and plant life. Because of the ubiquitous nature of this problem, holistic nurses need to understand the risks and exposure pathways as well as the environmental degradation and health risks of the common and pervasive pollutants that are present in every environment on the planet. Indoor air pollution comes from cooking and heating, chemicals and volatile organic compounds, as well as gases like radon (Rosário Filho et al., 2021). Outdoor air pollution comes from fossil fuel combustion, off-gassing from fossil fuel extraction, wildfires, chemicals, land contamination, and dust (Dominski et al., 2021). Air pollution impacts the respiratory system as well as the cardiovascular, neurological, and immune systems. It also causes generalized inflammation, respiratory distress, long-term damage to both tissues and organs, and is directly linked to multiple forms of cancer (Manisalidis et al., 2020). Both soil and water pollution come from heavy metals, chemicals and plastics, fossil fuel leaks and combustion, fires, pesticides, fertilizers as well as effluent, and sludge from sewage and animal waste (Maddela et al., 2022; Shetty et al., 2023). In addition to infectious diseases, these pollutants also carry risks for inflammation, neurodegenerative disorders, respiratory, genitourinary, reproductive, and dermatological illness (Myers & Frumkin, 2020). It is important for holistic nurses to understand how pollution in all forms impacts health. The Alliance of Nurses for Healthy Environments has a free eBook on *Environmental Health and Nursing* (McDermott-Levy et al., 2023a). In addition, holistic nurses can follow the advocacy and work of the Alliance of Nurses for Healthy Environments, the WHO, and their own local and regional environmental health divisions. These resources (available online) will assist them in understanding the specific air, soil, and water pollutants in their communities, the health impacts of these, and mitigation strategies to reduce health harms.

Chemical Pollution and Novel Entities

Chemical pollution and novel entities include endocrine-disrupting chemicals (EDCs), microplastics and nanomaterials, flame retardants, glyphosate, and contaminant metals (refer to **Box 20-2**). Emerging contaminants can be difficult to regulate, since they are relatively newer and understudied. As more data emerge, this may drive changes in policy for stricter contaminant levels for drinking water, food, etc. Toxicants can accumulate in plants and animals via food webs and can be contributing factors to long-term, predominantly chronic health impacts. In some instances, there can be acute, higher dose exposures; however, this may be due to occupational exposures for certain groups of people (e.g., military personnel, farm workers, miners).

Most of the toxicological concerns stem from low-level, but long-term exposures that may

Box 20-2 Chemical Pollution and Novel Entities

Endocrine-disrupting chemicals (EDCs) are toxic substances that are ubiquitous. They exist in the water, food, air, and soil and can interfere with the body's endocrine system. The endocrine system includes a network of glands and organs that are responsible for secretion and storage of hormones. Proper functioning of these hormones is essential for development, reproductive systems, mood, and metabolism. There are likely more than 1,000 chemicals that are classified as EDCs (Yilmaz et al., 2020). These EDCs can be lipophilic and can accumulate in adipose (fat) tissue over time. EDCs are known to cause some developmental and fertility issues, as well as contributing to cancer development. Understanding EDCs is both important for public health and for nursing practice, due to ubiquitous exposures that occur throughout the lifespan.

- ***Phthalates*** are a large group of compounds that can have estrogenic properties. One study found that reduction of daily-use parabens and phthalates reverses cancer-associated phenotypes and pro-carcinogenic endpoints (Dairkee et al., 2023). Phthalate biomarkers have been associated with prostate tumorigenesis in the United States (Guo et al., 2023). In one age-matched study, phthalate metabolites were detected in 82 percent of female participants and there was a strong association between breast cancer and urinary concentrations of phthalates, especially in premenopausal women (López-Carrillo et al., 2010).
- **Per- and polyfluoroalkyl substances (PFAS)** also known as "forever chemicals" were widely used in several industries in the United States and globally and is another class of EDCs. PFAS breakdown occurs very slowly and because of this, most of the ecosystem has been exposed to PFAS. PFAS blood levels are detectable through advanced analytical chemistry methods and can increase over time. One CDC study found that 97 percent of United States Americans have detectable blood levels of PFAS (Lewis et al., 2015). This same study found that exposure to PFAS may alter thyroid hormone homeostasis due to related increases in TSH among males and decreases in TSH in females exposed to PFAS.

  Several studies suggest that PFAS exposure may contribute to increasing rates of cancer, based on both cohort and case-control studies (Steenland & Winquist, 2021). Multiple cancers have been associated with PFAS exposure including testicular and kidney cancers, in addition to leukemias. One study found that serum perfluorooctanoic acid concentrations were positively associated with kidney cancer rates among women. However, this observation was not found in men (Winquist et al., 2023). One major study using U.S. National Health and Nutrition Examination Survey (NHANES) data sets used logistic regression analysis and found associations for increases in PFAS results in increased brain, esophageal, lung cancers, and melanoma (Moon & Mun, 2024). There was also a modest increase in prostate cancer (odds ratio 1.21) for every one unit increase of perfluorooctane sulfonate and perfluorononanoic acid.

  PFAS is an emerging toxicological concern, in which there are currently no approved medical treatments available. There are, however, commercially available filters that can be applied to residential water systems, if patients are concerned about their environmental exposures. In addition, it is important to note that while PFAS may be a contributing factor to disease states and outcomes, that health screenings beyond the standard of care are not typically warranted. In other words, PFAS blood levels should not be used to provide information about treatment or predict future risk of disease development. Holistic nurses can learn more about PFAS and how to reduce exposures through the Alliance of Nurses for Healthy Environments PFAS toolkit.

Microplastics and nanomaterials have been increasingly used in multiple applications since the 1950s. Plastics are cost-effective, versatile, stable, and lightweight. Unfortunately, these plastics, which are typically used and discarded, breakdown over time into micro (and nano) plastics. Due to oceanic, estuary, and atmospheric transport, these microplastics can aggregate and accumulate throughout the food web. Marine plastic pollution is to some extent irreversible. It is estimated that the amount of floating plastic in the ocean is approximately 236,000 tons (Wilcox et al., 2015). In humans, microplastics have been detected in stool samples (Schwabl et al., 2019), the gastrointestinal system (Ding et al., 2024), brain tissue (Nihart et al., 2025), and atheromas in the vasculature (Marfella et al., 2024). Microplastic exposure may enhance allergenic potentials of common allergens such as house dust mites, although further large-scale epidemiological studies are needed to validate this emerging information (Wu & Yang, 2025). Holistic nurses can guide their patients and communities on reducing exposures to plastics through information provided through the Environmental Working Group, which is based in Washington, D.C. This nongovernmental organization provides consumer guides to reduce exposures to a wide variety of environmental contaminants.

Flame retardants are compounds that are added to materials to prevent or slow down its flammability. Brominated flame-retardants (BFRs) and polybrominated diphenyl ethers (PBDEs) (another class of flame retardants) pose risks to human health. Fish and other marine products have the highest levels of BFRs due to their accumulation in the food web, and levels in North America are higher than Europe or Asian countries (Tao et al., 2024).

There is a link between flame retardant exposure and several chronic diseases. One study found an association between BFRs and Parkinson's disease in a cross-sectional study using the NHANES 2009-2016 data (Lv et al., 2024). Emerging data from NHANES demonstrates that BFR exposure may result in adverse effects on lung function (Mao et al., 2024), which may have implications for populations with preexisting airway disorders. PBDEs are known for disrupting metabolic processes associated with brain development, reproduction, and are also considered carcinogenic (Renzelli et al., 2023). Additionally, serum levels of PBDEs are associated with increased follicular-stimulating hormone and decreased inhibin-B in older men, which may influence reproductive health (Makey et al., 2016). One study found an association between serum PBDE and PBDE-associated DNA methylation changes that are linked to breast cancer risk (Ding et al., 2021). Further research is needed to fully understand the total impact of these compounds on human health. Holistic nurses can find information and prevention recommendations through the policy organizations Toxic-Free Future and the Safer States Alliance.

Glyphosate is a widely used broad-spectrum systemic herbicide that has been used globally. There is an established link, based on meta-analysis of human epidemiological studies suggesting an association between glyphosate-based herbicides and non-Hodgkin lymphoma (Zhang et al., 2019). One study found higher glyphosate exposure is linked to reduced grip strength in middle and older aged adults in the United States, based on an NHANES analysis and urinary glyphosate biomarkers (Jauregui-Zunzunegui et al., 2024). Exposure to this and other similar compounds may influence physical functional limitations, present with an aging population. Animal studies have shown a similar impact on muscle physiology and contractile strength following glyphosate exposures. Agricultural workers may be at the highest risk of glyphosate exposure due to ubiquitous usage of herbicides globally (Chang et al., 2023). There are several resources through state agriculture extension offices and national environmental agencies that holistic nurses can explore on pesticide safety and non-chemical alternatives for gardens and crop production.

Contaminant metals are ubiquitous and can occur from environmental or occupational exposures. Metals can target multiple organ systems including the brain, lungs, kidney, and blood. One study, using data from the Global Burden of Disease in 2019, identified that lead exposure is a significant burden to the development of chronic kidney disease, with the highest rates in Central Latin America and the lowest rates in Eastern Europe (Song et al., 2024). There may be socioeconomic factors that drive this impact. Chronic kidney disease is also very common in agricultural communities. Cadmium, another toxic heavy metal has been assessed as a possible molecular driver of breast cancer (Filippini et al., 2020), with a modest positive relationship between dietary cadmium and breast cancer. Arsenic exposure has consistently demonstrated increased cardiovascular disease risk. Findings from the Health Effects of Arsenic Longitudinal Study in Bangladesh suggest that well water arsenic was associated with an increase in pulse pressure (Farzan et al., 2015). Genetic variants such as the *AS3MT* mutation are associated with reduced arsenic metabolism efficiency (Delgado et al., 2021). Exposure to metal mixtures may increase parameters of oxidative stress, which can be positively associated with metals exposure (Pizent et al., 2022). Recent data suggest that children exposed to heavy metals in drinking water may have a greater cancer risk than adults (Emmanuel et al., 2022). Much of the longitudinal data from metals exposure originates from developing countries where water and food sources may be less regulated than in Western countries or the United States (Chowdhury et al., 2016). However, NHANES data suggests that approximately half of U.S. participants have multiple urinary metal biomarkers, which would indicate that metals exposure is still problematic even in Western countries such as the United States (Shim et al., 2017). The U.S. Environmental Protection Agency has guides for metals exposure prevention and screening recommendations in high-risk areas available on their website.

contribute to chronic health disease development and persistence. Other factors to consider may involve genetic susceptibility to toxicants; however, limited commercial testing is available. Toxicological exposures may also exacerbate susceptibility to other environmental exposures, such as allergens. As holistic nurses consider the future, it is important to consider susceptibility to environmental toxicants as a key factor in health and disease.

Biodiversity Loss

Biodiversity loss impacts human health in a myriad of ways. Arable land and local food systems rely on biodiversity to keep the soil healthy and nutrient dense and to pollinate fruits, as well as protect crops and ecosystems from harmful invasive species. As insect and animal systems are disrupted, the transmission of infectious diseases increases. Plants provide important sources of medicines, clean the air and process carbon dioxide, and secrete organic compounds that have microbiome and immune system benefits. Pollinators help with global food supplies, and many medicines that treat a large variety of illnesses are sourced in nature. As biodiversity and natural spaces are lost, humans experience grief and sadness, affecting mental health and well-being in large populations (Robinson et al., 2024). Holistic nurses can educate communities on the value and importance of biodiversity and give guidance and best practices for individual and community level care (avoiding pesticides and fertilizers, growing pollinator gardens and re-planting or repopulating biodiversity, etc.). To learn more, holistic nurses can visit the UN and WHO websites as well as the Planetary Health Alliance website.

Land Use, Land Cover

Land use, land cover, and changes made to environments for cities, industry, energy (e.g., damming rivers), and agriculture (e.g., deforestation) all impact human health. Urban developments can affect well-being and health, either positively or negatively (Mouratidis, 2021) including road design, the integration of nature, sound-reducing infrastructure, and exposure mitigation for urban heat islands (Kleinert & Horton, 2016). Mining activities and waste deposits that are not properly contained contaminate air, land, and water, and often leave long-term legacy waste that is harmful to human and ecosystem health. Deforestation contributes to loss of protective natural environments and plant life that absorbs greenhouse gasses and cleans the air. Holistic nurses can help patients and communities value and understand the health benefits of nature and the importance of conservation. They can also assess, at the local level, the health harms that their patients are experiencing or are at risk for. Holistic nurses can explore the multiple benefits of exposure to nature spaces and how this improves health. In addition, the WHO has guidance on how urban spaces can be designed to bolster health outcomes.

Climate Change

Climate change is the planetary-scale ecological driver that most people are familiar with. Climate change is affecting every latitude, leading to longer, hotter summers and shorter, warmer winters. As a result, humanity is witnessing the depletion of glaciers and snowpack, which is impacting freshwater supplies, contributing to sea-level rise and changing ocean circulation patterns. As temperatures rise, and temperate zones shift, changes in animal, plant, and insect populations occur. This contributes to shifts in food resources (including scarcity), as well as infectious disease patterns and frequency. Climate change is altering global weather patterns and intensifying weather-related natural disasters. This includes torrential rain/flooding, hurricanes, drought, and wildfires and extreme heat. Climate change also impacts health through weather-related climate shocks that temporarily or permanently displace people, disrupt access to food and clean water, and cause floods or fires that expose individuals to disease from air, land, and water pollutants. In addition, climate change profoundly impacts the mental health and well-being of all people, especially frontline communities, youth, and pregnant and childbearing individuals (Lee et al., 2023). Holistic nurses have a pivotal role in understanding and addressing climate change as well as the health impacts from climate change. They need to understand what their local issues are and educate their patients and communities on reducing health harms through disaster preparedness, local pollution mitigation efforts, and resilience building.

Nutrient Overloading and Cycling

Nutrient overloading and cycling occurs as the essential elements of carbon, hydrogen, nitrogen, oxygen, phosphorus, and sulfur shift and move around the systems and environments on Earth. Humans impact these biological, geological, and chemical processes in a variety of ways; through the combustion of fossil fuels, industrial practices and waste, agriculture practices, including the application of fertilizers and manure to crops, land use decisions, forest clearing, and management of water and wastewater systems. This impacts air, soil, and water quality, the quality and quantity of food, and ultimately the ability to sustain life. It is important for nurses to understand how these cycles work, and the various health hazards that result from imbalances in these cycles. Health harms include immunological and endocrine disorders, cancer, infectious diseases, and nutrient imbalances (Penuelas & Sardans, 2023). Holistic nurses need to understand their local risks and educate patients and communities about the care of the environment as well as the ongoing health hazards that are present. The Planetary Health Alliance has resources that holistic nurses can explore to explain these concepts and the possible solutions in more detail.

Ocean/Marine Degradation

Ocean/marine degradation from nonpoint sources (e.g., runoff from land), chemicals, fertilizers, plastic and other fossil fuel products, air pollution, and sewage have jeopardized the health of plant and animal life in the planet's oceans. Contaminated fish, overfishing, and marine dead zones (from chemical, oil, and fertilizer contamination) are impacting primary food sources for billions of people globally. Contaminated marine food supplies are causing significant human health problems with toxins, heavy metals, carcinogens, and endocrine- and reproductive system–disrupting chemicals (Landrigan et al., 2020). Holistic nurses can educate their patient populations on fish contamination, sustainable fishing practices, and sea foods to avoid. In addition, anything that reduces runoff from land, including sewage, effluent, waste (and single-use plastic waste) will help to reduce the impacts of pollution in the oceans. Holistic nurses can work with local communities to identify the community-specific health issues from ocean degradation, and how to prevent further damage through good community environmental stewardship. The Planetary Health Alliance and the National Oceanic and Atmospheric Administration in the United States, as well as similar national-level organizations worldwide, have resources that can help holistic nurses understand and reduce the health harms from marine degradation.

Resource Scarcity

Resource scarcity has an impact on health. Freshwater and arable land supplies are dwindling from climate change, poorly planned urban/rural water infrastructure, and contamination from pollution. Holistic nurses need to recognize the importance of water conservation, equitable water infrastructure, and the value of local regenerative agriculture practices, as well as local food security. Freshwater and healthy food are fundamental to human health and community resilience. In the planetary health model, nurses can promote sustainable, locally-grown food and advocate to ensure adequate, safe, and smart water access. Holistic nurses can follow the advocacy and work of The Nature Conservancy, the Sierra Club, and the U.S. Water Alliance as a few of many ways to become better informed about the health of water and land.

Planetary health can be used to guide holistic nurses in their work to advocate for the health and well-being of their patients and communities, as well as for future generations. This approach promotes the understanding that health is interconnected and that sustainable health practices, educate patients about the interconnectedness of human and environmental health, and contribute to a global movement aimed at healing both people and the planet. Holistic nurses can increase their "Planetary Health Literacy" (Jochem et al., 2023) through spending time understanding their local social and ecological determinants that impact the health and well-being of their patients and communities.

Nesting the various *socioecological and environmental determinants of health* helps to narrate the symbiotic relationships between individual health, community health, public health, environmental health, global health, and planetary health. Global health initiatives often reflect broader environmental shifts, prioritizing improved health and health equity for all people worldwide. Public health strategies are shaped by community-specific environmental factors, and community health is influenced by local ecological conditions, emphasizing the importance of sustainable living practices. Environmental health underpins all these facets by ensuring that the natural world remains a supportive habitat for human life. This interconnection echoes the profound wisdom of Indigenous and traditional health models, which have long recognized the necessity of living in harmony with the Earth and should guide the work of planetary health (Redvers et al., 2022) underscoring the importance of respecting and preserving the environment as a foundation for robust health across all levels of society (Brand et al., 2023).

Holistic nurses can combine the multiple determinants of health frameworks to understand the various ways to explore health impacts and strategies to promote health and well-being through practice, leadership, education, advocacy, scholarship and research, and engagement in community.

Nested Determinants of Health

Genetics and Microbiome

Holistic nurses recognize how genetics, epigenetics, genomics, and the health of microbiomes can be impacted over time by diseases, infections, and exposure to pollutants and disasters. The quality of food and water, and access to healthy nature, improves the microbiome; as nature and the environment experience degradation and people consume food that interferes with a healthy microbiome, disease and immune system dysfunction occurs. Holistic nurses can recognize and research these cellular level determinants and drivers of health. Their work is to advocate for safety from harmful exposures, provide education for patients and communities about these, conduct screening for risks and exposures, and advocate for safer environments and better protections.

Individual/Personal

Holistic nurses can help educate people to gain skills and adopt behaviors to promote health in the context of their unique physical, emotional, and spiritual needs. Additionally, they can educate patients about environmental health risks and sustainable living practices. They can empower them to recognize the importance of nature on their health, and to provide knowledge and promote skills for health. Holistic nurses can also help guide patients on how to reduce their exposures to environmental contaminants and chemicals, and their consumption of unhealthy processed food and products that contribute to disease.

Interpersonal

Holistic nurses can foster strong, supportive relationships between healthcare systems and patients to build trust and improve health outcomes. Holistic nurses can engage in outreach programs and partnerships to educate the public about holistic health, preventive care, and environmental health issues. They can develop and facilitate peer support groups where patients can share experiences and encourage each other.

Community

Holistic nurses can help support community relationships to connect people with each other and community resources. They can influence their local community environments/microsystems to promote health and well-being through supporting resilient infrastructure and promoting preparedness in the context of environmental degradation and extreme weather, drought, wildfires, flooding, etc.

Supportive community resources include local sustainable food systems, emergency preparedness planning, and well-designed and safe places to learn, live, and work. Communities can support access to natural spaces and integrate trees and pedestrian walkways into urban design. Community members can collaborate with local organizations, schools, and businesses to create health-promoting environments and resources, such as community gardens, clean-up initiatives, and educational workshops on sustainability and environmental stewardship.

Social/Cultural

Holistic nurses can support a culture of interconnection within nature and collective well-being through their thoughtful presence, advocacy, and community engagement work. As nurses connect their values for mutual flourishing, partnership, and connection, they can inform the values and social practices in their surroundings.

Organizational/Structural

Within organizational settings, holistic nurses can advocate for and support policies and practices that focus on health equity and mutual flourishing. In health care, they can cocreate systems that integrate holistic health sensibilities and wellness promotion into standard care. They can encourage responsible and sustainable practices like reducing waste, conserving energy, and promoting a healthy indoor environment by improving air quality and reducing the use of harmful chemicals.

Societal

Holistic nurses can advocate for public policies that address the socioecological and structural determinants of health and the SDG initiatives. Holistic nurses can advocate for access to clean water, nutritious food, safety, affordable housing, adequate income, and nature connection. They can work toward reducing health disparities by supporting initiatives that promote community health and health infrastructure and advocating for health equity and access to care. They can also promote environmental health policies that ensure communities have clean air, safe drinking water, healthy land, and protected natural spaces.

Planetary

Holistic nurses can work with their communities and across sectors and disciplines to follow the Planetary Health Alliance Global Planetary Health Road Map and Action Plan and heed the call of the Planetary Health Alliance Sao Paulo Declaration, which states:

> We need a fundamental shift in how we live on Earth, what we are calling the Great Transition. Achieving the Great Transition will require rapid and deep structural changes across most dimensions of human activity. This includes how we produce and consume food, energy, and manufactured goods; how we construct and live in our cities; and how we consider and measure growth, progress and development, and govern ourselves. It will also require rethinking our values and relationship within Nature and to each other from human exceptionalism, domination, and scarcity to interdependence, equity, and regeneration. The Great Transition offers the possibility of greater richness of experience, greater well-being, and an enhanced opportunity for all beings to thrive. It will take practitioners, scholars, and policy makers across every dimension of human activity working together. It will require listening to, integrating, and amplifying voices in every community from Indigenous Peoples, faith traditions, artists, entrepreneurs, to scientists. Every person, in every place, from every calling, has a role to play in safeguarding the health of the planet and people for future generations. (Planetary Health Alliance, 2021)

Special Considerations for Health Equity

Children

Children are a vulnerable, high-risk population. Each age group has its own vulnerabilities due to anatomical, physiological, and developmental factors. Children are affected by environmental pollution and climate change at every stage of development. Children with complex medical needs are at an even greater risk and need special attention (Cowen et al., 2023). Holistic nurses can approach care of the child and family through the lens of the child's personal environment, local environmental and climate challenges, and the greater global environmental perspective. This holistic approach can be implemented at every level of care and setting.

Areas of focus when caring for children's health with environmental considerations are as follows:

- Air quality and air pollution has shown to have effects on those with asthma and an association with autism spectrum disorder (ASD), lowbirth weight, and preterm births (Bekkar et al., 2020; McDermott-Levy et al., 2023b; National Institute of Environmental Health Sciences [NIEHS], 2024).
- Water quality and availability impacts hydration and hygiene (Cook et al., 2022; WHO, 2023).
- Soil quality and food source acquisition have potential effects to gut health, nutrition, and neurodevelopment (WHO, 2019).
- Heat-related illness affects children, who are prone to dehydration and heat exhaustion (Mangus & Canares, 2019).
- Loss of biodiversity in ecosystems affects mental well-being and can cause eco-anxiety (Clayton, 2020; Prescott et al., 2022).
- Disasters and extreme weather events are linked to stress, depression, displacement, loss of healthcare access, lack of access to basic survival resources, and loss of routine with school, recreation, and peers (Romanello et al., 2022).
- Exposure to toxins, pesticides, and heavy metals (lead and mercury) has adverse health effects to growth and development. There is also a link to an increase in autism with exposure in utero (NIEHS, 2024).
- Increase in emerging infectious disease affects children, who are susceptible due to compromised immune systems (Ostfeld & Keesing, 2020).

Children and adolescents may find that involvement in activism is beneficial. Websites like Talk Climate offer age-appropriate resources.

Black, Indigenous, and Other Historically Marginalized Communities

Black, Indigenous, and other historically marginalized communities in the United States and internationally often bear a disproportionate burden from environmental degradation and health disparities, which makes the connection between environmental and planetary health and holistic nursing crucial. These communities experience high rates of pollution-related illnesses, limited or lacking access to safe water and food, and are often more vulnerable to climate change–mediated disasters. By adopting a holistic approach, nurses can integrate environmental justice and leadership into their practice by advocating for healthier environments, food and water security, and disaster-resilient infrastructure. Environmental justice is when all people have the same protections from environmental health hazards. The Climate and Health Outlook Portal and Agency for Toxic Substances and Disease Registry are useful resources to help identify areas and populations that need attention.

Aging Populations

Aging populations can be particularly vulnerable to the impacts of environmental degradation and planetary health issues, such as extreme weather events, pollution, and the loss of natural resources, which can exacerbate chronic health conditions and limit their mobility. Holistic nursing addresses these challenges by considering the interconnectedness of environmental and human health, advocating for sustainable practices that protect both the planet and the well-being of the aging population. Through holistic care, nurses can support the older adult in adapting to environmental changes, promote healthy aging, and ensure continued access to safe, clean, and sustainable living environments.

Pregnancy

Pregnancy is also a critical period during which the health of both the mother and the developing fetus is intricately linked to the environment. Environmental pollutants, such as pesticides, heavy metals, and air pollution, negatively impact maternal and fetal health. These exposures lead to complications such as preterm birth, low birth weight, and developmental disorders. Holistic nursing plays a vital role in promoting environmental and planetary health by advocating for safe, responsible environmental policies and practices that reduce exposure to harmful toxins. By integrating these sensibilities into prenatal care, holistic nurses can implement programs that educate and provide adequate support for expectant mothers so that they can minimize their exposure to environmental hazards. Holistic nurses can also promote access to safe, nutrient dense, fresh, healthy diets. This approach not only promotes the well-being of the mother and child but also contributes to the broader goal of creating healthier environments for future generations.

Mental Health

Mental health is profoundly affected by environmental and planetary health issues, such as climate change, pollution, and the loss of natural spaces. These environmental stressors can contribute to increased rates of anxiety, depression, and other mental health disorders. Holistic nursing recognizes the deep connection between the environment and mental and emotional well-being. Holistic nurses can help with this problem through advocacy for interventions that promote both planetary and mental health. By incorporating nature-based therapies, such as ecotherapy and mindfulness practices in natural settings, holistic nurses can help individuals manage stress and improve their mental health. They can also advocate for policies that protect natural environments, ensuring that communities have access to green spaces that support mental wellness. Through a holistic approach, nurses can address the environmental determinants of mental health, fostering resilience, and promoting overall well-being in the face of planetary health challenges.

Within a holistic paradigm, mental health is seen in conjunction with the whole. As the global climate crisis grows, there will likely be a greater mental health effect on the general population. The WHO (2024b) is urging countries to include mental health support in their climate crisis response. Many emotions can interplay as society experiences the effects of climate change, such as sadness, hopelessness, anger, fear, guilt, and insecurity. Words such as *eco-anxiety*, *eco-grief*, and *solastalgia* are mental health terms used to describe emotions people may feel in response to disruption and loss resulting from ecological changes in the planet. Evidence has shown both direct and indirect linkages between changes in climate and human behavior, including adverse mental health disorders (Ingle & Mikulewicz, 2020). Future generations are especially at risk, as they will be chronologically more exposed to climate change effects. Holistic nurses can assist individuals and communities with coping behaviors by using the holistic nursing process to assess, educate, advocate, and offer health promotion strategies to enhance mental well-being.

Nurses on the Frontlines

Nurses on the frontlines bear witness to the stark health disparities faced by vulnerable populations, including children, BIPOC communities, and older adults. These dedicated professionals often witness firsthand the profound effects of socioeconomic inequality, lack of access to health care, and environmental degradation. They encounter patients whose conditions are exacerbated by inadequate living conditions, poor nutrition, and limited access to medical resources. These experiences highlight the immense strain on health systems and the physical and emotional toll on nurses who strive to provide compassionate care amidst these challenges. Health systems struggle to meet the growing demands of underserved communities, often with insufficient resources, compounding the difficulties faced by these vulnerable groups. These realities call for a collective reimagining of sensibilities and responsibilities toward health and well-being. It is an invitation to redesign the approach to healthcare, emphasizing equity, sustainability, and a commitment to addressing the root causes of health disparities including the environmental and planetary-scale ecological determinants of health. By fostering a more inclusive and resilient health system, all individuals, regardless of their circumstances, can achieve optimal health and well-being.

Disaster Preparedness in the Context of Climate Change

As healthcare leaders and trusted professionals, holistic nurses can lead the charge for community resilience in the wake of increased frequency and intensity of disaster-related weather events driven by climate change. Holistic nurses understand the significance of the public's health in the preparation and aftermath of these events. Holistic communication, education, and dissemination of accurate information to the public is essential to prepare communities to either weather the event in a safe manner or evacuate as necessary. In the aftermath, holistic nurses may volunteer through the American Red Cross, state and regional government agencies, or other emergency preparedness organizations. They may also work within their own healthcare systems to triage and treat those affected. Using the holistic principles of relationship-centered care and the human health experience, holistic nurses play an integral part in the healing process of communities experiencing disasters.

Extreme Heat

The risk of heat-related illness (HRI) is driven by heat exposure, individual susceptibility, and sociocultural factors. As HRI is preventable, holistic nurses play a role in identifying those at risk and providing education and strategies to prevent exposure. Populations particularly at risk of HRI include those of advanced age, infants and children, pregnant mothers, those with disabilities or chronic medical conditions, outdoor workers, athletes, people experiencing homelessness, low-income households or those without air conditioning. Actions for holistic nurses include the following:

- Be aware of state and local health advisory alerts.
- Screen patients for heat risk using assessments such as the HeatRisk tool by the Centers for Disease Control and Prevention that displays a map of daily heat risk across the United States with actions to take.
- Assist patients to develop and implement a heat action plan.
- Review any conditions or medications that put patients at risk for HRI. People with cardiovascular, respiratory, and renal conditions are at risk for exacerbations. Medications such as antidepressants, central nervous system stimulants, anticholinergics, antipsychotics, insulin, and cardiac drugs can increase the risk of HRI.
- Understand signs and nursing management of HRI, such as heat exhaustion and heat stroke.
- Determine safe discharge planning during extreme heat through electronic health record triggers.
- Inform patients how to find cooling centers in their vicinity.
- Promote the use of "check on your neighbor" programs (Sorensen & Hess, 2022).

Flooding

Floods are the most common disaster in the United States. Flooding results from an overflow of water from rain, snow, or storm surge that develops slowly or quickly. Holistic nurses can promote health before a flooding event through strategic planning, scenario review, and education efforts such as:

- Help patients to determine their flood risk and make a plan for a flood response. Note evacuation routes to higher ground.
- Preparing a flood kit that contains non-perishable foods, drinking water, cleaning

supplies, and medications for several days. For patients that are technology dependent, prepare a "to-go" bag with back-up batteries.

- Flood waters that remain in homes for more than 24–48 hours can result in mold formation, which affects indoor air quality. Inhaling mold can have adverse health effects.
- Avoid contact with flood water, as it may contain bacteria, chemicals, or hazardous materials that are harmful.
- Generator exhaust is toxic due to carbon monoxide. Implement safety measures with generators.
- Have drinking water available and follow local boil advisories.
- Help prevent the spread of mosquito-borne disease (Environmental Protection Agency [EPA], 2024a; U.S. Department of Homeland Security, 2024).

Wildfires

In 2022 in the United States, 66,255 fires burned 7,534,403 acres (National Centers for Environmental Information, 2022). Wildfire smoke is a mix of gases and particles from burning trees, plants, buildings, and other materials. Wildfire season is usually in the summer and early fall, although wildfires are unpredictable and can spread rapidly. To promote health in the event of a wildfire, holistic nurses can follow these recommendations:

- Encourage patients to stay informed by signing up for air quality alerts on their mobile devices. Additionally, ensure they have a planned evacuation route in case of emergencies.
- Be aware of the air quality index, especially for those with chronic respiratory disease. Indoor air quality can also be impacted, as smoke may enter homes.
- Educate patients on the health effects of particle pollution. Particulate matter from dust, soot, and smoke produced by wildfires can cause health problems depending on the size of the particles. Small particles less than 10 micrometers pose the greatest problem, as they can get into the lungs and bloodstream, leading to pulmonary and cardiovascular effects.
- Inhaling wildfire smoke can irritate the eyes, nose, and throat and cause wheezing, coughing, or difficulty breathing. Inhalation can exacerbate existing lung and heart disease.
- Educate patients to stay indoors, close windows and vents, use a MERV 13 or higher filter for HVAC systems, use an air HEPA filter, and use an N95 respirator outdoors (Colorado Department of Public Health and Environment, 2024; EPA, 2024b).

Healthcare System Sustainability

The healthcare sector emits approximately 8.5 percent of U.S. carbon emissions. Healthcare organizations have huge potential to have sociopolitical influences on decarbonization. The National Academy of Medicine (2024) has established a Climate Collaborative with the goal of decarbonizing the U.S. health sector. Members include hospital systems, clinicians, pharmaceuticals, academia, private payers, nonprofits, and the federal government. Areas of focus include supply chain, infrastructure, healthcare delivery, education, policy, and finance. For healthcare organizations, the process starts with establishing a sustainability team, performing a greenhouse gas inventory, setting goals, and implementing a plan toward decarbonization. Emissions can be reduced in the following areas: sustainable building design, anesthetic gasses, pressurized metered-dose inhalers, physical waste, single-use plastics, food services, and transportation.

Values and Ethics of Planetary and Environmental Health for Holistic Nurses

Healthcare professionals have a moral responsibility to act to protect all living things on the Earth. They do this by reducing overconsumption and making mindful, conscientious decisions when using resources. They also have an intergenerational responsibility to be a custodian of the Earth by leaving it in a viable condition for future generations (Foster et al., 2020). The ethical principles of benevolence, nonmaleficence, autonomy, veracity, and justice all apply to the field of planetary health. Using these principles, humans must respect nature and Indigenous wisdom when caring for the planet, do no more harm, give people the right to know and choose, uphold the truth, and advocate for equity. It is well known that those who contribute least to the degradation of the planet suffer the most, referred to as the "downstream effect." For example, the top 10 percent of global income earners produce almost 50 percent of total carbon emissions per person, while the bottom 50 percent produce only 7 percent (Howard et al., 2023). Holistic nurses must advocate for social justice. Holistic nurses can convey the importance of ethical stewardship through story. Using story helps to communicate a message of loving kindness and compassion toward the Earth and all who inhabit here. As Howard et al. (2023) described:

> Stories can transform values into the emotions needed to drive change, with anger helping overcome apathy, hope conquering fear, solidarity alleviating isolation, and inspiration found in stories of successful change making, which yield the sense that individuals can make a difference. (p. e260)

Integration of Planetary Health into the Domains of Nursing

Practice

Holistic nurses can:

- Play a key role in educating patients, families, and communities about the impact of environmental health on human well-being. They can advocate for policies and practices that protect natural ecosystems and promote sustainable living in both their workplaces and personal lives.
- Deepen their knowledge of the connection between ecosystems and human health by exploring resources like the EnviroAtlas Eco-Health Relationship Browser. This knowledge supports informed advocacy and patient education.
- Encourage healthy, sustainable eating habits by advocating for the consumption of locally sourced, organic, and plant-based foods. They can also educate patients on how food choices impact the environment and the benefits of supporting sustainable agriculture.
- Help communities prepare for environmental disasters and the impacts of climate change. By understanding these health risks, they can support emergency preparedness, build community resilience, and advocate for policies that protect vulnerable populations.
- Create healing spaces in healthcare settings by reducing waste, minimizing harmful chemicals, and adopting green healthcare practices. Emphasizing self-care and mindfulness for both nurses and patients supports sustainable well-being, reinforcing that environmental health begins with personal health.

Leadership

Holistic nurses can:

- Take the Planetary Health Pledge for Healthcare Professionals in the Anthropocene (LeClair & Potter, 2022; Wabnitz et al., 2020) to commit to sustainable and equitable health practices.
- Partner with global Indigenous communities. Holistic nurses can draw upon these partnerships to enrich environmental and planetary health initiatives with traditional ecological knowledge and practices.
- Integrate nature-based therapies into care plans. Holistic nurses can recommend activities like spending time outdoors, gardening, or incorporating natural elements such as plants, water features, and natural light in healthcare settings to support healing and well-being.
- Participate in nursing work groups focused on environmental health at local, state, national, and international levels to influence health policy efforts.

- Apply the principles of planetary health in both hospital and community settings, leading initiatives for environmentally sustainable practices and raising awareness of current environmental challenges.
- Form interdisciplinary "green teams." Holistic nurses can collaboratively address climate change and sustainability efforts within healthcare facilities.

Education

Holistic nurses can:

- Embed planetary health concepts into all levels of nursing education so that nurses understand and address the complex interconnections between human health and the environment. By incorporating topics such as environmental sustainability, climate change, and health equity into their educational programs, holistic nurses can raise awareness and educate both their peers and the communities they serve about the significance of planetary health.
- Design courses in planetary health or integrate these concepts into existing curricula. This includes developing standalone courses focused on planetary health as well as infusing relevant topics into courses on public health, nursing ethics, and community health to ensure a comprehensive understanding of the interconnectedness of health and the environment.
- Emphasize the importance of planetary health as part of professional development. Nurses should be encouraged to pursue ongoing education and training in planetary health, including workshops, seminars, and conferences that focus on the latest research and practices in this field.
- Partner with organizations that have developed open-access educational materials on climate change and planetary health, such as the Alliance of Nurses for Healthy Environments, the Global Consortium on Climate and Health Education, and the Planetary Health Alliance, to enhance educational offerings and promote interdisciplinary learning.
- Offer experiential educational opportunities, either through simulated activities or community service learning (National League for Nursing, 2022), allowing students to apply their knowledge in real-world contexts and engage directly with environmental health issues in their communities.

Advocacy

Holistic nurses can:

- Advocate for policies and practices that promote environmental responsibility in healthcare settings, such as reducing waste, conserving resources, and supporting sustainable healthcare initiatives.
- Study the connections between environmental health and human health. By integrating findings into practice, they can examine the effects of pollution, climate change, and biodiversity loss on health and develop interventions to mitigate these impacts.
- Recognize the therapeutic benefits of nature and encourage patients to spend time in natural settings. This approach can help reduce stress, improve mood, and enhance overall mental health through practices like forest bathing, mindfulness in nature, and outdoor physical activities.
- Participate in community outreach programs that educate the public on the importance of environmental health and wellness. By organizing workshops, health fairs, or informational sessions, they can empower communities to make informed choices that promote both personal and planetary health.

Scholarship

Holistic nurses can:

- Collaborate with other healthcare professionals, environmental organizations, and community groups to develop and implement initiatives that promote environmental health and sustainability.
- Join the collective voice advocating for the planet's health. Some global nurse advocacy groups include Nurses Drawdown, the International

Council of Nurses, and the Global Consortium for Climate and Health Education.
- Integrate planetary health concepts into individual and community assessments and interventions.
- Participate in research initiatives to explore the impacts of environmental factors on health outcomes, contributing to the body of knowledge in planetary health and influencing best practices in nursing.
- Publish their findings and best practices through journals, conferences, and community workshops to share valuable insights and advancements in the field of planetary health, fostering a culture of inquiry and ongoing education among peers. Potential areas for nursing scholarship and science include:
    - Human causes and health implications of climate change.
    - Mitigation and adaptation strategies.
    - Factors or experiences that influence the human need for interconnectedness with the planet .
    - How being in nature fosters healing in the human body.
    - Climate justice.
    - Identifying barriers to implementation of environmental health practices and strategies to overcome perceived barriers (Woychik et al., 2022).

Engagement (Personal and Community)

Holistic nurses can:

- Engage with local communities in activities that connect people with nature, such as organizing nature walks, community gardening projects, or educational workshops on environmental stewardship and sustainable living, making a significant impact.
- Foster partnerships with local schools or universities and community organizations to promote environmental health education, empowering individuals to take an active role in protecting their surroundings.
- Participate in public forums and community events to raise awareness about the importance of planetary health, sharing knowledge and resources that inspire collective action for a healthier environment.
- Support nursing organizations in their commitment to the urgency of educating nursing students, practicing nurses, and the public on planetary health concepts. In addition to the American Holistic Nurses Association, organizations include the American Nurses Association, National League for Nursing, American Association of Colleges of Nursing, and Sigma. Implications for education include:
    - Integrating planetary health topics into nursing curricula to highlight the links between environmental health and patient well-being.
    - Offering professional development programs focused on planetary health to enhance the skills of practicing nurses.
    - Creating community outreach initiatives that engage nursing students in promoting environmental health awareness.
    - Supporting research on effective teaching strategies for conveying planetary health concepts in nursing education.
    - Encouraging collaboration with interdisciplinary programs to broaden the scope of planetary health education.

Conclusion

Holistic nurses can cultivate a sense of responsibility and solidarity with the planet, its natural systems, and its diverse peoples, helping to drive the systemic changes needed for a fair and sustainable future for all life. The Great Transition (Planetary Health Alliance, 2021) represents a regeneration for humanity on Earth. Indifference is not an option; people must consider substituting "stewardship for domination, reverence for arrogance, and coexistence for conquest" (Frumkin & Myers, 2020, p. 492). Holistic nurses empower their patients with hope as they move from a state of decline toward a future where humans engage with the planet in reciprocity and openness to new ways of knowing (Foster et al., 2020). Humanity has a responsibility to redesign the systems and sensibilities that will shape a better future.

References

Albert, N. M., Pappas, S. H., Porter-O'Grady, T., & Malloch, K. (2022). *Quantum Leadership: Creating sustainable value in healthcare* (6th ed.). Jones & Bartlett Learning.

Bekkar, B., Pacheco, S., Basu, R., & DeNicola, N. (2020). Association of air pollution and heat exposure with preterm birth, low birth weight, and stillbirth in the US: A systematic review. *JAMA Network Open, 3*(6). https://doi.org/10.1001/jamanetworkopen.2020.824

Brand, G., Wise, S., Bedi, G., & Kickett, R. (2023). Embedding Indigenous knowledges and voices in planetary health education. *The Lancet Planetary Health, 7*(1), e97–e102.

Chang, V. C., Andreotti, G., Ospina, M., Parks, C. G., Liu, D., Shearer, J. J., Rothman, N., Silverman, D. T., Sandler, D. P., & Calafat, A. M. (2023). Glyphosate exposure and urinary oxidative stress biomarkers in the Agricultural Health Study. *JNCI: Journal of the National Cancer Institute, 115*(4), 394–404.

Chowdhury, S., Mazumder, M. J., Al-Attas, O., & Husain, T. (2016). Heavy metals in drinking water: Occurrences, implications, and future needs in developing countries. *Science of the Total Environment, 569*, 476–488.

Clayton, S. (2020). Mental health on a changing planet. In S. Myers, & H. Frumkin (Eds.), *Planetary health: Protecting nature to protect ourselves* (pp. 221–259). Island Press.

Colorado Department of Public Health and Environment. (2024). *Wildfire smoke and health.* https://cdphe.colorado.gov/outdoor-burning/wildfire-smoke-and-health

Cook, C., Huffling, K., Hulick, A., & Blake, S. B. (2022). *Water and health: Opportunities for nursing action*. Alliance of Nurses for Healthy Environments. https://envirn.org/water-and-health/

Cowen, K., Wisely, L., Dawson, R., Ball, J., & Bindler, R. (2023). *Principles of pediatric nursing: Caring for children* (8th ed.). Pearson.

Dairkee, S. H., Moore, D. H., Luciani, M. G., Anderle, N., Gerona, R., Ky, K., Torres, S. M., Marshall, P. V., & Goodson III, W. H. (2023). Reduction of daily-use parabens and phthalates reverses accumulation of cancer-associated phenotypes within disease-free breast tissue of study subjects. *Chemosphere, 322*, 138014.

Delgado, D. A., Chernoff, M., Huang, L., Tong, L., Chen, L., Jasmine, F., Shinkle, J., Cole, S. A., Haack, K., & Kent, J. (2021). Rare, protein-altering variants in AS3MT and arsenic metabolism efficiency: A multi-population association study. *Environmental Health Perspectives, 129*(4), 047007.

Ding, R., Chen, Y., Shi, X., Li, Y., Yu, Y., Sun, Z., & Duan, J. (2024). Size-dependent toxicity of polystyrene microplastics on the gastrointestinal tract: Oxidative stress related-DNA damage and potential carcinogenicity. *Science of the Total Environment, 912*, 169514.

Ding, Y. C., Hurley, S., Park, J.-S., Steele, L., Rakoff, M., Zhu, Y., Zhao, J., LaBarge, M., Bernstein, L., & Chen, S. (2021). Methylation biomarkers of polybrominated diphenyl ethers (PBDEs) and association with breast cancer risk at the time of menopause. *Environment International, 156*, 106772.

Dominski, F. H., Branco, J. H. L., Buonanno, G., Stabile, L., da Silva, M. G., & Andrade, A. (2021). Effects of air pollution on health: A mapping review of systematic reviews and meta-analyses. *Environmental Research, 201*, 111487.

Emmanuel, U. C., Chukwudi, M. I., Monday, S. S., & Anthony, A. I. (2022). Human health risk assessment of heavy metals in drinking water sources in three senatorial districts of Anambra State, Nigeria. *Toxicology Reports, 9*, 869–875.

Environmental Protection Agency. (2024a). *Flooding*. https://www.epa.gov/natural-disasters/flooding

Environmental Protection Agency. (2024b). *Wildfires*. https://www.epa.gov/natural-disasters/wildfires#prepare

Farzan, S. F., Karagas, M. R., Jiang, J., Wu, F., Liu, M., Newman, J. D., Jasmine, F., Kibriya, M. G., Paul-Brutus, R., & Parvez, F. (2015). Gene–arsenic interaction in longitudinal changes of blood pressure: Findings from the Health Effects of Arsenic Longitudinal Study (HEALS) in Bangladesh. *Toxicology and Applied Pharmacology, 288*(1), 95–105.

Filippini, T., Torres, D., Lopes, C., Carvalho, C., Moreira, P., Naska, A., Kasdagli, M.-I., Malavolti, M., Orsini, N., & Vinceti, M. (2020). Cadmium exposure and risk of breast cancer: A dose-response meta-analysis of cohort studies. *Environment International, 142*, 105879.

Foster, A., Cole, J., Petrikova, I., Farlow, A., & Frumkin, H. (2020). Planetary health ethics. In S. Myers, & H. Frumkin (Eds.), *Planetary health: Protecting nature to protect ourselves* (pp. 453–473). Island Press.

Frumkin, H., & Myers, S. (2020). Afterword: Coronavirus and planetary health. In S. Myers & H. Frumkin (Eds.), *Planetary health: Protecting nature to protect ourselves* (pp. 487–495). Island Press.

Guo, T., Meng, X., Liu, X., Wang, J., Yan, S., Zhang, X., Wang, M., Ren, S., & Huang, Y. (2023). Associations of phthalates with prostate cancer among the U.S. population. *Reproductive Toxicology, 116*, 108337.

Guzmán, C. A. F., Aguirre, A. A., Astle, B., Barros, E., Bayles, B., Chimbari, M., El-Abbadi, N., Evert, J., Hackett, F., Howard, C., Jennings, J., Krzyzek, A., LeClair, J., Maric, F., Martin, O., Osano, O., Patz, J., Potter, T., Redvers, N., ... Zylstra, M. (2021). A framework to guide planetary health education. *The Lancet Planetary Health, 5*(5), e253–e255.

Howard, C., MacNeill, A. J., Hughes, F., Alqodmani, L., Charlesworth, K., de Almeida, R., Harris, R., Jochum, B., Maibach, B., Maki, L., McGain, F., Miller, J., Nirmala, M., Pencheon, D., Robertson, S., Sherman, J., Vipond, J., Yin, H., & Montgomery, H. (2023). Learning to treat the climate emergency together: Social tipping interventions by the health community. *The Lancet, 7*, e251–e264.

Ingle, H. E., & Mikulewicz, M. (2020). Mental health and climate change: Tackling invisible injustice. *The Lancet, 4*(4), e128–e130.

Jauregui-Zunzunegui, S., Rodríguez-Artalejo, F., Tellez-Plaza, M., & García-Esquinas, E. (2024). Glyphosate exposure, muscular health and functional limitations in middle-aged and older adults. *Environmental Research*, *251*, 118547.

Jochem, C., von Sommoggy, J., Hornidge, A. K., Schwien horst-Stich, E. M., & Apfelbacher, C. (2023). Planetary health literacy: A conceptual model. *Frontiers in Public Health*, *10*, 980779.

Kleinert, S., & Horton, R. (2016). Urban design: an important future force for health and wellbeing. *The Lancet*, *388*(10062), 2848–2850.

Landrigan, P. J., Stegeman, J. J., Fleming, L. E., Allemand, D., Anderson, D. M., Backer, L. C., Brucker-Davis, F., Chevalier, N., Corra, L., Czerucka, D., Bottein, M.Y. D., Demeneix, B., Depledge, M., Deheyn, D. D., Dorman, C. J., Fénichel, P., Fisher, S., Gaill, F., Galgani, F., … Rampal, P. (2020). Human health and ocean pollution. *Annals of Global Health*, *86*(1), 151. https://doi.org/10.5334/aogh.2831

LeClair, J., & Potter, T. (2022). Planetary health nursing: Practical implications for research, education advocacy, and practice. *American Journal of Nursing, 122*(4), 47–52.

Lee, H., Romero, J., Arora, M., Birt, A., Drost, E., Flato, G., Forster, P., Friedlingstein, P., Fuglestvedt, J., Hawkins, E., Jotzo, F., Li, M., Masson-Delmotte, V., Meinshausen, M., Mulugetta, Y., Pathak, M., Pereira, J., Pirani, A., ... Skea, J. (2023). *Climate change 2023 synthesis report summary for policymakers*. Intergovernmental Panel on Climate Change.

Lewis, R. C., Johns, L. E., & Meeker, J. D. (2015). Serum biomarkers of exposure to perfluoroalkyl substances in relation to serum testosterone and measures of thyroid function among adults and adolescents from NHANES 2011–2012. *International Journal of Environmental Research and Public Health*, *12*(6), 6098–6114.

López-Carrillo, L., Hernández-Ramírez, R. U., Calafat, A. M., Torres-Sánchez, L., Galván-Portillo, M., Needham, L. L., Ruiz-Ramos, R., & Cebrián, M. E. (2010). Exposure to phthalates and breast cancer risk in northern Mexico. *Environmental Health Perspectives*, *118*(4), 539–544.

Lv, J.-j., Zhang, Y.-c., Li, X.-y., Zhang, L.-J., Yixi, Z.-M., Yang, C.-H., & Wang, X.-H. (2024). The association between brominated flame retardants exposure with Parkinson's disease in U.S. adults: A cross-sectional study of the National Health and Nutrition Examination Survey 2009–2016. *Frontiers in Public Health*, *12*, 1451686.

Macy, J., & Johnstone, C. (2022). *Active hope (revised): How to face the mess we're in with unexpected resilience and creative power*. New World Library.

Maddela, N. R., Ramakrishnan, B., Kakarla, D., Venkateswarlu, K., & Megharaj, M. (2022). Major contaminants of emerging concern in soils: A perspective on potential health risks. *RSC Advances*, *12*(20), 12396–12415.

Makey, C. M., McClean, M. D., Braverman, L. E., Pearce, E. N., Sjödin, A., Weinberg, J., & Webster, T. F. (2016). Polybrominated diphenyl ether exposure and reproductive hormones in North American men. *Reproductive Toxicology*, 62, 46–52.

Mangus, C. W., & Canares, T. L. (2019). Heat-related illness in children in an era of extreme temperatures. *Pediatrics in Review*, 40(3), 97–107.

Manisalidis, I., Stavropoulou, E., Stavropoulos, A., & Bezirtzoglou, E. (2020). Environmental and health impacts of air pollution: A review. *Frontiers in Public Health*, *8*, 14.

Mao, H., Lin, T., Huang, S., Xie, Z., Jin, S., Shen, X., Jin, Y., & Ding, Y. (2024). The impact of brominated flame retardants (BFRs) on pulmonary function in U.S. adults: A cross-sectional study based on NHANES (2007–2012). *Scientific Reports*, *14*(1), 6486.

Marfella, R., Prattichizzo, F., Sardu, C., Fulgenzi, G., Graciotti, L., Spadoni, T., D'Onofrio, N., Scisciola, L., La Grotta, R., & Frigé, C. (2024). Microplastics and nanoplastics in atheromas and cardiovascular events. *New England Journal of Medicine*, *390*(10), 900–910.

McDermott-Levy, R., Jackman-Murphy, K., Leffers, J., & Cantu, A. G. (Eds.). (2023a). *Environmental health in nursing* (3rd ed.). Alliance of Nurses for Healthy Environments.

McDermott-Levy, R., Pennea, E., & Moore, C. (2023b). Protecting children's health: Asthma and climate change. *The American Journal of Maternal Child Nursing*, *48*(4), 188–194. https://doi.org/10.1097/NMC.0000000000000927

Moon, J., & Mun, Y. (2024). The association between per-and polyfluoroalkyl substances (PFASs) and brain, esophageal, melanomatous skin, prostate, and lung cancer using the 2003–2018 U.S. National Health and Nutrition Examination Survey (NHANES) datasets. *Heliyon*, *10*(2).

Mouratidis, K. (2021). Urban planning and quality of life: A review of pathways linking the built environment to subjective well-being. *Cities*, *115*, 103229.

Myers, S., & Frumkin, H. (2020). *Planetary health: protecting nature to protect ourselves*. Island Press.

Myers, S. S., Pivor, J. I., & Saraiva, A. M. (2021). The São Paulo declaration on planetary health. *The Lancet*, *398*(10308), 1299.

National Academy of Medicine. (2024). *Action collaborative on decarbonizing the U.S. health sector.* https://nam.edu/programs/climate-change-and-human-health/action-collaborative-on-decarbonizing-the-u-s-health-sector/

National Centers for Environmental Information. (2022). *Monthly wildfires report for annual 2022*. https://www.ncei.noaa.gov/access/monitoring/monthly-report/fire/202213.

National Institute of Environmental Health Sciences. (2024). *Autism.* https://www.niehs.nih.gov/health/topics/conditions/autism#:~:text=Air%20pollution%20%E2%80%93%20Researchers%20found%20early,as%20likely%20to%20develop%20ASD.

National League for Nursing. (2022). *NLN vision statement: Climate change and health.* https://www.nln.org/docs/default-source/default-document-library/vision-series-climate-change-health.pdf?sfvrsn=86ee3340_3

Nihart, A. J., Garcia, M. A., El Hayek, E., Liu, R., Olewine, M., Kingston, J. D., Castillo, E. F., Gullapalli, R. R., Howard, T., & Bleske, B. (2025). Bioaccumulation of microplastics in decedent human brains. *Nature Medicine*, 1–6.

Ostfeld, R. S., & Keesing, F. (2020). Planetary health and infectious disease. In S. Myers & H. Frumkin (Eds.), *Planetary health: Protecting nature to protect ourselves* (pp. 141–164). Island Press.

Penuelas, J., & Sardans, J. (2023). Human-driven global nutrient imbalances increase risks to health. *Eco-Environment & Health*, *2*(4), 246–251.

Pizent, A., Anđelković, M., Tariba Lovaković, B., Živković Semren, T., Buha Djordjevic, A., Gamulin, M., Bonderović, V., Aćimović, M., & Bulat, Z. (2022). Environmental exposure to metals, parameters of oxidative stress in blood and prostate cancer: Results from two cohorts. *Antioxidants*, *11*(10), 2044.

Planetary Health Alliance. (n.d.). *Our health depends on our environment.* https://planetaryhealthalliance.org/#

Planetary Health Alliance. (2021). *The Sao Paulo declaration of planetary health.* https://www.planetaryhealthalliance.org/sao-paulo-declaration

Prescott, S. L., Greeson, J. M., El-Sherbini, M. S., & The Planetary Health Community Convened by the Nova Institute for Health. (2022). No health without mental health: Taking action to heal a world in distress—with people, places, and planet 'in mind'. *Challenges, 13*, 37. https://doi.org/10.3390/challe13020037

Redvers, N., Celidwen, Y., Schultz, C., Horn, O., Githaiga, C., Vera, M., Perdrisat, M., Mad Plume, L., Kobei, D., Kain, M. C., Poelina, A., Rojas, J. N., & Blondin, B. (2022). The determinants of planetary health: An Indigenous consensus perspective. *The Lancet Planetary Health*, *6*(2), e156–e163. https://doi.org/10.1016/S2542-5196(21)00354-5

Renzelli, V., Gallo, M., Morviducci, L., Marino, G., Ragni, A., Tuveri, E., Faggiano, A., Mazzilli, R., Natalicchio, A., & Zatelli, M. C. (2023). Polybrominated diphenyl ethers (PBDEs) and human health: Effects on metabolism, diabetes and cancer. *Cancers*, *15*(17), 4237.

Ripple, W., Wolf, C., Gregg, J., Rockström, J., Newsome, T., Law, B., Marques, L., Lenton, T., Xu, C., Huq, S., Simons, L., & King, D. (2023). The 2023 state of the climate report: Entering uncharted territory, *BioScience*, *73*(12), 841–850. https://doi.org/10.1093/biosci/biad080

Robinson, J. M., Breed, A. C., Camargo, A., Redvers, N., & Breed, M. F. (2024). Biodiversity and human health: A scoping review and examples of underrepresented linkages. *Environmental Research*, *246*. https://doi.org/10.1016/j.envres.2024.118115

Romanello, M., DiNapoli, C., Drummond, P., Green, C., Kennard, H., Lampard, P., Scamman, D., Arnell, N., Ayeb-Karisson, S., Ford, L., Belesova, K., Bowen, K., Cai, W., Callaghan, M., Campbell-Lendrum, C., Chambers, J., Daalen, K., Dalin, C., Dasandi, N., ...Costello, A. (2022). The 2022 report of the Lancet Countdown on health and climate change: Health at the mercy of fossil fuels. *The Lancet*, *400*(10363), 1619–1654. https://doi.org/10.1016/S0140-6736(22)01540-9

Rosário Filho, N. A., Urrutia-Pereira, M., D'Amato, G., Cecchi, L., Ansotegui, I. J., Galán, C., Pomés, A., Murrieta-Aguttes, M., Caraballo, L., Rouadi, P., Annesi-Maesano, I., Pawankar, R., Chong-Neto, H. J., & Peden, D. B. (2021). Air pollution and indoor settings. *World Allergy Organization Journal*, *14*(1). https://doi.org/10.1016/j.waojou.2020.100499

Schwabl, P., Köppel, S., Königshofer, P., Bucsics, T., Trauner, M., Reiberger, T., & Liebmann, B. (2019). Detection of various microplastics in human stool: A prospective case series. *Annals of Internal Medicine*, *171*(7), 453–457.

Shetty, S. S., Deepthi, D., Harshitha, S., Sonkusare, S., Naik, P. B., & Madhyastha, H. (2023). Environmental pollutants and their effects on human health. *Heliyon*, *9*(9).

Shim, Y. K., Lewin, M. D., Ruiz, P., Eichner, J. E., & Mumtaz, M. M. (2017). Prevalence and associated demographic characteristics of exposure to multiple metals and their species in human populations: The United States NHANES, 2007–2012. *Journal of Toxicology and Environmental Health, Part A*, *80*(9), 502–512.

Song, J., Pan, T., Xu, Z., Yi, W., Pan, R., Cheng, J., Hu, W., & Su, H. (2024). A systematic analysis of chronic kidney disease burden attributable to lead exposure based on the global burden of disease study 2019. *Science of the Total Environment*, *908*, 168189.

Sorensen, C., & Hess, J. (2022). Treatment and prevention of heat-related illness. *The New England Journal of Medicine, 387*(15), 1404–1413. https://doi.org/10.1056/NEJMcp2210623

Steenland, K., & Winquist, A. (2021). PFAS and cancer, a scoping review of the epidemiologic evidence. *Environmental Research*, *194*, 110690.

Stockholm Resilience Centre. (n.d.). *Planetary boundaries.* https://www.stockholmresilience.org/research/planetary-boundaries.html

Tao, W., Nian, W., & Li, L. (2024). Analysis of brominated flame retardants exposure-associated chronic kidney disease risk in the U.S. population from the NHANES. *Ecotoxicology and Environmental Safety*, *286*, 117159.

United Nations (UN). (n.d.). *The 17 goals: Sustainable development.* https://sdgs.un.org/goals

United Nations (UN). (2024). *The Sustainable Development Goals Report 2024.* https://unstats.un.org/sdgs/report/2024/The-Sustainable-Development-Goals-Report-2024.pdf

United Nations General Assembly Economic and Social Council. (2024). *Progress toward the sustainable development goals.* https://unstats.un.org/sdgs/files/report/2024/SG-SDG-Progress-Report-2024-advanced-unedited-version.pdf

United States Department of Homeland Security. (2024). *Floods.* https://www.ready.gov/floods

Wabnitz, K. J., Gabrysch, S., Guinto, R., Haines, A., Hermann, M., Howard, C., Potter, T., Prescott, S. L., & Redyers, N. (2020). A pledge for planetary health to unite health professionals in the Anthropocene. *The Lancet, 396*(10261), 1471–1473. https://doi.org/10.1016/S0140-6736(20)32039-0

Whitmee, S., Haines, A., Beyrer, C., Boltz, F., Capon, A. G., de Souza Dias, B. F., Ezeh, A., Frumkin, H., Gong, P., Head, P., Horton, R., Mace, G. M., Marten, R., Myers, S. S., Nishtar, S., Osofsky, S. A., Pattanayak, S. K., Pongsiri, M. J., Romanelli, C., … Yach, D. (2015). Safeguarding human health in the Anthropocene epoch: Report of The Rockefeller Foundation–Lancet Commission on planetary health. *The Lancet, 386*(10007), 1973–2028. https://doi.org/10.1016/S0140-6736(15)60901-1

Wilcox, C., Van Sebille, E., & Hardesty, B. D. (2015). Threat of plastic pollution to seabirds is global, pervasive, and increasing. *Proceedings of the National Academy of Sciences, 112*(38), 11899–11904.

Winquist, A., Hodge, J. M., Diver, W. R., Rodriguez, J. L., Troeschel, A. N., Daniel, J., & Teras, L. R. (2023). Case–cohort study of the association between PFAS and selected cancers among participants in the American Cancer Society's Cancer Prevention Study II LifeLink Cohort. *Environmental Health Perspectives, 131*(12), 127007.

World Health Organization (WHO). (2019). *Healthy environments for healthier populations: Why do they matter and what can we do?* WHO-CED-PHE-DO-19.01-eng.pdf

World Health Organization (WHO). (2023). *Water, sanitation, and hygiene (WASH).* https://www.who.int/health-topics/water-sanitation-and-hygiene-wash#tab=tab_1

World Health Organization (WHO). (2024a). *The Sustainable Development Goals Report 2024.* World Health Organization.

World Health Organization (WHO). (2024b). *Why mental health is a priority for action on climate change.* https://www.who.int/news/item/03-06-2022-why-mental-health-is-a-priority-for-action-on-climate-change

Woychik, R. P., Bianchi, D. W., Gibbons, G. H., Glass, R. I., Gordon, J. A., Perez-Stable, E. J., & Zenc, S. N. (2022). The NIH Climate Change and Health Initiative and Strategic Framework: Addressing the threat of climate change to health. *The Lancet, 400*(10366), 1831–1833.

Wu, Y., & Yang, F. (2025). Co-exposure to microplastics enhances the allergenic potentials of house dust mite allergen Der p 1. *Environmental Research, 277.* https://doi.org/10.1016/j.envres.2025.121613

Yilmaz, B., Terekeci, H., Sandal, S., & Kelestimur, F. (2020). Endocrine disrupting chemicals: Exposure, effects on human health, mechanism of action, models for testing and strategies for prevention. *Reviews in Endocrine and Metabolic Disorders, 21,* 127–147.

Zhang, L., Rana, I., Shaffer, R. M., Taioli, E., & Sheppard, L. (2019). Exposure to glyphosate-based herbicides and risk for non-Hodgkin lymphoma: A meta-analysis and supporting evidence. *Mutation Research/Reviews in Mutation Research, 781,* 186–206.

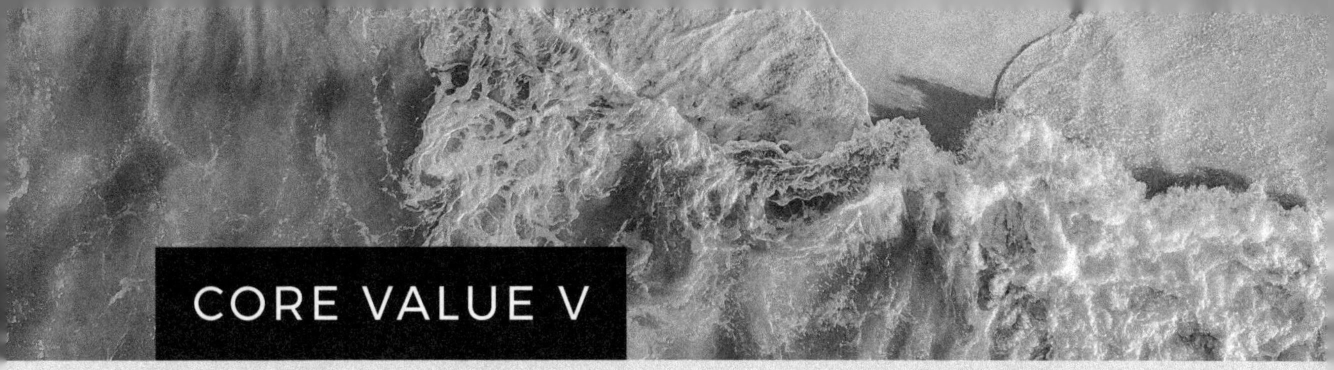

CORE VALUE V

Holistic Education and Research

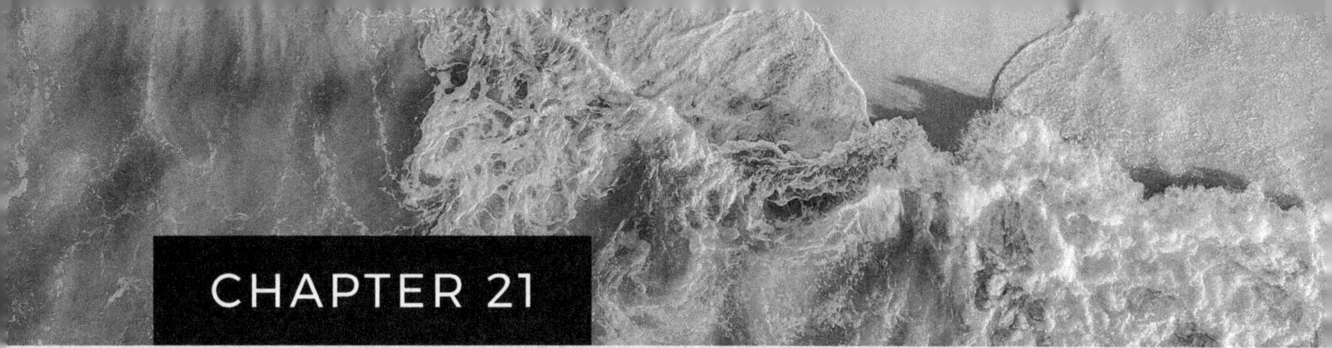

CHAPTER 21

Holistic Nursing Education: Self-Reflection, Growth, Development, and Lifelong Learning

Deborah A. Shields and Margaret E. Erickson

NURSE HEALER OBJECTIVES

- Reflect on the relationship between lifelong learning and holistic self-development.
- Examine current trends in nursing education.
- Explore education within the context of nursing's social and moral imperative to care (Fowler, 2015).
- Value holism as the essential philosophical foundation of all nursing education opportunities.
- Envision strategies/pathways designed to create pre- and post-licensure holistic education programs.

DEFINITIONS

Curriculum: A set of courses constituting an area of specialization (Merriam-Webster, 2019).

Education versus learning: Education is a process through which a society passes on knowledge, values, and skills from one generation to another. Learning is the acquisition of new skills, knowledge, and values (Prabhat, 2011).

Experiential learning: Learning by doing; it is an active process that engages the learner, not a passive one that happens to the learner. In experiential learning, the experience provides the platform for learning, and the careful analysis and reflection of the experience develop the learning. Individuals are encouraged to work things out for themselves; they are guided to and through their learning rather than being taught. (MTa Learning, n.d.)

Interprofessional education: "Interprofessional education occurs when learners of two or more health or social care professions engage in learning with, from, and about each other to improve collaboration and the delivery of care." (Institute of Medicine, 2015, p. xi)

Professional development: The process of improving and deepening practice by participating in continuing education and involvement in other professional activities in which knowledge, skills, and attitudes are learned and/or enhanced. In nursing, this lifelong journey integrates role-specific and professional education; the foundation must be the philosophy of holism and nursing knowledge.

Introduction

Educating the mind without educating the heart is no education at all.

—Aristotle

Learning is a lifelong process, beginning with our first breath and ending with our last one. As young children, we learn to take our first step, say our first word, and acquire the knowledge and skills needed to be successful in our lives. Learning involves affective, cognitive, and psychomotor attributes, and occurs through stories, encounters, communications, and other lived experiences with our environment and those around us. It does not occur in a vacuum and must hold personal meaning for the learner. Learning is a "transformative process of taking in information that—when internalized and mixed with what we have experienced—changes what we know and builds on what we do" (Bingham & Conner, 2015, p. 32). As we gain a greater understanding of the world we live in and those around us, we transform, evolve, and reach higher levels of self-awareness and growth in all aspects of our being.

Holistic nurses are committed to and engaged in the acquisition of knowledge, skills, attitudes, beliefs, and values through lifelong learning processes (American Holistic Nurses Association [AHNA], 2019). Underlying and essential to this commitment is an inherent understanding of the importance of personal self-reflection, self-assessment, self-development, and self-care. Through self-care, professional education and practice, and lived experiences, holistic nurses develop skills of authentic self-reflection essential to lifelong learning. This process creates opportunities that allow them to change how they think, feel, and practice. Continuing education, publishing, participating in professional associations, opportunities that facilitate self-study and awareness, networking with holistic nursing colleagues, achieving certification in Holistic Nursing and Nurse Coaching, and acquiring advanced degrees grounded in holism all provide possible options to facilitate personal and professional development.

Nursing education is frequently viewed within the context of the academic arena, specifically regarding university or college-based nursing programs. Education, however, occurs through multiple pathways, and learning often happens outside of a classroom (**Figure 21-1**).

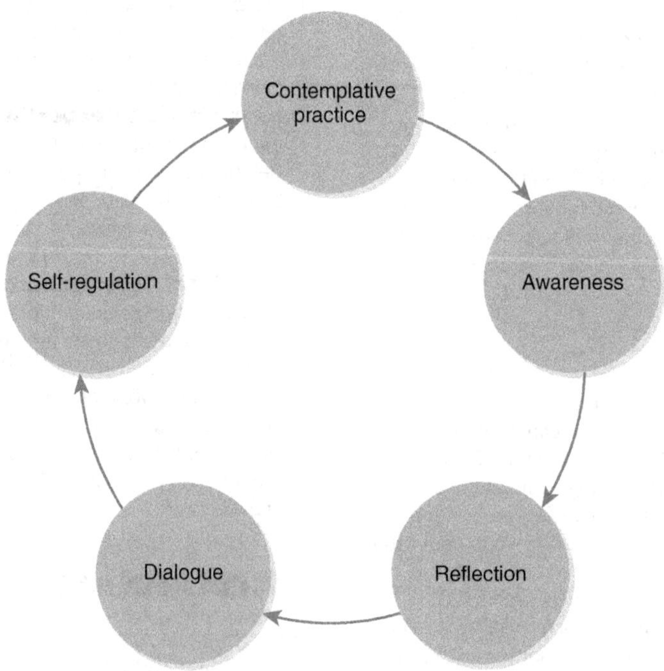

Figure 21-1 Holistic self-development in education

These opportunities, both formal and informal, may be self-initiated and/or facilitated by others. As people reflect, learn, and grow, they acquire new knowledge, abilities, and expertise that can be applied and utilized. Stout-Shaffer and Shields (2016) proposed a model of holistic self-development in education based on their earlier work. When applied to education, this continuous circular process of contemplative practice, awareness, reflection, dialogue, and self regulation offers a foundation that supports holistic nurses in providing care that meets their moral and social imperative to care. Refer to Chapter 10 for a discussion of holistic self-development.

A Social and Moral Imperative to Care

Florence Nightingale (1859) first described the relationship or social contract between nursing and society. She focused on society's charge that nurses facilitate health, healing, and recovery from disease through caring that would facilitate a greater state of well-being. Today, the American Nurses Association (ANA)'s (2025) *Code of Ethics for Nurses* and Fowler's (2015) *Guide to Nursing's Social Policy Statement 11* continue to support this charge and nursing's social imperative to care for all people.

According to Fowler (2015), the nursing profession has a social contract that explicates the reciprocal relationship between nursing and society as a whole. These reciprocal expectations authorize nurses to meet the healthcare needs of society and articulate nursing's expectations of society. Through this agreement, nurses provide compassionate care that addresses the individual's need for protection, advocacy, empowerment, optimization of eudemonistic health, prevention of illness and injury, alleviation of suffering, comfort, and well-being. This contractual arrangement also guides nurses in engaging in political and legislative action needed to support nursing practice, education, and research to achieve better healthcare-based outcomes at the individual, community, and global levels.

As would be expected, nursing's social contract and moral imperative to care also inform every aspect of lifelong learning and professional development for both educator and learner. Recognizing that teaching/learning is a reciprocal process of cocreating communities of engagement and growth and that the philosophy of holism is key in the development of nursing knowledge, this chapter explores the pathways to nursing professional development. Readers are invited to reflect on the broad spectrum of educational opportunities and contemporary trends and envision what might best serve them in their journeys of living nursing's social and moral imperative to care.

The Pathway to Professional Development

Historical Background

Nightingale (1859), recognized by many as the founder of modern nursing, believed that our responsibility was to "put the patient in the best condition for nature to act upon him" (p. 28). She recognized that the environment (i.e., fresh air, clean water, warm and clean accommodations, and healthy foods) was important and supported the healing process. She also recognized that issues such as feeling safe and secure and having access to beauty, comfort, and support services were equally important in helping people acquire a greater state of well-being. Early nursing curriculum, based on Nightingale's model, became more structured, and nurses were taught both the art and science of nursing. Attention to the whole person was foundational to nursing care. Refer to Chapter 2 for a discussion of early nurse training programs and schools.

In 1965, the U.S. Medicare program was implemented, providing care to anyone over 65 or who had permanent disabilities or end-stage renal disease. Hospital occupancy increased in alignment with the new reimbursement options, and nursing practice moved from more community-based to hospital settings. Nursing care has become more focused on medical issues. The diagnosis-related group (DRG) system was implemented in 1983 to control rising healthcare costs, and individuals were cared for based on their medical DRG. With these legislative changes, nursing began to align more closely with the biomedical model; curriculum hours devoted to public and community health decreased, and those related to hospital-based practice increased (Cherry & Jacobs, 2017). The nursing curriculum became less focused on the whole, the art and science of nursing, and more reductionistic. Emphasis was placed on *medical* care and promoting and maintaining physical health. Curing illnesses and diseases became the primary goal of nursing care. The *art of nursing* became less important, and the focus of care was directed toward the maintenance and resolution of illness and disease.

The call for curriculum revolution from reductionist, empirical paradigms to pedagogies that integrate technical competence into nursing's values and the ethic of whole-person care began in the 1980s. Bevis, Moccia, Munhall, Roach, Tanner, and Watson were among the early nursing scholars who led this charge as an imperative in transforming nursing education (Hills et al., 2021). With the desire to return to a paradigm that integrated nursing's values and the ethic of whole-person care, a movement to reconnect with nursing's earlier values and roots began.

During this time, a group of nurses dedicated to the philosophy of holism and the original roots of nursing convened and founded the American Holistic Nurses Association (AHNA). The organizers believed that the core of nursing is based on holism and that our social mandate requires that nurses care for all aspects of the human being. They questioned the assumption that the knowledge and skills based on the biomedical paradigm included both the art and science of nursing. Further, they articulated that nursing curriculum must include holistic, humanistic content and that it be taught within the context of holism. Interestingly, these nurses were reconnecting with and affirming the roots of professional nursing initiated by Florence Nightingale in the 1800s. However, because of differences in philosophy among nurses that had begun to evolve over time, a chasm in nursing began to emerge.

Philosophical Differences Between the Paradigms Emerge

Based on different philosophical perspectives, a major division within nursing occurred as two distinct paradigms—biomedical and holistic—began to emerge. Each paradigmatic approach arises from a different worldview; thus, the practice focus and outcomes, knowledge priorities, and competencies are not the same. The biomedical or wholistic paradigm views the whole of the human being as the sum of the parts. It posits a curative model, with a focus on physical health, illness and disease, and maintenance and prevention. The holistic paradigm views the whole of the human being as greater than the sum of the parts, giving rise to a model focused on caring for the *entire person* with an emphasis on facilitating healing and mind-body-spirit integration (Erickson, 2007; Fawcett, 1995, 2005; Newman, 1992; Newman et al., 2008; Parse, 1987, 2000).

Table 21-1 presents a brief outline of the major components of the two paradigms. Reviewing Table 21-1 will help the reader better understand the differences between the paradigms and the potential implications for education and practice. For information about the complete paradigm table, readers may contact the authors.

While Table 21-1 presents what seem to be opposing approaches to care, holistic nurses realize that both approaches are essential in cocreating, with clients, integrative plans of care that best meet their needs, goals, and life desires. Lifelong nursing education, then, must provide learning experiences designed to increase the knowledge, skills, and competencies related to both paradigms.

Holistic Nursing Education Unfolding

Nursing educators live in a world filled with exciting opportunities and complex challenges. Despite the call for curriculum change four decades ago, there continues to be a struggle to include humanistic, caring/healing content into

Table 21-1 Paradigms Driving Nursing Education and Related Practice Models

	Wholistic (Biomedical)	Holistic (Health, Wellness, Well-Being)
Essence of human nature	Creation of a whole person by the subsystems together	Person greater than the sum of his or her parts
Definition of health	Absence of illness or disease Management of conditions, illness, and disease	Eudaemonistic; harmony and balance among subsystems
Focus of care	Focus on prevention, maintenance, illnesses, and disease/conditions of the person.	Focus on maintaining and restoring the balance among the interacting, synergistic dimensions of the person
Goals of care	Curative, palliative Relief of symptoms	Healing, balance, harmony Achieve a sense of well-being
Caring definition	Doing for or to the patient/ person/family	Cocreated connection, relational presence; being with
Self-care	Predominant emphasis on care of the body; e.g., exercise, nutrition, and stress management	Predominant emphasis on care of the being as *Beingcare*; e.g., contemplative practice; intentional action that facilitates rejuvenation, balance, harmony, growth, and development
Sciences and philosophical foundations	Biomedical science	Science of holism

Data from models created by Shields & Schaffer and Erickson, H.].

a curriculum primarily focused on biomedicine. It is time to transform our sick care system into one grounded in holistic health and wellness. Essential to this shift, nurses must be prepared for full engagement in the process and represented in all matters of health. As experts in the science of health, wellness, and well-being, nurses bring an invaluable knowledge base and perspective of whole-person quality care to the healthcare team. The knowledge, skills, and competencies of holistic nursing practice must be the "DNA" of every nurse.

This transformation begins with nursing education. Educators are called to create caring/teaching–learning environments that support the development of a healing consciousness, the cultivation of compassionate presence, core strength and resilience, and the wisdom needed to build up the next generation of holistic nurses.

Foundational Principles

Holistic nursing education arises from the *Holistic* paradigm, in which the individual is viewed as a unitary, indivisible whole, energetically connected to all living beings, the environment, and the universe. It begins with the novice learner and extends to those who seek the terminal degree of Doctor of Nursing Practice (DNP) and/or Doctor of Philosophy (PhD) (Erickson et al., 2017). It is a process of deepening the art and science of nursing within the context of the philosophical foundations of holism. The integration of the core values, science, and the art of nursing is fundamental to the practice of holistic nursing, and these serve as benchmarks in holistic nursing education. The sophistication of core value interpretation, sciences required, and artistic applications increases with education; *all holistic nurses* practice from basic premises, and all increase their knowledge, skills, and attitudes as they increase their formal education. Holistic nursing education integrates professional practice experiences and formal and informal educational activities based on the AHNA core values, directed by the *Holistic Nursing: Scope and Standards of Practice*, and specified by the competencies required for practice. Competencies are the required behaviors identified by holistic nurses that are necessary for professional holistic nursing practice. They emerge from holistic nursing's core values and are specific to *Holistic Nursing: Scope and Standards of Practice*. As such, holistic nursing competencies are the result of integrating philosophy, core values, and science (Erickson et al., 2017; Shields & Erickson, 2017).

Hills et al. (2021) posited that there have been three "detours along the way" (p. 4) in the transformation of nursing curricula. The notion that nursing is an art and a science has resulted in a false dichotomy in which the art is caring, and the biomedical knowledge is science. This belief is reinforced by attitudes of singular, rational, quantifiable, and controlled approaches to illness. In truth, one might view "artscience" as a unified approach to health and wellness in which nurses envision creative, integrative strategies to promote health. A second detour is the ongoing challenges within the relationship between nursing and medicine, one that Hills et al. described as "ambivalent" (p. 6). While both professions have a knowledge base, they are not the same. The focus of medicine is on curing disease, whereas nursing expertise is health, wellness, and caring for people who are experiencing any number of health challenges. Currently, the nursing curriculum remains deeply ingrained in medical science and care. Both professions need each other's wisdom, and it would be beneficial to cultivate respectful, shared, and complementary relationships. Today's movement toward interprofessional education may be a positive step in cultivating shared disciplinary respect. Finally, Hills et al. asserted that the evidence-based (EBP) movement contributes to the challenges of transforming nursing curricula, writing "…it {EBP}is not oriented to include the more complex and sophisticated aspects of nursing's focus: people and inner meaning, perceptions, feelings, and the complex relational, experiential, contextual aspects of health and healing" (p. 8). While there is no question regarding the importance of evidence in the practice of nursing, they reminded us that nursing's continued evolution as a unique discipline requires us to "critically examine our caring knowledge and practices and develop ways of revealing evidence that are consistent with the philosophical and theoretical foundations of a mature discipline and profession distinct from, but complementary to, medicine and all health professions" (p. 9). Holistic nurses utilize evidence-informed practice, a process of seeking meaningful evidence using philosophy and theories, information and resources, research, practitioner expertise, traditional and historical data, and individual/patient preferences in person-centered shared decision making.

Building a Community of Transformation

The goal of holistic nurse educators is to develop educational programs that ensure students acquire and can apply knowledge, skills, and attitudes of the holistic nursing discipline in their practice. This can be, at times, a daunting undertaking, but pausing and reflecting on holistic self-development in the education model may offer a first step in this quest. Coming together as a faculty to stop and breathe can create a space for open, honest dialogue. Salient questions about the why and the how of revising existing programmatic activities must be examined. What challenges might be encountered? What supports are available to faculty? What makes an educational community caring?

Caring/healing educational communities are those where students, faculty, and staff feel nurtured, cared for, and valued. They are innovative spaces where reaching, stretching, and growing are embraced. Within these communities, learning unfolds in the creative weaving of a tapestry enfolding all ways of knowing. Creativity and dialogue are encouraged, and all members feel safe, respected, and heard.

However, no path is without some bumps. As a faculty, it is important to be aware of these and envision strategies to address them. Contemporary realities may include the following challenges: university, student, and stakeholder expectations; societal trends; and requirements of regulatory and accrediting bodies.

University, Student, and Stakeholder Expectations

Universities and colleges have expectations that are often challenging to meet. As societal needs grow and nursing education adjusts to accommodate the increasing societal needs and demands, different factors must be considered. Academic institutions demand that enrollment numbers be maintained or grow, and financial security is expected. Program quality must be consistent and/or improved; meeting benchmark outcomes (e.g., National Council Licensure Examination [NCLEX] pass rate) is critical. Student retention and progression are monitored, and successful completion and graduation within a specified timeline are expected. Graduates are to be respected and sought after, affirming the excellence and integrity of the academic programs. Despite the increased needs and expectations, there exists the pervasive reality of doing more with fewer resources—fewer faculty, fewer dollars, and often decreasing infrastructure and material resources.

Simultaneously, students also have high expectations of the faculty and the nursing programs in which they enroll. Students (and often parents) seek quality programs that are timely and affordable and do not result in postgraduation loans and debts. Curricula are expected to offer opportunities that support and facilitate professional growth and advancement; infrastructure support is essential. Students want qualified, caring, responsive, and respectful faculty available to facilitate their learning. This factor alone is extremely problematic, as there is currently a shortage of nursing faculty in the United States, which has resulted in a decline in nursing school admissions. According to the American Association of Colleges of Nursing (AACN, 2024), enrollment in nursing programs is "not growing fast enough to meet the projected demand for RN and APRN services." They go on to suggest that these trends raise concerns about the capacity of nursing schools to meet the projected demand for nursing services and that a shortage of nursing school faculty is restricting nursing program enrollments. According to AACN's (2024) report on 2023–2024 Enrollment and Graduations in Baccalaureate and Graduate Programs in Nursing, U.S. "nursing schools turned away 65,766 qualified applications (not applicants) from baccalaureate and graduate nursing programs in 2023 due to insufficient number of faculty, clinical sites, classroom space, and clinical preceptors, as well as budget constraints."

Regulatory and Accrediting Bodies' Expectations

Expectations and requirements of the regulatory and accrediting bodies for nursing have an enormous impact on nursing education. These include the National Council of State Boards of Nursing (NCSBN), state boards of nursing, and state, regional, and federal accrediting bodies.

Regulatory Bodies

The NCSBN is responsible for overseeing the development of the National Council Licensure Examination for Registered Nurses (NCLEX-RN), which serves to validate safe practice for entry-level nurses. A new test blueprint was implemented in April 2023, and it has significantly influenced the curriculum, particularly in testing. The implementation of the Consensus Model (CM) by the NCSBN has profoundly affected graduate nursing education. Requirements outlined by the CM dictate faculty qualifications; curricular requirements specific to populations, settings, and roles; what courses are taught; and who can practice at the advanced practice level. For further understanding about the implications of the CM on nursing education and practice, the reader is referred to Chapter 23.

Accrediting Bodies

The AACN serves as the collective voice for academic nursing, supporting and advancing excellence and innovation in nursing education, practice, and research. AACN goals include establishing quality nursing education standards; assisting in implementing those standards and required curriculum; influencing the nursing profession to improve health care; and promoting public support for professional nursing education, research, and practice. In 2021, AACN published the *Essentials: Core Competencies for Professional Nursing Education* 2020–2030, which outlines the necessary curriculum content and expected competencies of graduates from baccalaureate, master's, and Doctor of Nursing Practice programs. The *Essentials* are having a profound impact on nursing faculty as they revise the curriculum and transition to a competency-based model of education. Currently, AACN is working to develop a national consensus for progression indicators—the expected behaviors that demonstrate competency—for the competencies and sub-competencies outlined in the *Essentials* (AACN, 2021). It will be interesting to evaluate the outcomes of this shift to a competency-based curriculum and how it impacts the profession of nursing. Holistic educators are mindful of the importance of ensuring that the philosophy of holism underpins all nursing curricula.

The Commission on Collegiate Nursing Education (CCNE), an autonomous arm of AACN, validates the excellence and integrity of academic nursing programs through an independent accreditation process, ensuring the public that nursing programs demonstrate acceptable educational practices and continued growth and improvement. The National League for Nursing (NLN) offers programs to support faculty development, testing services, nursing research grants, and public policy. Accreditation services, offered through the NLN Commission for Nursing Education Accreditation, serve to promote excellence in pre- and post-licensure nursing education programs to prepare caring, competent nurses.

In the Blink of an Eye

On March 11, 2020, the World Health Organization (WHO) declared that COVID-19 was a pandemic (Ghebreyesus, 2020). Thousands of people all over the world were dying from this highly contagious disease. While everyone was affected by this, certain sectors were affected more heavily. Healthcare professionals, specifically nurses, found themselves central to the care of this population. The nursing shortage, well known before 2020, would feel the impact of the pandemic on practicing nurses and on the future of nursing (AACN, 2024; Farahani et al., 2024; Health Resources and Services Administration [HRSA], 2024b).

Nursing education was profoundly impacted as, almost overnight, faculty and students were called to recreate learning communities and, in general, reimagine how they conducted business. Courses rapidly shifted from live to online. Clinical experiences became simulations. Gone were the days of in-person support systems. The effects were felt by nursing students, faculty, and administrators. Barrett (2022) reported that students faced enormous pressures and anxieties. From the fear of contracting COVID-19 and/or passing the disease on to someone they care about, to having to manage online technicalities, students faced numerous stressors. Barrett went on to report that the majority of students met the challenges, and perhaps, a positive effect was increased resilience.

Head et al. (2022) posited that the rapid transition to remote learning created challenges to learning (e.g., online classes, internet difficulty, clinical—virtual or lost), challenges to living (e.g., physical health, mental health, isolation, Zoom fatigue), and challenges to professional commitment (e.g., readiness to assume professional role, burnout, heavy workloads) for nursing students. The team conducted 40 interviews in two midwestern nursing schools. For each of the categories of challenges, they explored the disruptions and the student responses. From that, they identified opportunities that students took to develop interventions and improve their experience, including changing the environment, learning via virtual gatherings, responding to the flexibility of faculty, pursuing intentional self-care, and undertaking supplemental learning. They concluded that the challenges of the COVID-19 pandemic helped these nursing students grow and become more resilient, and acknowledged the importance of timely communication, reliable faculty support, and mental health resources in achieving this outcome.

In a mixed-methods, 4-phase longitudinal study conducted by the NCSBN, Martin et al. (2023) assessed the "impact of institutional, academic, and demographic characteristics on prelicensure nursing students' academic, initial postgraduation, and early career outcomes during the COVID-19 pandemic" (p. 83). They were interested in better understanding how the rapid shift to online and simulation-based teaching methods affected new graduates' clinical preparedness, which is critical to patient safety. A combination of real-time student and faculty self-report data, including externally validated instruments, within and end-of-program standardized test scores, and focus group findings were used to collect data from the >1,100 student and faculty participants affiliated with 51 prelicensure RN programs located across 27 states. The results demonstrated the "breadth, scale, and ever-evolving nature of prelicensure RN programs' efforts to maintain the continuity of nursing students' education during the public health crisis" (Martin et al., 2023, p. 83). Participants' engagement in their learning increased over time. However, they also found that today's new graduates' perceived clinical deficiencies contribute to their feeling that they are in a more precarious position than their predecessors. Ultimately, the lessons learned in this study are useful in planning nursing education for the future.

Consideration of all these realities in nursing—and nursing education—leads us to ask how nurse educators should proceed to prepare nurse graduates to meet the needs of society. According to an updated Health Workforce Analysis published by HRSA (2024a), federal authorities predict that if labor force patterns remain the same as today, the demand for RNs in 2036 will exceed supply by 9 percent, resulting in a national shortage of 337,970 full-time equivalent RNs. Key findings of the National Sample Survey of Registered Nurses (NSSRN) show that the nursing workforce is becoming more diverse, more highly educated, but less satisfied with their job. Globally, the nursing shortage stands at ~5.9 million nurses, predominantly in low- and middle-income countries. Buchan and Catton (2023) stated that "there must be a coordinated effort by international stakeholders and countries to develop a long-term, ten-year plan to aim for a sustainable global nursing workforce" (p. 17).

The pandemic has irrevocably changed healthcare and nursing education. Administrators, educators, and students were nimble, creative, innovative, and courageous. While education will look different in the future, caring will remain at the heart of nursing. Leaver et al. (2022) suggested the following curricular recommendations: increase content related to public health, disaster preparedness, health equity, mental health, and technology; establish strong academic–practice partnerships, including telehealth; develop new teaching methodologies and learner engagement strategies; and research to evaluate what is working and what is not. Indeed, in the blink of an eye, life can change forever.

Beyond Boundaries: Holistic Nursing Education in the 21st Century

In 2017, the American Holistic Nurses Credentialing Corporation (AHNCC) published the *Foundations, Competencies and Curricular Guidelines for Basic to Doctoral Holistic Nursing Education, 1st Edition*, also known as the *2017 Curricular Guidelines (CG)*. This work clarified and standardized the required foundations and competencies of holistic nursing and provided a formalized structure for educational curricula needed to seamlessly prepare holistic nurses across all levels of education. In 2022, the Global Academy of Holistic Nursing assumed ownership of the *CG* and, in 2025, finalized *Beyond Boundaries: Holistic Nursing Education in the 21st Century* Erickson et al. (2025). This publication, synchronous with the times, can be used by educators aiming to embark on individual course or curriculum development and/or revision; its applicability stretches across all academic programs and, as well, in continuing nursing professional development.

Curriculum threads are concepts interwoven into every course in a curriculum. They provide a substance and a structure, and they identify those ideas deemed important by the faculty to achieve program outcomes. The following are the five curricular threads for basic and advanced nursing programs:

1. Enculturation: The assimilation of an integral sense of self with the unique attributes of the profession.
2. Assimilation of knowledge, skills, and attitudes of holistic nursing.
3. Articulation of holistic nursing praxes as scholarship.
4. Recognition of self as a professional scholar with a social commitment.
5. Declaration of self as a leader in health care with the perspective of a holistic nurse as a scholar and advocate for society.

The philosophy of holism views the individual as an integrated body, mind, emotional, social, spiritual, energetic totality. Conventional and complementary/integrative healthcare approaches are utilized in supporting the individual's wholeness, health, well-being, and quality of life. Curricular threads provide a foundation and, interwoven with the *Essential Requirements for Holistic Nursing*, articulate this educational focus. The *Essential Requirements for Holistic Nursing* include:

- Philosophical and Scientific Underpinnings
- Clinical Scholarship and Analytic Methods for Evidence-Informed Practice
- Diversity, Equity, Inclusion, and Social Justice
- Organizational, Systems, Caring Leadership for Person-Centered Quality Improvement and Safety
- Holistic Education and Research Supporting Dynamic Changes in Healthcare
- Informatics, Technology, and Person-Centered Care for the Improvement and Transformation of Holistic Healthcare
- Ethics, Policy, and Advocacy in Holistic Healthcare
- Interprofessional Collaboration for Improving Patient and Population Health Outcomes

All *prelicensure* nursing curricula preparing students for RN licensure include basic content on physiological, psychological, emotional, and spiritual processes with populations across the life span, conventional care and treatment approaches, and clinical experiences in both acute care and community practice settings. The focus is often on specialties (e.g., pediatrics, medical–surgical, critical care, psychiatric) and, as previously discussed, emphasize cure. One expected outcome for graduates from an entry-level holistic nursing program is that the graduate will have the ability to apply the knowledge, skills, and attitudes of the holistic nursing discipline in their practice. Achieving this outcome is supported by creating educational experiences designed to help students embrace holistic nursing principles and philosophy, understand how they relate to nursing theories, and understand the implications for practice.

There are several ways *post-licensure* registered nurses (academic and professional development) can acquire additional specialized knowledge and skills that prepare them for advanced holistic nursing practice. They might enroll in a Master's Degree in Nursing (MSN) program, a post-MSN program that prepares them for advanced holistic nursing or advanced practice holistic nursing certification, and/or they might pursue doctoral degrees (Doctor of Nursing Practice or Doctor of Philosophy in Nursing), which include a range of options (e.g., Bachelor of Science in Nursing to DNP). Core coursework in all graduate nursing programs should include nursing theory, nursing research, evidence-informed practice and quality science; health ethics and policy foundations; and nursing informatics. Most graduate students must also complete advanced physical assessment, pathophysiology, and pharmacology courses.

In a graduate nursing program with a holistic focus, core courses should include an introduction to holism (holistic philosophy, nursing theory, core values, reflection as inquiry, and approaches to personal and professional self-development through self-care, aesthetics, and scholarship); advanced sciences of health and holism; advanced holistic health assessment; and pharmacotherapeutics (including natural herbs and dietary supplements).

Other courses included in the graduate curriculum reflect developing knowledge, competence, and skills related to the intended nursing role (e.g., educator, administrator, and advanced practice nurse). Students also benefit from a wide range of experiential and clinical activities important to their concentration and overall professional development.

Expected outcomes for the Advanced Holistic Nurse graduate include the demonstration of a greater depth and scope of knowledge, a greater integration of information, increased complexity of skills and interventions, and notable role autonomy. Advanced holistic nurses are expected to provide transformational leadership and serve as role models in practice, teaching, research, consultation, management, advocacy, and/or policy formation in advancing holistic nursing to improve the holistic health of people and organizations.

This brief overview is designed to be an introduction to the nursing education curriculum. For an in-depth, comprehensive discussion, the reader is referred to *Beyond Boundaries: Holistic Nursing Education in the 21st Century*.

Onward the Journey–Professional Development After Graduation

After completing nursing education, nurses enter the wide world of practice—a world that is exciting, frightening, and filled with possibilities. Most decisions about lifelong learning reside with the nurse, and the opportunities are endless. Nurses must demonstrate currency and competence in their chosen practice; many healthcare systems have developed competence-based education that includes both required topics (e.g., the Health Insurance Portability and Accountability Act and fire safety) and practice-specific modules (e.g., Advanced Cardiac Life Support and administration of chemotherapy). Additionally, nurses must be current with the state of the profession—for example, their state's Nurse Practice Act, nursing scope and standards of practice, and relevant practice issues and legislative initiatives in their state, nationally, and globally. Holistic nurses must be cognizant of the movements in place designed to ensure holism is the philosophical foundation of care.

There are numerous educational venues and delivery options available to nurses, and each nurse must choose what is best suited to meet their learning needs and life situation. Will it be a self-read journal article, a journal/research club, a short didactic program, a one- or multiple-day conference, or something else? Will it be live, synchronous online (e.g., a webinar), or asynchronous (e.g., a recorded webinar)? What are the benefits and challenges of each? What about cost—and who will pay? There is a lot to consider, but, regardless of the choice, holistic nurses seek lifelong opportunities that support the deepening of their holistic nursing practice. In planning postgraduate holistic professional development, it is interesting to briefly explore the past.

A Peek into Yesteryear

Nurses have always been committed to learning and being current in their practice. From the earliest history, there have been journals (e.g., the *American Journal of Nursing*, first published circa 1900), in-service training sessions, and, importantly, opportunities where information, knowledge, and skills were shared on the spot.

Jones-Shenk (2019) and Brunt and Morris (2025) offer a glimpse into the past. In 1893, The American Society of Superintendents for Training School Nurses established the first national nursing organization focusing on education. During the 1960s, nursing concentrated on "organizing and standardizing nursing education to improve the development of new nurses (Jones-Shenk, 2019, p. 143). In 1965, the ANA, with the support of the NLN, issued a position paper that called for entry-level nurses in the future to hold a bachelor's degree. While the academic landscape was changing (fewer diploma, more baccalaureate programs), practicing nurses were tasked with remaining current amidst rapid growth, advancement, and increasingly complex care needs. Veterans returning from Vietnam presented new challenges. According to Jones-Shenk, the "need and demand for additional education for nurses in practice were growing and the lack of structures to support consistency and quality of the education [was] increasingly evident" (p. 143).

In-service education was the primary vehicle for education. In 1970, the ANA received a one-year $42,000 grant for a project entitled *Identification of Need for Continuing Education for Nurses* by the National Professional Organization. Educational approaches shifted and became more comprehensive; the term *in-service education* evolved into continuing education, and in 1974, the ANA published the *Standards for Continuing Education in Nursing and ANA Continuing Education Guidelines for State /Nurses Associations*. In the same year, Helen Tobin, often referred to as the "Godmother of Staff Development," published *The Process of Staff Development: Components for Change*. The *Journal for Nurses in Staff Development* (now known as the *Journal for Nurses in Professional Development*) was published in 1985.

Continuing education flourished during the late 1900s. Advances in health care were occurring at breakneck speed. Nursing practice also expanded, with increased roles, opportunities, and the need for additional education and credentialing. The American Nurses Credentialing Corporation (ANCC), the accrediting and certifying arm of the ANA, was established in 1991. Almost simultaneously, the American Holistic Nurses Association began a four-phase AHNA Certificate Program in Holistic Nursing. In 1997, the AHNA Certification Board established a separate 501(c)(6) organization, the AHNCC, to serve as the credentialing body for the Holistic Nursing Certification Examination.

Today, nursing professional development is recognized as a practice specialty. In 1989, Belinda Puetz led efforts to establish and incorporate the National Nursing Staff Development Organization (NNSDO). NNSDO transformed into the Association for Nursing Professional Development (ANPD) in 2012. "ANPD's mission is to advance quality health care by defining and promoting nursing professional development practice. The goal of ANPD is to be acknowledged as the expert voice, advocate, and leading resource for nursing professional development practice (Brunt & Morris, 2025, p. 1).

The term *in-service* transitioned to continuing education, then to staff development, and eventually to continuing nursing professional development. While the names have changed and the organization and delivery of education have expanded, and in some ways become more complex, the aim has remained consistent—to provide education that ensures person-centered, safe, quality, knowledgeable, and excellent nursing care.

Deepening Holistic Practice: Touchstones on the Journey

Introduced earlier in this writing, holistic nursing practice is the lived experience of deepening knowledge, skills, and expertise that unfolds within all patterns of knowing. There are numerous touchstones on this journey, some affecting every nurse and others unique to the nurse's personally defined professional goals. Let us briefly consider.

Shifting from Teacher-Centric to Learner-Centric Professional Development

The planning, implementation, and evaluation of holistic learner-centric educational activities is a touchstone that invites educators to envision a world of possibilities and may require that they move out of their comfort zone. Gone are the days of a teacher droning away while students sit passively unengaged. Educators are challenged to cocreate caring/learning communities where everyone is both teacher and learner. The emphasis is on experiential learning and learner engagement; strategies and delivery options are abundant. Let us explore this exciting, complex world of developing meaningful, relevant educational activities for holistic nurses, beginning with the theoretical foundations of adult learning.

While numerous adult learning theories provide ideas and insight into the ways that adults learn, no single theory can be universally applied. Malcolm Knowles's widely known work (ca. 1968) in differentiating andragogy (helping adults learn) and pedagogy (helping children learn) posited key assumptions about adult learners as:

1. having a self-concept: being autonomous, self-directed, and independent;
2. able to draw on life experiences;

3. internally motivated; and
4. ready to learn and apply that learning immediately.

Their work was met with some criticism, but it did open a conversation about the importance of educational approaches that meet people where they are. Andragogical principles require the collaboration of both educators and learners to actively carry out learning processes (Bouchrika, 2025).

Today, the emphasis in professional development focuses on experiential learning—learning by doing. Kolb, with Fry, brought forward ideas from earlier work by Dewey and Piaget and developed the *experiential learning theory*. This theory, based on the belief that "learning is the process whereby knowledge is created through the transformation of experience," (McLeod, 2025, p. 38) works on a four-stage learning cycle and four distinct learning styles. The learning cycles include:

1. Concrete experience, a new or reinterpreted experience or situation.
2. Reflective observation on the experience, particularly noticing inconsistencies between the experience and understanding.
3. Abstract conceptualization, giving rise to a new idea, or modifying an existing abstract concept.
4. Active experimentation, applying ideas to see what happens.

Importantly, movement through these stages is dynamic and continuous, and Kolb posited that effective learning requires that the learner engage in all of them. Learning styles include doers (hands-on), reflectors (view situations from a variety of perspectives), assimilators (pull a wide range of information into concise form), and convergers (find uses for ideas and theories). Of course, there is much more to each of these, and humans are unique, unitary beings, but exploring these ideas is helpful in planning activities.

Holistic educators benefit from knowledge of the adult learning theories, but one, Donald Schon (1983), resonates within holistic approaches to learning. His work on reflection expanded ideas about the possibilities of cultivating reflective practice as an important way of knowing. He argued that the rigor of reflection is both like and unlike that of controlled research, and he believed it to be the heart of professional artistry. Schon differentiated reflection-in-action (reflecting while something is happening) from reflection-on-action (reviewing, analyzing, and evaluating what has happened). His work is profound and includes many ideas worth exploring. Holistic educators incorporate reflective practice into experiential learning activities for its beauty and power to sit compassionately with self, not judging but rather noticing and deepening practice. According to Johns (2022), reflective practice is:

> Being mindful of self, either within or after experience, as if a mirror in which the practitioner can view and focus self within the context of a particular experience in order to confront, understand, and become empowered towards holding and resolving the creative tension between one's vision of desirable practice and one's actual practice, to gain insight within a reflexive spiral towards realising one's vision of practice as a lived reality. (p. 8)

Reflection, then, is the foundation of reflective practice. In building educational activities, the enduring threads include *nursing knowledge, holistic self-development and self-care,* and *reflective practice*. Regardless of the aim, content, or delivery, these threads should be interwoven structural supports.

Building activities generally include three processes: planning, implementation, and evaluation. The first steps in activity *planning* involve clearly defining the educational need. Pilcher and Graebe (2018) discussed the importance of identifying the practice gap to discern whether the need is knowledge, skill, application to practice, a combination, or something completely different. From there, educators can envision an activity designed to meet the learning outcome—what the learner will be able to do and/or do differently because of participating in the educational activity. Learner engagement strategies are the ways the educator brings the content to life, and there are many. The onus is on creatively integrating those most appropriate for the audience and the educational need, which support meeting the learning outcome and are interactive and fun. Examples of learner engagement strategies include gaming, nursing situations, hands-on activities, role playing, aesthetic/creative activities, and simulation.

The *implementation* of educational activities may be live or online. Online delivery might be synchronous (e.g., live presentation), asynchronous (e.g., recorded lecture), or a combination. Delivery platforms are numerous; many have recording capabilities so those not attending can still see and hear what happened. We are living more and more in a virtual world—an interesting thought for holistic educators. Examples of holistic implementation strategies include opening meditations before being able to begin the lesson, virtual cafes, art museums and concerts, group activities, and interactive blogs.

Evaluation of the activity closes the loop, yet, in reality, keeps it continuous as the educator determines the extent to which the learning outcome has been met and then revises the activity as indicated. This is the circular holistic caring process as applied to education: assessing, planning, determining outcomes, implementing, evaluating, reassessing = being dynamic and enduring.

It is beyond the scope of this chapter to examine all of the touchstones that inform nursing practice. Transition into practice and transitions while in practice are both pivotal moments in time for a nurse. Both new graduates and experienced nurses transitioning to different population foci or roles require support. There is no right or standard orientation process: some systems have more formalized transition programs (e.g., nurse residencies, mentorship, bridging programs); some have a less formal process. Regardless, it is important to welcome new people and make them feel like part of the team.

Other touchstones are related to workload, feeling safe at work, being treated with respect, having role autonomy, and system resources and supports. Much of what happens will affect the nurse's growth and their desire to remain in nursing.

At the End of the Day

Holistic nurses are committed to continuous lifelong learning and personal growth for self and others. As role models, they engage in self-assessment and self-reflection and commit to practicing self-development and self-care to enhance their wholeness. ANA and AHNA (2019) define the holistic nurses' responsibility for professional development in the *Holistic Nursing: Scope and Standards*. Standard 12, Education, states: "The holistic registered nurse attains knowledge and competence that reflect current nursing practice and promotes futuristic thinking" (p. 100). Standard 15, Professional Practice Evaluation, states: "The holistic registered nurse evaluates one's own and others' nursing practice" (p. 106). Provision 7 of the ANA (2025) *Code of Ethics for Nurses* states, "Nurses advance the profession through multiple approaches to knowledge development, professional standards and the generation of policies for nursing, health, and social concerns" (p viii). Holistic nurses' commitment to living in concert with the profession's scope and standards of practice and ethical code illuminates their commitment to live their social and moral imperative to care.

Integration

There are widespread implications related to transforming nursing education. Educators must be willing to try new ways of being and doing to make this shift happen. One example is completing the requirements for endorsement as a holistic nursing academic-based program. Achieving endorsement signifies that the curriculum has been evaluated and found to be based on the philosophy of holism and is consistent with *Holistic Nursing: Scope and Standards of Practice*. Endorsement is received from the AHNCC; full details about the process can be found on the AHNCC's website. Researchers must explore diverse educational approaches and study the impact that holistic nursing education has on the nurse, the recipient of care, and the healthcare system (e.g., retention, less burnout); additionally, research must remain a solid core course in all nursing programs. We must shift from evidence-based to evidence-informed practice. Policymakers must devise ways to support resource acquisition. All nurses should advocate for Title 8 funding for nursing education and for maintaining the National Institute of Nursing Research as a standalone institute. At the time of this writing, both of these are at risk. Practicing nurses must carry the foundation of holism forward into the entirety of their lifeway. Ultimately, every nurse in every arena must be present, informed, courageous, and find and use their voice.

Conclusion

Ideas that are unfolding in education have been introduced and discussed in this chapter, but there are others yet to be discovered and explored. Imagine a world where interprofessional education and practice are the norm—where healthcare professionals know about, value, and communicate with clarity and respect, enhancing whole-person care. Imagine a world where the culture of health care focuses on health instead of illness—where people, not diseases, receive care. Imagine a world where the threads of nursing knowledge, holistic self-development and self-care, and reflective practice are integrated into every nursing professional development activity—where every nurse is a certified Holistic Nurse. Imagine it—believe it can happen, and it will!

References

American Association of Colleges of Nursing. (2021). *The essentials: Core competencies for professional nursing education 2020–2030*. https://www.aacnnursing.org/Portals/42/AcademicNursing/pdf/Essentials-2021.pdf

American Association of Colleges of Nursing. (2024). *Nursing faculty shortage fact sheet*. http://www.aacnnursing.org/portals/42/news/factsheets /faculty-shortage factsheet /pdf

American Holistic Nurses Association. (2019). *Holistic self-care for nurses*. https://www.ahna.org/Membership/Member-Advantage/Whatisselfcare

American Nurses Association. (2025). *Code of ethics for nurses*. Nursesbooks.org.

American Nurses Association & American Holistic Nurses Association. (2019). *Holistic nursing: Scope and standards of practice* (3rd ed.). Nursesbooks.org.

Barrett, D. (2022). Impact of COVID-19 on nursing students: What does the evidence tell us? *Evidence Based Nursing, 25*(2), 37–38. https://doi.org/10.1136/ebnurs-2022-103533

Bingham, T., & Conner, M. (2015). *The new social learning: Connect, collaborate, work* (2nd ed.). ATD Press.

Bouchrika, I. (2025). *The andragogy approach: Knowles' adult learning theory principles for 2025*. https://www.learning-theories.com/andragogy-adult-learning-theory-knowles.html

Brunt, B., & Morris, M. (2025). *Nursing professional development*. StatPearls Publishing

Buchan, J., & Catton, H. (2023). *Recover to rebuild*. International Council of Nurses. ICN_Recover-to-Rebuild_report_EN.pdf

Cherry, B., & Jacobs, S. (2017). *Contemporary nursing, issues, trends, & management*. Elsevier

Erickson, H. (2007). Philosophy and theory of holism. *Nursing Clinics of North America, 42*, 139–163.

Erickson, H., Erickson, M., Enzman-Hines, M., Sandor, M. K., Shields, D., & Southard, M. E. (2017). *Foundations, competencies, and curricular guidelines for basic to doctoral holistic nursing education*. American Holistic Nurses Credentialing Corporation in concert with the American Holistic Nurses Association.

Erickson, H., Shields, D., Enzman-Hines, M., Erickson, M., & Hanley, M. A. (2025). *Beyond boundaries: Holistic nursing education in the 21st century*. In press. Kendall Hunt Publishing.

Farahani, M., Nargesi, S., Saniee, N., Dolatshahi, Z., Beni, F. H. & Shariatpanahi, S. (2024). Factors affecting nurses retention during the COVID-19 pandemic: A systematic review. *Human Resources for Health, 22*(78), 2–21. https://doi.org/10.1186/s12960-024-00960-7

Fawcett, J. (1995). *Analysis and evaluation of conceptual models of nursing* (3rd ed.). F. A. Davis.

Fawcett, J. (2005). The structure of contemporary nursing knowledge. In J. Fawcett & S. Desanto-Madeya (Eds.), *Contemporary nursing knowledge: Analysis and evaluation of nursing .models and theories* (pp. 3–30). F. A. Davis.

Fowler, M. (2015). *Guide to nursing's social policy statement. Understanding from social contract to social covenant*. Nursesbooks.org

Ghebreyesus, T. (2020, March 11). WHO Director-General's opening remarks at the media briefing on COVID-19. 11 March 2020

Head, M., Acosta, S., Bickford, E., & Leatherland, M. (2022). Impact of COVID-19 on undergraduate nursing education: Student perspectives. *Academic Medicine, 97*(3), S49–S54.https://doi.org/10.1097/ACM.0000000000004530

Health Resources & Services Administration. (2024a). *2022 national sample survey of registered nurses snapshot*. https://bhw.hrsa.gov/sites/default/files/bureau-health-workforce/data-research/nssrn-covid-impact-report.pdf.

Health Resources & Services Administration. (2024b). *Experience of nurses working during the COVID pandemic – data from the 2022 NSSRN.* https://bhw.hrsa.gov/sites/default/files/bureau-health-workforce/data-research/nssrn-covid-impact-report.pdf

Hills, M., Watson, J., & Cara, C. (2021). *Creating a caring science curriculum: An emancipatory relational pedagogy for nursing* (2nd ed). Springer.

Institute of Medicine. (2015). *Measuring the impact of interprofessional education on collaborative practice and patient outcomes.* National Academies Press.

Johns, C. (2022). *Becoming a reflective practitioner* (6th ed.). Wiley-Blackwell.

Jones-Shenk, J. (2019). From in-service education to continuing education in nursing: A brief historical journey. *The Journal of Continuing Education in Nursing, 50*(4), 143–144.

Leaver, C., Stanley, J., & Veenema, T. G. (2022). Impact of the COVID-19 pandemic on the future of nursing education. *Academic Medicine, 97*(3), S82–S89. https://doi.org/10.1097/ACM.00000000000

Martin, B., Kaminsky Ozturk, N., Smiley, R., Spector, N., Silvestro, J., Bowles, W., & Alexander, M. (2023). National Council of State Boards of Nursing. Assessing the impact of the COVID-19 pandemic on nursing education: A national study of prelicensure RN programs. *Journal of Nursing Regulation, 14*(1), S1–S67. https://doi.org/10.1016/S2155-8256(23)00041-8

McLeod, S. (2025). Kolb's learning styles and experiential learning cycle. https://www.simplypsychology.org/learning-kolb.html

Merriam-Webster. (2019). *Curriculum.* In Merriam-Webster.com dictionary. https://www.merriam-webster.com/dictionary/curriculum

MTa Learning. (n.d.). *What is experiential learning?* https://www.experientiallearning.org/about-mta/what-is-experiential-learning

Newman, M. A. (1992). Prevailing paradigms in nursing. *Nursing Outlook, 40*(1), 10–13, 32.

Newman, M. A., Smith, M. C., Pharris, M. D., & Jones, D. (2008). The focus of the discipline revisited. *Advances in Nursing Science, 31*(1), E16–E27.

Nightingale, F. (1859). *Notes on nursing.* Dover Publications.

Parse, R. R. (1987). *Nursing science major paradigms, theories, and critiques.* W.B. Saunders.

Parse, R. R. (2000). Paradigms: A reprise. *Nursing Science Quarterly, 13*(4), 275–276.

Pilcher, J., & Graebe, J. (2018). Strategies to promote learning and engage participants. *The Journal of Continuing Education in Nursing, 49*(5), 197–199.

Prabhat, S. (2011). *Difference between education and learning.* http://www.differencebetween.net /miscellan0eous/difference-between-education-and-learning/

Schon, D. (1983). The reflective practitioner—How professionals think in action. *Basic Books.* https://sopper.dk/speciale /arkiv/book49.pdf

Shields, D., & Erickson, M. (2017). Learning and living nursing's moral/social imperative to care. *Beginnings, 37*(5), 6–7, 20–21.

Stout-Shaffer, S., & Shields, D. (2016). *Holistic self-development in education.* Unpublished model.

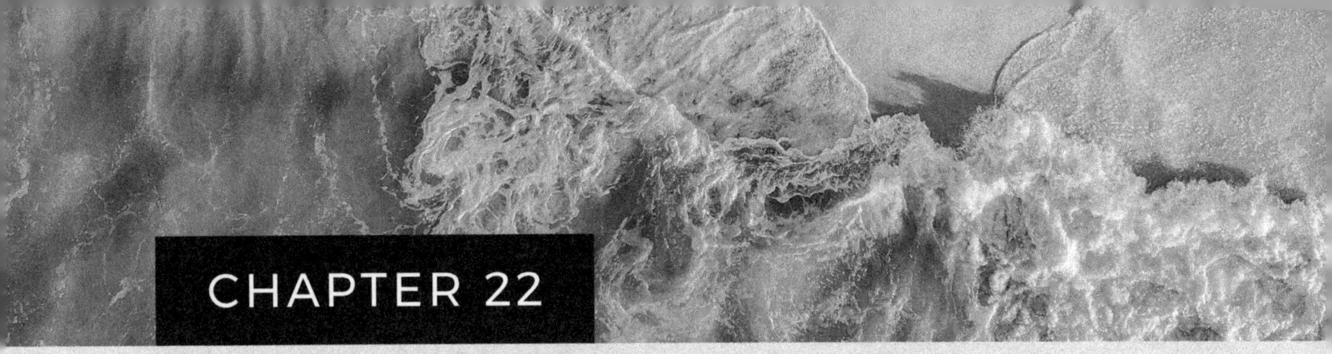

CHAPTER 22

Exploring, Applying, Creating, and Disseminating Evidence to Enhance Holistic Nursing Practice

Wyona M. Freysteinson

NURSE HEALER OBJECTIVES

- Discuss methods of exploring the evidence.
- Review the application of holistic nursing evidence into practice.
- Identify methods for generating holistic nursing evidence.
- Examine innovative approaches for disseminating holistic nursing evidence.
- Reflect on a research trajectory.

DEFINITIONS

Holistic nursing evidence: The body of knowledge and research that supports the practice of holistic nursing and emphasizes the care of the whole person—mind, body, spirit, and environment.

Literature reviews: Comprehensive analyses of existing research that summarize findings related to holistic nursing practices.

Evidence-based practice: A synthesis of the best available research evidence, clinical expertise, and patient experiences and preferences to inform and guide holistic nursing care.

Quality improvement: Using systematic methods to ensure quality by continually assessing and refining processes.

Disseminating evidence: The strategic processes used to share holistic nursing knowledge with the audiences who will most benefit from the information.

Research trajectory: The unwavering evolving research journey of a researcher's focused holistic inquiry over time.

Introduction

Numerous intriguing and perplexing mysteries arise in the daily practice of nursing. Holistic nurses are encouraged to reflect on these experiences, contemplate the mysteries, and derive insights to shape and focus nursing questions. The primary goal of holistic nursing scholarship is to explore, expand, create, apply, and share holistic nursing expertise to expand the knowledge base of healing and holism for nursing practice.

Holistic nursing research provides a window into unique aspects of human healing, nursing ways of being, and interventions to optimize human health.

- The goal of holistic nursing research is to advance a person-centered, philosophical, theoretical, and practice knowledge base that positively transforms human health.
- The reach of holistic nursing research extends to all people, including minoritized and diverse communities, all disciplines, and all healthcare and policy settings, to make the world a better place.
- All modes of holistic nursing inquiry are encouraged, including those that are boundaryless and limitless (Freysteinson et al., 2024).

Exploring the Evidence: A Guide for Holistic Nurses

Your contribution to applying holistic nursing evidence into practice is highly valued. Key priorities for holistic nursing are to (1) enhance the well-being of nurses; (2) create unique holistic nursing practices; (3) mitigate pain that is physical, psychosocial, or spiritual; (4) delve into understanding and reducing health inequities; and (5) develop nature and environmental studies (Freysteinson et al., 2024). Understanding and application of evidence directly impacts patient care and outcomes. Finding and understanding the literature on a specific topic can initially feel overwhelming. Here is a step-by-step approach to help one navigate and gather evidence that supports holistic nursing practice:

1. **Start with a Question**: Research questions about healing, ways of being, and health-improving interventions often originate from real-world patient dilemmas or a broad area of interest. Developing a research question is like putting a puzzle together: it is an ongoing process of revising and adjusting as one delves into the knowledge of what is and is not known. Initially, one may engage with those who have had similar puzzling experiences or uncertainties. Patients, clients, and nurses can provide valuable perspectives. A thorough review of existing literature helps clarify what is already known and highlights gaps in knowledge. The question evolves into a feasible and meaningful contribution to the field through iterative refinement and incorporating feedback.
2. **Databases:** A database, search engine, and browser are programs that allow users to navigate websites on the internet. Worldwide, there are over 1,500 databases. Popular browsers are Google, Chrome, Bing, Safari, Edge, and Firefox. Use DuckDuckGo for more academic browsing, as this browser allows for private searches and blocks cookie pop-ups. PubMed, CINAHL, and Scopus are common databases that healthcare organizations subscribe to for academic literature on health and holistic care topics. Google Scholar is intuitive (easy to use) and does not require specialized key terms. What sets this database apart is that it includes the number of times an article has been cited, providing a quick measure of the work's academic impact. However, users should be cautious, as this database includes predatory or non-peer-reviewed works, which can compromise the reliability of search results. The database redeems itself in that search results typically highlight articles from reputable publishers first.
3. **Search Using Key Words**: Think of a few keywords or phrases related to a question or topic or consult with a librarian. Key terms are the foundational concepts or phrases that define and clarify the focus of a study or discussion, particularly in holistic nursing. In holistic nursing, key terms might include concepts like "healing," "integrative care," "mind–body connection," or "patient-centered care." These terms can be used to refine the search and find literature directly relevant to your area of interest.
4. **Explore Different Types of Information**:
    - **Review Articles**: When one begins to search for academic literature to learn about a topic, the best place to start is by searching for literature review articles. These studies provide summaries of the

findings of multiple research studies on a single topic. Several review articles will provide a broad understanding of the evidence. To find review articles, include "review" as a search term. For example, the terms "compassion" AND "review" AND "nursing" led to a literature review of compassionate care interventions (Robinson et al., 2023).
- **Research Articles:** These offer detailed insights from individual studies and help understand specific interventions, results, and outcomes. For example, the words "therapeutic touch" AND "randomized control trial" will unearth multiple research studies.

5. **Credibility and Reliability**: Assess each article for trustworthiness. Examine the author's credentials, where the study was published, and if it comes from a credible journal or website. Quality sources strengthen your knowledge of the subject and ensure one is guided by trustworthy evidence.
6. **Check for Predatory Works:** Be cautious when selecting journals for publishing or referencing, as predatory journals are rising. These profit-driven publications often lack peer review, publish poor-quality research, and charge high fees. These journals may promise rapid publication or mimic reputable journals, risking one's professional reputation (Oermann et al., 2021). To avoid predatory articles, research the journal's background, check its impact factor and indexing, and consult trusted resources, i.e., your organization's librarian, Directory of Open Access Journals or Beall's list.
7. **Broaden One's Perspective:** Holistic nurses can explore various resources to deepen their understanding. Professional organizations like the American Holistic Nurses Association and the Global Association of Holistic Nurses offer access to white papers and holistic researchers. Networking with interdisciplinary teams, including wellness practitioners, can provide valuable insights into diverse healing modalities. By collaborating with professionals from different fields, holistic nurses can gain a broader perspective on patient care and learn about complementary therapies that can enhance their practice.
8. **Organize Findings**: Keep notes on each source as you gather information. Record the key points: who authored it, method, population, sample, data collection, and results. Consider automating these research tasks with an AI generator to search for and obtain instant summaries of research papers. Elicit AI provides an Excel spreadsheet (matrix) with multiple columns (e.g., summary, methodology, intervention, findings) that can be downloaded. Elicit, and most AI generators, do not access all databases; however, articles from searches obtained in other databases can be added to the matrix.
9. **Make Sense of What You Found**: Search for patterns or themes in the literature. Several research studies may have similar findings, or there may be gaps where more research is needed (significant gaps are exciting research deserts and an ocean of possibilities). Recognizing these patterns can guide your future project. Following these steps will build a solid foundation of evidence-based knowledge, allowing one to bring the best of holistic, research-supported practices to your patients.

Evidence-based Practice

Evidence-based knowledge in holistic nursing means integrating the best available research with clinical expertise and patient preferences to make informed, compassionate care decisions. It involves recognizing the whole person—mind, body, spirit, and environment—and using research to guide care that nurtures all these dimensions. For instance, if research shows that a particular therapeutic touch promotes relaxation and reduces pain, holistic nurses may integrate this practice to support physical healing and emotional comfort. The process of building evidence-based knowledge in holistic nursing involves:

1. **Identify relevant, holistic questions** using what, when, or why.

2. **Review research** from academic databases and credible websites.
3. **Evaluate and apply findings** to fit each patient's values and lifestyle.
4. **Observe and assess outcomes** holistically, examining the impact on physical, emotional, and spiritual well-being.

Evidence-based knowledge in holistic nursing is patient-centered, fostering clinically effective care and deeply respecting each patient's values and preferences.

Quality Improvement

Quality improvement (QI) in holistic nursing is a continuous process of enhancing patient care by examining and refining the methods used in practice. It involves recognizing areas where holistic care delivery can be optimized, such as reducing wait times for complementary therapies, improving communication between care providers, or streamlining processes to make them more patient centered. In holistic nursing, the QI process includes:

1. **Apply a QI methodology** to organize a project. Plan, Do, Study, Act (PDSA) is a widely used framework for improving processes (Leis & Shojania, 2017). It involves a cyclical, iterative process.
2. **Identify** areas for improvement.
3. **Collect** data on current practices, such as patient feedback on integrative care experiences and academic literature.
4. **Test** small changes in a structured way.
5. **Review** results and gather insights on what fosters patient healing.

Evidence-based knowledge and quality improvement complement each other in holistic nursing practice. Evidence-based knowledge provides a research-backed foundation, while quality improvement ensures that care is continuously adapted to meet patient needs holistically person-centered. Together, EBP and QI create a cycle of learning and growth that fosters higher-quality, integrative care that aligns with the principles of holistic nursing—addressing physical symptoms and emotional, social, and spiritual well-being.

Creating Holistic Nursing Evidence

Innovative holistic nursing interventions must be developed, researched, and shared with the greater holistic nursing community. Similarly, innovative interventions that have already been developed and are being used must be studied and disseminated to enhance patient care. Innovations in holistic nursing care begin, metaphorically, "at the bedside": innovations can occur anywhere there are holistic nurses. Holistic nurses are highly attuned to subtle changes in their patients, often reflecting silently, "What is this patient experiencing?" or "What is the best way to approach this situation?" When little is known about a specific experience or when implementing a novel intervention, these observations become the foundation for generating evidence. Use your imagination to uncover an intervention you have been using or create new interventions. Examples

- Patients, families, and team members in Magee and Raines' caring arts program chose drawing, collage, painting silk scarves, and bottle cap art (Magee & Raines, 2022).
- Ku, Chua, and Shorey conducted a meta-analysis of storytelling in eight studies and found a significant decrease in anxiety and fear for hospitalized children (Ku et al., 2025).
- Nurses are collaborating with a music therapist to decrease pain, anxiety, and agitation in critical care patients (Golino et al., 2019, 2023).
- Oktri and Lorica did a systematic review of healing gardens and found that healing gardens provide positive energy, protected self-expressions of healing, and improved quality of life for patients (Oktri & Lorica, 2020).

Research Methods

Polit and Beck's research textbook is authored by Jane Flanagan and Cheryl Beck, both holistic nurses (Flanagan & Beck, 2024). Their book provides an excellent overview of research methodology. Examples of research methods that align with holistic nursing practices are:

1. **Case Studies**: A case study thoroughly examines a patient's experience. Consider a case study of a unique patient experience where one intuitively intervenes with a unique holistic approach.
2. **Questionnaires**: Survey questionnaires are a helpful way to gather data from many people on their thoughts and experiences.
3. **Phenomenology**: This is an approach where individuals share their thoughts, feelings, and emotions about an experience that has not been studied from people's perspective. The data is analyzed and shared in a descriptive style.
4. **Hermeneutical Phenomenology**: Hermeneutics is the interpretive study of an individual's words about an experience. Watson discusses the philosophy underlying between descriptive and interpretative phenomenology (Watson, 2024).
5. **Story Telling**: Story-theory-guided research and practice is a nursing midrange theory that reflects Liehr and Smith's journey. This gentle research technique of gentle discussion and profound listening in true presence brings health challenges to light (Liehr & Smith, 2020).
6. **Small Pilot or Feasibility Studies**: Large funding agencies place great value on feasibility studies. These studies do not explore effects or outcomes; rather, these studies determine the feasibility of the intended research methodology (i.e., how difficult was it to recruit individuals, and could the intervention be replicated precisely by each nurse?) On the other hand, there are pilot studies. These studies are preliminary studies that explore the effects of a holistic intervention on a specific group of patients.

The world of holistic nursing research begs expansion. By evaluating outcomes of health practices, holistic nurses can generate evidence that supports and advances the field, encouraging broader acceptance and integration of their holistic interventions.

Developing Theory

Holistic nursing theory involves addressing gaps in understanding and practice through systematic inquiry. It is grounded in the holistic care philosophy of treating the whole person. By drawing from clinical observations and qualitative studies of patient experiences, theories provide a framework for compassionate, holistic nursing care.

Disseminating Holistic Nursing Evidence

Sharing our work in evidence-based practice, quality improvement, and research with the greater world of holistic nurses and others is essential to advancing the knowledge and practice of holistic care. Without consistent efforts to share findings, much of the valuable insight gained through holistic nursing may remain localized, with only small portions shared sporadically across the globe. This fragmented dissemination limits the potential for holistic nursing to grow as a unified, evidence-based practice and reduces opportunities for collaboration and innovation within and beyond the field. By prioritizing the sharing of holistic nursing research, we can ensure that this valuable knowledge reaches a broader audience and contributes to improving patient care worldwide.

- **Holistic Nursing Journals**: Publishing evidence in journals specifically focused on holistic nursing, such as the *Journal of Holistic Nursing* or *Holistic Nursing Practice,* ensures that research reaches an audience dedicated to holistic nursing care.
- **Other Nursing, Multi-disciplinary Journal, and Non-Academic Journals**: Whether to publish in a holistic nursing journal or another journal is a question that is often asked. There is value in both options: publishing in holistic nursing journals reaches an audience of holistic nurses. Publishing in other journals communicates the value of holistic nursing to the world.
- **Blogs:** New authors may consider writing short blogs for Nursology.net, as there is a

team who provide assistance to first-time blog users.

- **Holistic Nursing Conferences**: Presenting at events organized by associations like the American Holistic Nurses Association (AHNA) or other holistic health conferences allows nurses to connect with like-minded professionals. These gatherings provide a supportive environment for sharing evidence.
- **Holistic Nursing Associations**: Leveraging associations like AHNA can amplify research dissemination through newsletters, online resources, and member-exclusive events. Publishing in association newsletters or presenting at local chapter meetings allows holistic nurses to reach practitioners who prioritize holistic, patient-centered approaches.
- **Website**: Creating a website offers a dedicated space to showcase work expertise and build one's professional presence. It is a hub for connecting with the community and promoting holistic nursing.
- **Webinars**: Hosting webinars or online sessions can reach a broad audience of holistic practitioners and community members.
- **Video**: Using video to disseminate research is an engaging and accessible way to share findings with diverse audiences. Videos can effectively communicate complex ideas through visuals, storytelling, and demonstrations, making research more relatable and impactful for practitioners, policymakers, and the public.
- **Clinical In-Services**: Offering in-service training in healthcare settings on holistic topics helps nurses learn about the details of holistic practices and interventions they can bring directly to patient care.
- **Patient-Centered Education Materials**: Developing pamphlets, handouts, and videos incorporating holistic research is another approach to reach the individuals who need it most.
- **Social Media**: Sharing holistic research through social media channels can reach a diverse audience, spreading awareness of holistic practices beyond the nursing community. Platforms like Instagram, Facebook, and LinkedIn provide opportunities to discuss the benefits of holistic nursing and engage directly with a wide range of followers interested in integrative care.
- **Infographics and Visual Storytelling**: Share infographics or other visual materials that break down complex holistic research into accessible, visually appealing content that can be used in healthcare settings, community spaces, or online. Visual summaries emphasizing holistic concepts—like mind-body-spirit balance or natural healing practices—make research findings more approachable and meaningful to diverse audiences.
- **Open Access Repositories**: Uploading research to open-access repositories focused on integrative health and nursing increases accessibility and ensures that holistic evidence is freely available to a broader audience. Platforms like ResearchGate and institutional repositories make it easy for holistic nurses and other professionals to apply research findings in practice.
- **Continuing Education (CE) in Holistic Topics**: Developing CE modules based on holistic research, such as the benefits of therapeutic touch or stress reduction through breathwork, allows nurses to expand their knowledge and skills in integrative care. Nursing associations and holistic organizations can offer CE courses with a holistic focus.

Nursing Research Trajectory

When we see the words *research trajectory*, we may envision a well-written action plan; however, this seldom occurs. A holistic nursing research trajectory is more like a spur-of-the-moment journey to anywhere that the head or heart takes us. In one's mind's eye, there is a vague notion, an inkling of what may lie ahead on the next step or at the journey's end. The path alternates between being smooth and rugged. There are many potholes and pitfalls, some of which bring one to a jolting halt with the worry that the journey is lost. There are numerous forks in the road, some of which require asking those who may know and other paths where an unseen but loving force leads one. The journey may begin with a whisper of energy, a gut feeling, or a sudden realization that one is facing an unknown. Doing something about that feeling (i.e., asking other holistic nurses or searching the literature) begins the research journey.

My Research Trajectory

My journey was an ever-evolving journey of inquiry into the complexities of mirror-viewing.

Over 60 years ago, I decided to be a nurse. At age three, I was my great-grandmother's nurse. Grandma had diabetes. I loved testing her urine for ketones and learning the good and bad colors. By four, I was giving her insulin injections, and at five, I was drawing up her insulin. I learned about her diet—all we knew then was to avoid sugar. Every day, Grandma would sit in front of the mirror in her bedroom as I combed her hair. When she was terminally ill, her last wish was her hand mirror so that she could see her face.

When I turned 16 years old, I started work as a nursing aide in a nursing home where my orientation consisted of "feed, wash, and put them (12 people) to bed." Every day was unique as I cared for individuals in different units. One day, I walked into a room and was shocked to find the *ugliest person* this 16-year-old had ever laid eyes on. A woman lay on the bed: she weighed as little as 80 pounds, her face was in agony, and her fingers and limbs were severely distorted. She ate one or two bites of food and offered me her tea. After eating, I wiped her face, and she asked for her hand mirror. As I brought the mirror toward her face with shaking hands, a hundred thoughts went through my mind (i.e., I will lose my job for doing this; we will need an ambulance; she may die of shock when she peers into the mirror). The agony and ugliness left her face as she gazed into the mirror. I call her Miss Peace.

In nursing school, during the bed bath lab, and although the instructor did not comment on it, I noticed a mirror on an overbed table and spontaneously thought, "Nurses should use mirrors." When I began my nursing career (approximately 50 years ago), we bathed our patients, and I would offer the mirror after a bed bath. I carried a pocket mirror. The response I would see as others viewed themselves in a mirror was like that of Miss Peace.

Clinical Fright

I gently offered a mirror to patients with minor wounds and traumatic injuries. Only one older gentleman uttered "no" as I offered a mirror. I would later realize that many people do not use mirrors, a concept that I call mirror avoidance. Others would peer with curiosity at their wounds. One day, I offered my mirror to a teenager in a neurosurgery unit. He had recently had brain surgery and as a result, the hair on one side of his head had been shaved off. The teen's reaction was one of pure panic and a moment of mirror terror. That moment was pivotal—it sparked a research journey of mirrors and holistic nursing care. I needed to understand what happened to my patients when they gazed into mirrors, how and when, and even if nurses should use mirrors. And if not nurses, who would support patients in mirror-viewing?

Mirror Taboo

When I proposed studying mirror-viewing for my master's thesis, I encountered resistance at nearly every turn. Some colleagues were horrified by the idea, while others dismissed it entirely. A social worker pulled me aside and uttered, "Nurses should not use mirrors with patients." My dean, a nurse, said: "People who are sick and dying in hospitals do not look in mirrors." This statement, made by someone who was an authority, was the jolting moment that almost ended my research trajectory. That night, I began to count the number of patients I may have had over 13 years who viewed their faces or wounds in my pocket or a bedside table mirror: hundreds of images flashed through my mind as I relived precious moments of supporting individuals in this sacred moment. Although mirrors are ordinary, giving voice to the mirror experience was taboo. A taboo is something uncanny, forbidden, or sacred.

Death, for example, was at one time something we could not discuss when someone was dying: holistic nurses gently eased society away from this taboo. Nurses too, could demystify this mirror taboo that had been unearthed.

Hermeneutic Phenomenology

Despite objections, I was led by an unseen force or serendipitously found a philosopher on campus who had been a student of the philosopher Paul Ricoeur. This philosopher was fascinated by understanding the experience of viewing self in the mirror and became a member of my thesis committee. Seven women who perceived themselves to be terminally ill (one died three days after our interview) consented to sharing their mirror experiences. Their stories of viewing self in the mirror were intimate, spellbinding, and healing. The woman who died three days after our interview said people feel curious and compelled to check their body: "you just gotta do that." My findings revealed two prerequisites for mirror viewing: one must have access to a mirror, and some require assistance in using a mirror. I learned that experience is a decision, the act of seeing and consenting to what one has observed (i.e., wondering what one may appear like in a coffin). I also discovered the profound emotional impact of seeing oneself after a significant physical change, from shock and horror to moments of self-acceptance.

Surveys

I visited 10 hospitals and surveyed the mirrors in one empty patient room at each facility. Seven of the hospitals lacked bed-table mirrors. In three hospitals, a small mirror was mounted above a sink, seemingly intended for nurses to use as they entered the room. I found similar disappointing results in nursing homes. In one nursing home, the only mirrors were small and mounted so high in the bathrooms that it would be impossible for individuals in wheelchairs to see their faces. The residents were disheveled, depressed, and despondent. The only full-length mirror I observed in 10 nursing homes was in the front lobby of one nursing home. As I quietly sat in a lobby chair, I noticed many older individuals, some were walking and others were in wheelchairs, checking their reflections, turning about, and adjusting their clothing to ensure they appeared presentable. The nursing home office door was beside that mirror: the administrator exited the office in a wheelchair.

Storytelling

As I continued my research, I explored mirror-viewing stories with my graduate PhD nursing students in various patient populations, including relatives of individuals with dementia, those recovering from mastectomies, amputations, and flat closures. Each group had unique experiences, but common themes emerged: decision, action, and consent. Mastectomy patients described a mix of curiosity and distress when seeing their surgical sites for the first time. Amputees who have lower limb amputations often shared that mirror-viewing is a necessary step in adjusting their prostheses, and accepting a new reality, though overwhelming emotions often accompany it. These experiences showed me how profoundly mirrors influence body image and emotional well-being.

The mirror-viewing theory, which took 30 years to develop, explores the neural processes underlying self-recognition and the disruptions caused by visible bodily changes.

Integration

The findings of eight research studies, a literature review, and community consultation led to the development of the Neurocognitive Theory of Mirror-Viewing (Freysteinson, 2020), supportive mirror interventions, an instrument to measure mirror-viewing, and tailored education.

Clinical Practice

When a hospital in Texas uncovered no private full-length mirrors for individuals undergoing lower limb amputation, management purchased 140 mirrors (small two-sided magnification and full-length rolling mirrors) to implement supportive nursing interventions. The materials department swiftly returned the mirrors. When asked about this, the researchers were informed that mirrors were unsafe and patients did not need mirrors (echoes of the mirror taboo). Once the mirrors were sent (again), researchers found that mirror-viewing education significantly improved the confidence and frequency of nurses supporting patients in mirror-viewing following visible disfigurement (Freysteinson et al., 2021).

Education

The renowned Texas Rehabilitation and Research Memorial Hospital incorporated this education into its nursing orientation program and released the training module to 17 hospitals. A YouTube video designed to teach nurses why, when, and how to support an individual with mirror-viewing after amputation and other disfigurement has received over 21,000 views. Educational events have opened an unacknowledged phenomenon of mirror discomfort, mirror avoidance, and intrusive traumatic mirror-image memories, prompting many individuals, including nurses, to share their own distressing mirror-viewing experiences after a traumatic surgery or accident.

Global Health

Consultations with psychologists in the United Kingdom have led to the introduction of mirrors and mirror-viewing support in burn and intensive care units. This work has been presented in Africa, Australia, Canada, Ireland, South Korea, the United Kingdom, and the United States through over 50 presentations and 25 posters to more than 5,000 nurses and interdisciplinary team members. My mirror-viewing publications have been cited over 800 times by authors in 28 countries and used as a research highlight in nursing textbooks. The diversity of cited work extends to birthing, dementia, endotracheal tube experience, and healing environments. Recently, two young design students in Denmark developed a sleek wall with mirrors of various sizes for hospital rooms. The application of mirror-viewing theoretical concepts is increasingly becoming routine in caring for individuals with disfigurement.

Concluding Words

This journey has taught me the importance of addressing the mirror taboo in health care and providing patients with the support they need to choose to gaze at their reflections rather than seeing themselves for the first time in a hospital elevator or lobby mirror. I am honored to contribute to holistic nursing by offering insights into a tool as simple yet profound as a mirror. The research world of holistic nursing is rich with possibilities. We must explore, apply, and disseminate our knowledge to enhance holistic nursing practice. Our work will be filled with potholes and pitfalls; however, as holistic nurses, we have the wisdom to walk through and around almost anything.

References

Flanagan, J. M., & Beck, C. (2024). *Polit and Beck's nursing research: Generating and assessing evidence for nursing practice* (12th ed.). Wolters Kluwer.

Freysteinson, W. M. (2020). Demystifying the mirror taboo: A neurocognitive model of mirror viewing self in the mirror. *Nursing Inquiry, 27*(4), e12351. https://doi.org/10.1111/nin.12351

Freysteinson, W. M., Enzman Hines, M., Wardell, D., Friesen, M., Conrad, S., Zahourek, R., Gallo, A., & Prather, J. (2024). Identifying holistic nursing research priorities for 2023–2026. *Journal of Holistic Nursing, 42*(2), 182–201. https://doi.org/10.1177/08980101231213725

Freysteinson, W. M., Sarbacker, L., Gobeli, L., Tristan, K., Esquela, M. A., Wellington, C., Gonzalez, K., Thayer, B., & Yeatts, P. (2021). Educating nurses on supported mirror viewing for patients after amputation and other visible disfigurements. *Rehabilitation Nursing Journal, 46*(1), 43–51. [2.5 CEU]. https://doi.org/10.1097/RNJ.0000000000000287

Golino, A. J., Leone, R., Gollenberg, A., Christopher, C., Stanger, D., Davis, T. M., Meadows, A., Zhang, Z., & Friesen, M. A. (2019). Impact of an active music therapy intervention on intensive care patients. *American Journal of Critical Care*, 28(1), 48–55. https://doi-org.ezp.twu.edu/10.4037/ajcc2019792

Golino, A., Leone, R., Gollenberg, A., Gillam, A., Toone, K., Samahon, Y., Davis, T., Stanger, D., Friesen, M. A., & Meadows, A. (2023). Impact of a receptive music therapy intervention on mechanically-ventilated patients in the ICU: A randomized controlled trial. *American Journal of Critical Care*, *32*(2), 109–115. https://doi:10.4037/ajcc2023499

Ku, S. H., Chua, J. S., & Shorey, S. (2025). Effect of storytelling on anxiety and fear in children during hospitalization. *Journal of Pediatric Nursing*, *80*, P 41–48. https://doi.org/10.1016/j.pedn.2024.11.006

Liehr, P., & Smith, M. J. (2020). Claiming the narrative wave with story theory. *Advances in Nursing Science*, *43*(1), 15–27. http://dx.doi.org/10.1097/ANS.0000000000000303

Leis, J. A., & Shojania, K. G., (2017). A primer on PDSA: Executing plan-do-study-act cycles in practice, not just in name. *BMJ Quality Safety, 26*, 572–577. http://dx.doi.org/10.1136/bmjqs-2016-006245

Magee, P., & Raines, D. (2022). Building a caring arts program with oncology patients: From inception to impact. *Journal of Holistic Nursing, 40*(3), 238–254. https://doi-org.ezp.twu.edu/10.1177/08980101211037489

Oermann, M., Wrigley, J., Leslie H., Ledbetter, L., Carter-Templeton, H., & Edie, A. (2021). Integrity of databases for literature searches in nursing: Avoiding predatory journals. *Advances in Nursing Science, 44*(2), 102–110, https://doi.org/10.1097/ANS.0000000000000349

Oktri, A. H., & Lorica, J. (2020). The effect of healing garden to improve the patients healing: An integrative literature review. *Journal of Health and Caring Sciences*, 2(1), 34–47. https://doi-org.ezp.twu.edu/10.37719/jhcs.2020.v2i1.ra001

Robinson, J., Raphael, D., Moeke-Maxwell, T., Parr, J., Gott, M., & Slark, J. (2023). Implementing interventions to improve compassionate nursing care: A literature review. *International Nursing Review*, *71*(3), 457–467. https://doi.org/10.1111/inr.12910

Watson, A. A. (2024). A postmodernist qualitative research approach: Choosing between descriptive and interpretive phenomenology. *Journal of Advanced Nursing*. https://doi.org/10.1111/jan.16730

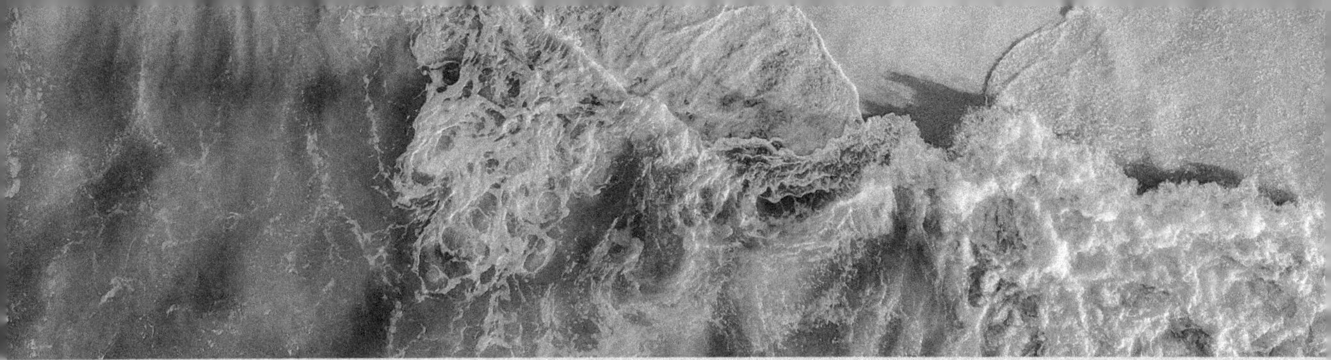

Advanced Concepts

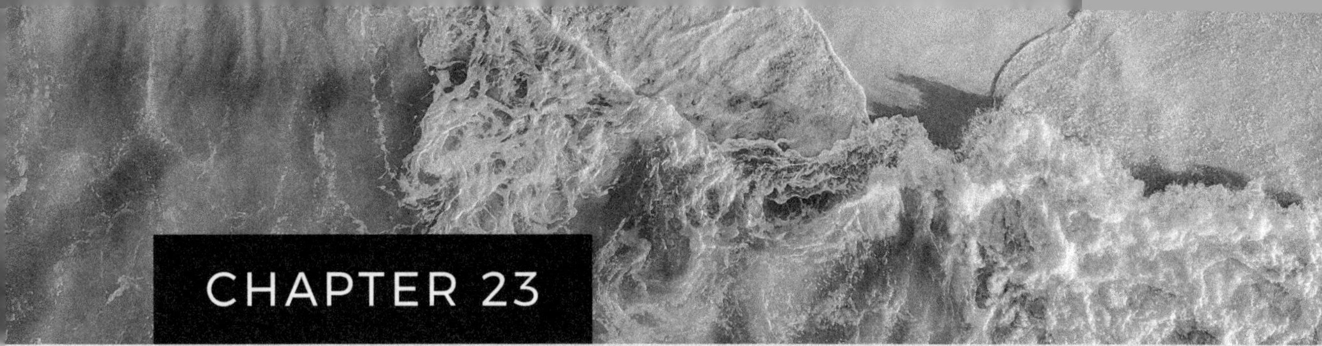

CHAPTER 23

Opportunities and Challenges in Advanced Holistic Nursing

Mary Enzman Hines

NURSE HEALER OBJECTIVES

- Explore the worldview, theories, and models embraced by advanced holistic nurses.
- Explicate the foci of care for advanced holistic nurses.
- Analyze the consensus model and its potential effect on advanced holistic nurses.
- Analyze the complementary aspects of advanced holistic and integrative care related to patient-centered treatment.

DEFINITIONS

Advanced holistic nurse by certification (AHN-BC): A certified advanced holistic nurse who synthesizes multiple sources of knowledge and therapies, including patient self-knowledge, and develops holistic care plans cocreated with patients. Certified advanced practice holistic nurses have the skills, knowledge, and education to provide patients, peers, and colleagues with information and care promoting health, wellness, and well-being and partner with patients to ensure person-centered care. These advanced practice nurses work in a variety of nursing settings including clinical settings, education, coaching, and administration (AHNCC, 2017a).

Advanced practice holistic nurse by certification (APHN-BC): Performs all tasks that the AHN-BC carries out with the added responsibilities of prescribing holistic treatments; developing holistic care plans cocreated by partnering with the patient; and prescribing pharmacologic agents based on current knowledge of pharmacology/herbology, homeopathy, psychoneuroimmunology and bio-psycho-physiology, clinical indicators, age, holistic status/needs, results of diagnostic labs, and the person's beliefs, values, and choices. Certified advanced practice holistic nurses have the skills and education to evaluate and analyze the therapeutic effects, possible side effects, and interactions of all prescribed treatments; provide patients with information about cost and expected outcomes of planned treatment and integrative options; partner with others to create an interprofessional plan that focuses on safe, effective holistic outcomes; document collaborative discussions, including holistic plan changes, communications, and rationale; and document referrals, including provisions for continuity of holistic care (AHNCC, 2017a).

Advanced practice holistic nurses: A unique group of nurses weaving a tapestry of body-mind-emotion-spirit-energy-cultural-environmental approaches to promote caring–healing within self and others. As advanced practice holistic nurses engage in a caring–healing process, it is a journey of changing and evolving of self and others and providing care aimed at promoting the health and well-being of populations across the life span (AHNCC, 2017a).

Advanced practice nurse (APN): A registered nurse who has a master's degree, post-master's certificate, or practice-focused Doctor of Nursing practice degree. APNs employ expert knowledge, complex decision-making skills, and clinical competencies necessary for expanded practice and can take on complex caseloads with greater independence and discretion. APNs are licensed at the state level and certified by national nursing organizations (APRN Consensus Work Group and National Council of State Boards of Nursing APRN Advisory Committee, 2008).

Advanced practice registered nurse (APRN): APRNs include nurse practitioners, clinical nurse specialists, nurse anesthetists, and nurse midwives, who are often primary care providers and are at the forefront of providing preventive care services to the public. APRNs treat and diagnose illnesses, advise the public on health issues, manage chronic disease, and engage in continuous education to remain ahead of any technological, methodological, or other developments in the field. APRNs hold at least a master's degree, in addition to the initial nursing education and licensing required for all registered nurses (RNs) (APRN Consensus Work Group and National Council of State Boards of Nursing APRN Advisory Committee, 2008).

Certification: Credential that authenticates the specialty knowledge for specific areas of care and offers employers, healthcare organizations, and patients proof that certified advanced practice holistic nurses possess the specialty knowledge, skills, and experience to effectively deliver safe, quality care that promotes optimal health and wellness outcomes and maintains a detailed set of standards of practice that validate these professional competencies (AHNCC, 2017a).

Consensus model for APRN regulation: Document that provides guidance for the licensure, accreditation, certification, and education of APRNs (APRN Consensus Work Group and National Council of State Boards of Nursing APRN Advisory Committee, 2008). The consensus model defines APRN and classifies key requirements for APRN education.

Current procedural terminology codes: Codes that describe medical, surgical, and diagnostic services and are designed to communicate uniform information about medical services and procedures for financial and analytical purposes.

Integrative health care: An approach characterized by a high degree of collaboration and communication among health professionals. What makes integrative health care unique is the sharing of information among team members, while keeping the patient at the center of care and decision making. The plan of care for each patient addresses biological, psychological, spiritual, and social needs. The interdisciplinary healthcare team includes a diverse group of members (e.g., nurses, physicians, psychologists, social workers, nutritionists, occupational and physical therapists, energy therapists, chiropractors), depending on the needs of the patient.

Patient-focused/centered care: Care approach that embraces a disease treatment model and views the patient from a systems approach (Daley, 2012). Patient-centered care delineates eight dimensions of patient-centered care, including (1) respect for the patient's values, preferences, and expressed needs; (2) information and education; (3) access to care; (4) emotional support to relieve fear and anxiety; (5) involvement of family and friends; (6) continuity and secure transition between healthcare settings; (7) physical comfort; and (8) coordination of care (Cliff, 2012).

Person-centered care: Care approach that puts the patient at the center of care and partners with patients in more meaningful ways (Alexander & Shirey, 2020). According to the Institute of Medicine (IOM), person-centered care is the act of providing care that is respectful of, and responsive to, individual patient preferences, needs, and values, ensuring that patient values guide all clinical decisions and supports transparency, compassion, and empowerment (IOM, 2010). The rise of person-centered care makes way for healthcare systems designed to optimize the agency and comfort of the most important and vulnerable people: patients, families, and their communities. Person-centered care is a holistic approach that delivers respectful and individualized care, promoting negotiation of care and offering choices through a therapeutic relationship where persons are empowered to be involved in health decisions (Morgan & Yoder, 2012).

Praxis: The synthesis of thoughtful reflection, caring, and action within a theory- and research-driven practice (Enzman Hines, 2009).

The Evolving Role of the Advanced Practice Holistic Nurse

Change will not come if we wait for some other person or some other time. We are the ones we have been waiting for. We are the change that we seek.

—**Barack Obama** (2008)

Evidently, health care is in a time of change with holistic nursing at the center of that change. Emerging from the pandemic, healthcare organizations now recognize the contributions that holistic nurses, particularly advanced practice holistic nurses (APHNs), bring to health care with a focus on caring–healing expressed through authenticity, presence, compassion, knowing participation, cultural humility, reflection, and self-care practices. Holistic nurses engage in relation-based, person-centered care, negotiate for humanistic care, support care choices, and deliver respectful and individualized care where persons are empowered to be involved in all health decisions.

Globally, health care needs wise, visionary, creative leaders in advanced holistic nursing. In health care, the current state and pace of change has created unprecedented challenges for individuals, the nation, and the world (Broome & Marshall, 2017). In the United States, health care has undergone significant demographic, economic, social, and environmental changes that have created system complexity, financial instability, and an inequitable distribution of resources, disparity within the quality of care, and higher costs for services (IOM, 2010). This, in turn, has impacted how care is provided for individuals, families, and population-based health models. Complex health conditions plaguing individuals today require greater skills and knowledge for advanced practice nurses (APNs). Clinical expertise within holistic advanced practice nursing, whether it is in primary care, direct patient care, coaching, education, research, and/or administration, requires new ways of thinking about health, wellness, wellbeing, and wellbecoming.

Nursing has a rich history with diverse approaches to knowledge development, but ambiguity still exists about what is our unifying focus for the discipline, particularly practice (Willis et al., 2018). There is a great need for nurses, specifically advance practice nurses, to express a "coherent philosophical foundation" in our practice and nursing's survival as a healing practice discipline depends on being able to effectively communicate a unifying focus for nursing (Willis et al., 2018). The emerging paradigm for holistic nursing was developed by nurse theorists and leaders including Benner, Dossey, Erickson, Leininger, Newman, Ray, Rogers, Smith, and Watson. These theorists provide the nursing profession with concepts influencing holistic nursing including caring–healing, culture, consciousness, cocreative processes of human becoming, quality of life, humanistic existential concerns, interpersonal relationships, irreducible human–environment life processes, pattern, pattern recognition and energy, role and role modeling, and bureaucratic caring. Newman, Sime, and Corcoran-Perry presented us with a definition of *nursing* as "caring in the human health experience," providing us with a focus on caring, health, and wholeness that is studied from a unitary-transformative stance supporting the process of mutuality and creative unfolding (Newman et al., 1991, p. 38). Other scholars have proposed human living as a unifying concept (Kim, 2000), human flourishing (Willis et al., 2018), and human dignity (Jacobs, 2001; Willis et al., 2018) and contend that nursing knowledge needs to relate to the knowledge bases of other healthcare disciplines for the purpose of facilitating human flourishing, health, and healing. Newman called for a reconciliation of opposing perspectives in nursing and health care through a unitary perspective with various views of health and healing included within the whole (Newman, 2002, 2003). According to Willis, examples of nursing practice include (a) engaging in relations grounded in unconditional acceptance of the whole person; (b) recognizing values, knowing, supporting, empowering, and nurturing of all human beings; (c) engaging in therapeutic human-to-human relationships;

(d) helping individuals process meaning(s) and significance of life experiences and their health and healing; (e) recognizing, engaging, appreciating, and advocating for individuals in their personal choices, rights, and responsibilities; (f) exploring, respecting, and advocating an individual's ideas about quality of life; and (g) practicing, ensuring, and promoting meaning in health and healing, choice, and quality of life (Willis et al., 2018).

Nursing knowledge and practice advance as nurses conceptualize practice within a central unifying focus and the use of questions, evidence, and interventions from multiple patterns of knowing: personal, empirics, ethics, aesthetics, sociopolitical, unknowing, spiritual, reflexive, and emancipatory (Willis et al., 2018). When advanced nursing is practiced at the individual, family, organizational, community, society, and global levels, nursing research needs to address questions related to nursing's theoretical base of human care, meanings, choice, quality of life, and healing. Scholarly endeavors will develop and refine the knowledge essential to practice development. The future of nursing practice will be influenced by every nurse's understanding of the discipline as holistic, use of disciplinary philosophies, theories and practice knowledge, and contributions to meeting the goals of health, healing, well-being, and wellbecoming across society and practice settings (Willis et al., 2018).

Advanced holistic nursing needs leaders who can draw from their roots in nursing and clinical practice to collaborate with policymakers and members of the community to create new solutions for the issues and problems in health care to improve quality of life, transform the healthcare landscape, and inspire the next generation of APHNs (Salmond & Forrester, 2016). In an era of increasingly sophisticated healthcare technology and technical demands, holistic advanced practice nurses must preserve efforts to provide humanistic, compassionate, and holistic care (AHNCC, 2017a).

Given developments such as the Institute of Medicine's report *The Future of Nursing: Leading Change, Advancing Health* (Alexander & Shirey, 2020) and the 2010 healthcare reform law, the Patient Protection and the Affordable Care Act (Mach & Kinzer, 2018), legislation at the national level has expanded the role of APNs, specifically nurse practitioners, giving authority to order home care services and chronic care services in the primary care setting. These developments provide APNs and advanced practice registered nurses (APRNs) with opportunities to deliver care and contribute to roles that lead to change in the healthcare landscape. With the passage of the Affordable Care Act (Mach & Kinzer, 2018), the focus of national and international health care shifted from disease management and cure to wellness, health promotion, and disease prevention. This movement of a wellness model seeks to ensure that APNs are supported in practicing to their full potential.

The increasing globalization of health care, changing demographics and expanding diversity of populations, and rapid technological changes mandate that nurses possess a breadth of skills and competencies to provide holistic, culturally sensitive health care (Morgan & Yoder, 2012). Today, virtually every discussion of healthcare reform begins with multiple concerns: the rising cost of health care, the lasting effects of the COVID-19 pandemic on global health, an expanding aging population, rising mental health needs, the role of advanced technology in healthcare documentation and monitoring, and the rising numbers of uninsured Americans (Denisco & Stewart, 2024; Morgan & Yoder, 2012). Between 2010 and 2030, the older population will increase by 75 percent to 69 million in the United States. One in five Americans will be a senior citizen. In 2050, an estimated 88.5 million in the United States will be aged 65 and older, and by 2060, there will be about 98 million older persons. Statistics indicate that 80 percent of older adults have at least one chronic condition, while 68 percent have at least two chronic conditions. An estimated 18.1 percent (43.6 million) of U.S. adults aged 18 years or older experience mental illness, and 4.2 percent (9.8 million) experience a seriously debilitating mental illness (Esposito & Contreras, 2024). These statistics are driving a paradigm shift in the role of APHNs in primary care and entrepreneurial roles. These trends will shape and mold the APHN entrepreneur of the future. Increasing numbers of holistic advance practice nurses, specifically holistic NPs, will be needed to care for the growing number of U.S. adults with chronic conditions and geriatric syndromes.

Reforming health care to address these challenges requires a well-educated and informed nursing workforce (Rother & Lavizzo-Mourey, 2009). With millions of Americans now gaining access to health care, there is an appreciation for the roles of APRNs, APHC-BCs, and APHNs in meeting the critical healthcare needs of vulnerable populations (e.g., aging adults, women, children, individuals with mental health needs), as well as an increased mindfulness of the barriers that currently prevent many APRNs, APHN-BCs, and APHN-BCs from delivering care (Rother & Lavizzo-Mourey, 2009; Delaney & Barrera, 2012; Enzman Hines, 2012; Martin-Misener et al., 2024; Sangster-Gormley et al., 2011).

Holistic nursing integrates the art and science of unitary human caring–healing that is based in the belief that humans are unitary, energetic beings, open to and constantly interacting with the energy system of the universe (Rogers, 1989). The evolving pattern of the whole results in expanding consciousness (Newman, 2008). Holistic nursing interventions are the creation of artistic actions, based on the sciences of caring, health, well-being, wellbecoming, and healing. They are designed to facilitate the holistic person's growth, health, and healing (ANA & AHNA, 2019). Holistic nursing practice focuses on creating interpersonal relationships needed to facilitate and enhance the individual's healing with the goal of a maximum state of health, well-being, wellbecoming, and human betterment (ANA & AHNA, 2019; Phillips, 2018). Holistic APNs emphasize unity and wholeness where health patterning is dynamic, interactive, and in constant change. A unitary caring–healing worldview cannot be reduced or separated and is necessary for eudemonistic health, well-being, and wellbecoming (ANA & AHNA, 2019).

Holistic advanced practice nursing actions are designed to purposefully promote normal human abilities (e.g., growing, unfolding, healing, transitioning). Therefore, advanced holistic nurses use strategies that facilitate and guide these processes, protect individuals from elements in the environment that might impede their inherent abilities, and prevent exposure to factors that could cause further assault on the individual's natural abilities. Additionally, holistic APNs use presence (McKivergin, 2009) to initiate and facilitate energetically connected relationships (Slater, 2014); are compassionate, unconditionally accepting members of the human–caring relationship (Quinn, 2016); use self-care, self-reflection (Levin & Reich, 2013; Shields et al., 2016), and reflective practice (Johns, 2017) to reinforce their inherent and professional abilities; and use reflection as a way of being in practice to enhance patterns of knowing that include personal awareness and personal knowing (Johns, 2017; Erickson & Erickson, 2010). Holistic APNs create caring environments where patients/clients are valued, recognizing the worth in self and other, and reaching out to the other to create common goals over personal goals. Holistic APNs set intent to be energetically connected; facilitate growth, health, wellness, well-being, and healing; and to create, apply, and evaluate artistic strategies based on the sciences of growth, development, health, wellness, and healing (ANA & AHNA, 2019). Accessing the attributes of person-centered care, holistic APNs promote the healing of human beings, within a culturally sensitive, evidence-informed practice designed to promote infinite possibilities (Newman, 2008; Dossey & Keegan, 2016; Enzman Hines, 2016).

Complementary modalities (i.e., yoga, therapeutic touch, reiki, healing touch, meditation, tai chi) are increasing in popularity, as holistic APNs integrate holistic therapies into everyday care for both self and patient. Approximately 30 percent of adults and 12 percent of children are seeking and using complementary modalities, holistic approaches to stress management, and holistic treatment plans in addition to their allopathic care (National Center for Complementary and Integrative Health, 2018). Holistic and complementary modalities expand the experiences of the AHN/APHNs, patients/clients, changing the way the AHN/APHNs experiences practice and health care.

Holistic APNs use a holistic approach in health care, embracing a worldview emphasizing that caring–healing is always possible, no matter what the individual's situation (Enzman Hines, 2012). In the caring–healing process, patients draw on an inner strength with a goal to reach something that is intangible. One of the greatest challenges for holistic APNs is focusing on caring–healing within a healthcare system that predominantly embraces a biomedical/reductionistic view of individuals and health care. APNs can meet these challenges by expanding caring–healing approaches informed by research, education, and practice (praxis) (Enzman Hines, 2016). "To create a caring environment and engender an atmosphere of respect and compassion, nurses need to understand what caring is, how to be caring, and the impact of caring and non-caring on others" (National Center for Complementary and Integrative Health, 2018, p. 19). Praxis is the synthesis of thoughtful reflection, caring, and action within a theory and research-driven practice (Enzman Hines, 2009). Holistic APNs are a unique group of nurses weaving a tapestry of bio-psycho-social-spiritual-cultural elements to promote healing within self and others. As holistic APNs engage in this healing process, it is a journey of changing and evolving of self and others (National Center for Complementary and Integrative Health, 2018).

Practicing as an advanced holistic nurse (AHN-BC) or advanced practice holistic nurse (APHN-BC) in any nursing role and setting, whether in acute care, primary care, coaching, or academia, the AHN-BC's/APHN-BC's greatest influence is contributing to person-centered care and a whole-person approach based on a holistic philosophy of caring and healing. Advanced holistic nurses of any degree level and practice area are finding great satisfaction in providing care by embracing a holistic approach. Advanced holistic nurses graduating from programs with unitary/holistic conceptual frameworks and philosophies are uniquely prepared to assume leadership roles in the promotion of health and wellness, prevention of illness and complications, and the advancement of the health and well-being/wellbecoming of individuals, communities, and society. Advanced holistic nurses who do not graduate from a holistically based education program can further expand their knowledge through courses available in university and continuing education platforms. These courses include the 4 "Ps" of Philosophy and Theory of Holistic Nursing Advanced Practice, Advanced Practice Holistic Assessment, Psychobiology/Psychoneuroimmunology, and Pharmacotherapeutics of Holistic Care (i.e., pharmacology, nutritional therapies, homeopathy, herbs).

The American Nurses Association (ANA), in collaboration with the American Holistic Nurses Association (AHNA), published *Holistic Nursing: Scope and Standards of Practice,* 3rd ed., which defines the scope of holistic nursing practice and the expected level of care provided by basic and advanced holistic nurses (ANA & AHNA, 2019). Based on a philosophy that nursing is an art and a science, with the primary purpose of providing holistic care for the whole person, the scope and standards of holistic nursing practice support five core values.

Table 23-1 summarizes the personal–professional responsibilities of the APHN based on the five core values of advanced holistic nursing.

Currently, the American Holistic Nurses Certification Corporation (AHNCC) provides certification for advanced holistic nurses and advanced practice holistic nurses (AHNCC, 2017a). The certifications result in -BC (by certification) being added to the abbreviations for these positions (AHN-BC and APHN-BC).

Defining Advanced Practice Registered Nurses

Various definitions exist for APRNs but are delineated within roles of nurse practitioner, nurse midwife, clinical nurse specialist, or nurse anesthetist. In holistic advanced practice there are two certifications available: the AHN-BC, which includes the group of holistic nurses who hold an advanced degree and certification in advanced holistic nursing and work in education or clinical practice, and the APHN-BC, who has additional education to prescribe medications and treatments for a specified population (e.g., adult-gerontology,

Table 23-1 Personal–Professional Responsibilities of AHN-BC/APHN-BC Nurses Based on Core Values of Holistic Nursing

1. **Holistic Philosophy, Theories, and Practice** • Lead systemwide change through the integration of relevant theories/ethical frameworks • Serve as mentors and educators to improve access to the philosophy and worldview of holism • Contribute to the realization of a praxis based on the interconnectedness of all people • Strive to advocate for policy changes that reflect the healing needs of individuals, groups, communities, and nations 2. **Holistic Caring Process** • Role model relationship-based and human-centered care • Create safe and healing environments based on integrative assessments that incorporate mental-emotional-spiritual-energetic aspects of well-being • Promote caring as essential to vitality for both self and others 3. **Holistic Communication, Therapeutic Healing Environment, and Cultural Diversity** • Become ambassadors of cultural humility in understanding individual contexts of vulnerability • Engage global systems in the change process from medical to health/wellness model • Influence the healthcare infrastructure toward an experience of holistic health nursing from the current illness/sick nursing model	4. **Holistic Education and Research** • Lead and/or collaborate on research initiatives that promote the continued emergence of holistic nursing and related patient outcomes • Strive to integrate holistic values into curricula for all levels of nursing education • Advocate for the holistic nurse to become the forerunner of ethical education and research with continued emphasis on promoting and protecting human dignity 5. **Holistic Nurse Self-Reflection and Self-Care** • Guide the community of nursing in self and community care through teaching modalities and providing reflective and introspective opportunities • Encourage reflection that provides global healing through interprofessional collaboration and engagement • Educate nurses worldwide about the essential nature of self-care in providing responsible healthcare delivery to all populations

Reproduced from Rosa, W., & Lubansky, S. (2016). The advanced practice holistic nurse: A leader in the implementation of core values. *Beginnings, 36*(3), 13, 26.

women's health/gender care, family, pediatrics, neonatal, psychiatric/mental health) from a holistic knowledge base. The practice of AHN-BCs and APHN-BCs focuses on facilitating healing, health, and wellbecoming a holistic person throughout the life span (ANA & AHNA, 2019). Advanced holistic nurses honor the individual's subjective experience about health, health beliefs, and values. Embracing a holistic worldview, advanced holistic nurses engage in mutual relationship with individuals, families, communities, and populations, drawing on nursing knowledge, theories, research, expertise, intuition, and creativity and incorporating the roles of clinician, educator, consultant, coach, partner, role model, and ally/advocate. Holistic nursing practice encourages peer review of professional practice in various clinical settings and provides care based on current professional standards, laws, and regulations governing nursing practice (ANA & AHNA, 2019). Advanced holistic nurses embrace a holistic, person-centered approach to health care. Key elements in the scope of practice in patient care for holistic APNs are summarized in **Box 23-1**. *Holistic Nursing: Scope and Standards of Practice,* 3rd ed., further elaborates the competencies of advanced holistic nursing practice (ANA & AHNA, 2019).

Conventional/Biomedical Approach to Advance Practice Nursing

The dominant model for APRN practice, supporting the conventional model of health care

Box 23-1 Exemplar Competencies of the Advanced Practice Holistic Nurse in Patient Care

1. Collects comprehensive data pertinent to the healthcare consumer's health and situation
2. Analyzes data to determine the diagnosis or the issues by synthesizing data or information to identify patterns and variances with life content
3. Identifies expected outcomes for a plan individualized for consumer care by partnering with the client and/or healthcare provider, setting realistic time frames for achieving outcomes and documenting outcomes
4. Develops a plan that prescribes strategies and alternatives to attain expected outcomes
5. Implements identified plan
6. Coordinates care within nursing and across the interprofessional team
7. Provides clients with information regarding their health and wellness
8. Provides consultation to influence the identified plan, enhance the abilities of others, and effect change
9. Evaluates the progress of the caring process

Reproduced from ANA/AHNA. (2019). *Scopes and standards of holistic nursing* (p. 15).

(patient focused), is recognized by the American Academy of Colleges of Nursing, which endorsed the *Consensus Model for APRN Regulation: Licensure, Accreditation, Certification and Education* in 2008 (APRN Consensus Work Group and National Council of State Boards of Nursing APRN Advisory Committee, 2008). In this document, the APRN is defined as a nurse who has done the following:

1. Completed a graduate-level education program in preparation for one of four recognized APRN roles (i.e., Clinical Nurse Specialist, Nurse Practitioner, Nurse Midwife, and Nurse Anesthesiologist)
2. Passed a national certification examination and remain certified
3. Acquired advanced clinical knowledge and skills
4. Gained practice building on the competencies of registered nurses demonstrating greater knowledge, increased complexity of skills and interventions, and greater role autonomy
5. Prepared to assume responsibility and accountability for health promotion and/or maintenance and assessment, diagnosis, and management of patient problems, including prescription of pharmacologic and nonpharmacologic interventions
6. Performed sufficient clinical experience to reflect the intended license
7. Obtained a license to practice as an APRN in one of the four following roles: certified registered nurse anesthetist, certified nurse midwife, clinical nurse specialist, or certified nurse practitioner (**Table 23-2**).

APRNs are educated and certified in one of four roles and in at least one of the following six population foci:

1. Family/individual across the life span
2. Adult–gerontology
3. Pediatrics
4. Neonatal
5. Women's health/gender related
6. Psychiatric/mental health

In addition, APRNs may further specialize in practice beyond the role and population focus, including but not limited to oncology, orthopedics, nephrology, palliative care, pain management, cardiology, and gastroenterology (**Figure 23-1**). Specifically, the three criteria for APRN status are as follows:

1. The nurse to select one of four specified roles (CRNA, CNM, CNS, CNP)
2. A specific population
3. A formal education that includes three courses to acquire knowledge specific to these roles (advanced assessment, advanced pathophysiology, and advanced pharmacology).

Graduate nurses have also expanded roles into specialties, including health and wellness coaching, informatics, public health, administration, and education. Like APRNs, these roles have gained importance in providing high-quality

Table 23-2 Consensus Model of Advanced Practice Registered Nurse Roles

Role	Description
Certified Nurse Midwife (CNM)	The CNM provides a full range of primary health services to women throughout the life span, including gynecological care, family planning services, preconception care, prenatal and postpartum care, childbirth, and care of the newborn.
Clinical Nurse Specialist (CNS)	The CNS has a unique APRN role to integrate care across the continuum and throughout three spheres of influence: patient, nurse, and system. The three spheres are overlapping and interrelated, but each sphere possesses a distinctive focus. In each sphere, the primary goal is continuous improvement of patient outcomes and nursing care. Key elements of CNS practice are to create environments through mentoring and system change that empower nurses to develop caring, evidence-based practices to alleviate patient distress, facilitate ethical decision making, and respond to diversity.
Certified Nurse Practitioner (CNP)	CNPs provide care along the wellness–illness continuum as a dynamic process in which direct primary and acute care is provided across settings. CNPs are members of the health delivery system, practicing autonomously in areas as diverse as family, pediatrics, internal medicine, geriatrics, and women's health care. CNPs are prepared to diagnose and treat patients with undifferentiated symptoms as well as those with established diagnoses. This can be primary or acute care focused depending on the CNP's preparation.
Certified Registered Nurse Anesthetist	The certified registered nurse anesthetist is prepared to provide the full spectrum of patients' anesthesia care and anesthesia-related care for individuals across the life span, whose health status may range from health through all recognized levels of acuity, including persons with immediate, severe, or life-threatening illnesses or injury. The care is provided in diverse settings including hospitals, obstetrical delivery rooms, pain management centers, and ambulatory surgical centers.

Reproduced from AACN (2008). *Consensus model for APRN regulation: Licensure, accreditation, certification and education.* APRN Consensus Work Group & the National Council of State Boards of Nursing APRN Advisory Committee. http://www.aacn.nche.edu/education-resources/APRNReport.pdf

care in the reformed healthcare system. The distinction between these roles and specialties and the four APRN roles is the focus on direct care to individuals (Summers, 2011). Furthermore, these additional roles do not require regulatory licensure beyond the RN.

The Consensus Model

The model for APRN regulation is the result of the APRN Consensus Work Group and the National Council of State Boards of Nursing APRN Advisory Committee dialogue (APRN Consensus Work Group and National Council of State Boards of Nursing APRN Advisory Committee, 2008). The APRN Joint Dialogue Group recommended the APRN Regulatory Model for the licensure, accreditation, certification, and education of APRNs. Advanced practice registered nurse regulations identify four essential components—licensure, accreditation, certification, and education—giving rise to the acronym LACE. The model states that, for successful implementation, all four of the following elements must be present and working together to ensure appropriate regulations (AACN, 2012):

1. Licensure is the granting of authority to practice. The model requires state boards of nursing to license APRNs as independent practitioners.
2. Accreditation is the formal review and approval by a recognized agency of the

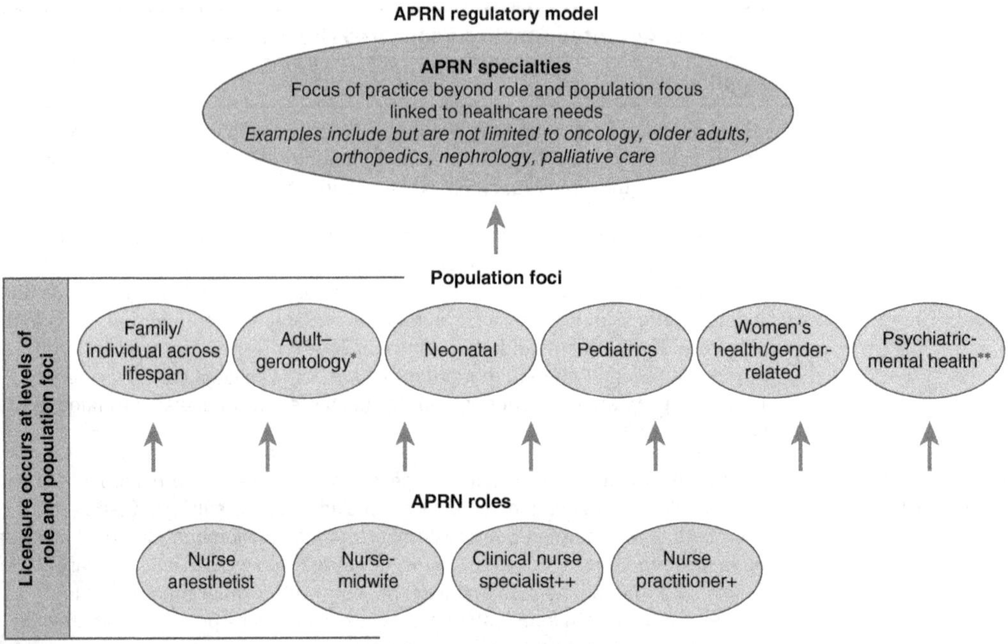

Figure 23-1 Advanced practice registered nurse regulatory model.

*The population focus *adult–gerontology* encompasses the young adult to the older adult, including the frail elderly. Advanced practice registered nurses educated and certified in the adult–gerontology population are educated and certified across both areas of practice and will be titled Adult-Gerontology CNP or CNS. In addition, all APRNs in any of the four roles providing care for the adult population (e.g., family or gender specific) must be prepared to meet the growing needs of the older adult population. Therefore, the education program should include didactic and clinical education experiences necessary to prepare APRNs with enhanced skills and knowledge.

**The population focus *psychiatric/mental health* encompasses education and practice across the life span.

Reproduced from AACN (2008). *Consensus model for APRN regulation: Licensure, accreditation, certification and education.* APRN Consensus Work Group & the National Council of State Boards of Nursing APRN Advisory Committee. http://www.aacn.nche.edu/education-resources/APRNReport.pdf

educational degree or certificate program in graduate nursing. The model requires accreditation standards and processes to assess APRN education programs to ensure that the APRN core, roles, and population core competencies are met and to monitor education programs throughout the accreditation period.

3. Certification is the formal recognition of the knowledge, skills, and experience identified by standards within the profession. Certifiers, accredited by a national certification body, are required to follow established testing and psychometrically based standards for an APRN exam. In addition, provisions ensure competence and maintenance of certification and participate in ongoing relationships and transparency to state boards of nursing.
4. Education is the formal preparation of the APRN within a graduate program granting a graduate degree or graduate certificate. APRN education programs/tracks must be accredited by a nursing accrediting organization recognized by the U.S. Department of Education and/or the Council for Higher Education Accreditation, be preapproved and preaccredited prior to the admission of students and ensure that graduates are eligible for national certification and licensure.

APRN Education

The consensus model classifies key requirements for APRN education. These requirements include recommendations for formal education with a graduate degree or postgraduate certificate awarded by an accredited academic institution. Academic institutions have also ensured that curricula comply with the model requirements for the three *Ps*: three separate comprehensive graduate courses (the APRN core) in advanced pathophysiology, advanced health assessment, and advanced pharmacology. Although there is a future recommendation that the entry level to APRN practice be the Doctor of Nursing practice, there presently is no consensus about this requirement (AACN, 2006). Many education institutions are converting both post-master's and Bachelor of Science in nursing programs to Doctor of Nursing practice programs to move the 2015 recommendation forward.

APRN Specialties

Preparation in specialty practice, an option for APRNs, represents a focused area of preparation and practice beyond the APRN role. Criteria for defining specialties as an APRN is informed by the ANA criteria for recognition as a nursing specialty and encompasses areas including but not exclusive of palliative care, cardiology, pulmonary medicine, oncology, nephrology, and pain management. A family nurse practitioner could specialize in nephrology, a pediatric nurse practitioner could specialize in pain management, and a clinical nurse specialist could specialize in palliative care. State licensing boards do not regulate APRNs at this level of specialization, but certification in a specialty area of practice is strongly recommended (AACN, 2012).

Implementation of the Consensus Model

The implementation of the consensus model has met with opposition. As state nursing board laws and regulations continue to vary, there has been a tendency to focus on those that will require careful analysis of each state's laws and regulations to determine which revisions are necessary. However, not all laws and regulations are legal or regulatory. The implementation of educational requirements continues to vary from state to state, specifically the work required to meet the three Ps in advanced practice (Summers, 2011). An interdependence of licensure, accreditation, certification, and education will require sequential implementation. After the Joint Dialogue Group agreed on the APRN consensus model, the LACE Network was formed as an implementation team. The APRN LACE Network is collaboratively working to produce a structure and process for the implementation of these recommendations (AACN, 2012). Stakeholders are now developing documents for clarifying the issues posed in the model. The American College of Nurse-Midwives, the Accreditation Commission for Midwifery Education, and the American Midwifery Certification Board recently published a white paper, *Midwifery in the United States and the Consensus Model for APRN Regulation* (ANA & AHNA, 2019). Several other specialty organizations are responding to the consensus model in a similar way, including the National Association of Clinical Nurse Specialists (NACNS), the AHNA/AHNCC, and the National Organization of Nurse Practitioner Faculties. Concerns have been voiced about the LACE Network focus on nurse practitioners (NPs) as the major role described for the APRN and the vanishing role of CNSs in some institutions secondary to the lack of certifications for CNSs in specialty and community settings (AHNCC, 2017a).

The differences between an APRN in conventional medicine and a holistic APRN are summarized in **Table 23-3**. The AHNCC has responded to the consensus model by stating that this document would limit the scope and practice of AHNs and APHNs.

Health care is occurring in a perplexing new environment of rapid change with fast-paced innovations occurring in the information and healthcare technologies along with expectations for better care for individuals and improved health for populations at lower costs (Summers, 2011). Within this lightning-quick, ever-changing environment, there is complexity, uncertainty, and tremendous opportunity for holistic APNs to lead the change. These holistic nurse leaders will have to be futuristic, highly intelligent, and politically aware as they address these evolving changes in health care and society (Enzman Hines, 2009). One of the major challenges as an advanced holistic nurse leader will be the shift from the perspective of individualized care to care of entire populations to global care. As this shift occurs, the scope of practice will broaden and will

Table 23-3 Comparison of Currently Recognized APRNs and Advanced Holistic Nurses: Description of Their Population, Setting, Subspecialty, Type of Care, and Type of Health Concern (Problem)

	APRNs Currently Recognized by Consensus Model	APRN Holistic Nurses (AHN-BC & APHN-BC)
Description	Experts in subspecialty, type of care, and/or problem focus who work in any setting where their role is mandated, needed or incorporated into a system.	Experts in holism, healing, health promotion, well-being, and illness prevention who work in any setting where a nurse–client professional relationship exists.
Population	pediatrics, geriatrics, women's health, community health, etc.	The population of holistic nursing consists of all persons who want or need to be facilitated with healing, health, or growth that results in mind-body-spirit synchrony and integration.
Setting	Critical care, emergency room, doctor's office, private practice settings, etc.	Holistic nurses practice in any setting where nurse and client establish a professional partnership.
Disease or Medical Subspecialty	Diabetes, oncology, renal, cardiology, etc.	Not applicable for holistic nurses. Holistic nurses are concerned with the integration of mind-body-spirit of all persons, including those who have a chronic or acute medical problem or disease. Although some holistic nurses work with a population of persons with diabetes or oncology problems (and may have advanced education in this area), their focus is on the entire person's need.
Type of Care	Psychiatric, rehabilitation, primary care, emergency care, etc.	Holistic nursing embraces all nursing that has the enhancement of healing the whole person from birth to death—and all age groups from infant to elder—as its goal. This means viewing the whole person and their needs in their entirety with integration as the goal. The holistic nurse creates a caring–healing space within herself/himself that allows the nurse to be an instrument of healing; shares authenticity of unconditional presence that helps to remove the barriers to the healing process; facilitates another person's growth (body-mind-emotion-spirit-energetic-environment connections); and assists with maintaining wellness, recovery from illness, or transition to peaceful death.
Type of problem or Practice focus	Diseases, pain, wounds, stress, chronic medical problems, etc.	Holistic nurses are concerned with their client's health and well-being needs, problems, and/or conditions.
Licensure/ Certification	Certified by American Nurses Credentialing Center. Examination is based on specialty Advanced Practice Competencies	Certified by the American Holistic Nurses Credentialing Corporation. Examination is based on Holistic Nursing Advanced Practice Competencies.

Reproduced from *A Position Statement on the APRN Model.* (March 12, 2013) AHNCC: American Holistic Nurses Credentialing Corporation. https://gahnscholars.org/wp-content/uploads/2021/02/APRN_Position_Statement_for_NCSBN.pdf; National Association of Clinical Nurse Specialists. (2022, 2023). *Statement on the APRN consensus model implementation.* https://nacns.org/wp-content/uploads/2023/12/NACNS-2022-Census-Results-Infographic.pdf; https://nacns.org/wp-content/uploads/2023/05/Position-Statement-CNS-Full-Practice-FINAL.pdf require new skills, particularly the ability to zoom in and out in the face of challenges. It will require courageous holistic nurse leaders who understand and embrace collaboration, partnerships, and an unwavering focus on excellence and patient-centered care. It is time for nursing to lead the revolution and for holistic nurse leaders to be the activists of change (Salmond & Forrester, 2016). Key to this new view is the transition from the doing aspects of care to the reflective elements of care (Broome & Marshall, 2017). Additionally, a shift from patient-focused/centered care to person-centered care will be paramount. Daley differentiated the two divergent views and contends that nursing needs to put the patient at the center of care and partner with patients in more meaningful ways. "We [nurses] have long understood that respect and relationship between the nurse and individual—not simply proximity and knowledge—are what engender trust and contribute to more positive individual experiences and better health outcomes" (Daley, 2012, p. 3).

Paradoxically, the current major regulatory initiative by nursing, the consensus model, is designed to position APRNs to provide leadership in the present healthcare transformation and does not consider the differences in the worldview for the formulation of guidelines (AACN, 2012). The current consensus model simultaneously emphasizes patient-focused/centered care and hinders person-centered care. In the consensus model, the role of the holistic APN will be considered an add-on specialty that forces education programs to adapt to patient-focused care guidelines dedicated to the management of illness/disease conditions rather than person-centered care that emphasizes health, wellness, and healing. This has the potential to create a barrier to those who practice advanced practice holistic nursing (Enzman Hines, 2012).

Education Programs for Advanced Practice Nurses

Graduate nursing programs integrate a worldview and conceptual framework that direct the development of curriculum. This curriculum is accredited by higher education nursing certifying groups, either the Commission on Collegiate Nursing Education or the National League for Nursing Accrediting Commission. Most graduate programs follow the *patient-focused/centered* rather than the person-centered care approach to APN education, supporting the process presented in the consensus model (refer to Figure 28-1). Specialty organizations, such as the National Organization of Nurse Practitioner Faculties and NACNS, work closely with nursing schools and colleges to develop curricula that will prepare APN students for the certification exam by specialty-certifying bodies in a population focus, including the American Association of Nurse Practitioners; the AHNCC; the American Nurses Credentialing Center, which has both population-based nurse practitioner certification and CNS certification in some specialty populations; and the Pediatric Nursing Certification Board. According to the consensus model and the NCSBN, APRN education must include the following components (APRN Consensus Work Group and National Council of State Boards of Nursing APRN Advisory Committee, 2008):

1. Formal education with a graduate degree or postgraduate certification (either post-master's or postdoctoral) that is granted by an academic institution and accredited by nursing or nursing-related accrediting organizations recognized by the U.S. Department of Education and/or the Council for Higher Education Accreditation.
2. Awarded preapproval, preaccreditation, or accreditation prior to admitting students, be comprehensive, and be at the graduate level.
3. Prepare the graduate to practice in one of four identified APRN roles (CNS, CNM, nurse practitioner, certified registered nurse anesthetist), and prepare the graduate with the core competencies for one of the APRN roles across at least one of the six population foci (adult–gerontology, pediatrics, neonatal health, women's health/gender related, family, psychiatric/mental health).
4. Minimally include three separate graduate-level courses (referred to as the *three Ps* or

APRN core) in advanced physiology/pathophysiology, including principles that apply across the life span; advanced health assessment, including assessment of all human systems, advanced assessment techniques, concepts, and approaches; and advanced pharmacology, including pharmacodynamics, pharmacokinetics, and pharmacotherapeutics of all broad categories of drugs. In addition, content specific to the role and population should be included in other role and population didactics and clinical courses; include a basic understanding of decision making in the identified role; prepare the graduate to assume responsibility and accountability for health promotion and/or maintenance, specifically assessment, diagnosis, and management of patient problems, including the use and prescription of pharmacologic and nonpharmacologic agents/interventions; and ensure that clinical and didactic coursework is comprehensive and sufficient to prepare graduates with the skills to practice in an APRN role that is population focused.

5. The consensus model requires that APHNs (AHN-BC and APHN-BC) take traditional courses (e.g., select three *Ps*) to acquire formal education based on precepts, knowledge, and skills associated with a *reductionistic view* of health care acquiring knowledge, skills, and experience within a biomedical model. This is inconsistent with the competencies essential to advanced practice holistic nursing (e.g., 4 *Ps* courses in Advanced Philosophy and Theory of Holistic Nursing, Pharmacotherapeutics of Holistic Care [including herbal, homeopathic treatments and nutritional supplements], Psychobiological/Psychoneuroimmunology, and Advanced Holistic Physical Assessment/Integrative Health Practices) (AHNCC, 2017a). Additionally, education in traditional programs prepares APNs with a problem-oriented, systems approach to care rather than a unitary/holistic, whole-person approach focused on aiding patient/clients in developing heath patterns that focus on human betterment and wellbecoming (Phillips, 2018).

Advanced Holistic Nursing Education

Nursing, a person-centered profession, has embraced two paradigms (Erickson, 2010; Parse, 1987). First described as models of holism versus wholism (Erickson, 2010) and then as the simultaneity and totality paradigms (Parse, 1987), nursing has been split between traditional and holistic approaches to health care. These paradigms differ in how the nurse views the world: Nurses who use science in the development of a nursing profession and carry out the roles and responsibilities of nursing or embrace nursing as a traditional science employ a systems model as their guide, and nurses who practice according to a holistic or simultaneity paradigm view health as a sense of well-being—a quality of life (Erickson, 2010). Advance practice holistic nurses focus on "protecting, promoting, and optimizing health and wellness; assisting healing; preventing illness and injury; alleviating suffering; and supporting people to find peace, comfort, harmony, and balance" (ANA & AHNA, 2019, p. 3). Advance practice holistic nurses fulfill one or more roles, depending on their educational preparation. They support individuals in making informed decisions about their personal health and well-being/wellbecoming; promote the health and well-being/wellbecoming of groups and society; provide leadership for groups or communities seeking to advance health within society; support and/or mentor colleagues who have an active role in the advancement of health within society; develop new programs based on the sciences of holistic health, wellness, and well-being; and creating new knowledge for the profession (Enzman Hines, 2016; ANA & AHNA, 2019). Advanced practice holistic nurses' professional activities are designed to comfort and empower the patient, facilitate patients in finding meaning and purpose in life experiences, foster growth and healing when needed, and transcend with grace and peace at the end of life. Advance practice holistic nurses also mentor and provide leadership and guidance for colleagues and interprofessional team members within a holistic healthcare model (Erickson (Ed.), 2010). Hills and Watson devoted an entire book to describing a caring curriculum for undergraduate and graduate holistic nursing programs (Hills & Watson, 2011). Promoting caring within advanced practice education, Enzman Hines provides a holistic framework for graduate education for an advanced practice program that provides the core elements of a holistic advanced practice curriculum (Enzman Hines, 2011). Concurrently, a task force was created as part of AHNCC in collaboration with the Global Academy of Holistic Nursing (GAHN), to create and revise the *Foundations, Competencies, and Curricular Guidelines for Basic to Doctoral Holistic Nursing Education* (AHNCC, 2017b) providing supportive materials (e.g., webinars and tool kits) to assist in the development of basic and graduate programs in holistic nursing.

Credentialing Advanced Practice Holistic Nurses

The AHNCC first started credentialing holistic nurses in 1997 and has since moved into credentialing AHNs and APHNs through a national certification process. The AHNCC Board of Directors provides specific guidelines for nursing programs. Most nursing programs are based on a mixture of paradigms, while others are based on a simultaneity (holistic) paradigm. The AHNCC contends that these conclusions were validated by reviewing hundreds of qualitative assessments submitted by candidates for certification (AHNCC, 2024). Many nurses prepared in the totality paradigm, or a program mixed with both paradigms, have a desire to practice holistically. As a result, after graduation, these nurses will need to seek additional education to gain the essential knowledge and skills to practice as a holistic nurse. Nurses who attend graduate programs based on the holistic/simultaneity paradigm are prepared to practice as advanced holistic nurses and are allies/advocates of the principles of holistic nursing (Enzman Hines, 2016), providing leadership for holism in the healthcare system. The AHNCC developed an Endorsement Program for nursing educational programs who support the simultaneity paradigm and provide education in holistic undergraduate and advanced practice (AHNCC, 2024). Endorsed programs in advanced practice holistic nursing provide a curriculum consistent with the AHNA core values and prepare graduates to practice within the AHNA scope and standards of advanced holistic nursing (ANA & AHNA, 2019), employ faculty certified as advanced holistic nurses who support the simultaneity paradigm, and advertise the school or college as one that prepares advanced holistic nurses qualified to sit for AHNCC certification as a AHN-BC or APHN-BC. A list of current AHNCC-endorsed programs can be found on the AHNCC website (www.ahncc.org). Endorsed holistic nursing educational programs have a school or college philosophy that reflects the AHNA's philosophy of nursing and code of ethics and core values. The school's or college's mission statements reflect goals consistent with preparing nurses based on *Holistic Nursing: Scope and Standards of Practice,* 3rd ed (ANA & AHNA, 2019). Both the philosophy and mission must be consistent with the level of the program being endorsed. The curriculum outline and all courses include course descriptions and objectives that evidence holistic nursing as a thread running throughout the program. A single elective course in the program is not sufficient to qualify as a holistic nursing program. Course content, threaded throughout the program, provides the knowledge and skills needed to practice holistic nursing at the appropriate level and demonstrates how the student is prepared to practice holistic nursing. Concepts such as presence, intentionality, unconditional acceptance (of the human), self-care, reflective practice, caring–healing, and other key holistic nursing concepts must be evident in the course content, descriptions, and practice experiences (Erickson, 2009). The lead faculty teaching the courses must be certified by AHNCC as either an AHN-BC or APHN-BC.

The Value of the Certification Process for AHN-BC and APHN-BC

Changes in the social and professional environment of nursing since 2000 have moved holistic nursing into mainstream health care and resulted in a call for national certification of holistic nurses

(Erickson, 2009). The AHNCC assumed the responsibility for this certification in 1997 and has expanded the certification for registered nurses to three levels: (1) the diploma/associate degree nurse, (2) the baccalaureate degree nurse, and (3) the nurse with a graduate degree preparing the APN as an AHN-BC or an APHN-BC. AHN-BCs demonstrate expertise in the basic practice of holistic nursing and perform the advanced competencies of AHN-BCs (refer to Table 28-3). APHN-BCs practicing in a bedside clinical setting, coaching, an educational setting, or an entrepreneurial practice setting often seek this certification. The AHN-BC often assists nurses in a variety of settings to integrate holistic core values and competences through mentoring and education.

Roles

Advance practice holistic nurses practice in a variety of settings (e.g., hospital-based care, primary care, private practice [health coach, home care, mental health practice, holistic health practice], community/public health care, research, education). AHN-BCs serve as educators, holistic nurse coaches, administrators, and nurse leaders in hospital settings and seek to integrate the simultaneity/unitary caring healing paradigm and concepts into clinical practice within the hospital, home-care, community, or society. In contrast, APHNs hold the credential APHN-BCs have obtained and demonstrate competencies in advanced knowledge of pharmacology (including herbal and homeopathic therapies, nutritional supplements), psychobiology/psychoneuroimmunology, integrative health practices, and advanced holistic philosophy and theory to plan and prescribe care consistent with patient needs, health issues, and problems. The APHN-BC also synthesizes multiple sources of knowledge and therapies, including patient self-knowledge, when prescribing holistic treatments; developing holistic care plans cocreated by partnering with the patient; and prescribing pharmacologic agents based on current knowledge of pharmacology and physiology, clinical indicators, age, holistic status/needs, results of diagnostic labs, and the person's beliefs, values, and choices. In addition, APHN-BCs evaluate and analyze the therapeutic effects, possible side effects, and interactions of all prescribed treatments; provide patients with information about cost and expected outcomes of planned treatment and integrative options; partner with others to create an interprofessional plan that focuses on safe, effective, holistic outcomes; document collaborative discussions, including holistic plan changes, communications, and rationale; and documents referrals, including provisions for continuity of holistic care (AHNCC, 2017a).

Holistic nurse coaching is a role that some APNs choose to expand their skill set. These nurses interact with intention, purpose, and skills to cocreate a plan of care with the purpose of promoting and facilitating the client in achieving their goals. These interactions are time-limited. A contract is developed between the client and nurse, which determines a focus in interaction. The outcomes are centered on attainable and specific goals developed by the coach and client. The skill set of the nurse coach includes building relationships; supporting, encouraging, challenging, motivating, observing, and analyzing the needs of clients; active and open listening; using motivational interviewing; appreciative discovery; and providing interventions and feedback (Southard et al., 2020). Several programs provide nurse coach education and can be found on the AHNCC website (www.ahncc.org). Once completing the course content to prepare the advance practice nurse as a holistic health and wellness nurse coach, they can seek certification as a holistic nurse coach (HWNC-BC) when certified as an AHN-BC or APHN-BC.

Why Should an Advanced Holistic Nurse Become Certified?

Professional nursing certification for AHN-BC and APHN-BC has established the importance of holistic nursing as a specialty. Certification assures employers, healthcare organizations, and patients that certified AHNs/APHNs possess the specialty knowledge, skills, and experience to effectively deliver safe quality care that promotes optimal health and wellness outcomes (AHNCC, 2017a).

Certification maintains a detailed set of standards of practice that ensure these professional competencies. Credentialing and certification provide consumers with increased choices when selecting healthcare providers, identify the level of care provided to patients, and assist in the evaluation of educational preparation of potential providers (Sharoff, 2008).

Who Are Certified Advanced Holistic Nurses?

Certified AHN-BCs and APHN-BCs integrate caring–healing, person-centered care; the dynamics of holism; and unity into an approach to practice. Person-centered care supports the essential stance that the patient is the primary source of information and the patient's self-knowledge must be a key consideration in care. Thus, AHN-BCs/APHN-BCs consider the patient's worldview as essential data. Input from many AHN-BCs/APHN-BCs reveal that nursing is not only a profession but also a calling and a way of being in the world (Smith et al., 2013). AHN-BCs/APHN-BCs provide healing work in health care and understand the importance of caring–healing environments, relationship-centered care, presence, intention, and the human spirit in healing. Holistic APNs identify opportunities for expanding practice (IOM, 2010). The AHNCC defines holistic nursing as all nursing practice that cares for the person as an integrated, holistic human being, inseparable and integral to the environment (AHNCC, 2017b). Holistic nurses recognize and honor the belief systems of others and have increased awareness of the interconnectedness of all living beings within the global community (Sharoff, 2008). "Holistic nursing practice is the science, art, and the 'creative fire' where holistic nurses uncover, recover, support and celebrate the creative self" (O'Grady, 2015, p. 15).

The AHNCC certification examinations for the AHN-BC and APHN-BC test the individual nurse's knowledge of advanced holistic nursing practice. Ongoing certification requires nurses to show evidence of continued efforts to enhance knowledge of advanced holistic nursing through continuing education. Once certified, AHN-BCs and APHN-BCs will be challenged to become lifelong learners, enhancing and expanding their knowledge and scholarship within holistic nursing.

Exemplars of Holistic Care in Advance Practice

Let us imagine what a truly holistic healthcare system looks like. The following is a nursing situation identifying how a patient followed by an FNP whose practice is informed by a holistic philosophy and theory approach to health care occurs.

Holistic health care uses a caring–healing approach to patient care and is a growing reality

Nursing Situation

Jane Worthington has been experiencing headaches for the past month that have begun to interfere with her daily activities and her life at home with her family. The headaches begin at any time of the day and often last for many hours. She has tried over-the-counter remedies such as acetaminophen and ibuprofen without relief. The headaches can bring nausea and dizziness at times, and she is having trouble sleeping because of the pain. Jane has experienced no changes in vision, but she does have neck pain at times with the headaches. She has been to her primary care provider who has not been able to diagnose the cause of her headaches: a CT scan was negative for brain lesion, her sinuses were normal, and her spinal X-ray showed no spinal problems. Jane has been reading about an integrative healthcare practice in her area, and, because they advertise patient-centered care and the use of alternative and complementary therapies to relieve problems, she decides to make an appointment.

When Jane arrives at the office, she is asked to complete the usual forms for insurance, but no health history forms are given to her. Instead, she is taken to a pleasant room where a nurse asks her about her health history, her life, her job, and her health beliefs and ideas about what she wants from her visits to the care center. The nurse asks Jane about the coping skills she uses when problems arise and about her beliefs related to spirituality. She also asks Jane about her living and working environments both in terms of physical requirements and stress level. Jane states that she has a very stressful job that requires at least 8 hours a day of prolonged sitting and use of media. She has two teenage children who need her guidance, and a spouse. She shares with the nurse practitioner (a holistic APN) that she began having headaches about 1 year ago. At that time, she would get a headache about once a month, but now she gets headaches almost every day. The headaches start at the base of her head and radiate up into her head. She has no problems with light or sound, but sometimes she has such pain with the headaches that she gets nauseous. Jane sometimes has a glass or two of red wine with dinner, but that only seems to increase the likelihood of headaches the next day.

Jane was sent to have blood work and a cervical spine X-ray and given a follow-up appointment in 2 days. The integrative team, made up of a nurse practitioner, physician, physical therapist, and nutritionist, meet to discuss her case. They propose a program including nutrition counseling and diet review to remove triggers for the headaches, massage and yoga to reduce muscle tension (if the cervical spine is not injured), meditation and training in mindfulness to reduce stress levels, and medication to manage the pain when the headaches appear. Jane returns in 2 days. Her cervical spine X-rays are normal, and her blood work is normal, except that her thyroid levels are elevated. After a discussion with the integrative team, Jane agrees to the plan that now includes thyroid hormone replacement. She is not sure about the meditation and mindfulness stress reduction but is willing to give them a try. She will return to the office in 2 weeks to reevaluate her therapies to determine if her goal of reduced headaches is reached.

In 2 weeks, Jane returns to the office and states that she feels much better. She has reviewed her diet history with the nutritionist and adjusted her diet in ways that were recommended. Jane is enthusiastic about these dietary changes and states that in her discussion with the nutritionist, she was given choices and options to still eat the foods she enjoys. Jane really liked the yoga and massage, is sleeping better, and is more relaxed after work and no longer drinks red wine to help her cope. The meditation and mindful stress reduction sessions are somewhat challenging for her at this time. She finds it hard to shift from a fast-paced work setting to being still and quiet; however, the instructor has given her some exercises to do on her way to the session that are helping her to calm her mind and prepare. Jane is willing to keep going to these classes for now and will report on her progress. Her most important goal has been reached. In the past 2 weeks, she has had only one headache. She used the visualization she learned in mindfulness stress reduction to relieve the pain, and the headache went away quickly. Jane states that she is very happy that her headaches are gone, and she did not need medication but could work on the problem with her team and resolve the headaches in a natural way.

in the United States. Cost-effective holistic health care puts patients in charge of their own health, allowing the patient and provider/team to be active partners in care. Holistic nurses are at the forefront of initiatives to promote integrative health. Creating a healthcare system that values the whole person and empowers each patient to make decisions based on health beliefs and a sense of wholeness will move our entire healthcare system away from a disease-oriented model to a wellness model.

Implications

Clinical Practice

Integrating a caring–healing philosophy, holistic APNs provide care that is patient-centered and focused on the health and well-being/wellbecoming of individuals and populations. Promoting, advocating, and protecting the rights, health, and safety of the patient, the holistic APN approaches care using an integrated and comprehensive caring approach. Holistic APNs take on a variety of roles in practice, including expert clinician/facilitator of healing, consultant/collaborator, educator, coach, administrator, leader and change agent, researcher, and advocate. Holistic APNs create authentic relationships with patients and populations, partnering to promote caring–healing outcomes. Current changes in the healthcare arena require the development of clinical skills that are patient-centered, holistic/integrative, and focused on health, well-being, and wellbecoming. Holistic APNs will be the leaders in these healthcare changes.

Education

Holistic APNs hold a master's or doctoral degree, AHN-BC or APHN-BC certification, demonstrate caring–healing skills and knowledge, an integration of a caring–healing philosophy, and an ability to assume a variety of roles in the ever-changing healthcare environment as educators, practitioners, researchers, consultants, managers, advocates, and policymakers. The work is aimed at advancing holistic nursing and assuming leadership roles in the provision of the holistic health care of individuals and organizations. Key coursework in graduate holistic nursing programs differentiates them from the graduate education of the biomedical educated APNs through the inclusion of courses in advanced foundations of holistic nursing, advanced nursing research and evidence-informed practice, advanced sciences of holistic health and holism (psychoneuroimmunology, biophysical health), advanced holistic health assessment, and pharmacotherapeutics. Guidelines have been developed that assist in the development of advanced holistic nursing programs through the collaboration of the Global Academy of Holistic Nursing (GAHN), AHNA, and AHNCC (AHNCC, 2017b). Nurses seeking to acquire holistic knowledge in advanced holistic practice can achieve this education through both academic and professional development.

Research

Holistic APNs are introduced to multiple sources of data, information, and outcomes within evidence-informed practice. There are many questions/ideas that emerge in practice within the roles of the holistic APN's role in clinical/research, including the following:

- Utilizing multiple patterns of knowing to research questions that will inform holistic nursing practice
- Examining the benefits of certified AHN-BCs and APHN-BCs providing care in our healthcare system
- Analyzing the outcomes of caring–healing practices for AHN-BCs and APHN-BCs providing holistic health care
- Comparing and contrasting the outcomes of care provided by certified holistic APNs and APRNs following the traditional biomedical model
- Investigating the successes of students graduating from holistic nursing programs
- Evaluating patient satisfaction with care provided by holistic APNs
- Describing and explicating patient experiences of holistic health care (e.g., Do patients follow the care plan more systematically when they feel as though they have been a part of the plan development)? How does that affect health outcomes?

Policy

Advanced holistic nurses are prepared to design, influence, advocate, and implement healthcare policy that facilitates holistic healthcare access, safety, quality and efficacy. The advanced holistic nurse is knowledgeable in the design and implementation of healthcare policy addressing issues of social justice and equity in holistic health care. Additionally, advanced holistic nurses identify and evaluate healthcare policies and processes and engage in politically competent action (O'Grady, 2015).

Conclusion

This chapter presents the multiple benefits of having a certified holistic APN with graduate holistic education and acquired advanced holistic knowledge and skills as the leader in providing caring–healing approaches in health care for multiple populations across the life span. Holistic APNs challenge the provision of nursing care from a reductionistic view to a view of caring–healing care focused on informing and supporting individuals and populations in achieving their healthcare goals. The foundations of advanced holistic nursing education provide a caring–healing philosophical framework that includes the essence of nurturing compassionate practice by nurses committed to society and prepared to address diverse healthcare challenges.

References

Alexander, S., & Shirey, M. (2020). Advanced nursing practice: Pathway to entrepreneurship. In J. Fulton, A. Goudreau, & L. Swartzell (Eds.), *Foundations of clinical nurse specialist practice* (3rd ed.). Spring Publishing.

American Association of Colleges of Nursing (AACN). (2006). *The essentials of doctoral education for advanced nursing practice.* AACN.

American Association of Colleges of Nursing (AACN). (2012, October). *Update on the LACE Network and implementation of the APRN consensus model.* AACN.

American Holistic Nurses Credentialing Corporation (AHNCC). (2017a, December). *Core essentials for the practice of advanced holistic nursing AHN-BC and APHN-BC.* www.ahncc.org/wp-content/uploads/2017/12/2017-ADVANCED-CORE-ESSENTIALS-DOCUMENT-Final-PDF.pdf

American Holistic Nurses Credentialing Corporation (AHNCC). (2017b). *Foundations, competencies, and curricular guidelines for basic to doctoral holistic nursing education.* https://www.ahncc.org/resources/curriculum-guidelines/

American Holistic Nurses Credentialing Corporation (AHNCC). (2024). *Endorsement program.* https://www.ahncc.org/school-endorsement-program/what-is-an-endorsed-school/

American Nurses Association & American Holistic Nurses Association (ANA & AHNA). (2019). *Holistic nursing: Scope and standards of practice* (3rd ed.). Nursesbooks.org.

APRN Consensus Work Group and National Council of State Boards of Nursing APRN Advisory Committee. (2008, July 7). *Consensus model for APRN regulation: Licensure, accreditation, certification and education.* AACN. www.aacn.nche.edu/education-resources/APRNReport.pdf

Broome, M., & Marshall, E. (2017). Expert clinician to transformational leader in a complex health care organization. In E. Marshall & M. Broome (Eds.), *Transformational leadership in nursing* (pp. 3–36). Springer Publishing.

Cliff, B. (2012). The evolution of patient-centered care. *Journal of Healthcare Management, 57*(2), 86–88.

Daley, K. A. (2012). Person-centered care. What does it actually mean? *The American Nurse, 44*(6), 3.

Delaney, C., & Barrera, C. (2012). Advanced practice nursing students' knowledge, self-efficacy, and attitudes related to depression to older adults. Teaching holistic depression care. *Holistic Nursing Practice, 26*(4), 210–220.

Denisco, S., & Stewart, J. (2024). Historical perspectives: The art and science of nurse practitionering and advanced practice nursing. In S. Denisco (Ed.). *Advanced Practice Nursing: Essential Knowledge for the Profession* (5th ed.) (pp. 21–41). Jones & Bartlett Learning.

Dossey, B., & Keegan, L. (2016). *Holistic nursing: A handbook for practice* (7th ed.). Jones & Bartlett Learning.

Enzman Hines, M. (2009). Reflective practice: How we know what we know. *Beginnings, 29*(2), 3–5.

Enzman Hines, M. (2011). Caring in advance practice education: A new view of the future. In M. Hills & J. Watson (Eds.), *Creating a caring science curriculum: An emancipatory pedagogy for nursing* (pp. 203–216). Springer.

Enzman Hines, M. (2012). Holistic nursing and healthcare reform: Challenges and opportunities. *Beginnings, 32*(4), 4–7.

Enzman Hines, M. (2016). Turning words into action: The emerging role of advanced holistic nurses. *AHNA Beginnings, 36*(3), 6-7, 32-3.

Erickson, H. (2009). Holistic nurses' examinations: Past, present, future. *Journal of Holistic Nursing, 27*(3), 186–202.

Erickson, H. (Ed.). (2010). *Exploring the interface between the philosophy and discipline of holistic nursing: Modeling and role-modeling at work.* Unicorns Unlimited.

Erickson, H., & Erickson, M. (2010). Ways of knowing and the metaparadigm. In H. Erickson (Ed.), *Exploring the interface between the philosophy and discipline of holistic nursing* (pp. 52–69). Unicorns Unlimited.

Esposito, C., & Contreras Sollazzo, L. (2024) Nurse entrepreneurs: The real independent practice of nursing. *Journal of the New York State Nurses Association, 46*(2), 26.

Hills, M., & Watson, J. (2011). *Creating a caring science curriculum: A Relational emancipatory pedagogy for nursing.* Springer.

Institute of Medicine (IOM). (2010). *The future of nursing: Leading change, advancing health.* The National Academies Press. http://www/iom.edu/Reports/2010/The-future-of-nursing-leading-change-advancing-health.asps

Jacobs, B. B. (2001). Respect for human dignity: A central phenomenon to philosophically unite nursing theory and practice through consilience of knowledge. *Advances in Nursing Science, 24*(1), 17–35.

Johns, C. (2017). *Becoming a reflective practitioner.* John Wiley & Sons.

Kim, H. S. (2000). An integrative framework for conceptualizing clients: A proposal for a nursing perspective in the new century. *Nursing Science Quarterly, 13*(1), 37–40.

Levin, J., & Reich, J. (2013). Self-reflection. In B. Dossey & L. Keegan (Eds.), *Holistic nursing practice: A handbook for practice* (6th ed., pp. 247–259). Jones & Bartlett Learning.

Mach, A. L., & Kinzer, J. (2018, June 27). *Legislative actions to modify the Affordable Care Act in the 111th–115th Congresses.* https://www.congress.gov/crs-product/R45244

Martin-Misener, R, Donald, F., Rayner, J., Carter, N., Kilpatrick, K., Ziegler, E., Bourgeault, I., & Bryant-Lukosius, D. (2024). Factors influencing nurse practitioner panel size in team-based primary care: A qualitative case study. *BMC Primary Care, 25*(1):304 https/doi.org/10.1186/s12875-024-02547-6

McKivergin, M. J. (2009). The nurse as an instrument of healing. In B. Dossey & L. Keegan (Eds.), *Holistic nursing: A handbook for practice* (5th ed., pp. 721–735). Jones and Bartlett Publishers.

Morgan, S., & Yoder, L. H. (2012). A concept analysis of person-centered care. *Journal Holistic Nursing. 30*(1), 6–15. https://doi.org/10.1177/0898010111412189

National Center for Complementary and Integrative Health. (2018). *The use of complementary and alternative medicine in the United States.* https://www.nccih.nih.gov/research/statistics-on-complementary-and-integrative-health-approaches

Newman, M. (2002). The pattern that connects. *Advances in Nursing Science, 24*(3), 1–7.

Newman, M. (2003). A world of no boundaries. *Advances in Nursing Science, 26*(4), 240–245.

Newman, M. (2008). *Transforming presence: The difference that nursing makes.* F. A. Davis.

Newman, M. A., Sime, A., Sime, M., & Corcoran-Perry, S. (1991). The focus of the discipline of nursing. *Advances in Nursing Science, 14*(1), 1–6.

O'Grady, E. (2015). The policy process. In D. Mason, E. Dickson, G. A. Perez, & M. McLemore (Eds.), *Policy and procedures in nursing and health care* (8th ed.). Elsevier; 2015.

Obama, B. (2008, Feb. 5). *Campaign speech.* Chicago, Illinois.

Parse, R. R. (1987). *Nursing science: Major paradigms, theories, and critiques.* Saunders.

Phillips, J. (2018). Nursing science, nursing theory: Nurse atheists, nurse agnostics, nurse theists. *Nursing Science Quarterly, 31*(2), 105–108.

Quinn, J. (2016). Transpersonal human caring and healing. In B. Dossey & L. Kegan (Eds.), *Holistic nursing: A handbook for practice* (7th ed., pp. 101–110). Jones & Bartlett Learning.

Rogers, M. (1989). Nursing: A science of unitary human beings. In J. P. Riehl-Sisca (Ed.), *Conceptual models for nursing practice* (3rd ed., pp. 181–188). Appleton & Lange.

Rosa, W., & Lubansky, S. (2016). The advanced practice holistic nurse: A leader in the implementation of core values. *Beginnings, 36*(3), 13.

Rother, J., & Lavizzo-Mourey, R. (2009). Addressing the nursing workforce: A critical element for health reform. *Health Affairs, 28*(4), 620–624.

Salmond, S., & Forrester. D. (2016). Nurses leading change: The time is now! In D. Forrester (Ed.), *Nursing's greatest leaders: A history of activism* (pp. 269–286). Springer Publishing.

Sangster-Gormley, E., Martin-Misener, R., Downe-Wamboldr, B., DiCenso, A. (2011). Factors affecting nurse practitioner role implementation in Canadian practice settings: An integrative review. *Journal of Advanced Nursing, 67*(6) 1178–1190

Sharoff, L. (2008). Exploring nurses' perceived benefits of utilizing holistic modalities for self and clients. *Holistic Nursing Practice, 22*(1), 15–24.

Shields, D. A., Levin, J., Reich, J., Murnane, S., & Hanley, M. A. (2016). Creative expressions in healing. In B. Dossey & L. Keegan (Eds.), *Holistic nursing: A handbook for practice* (7th ed., pp. 321–343). Jones & Bartlett Learning.

Slater, V. (2014). Energy healing. In M. Helming, C. Barrere, K. Avino, & D. Shields (Eds.), *Core curriculum for holistic nursing* (2nd ed., pp. 339–349). Jones & Bartlett Learning.

Smith, M. C., Zahourek, R., Enzman Hines, M., Engebretson, J., & Wind Wardell, D. (2013). Holistic nurses' stories of personal healing. *Journal of Holistic Nursing, 31*(3), 173–187.

Southard, M. E., Dossey, B. M., Bark, L., & Gulina Schaub, B. (2020). *The art and science of nurse coaching: The provider's guide to coaching scope and competencies.* (2nd ed.). American Nurses Association.

Summers, L. (2011). Coming to a consensus about APRN regulation. *Nursing Management, 42*(12), 10–14.

Willis, D., Grace, P., & Roy, C. (2018). A central unifying focus for the discipline: Facilitating humanization, meaning, choice, quality of life, and healing in living and dying. *Advances in Nursing Science, 31*(1), E28–E40. https://doi.org/10.1097/01.ANS.0000311534.04059.d9

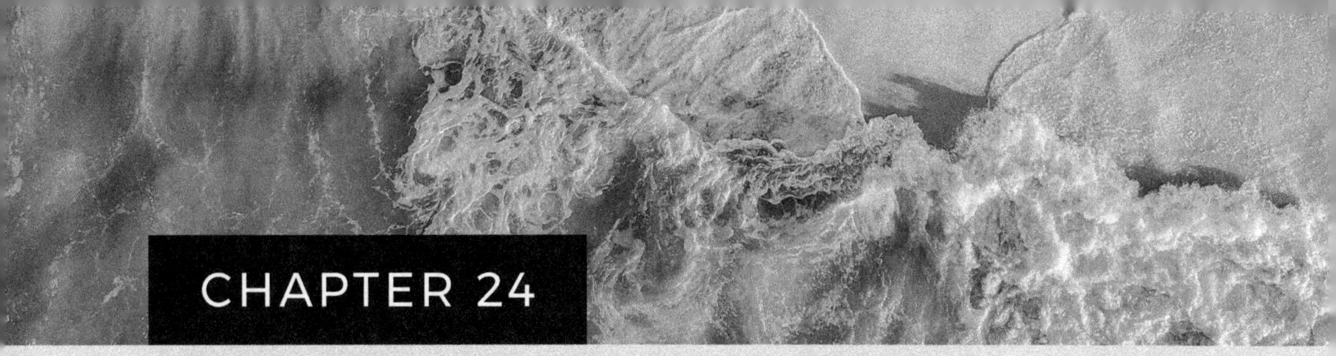

CHAPTER 24

Envisioning a Holistic Framework for Independent Practice

Mary Enzman Hines

HOLISTIC INDEPENDENT PRACTICE OBJECTIVES

- Create a holistic, integrative/healing practice model for advanced nursing practice.
- Identify entrepreneurial skills for developing holistic, integrative/holistic independent practice.
- Examine areas to assist in developing a viable holistic practice and obtaining resources for the development of this practice.
- Develop short- and long-term goals for implementing and sustaining an advanced holistic nursing practice.

DEFINITIONS

Business plan: A detailed plan setting out the objectives of a business, the strategy and tactics planned to achieve them, and the expected profits.

Entrepreneur: An individual who exercises initiative by organizing a venture that takes benefit of an opportunity. Nurse entrepreneurs fill the gaps in healthcare delivery by supporting the development of creative, innovative models and approaches to healthcare services, advancing and integrating technology, and addressing diverse populations. Nurse entrepreneurs provide opportunities for nurses to have a significant impact, achieve greater career and personal goals, and experience an enhanced sense of empowerment (Alexander & Shirey, 2021). Many of these trends have shifted models of care from an acute care focus to prevention and detection (Vannucci & Weinstein, 2017). The Institute of Medicine (IOM) challenged that nursing education programs and associations need to provide entrepreneurial professional development that enables nurses to initiate programs and businesses that will contribute to improving health and health care (Institute of Medicine, 2010).

Full Practice Authority (FPA): States with full practice authority allow advanced practice registered nurses (APRNs) to practice to the full extent of their training and education, including diagnosing, treating, and prescribing patient health conditions.

Holistic Nursing Practice: Holistic nursing practice focuses on creating interpersonal relationships needed to facilitate and enhance an individual's healing with the goal of a maximum state of health, well-being, wellbecoming, and human betterment (ANA & AHNA, 2019; Phillips, 2018). Holistic APNs emphasize unity and wholeness where health patterning is dynamic, interactive, and in constant change.

Integrative health care: An approach characterized by a high degree of collaboration and communication among health professionals.

What makes integrative health care unique is the sharing of information among team members while keeping the patient at the center of care and decision making. The plan of care for each patient addresses biological, psychological, spiritual, and social needs. The interdisciplinary healthcare team includes a diverse group of members (e.g., nurses, physicians, psychologists, social workers, nutritionists, occupational/physical therapist).

Independent Practice: Independent practice is an APN's ability to provide care without mandated supervision from a physician. An APN who lives in a state that has granted independence in its scope of practice can assess, diagnose, and treat health and illness conditions. In total, 27 states (and Washington D.C.) allow APNs to engage in independent practice. The American Academy of Nurse Practitioners (AANP) categorizes each state's degree of independence as full practice (entirely independent), reduced practice (partially independent), and restricted practice (non-independent) (AANP, 2025).

Praxis: The synthesis of thoughtful reflection, caring, and action with a theory and research driven practice (Enzman Hines, 2009). "A holistic framework for independent nursing practice integrates clinical expertise, patient-centered care, and evidence-based decision making to ensure comprehensive and effective healthcare delivery" (American Holistic Nurses Association (AHNA). *What is Holistic Nursing?* www.ahna.org).

Current Landscape of Advanced Practice Nursing

As of 2024, 28 states and the District of Columbia allow advanced practice nurses (APNs) to practice independently, while the remaining states requires some form of collaboration or supervision (AANP, 2025). APNs with independent practice authority provide a wider range of healthcare services including assessing and diagnosing patient health conditions, ordering and interpreting diagnostic tests, initiation, management of evaluation of treatment plans, providing health education, and counselling. Examples of independent practice include starting a nurse practitioner independent practice, working in a primary care setting with full practice authority, or providing care in rural or underserved areas. The benefits of full practice authority result in improved access to care, increased efficiency and reduced costs, and enhanced patient choice and satisfaction (Liu et al., 2020). APNs play a crucial role in health care, especially in rural and underserved populations, providing access and quality care.

Advanced Practice Holistic Nurses as Entrepreneurs

Traditionally, all nurses have worked for hospitals or physicians and have not seen themselves as entrepreneurs. This is changing, and nurse entrepreneurs in all areas of care are considering opening their own businesses. Businesses owned and operated by holistic nurses include home care, staffing, care navigation, wound care, holistic nurse coaching, holistic nurse practitioner care in private practice, and holistic services. Entrepreneurial holistic APNs across all healthcare settings are a positive force for a wider scope of practice to fill the gaps in health care. Nurses in advanced practice have a deep understanding of the healthcare needs and gaps evident in today's healthcare system, combining clinical expertise and knowledge with a willingness to embrace new ways of thinking, a sense of empowerment, and the courage to consider options outside of the status quo. Holistic APNs have the capacity and talent to create new and creative models of care (Alexander & Shirey, 2021). Holistic APNs who establish their own business use nursing and holistic visions and values, expanding the human influence and use of whole-person knowledge and skill in health care (Bagheri & Akbair, 2018).

Entrepreneurial actions in nursing education and practice have created a movement that has expanded over the last two decades. Researchers and leaders have urged healthcare professionals, specifically nurses, to adopt creative, innovative, and entrepreneurial approaches to address emerging healthcare needs of individuals, communities, and society (Alexander & Shirey, 2021; Darbyshire, 2014; Darbyshire et al., 2005; Institute of Medicine, 2001; McDonald, 2011).

Florence Nightingale was identified as a social entrepreneur who had a positive impact on health and society, Lillian Wald was a public health innovator who founded the famous Henry Street Settlement and was a leader of the American Public Health Nursing movement, and Clara Barton established the American Red Cross (Gillis, 2011). Social entrepreneurs are the creators of innovative ideas and practical models for social good (Gillis, 2011). Social, economic, political, leadership, demographics, and technology are creating demands on health care that increase the need for entrepreneurialism in nursing (Darbyshire, 2014). Entrepreneurial nurses focus on innovation and evidence-informed interventions, effectiveness, and efficiency, leading to change and modernization of health systems (Bagheri & Akbair, 2018). Holistic entrepreneurial nurses fulfill a leadership role that focuses on health, well-being, and well-becoming rather than disease. Able to develop new ideas and creative strategies combined with specialists' skills and knowledge, holistic nurses create new and exciting products and services to improve the health of patients and provide a meaningful and satisfying professional opportunity for nurses.

The World Health Organization (WHO) has reviewed the use of APNs in health care around the globe and found that they are under deployed, and their knowledge and services are underutilized (WHO, 2008). A paucity of research is available to provide practical guidelines for entrepreneurial nursing while barriers to practice remain. One of the barriers to entrepreneurial nursing historically begins with nursing education that has focused on acceptance, standardization, and prescription rather than on innovation and leadership (American College of Nurse-Midwives, Accreditation Commission for Midwifery Education, and American Midwifery Certification Board, 2014). As U.S. health care rapidly changes, a shift is occurring to a team approach on health, health promotion, and disease prevention. This system is poised for innovation and creativity that directly affects health care.

Holistic APNs practicing in a variety of practice settings (e.g., primary care, community health, public health, mental health, end-of-life care) are creating successful models of care and delivering innovative, holistic caring–healing to a variety of clients and populations. There are several approaches to developing successful independent healthcare practices (Bagheri & Akbair, 2018); however, nursing education lacks focus on developing entrepreneurial skills. When holistic APNs consider developing independent healthcare practices/businesses, several steps must be considered to establish a plan, identify a target population/client base, implementing the plan, and setting and reassessing goals for success. Steps to consider include:

Getting Started: Reflecting on your reasons for starting a business. Be clear right from the start on what your business will provide and where your skills are best used. Ask yourself the following questions:

- Who is my target population?
- Who are the stakeholders (e.g., business coach, similar practice owners, local small business resources) who will provide information key to getting started?
- What are the comprehensive services that will be offered?
- What are the finances that will be required for startup and ongoing operations?
- What are potential funding sources?
- How will the business be advertised and marketed (e.g., website, colleague connections, google, community groups) and costs related to marketing?
- What are the immediate barriers?
- Clarifying your goals and developing a business plan?

Develop an Organized Plan: How do you want your business to operate? The clearer you are with the focus of your business, the better your business function.

- Identify the hours and format of services you will offer.
- Identify ways to connect with potential clients (e.g., word of mouth,

Google, professional connections, formal advertising).

- Connect to your target professional group and create meaningful collaborations. Quality connections create more value than sheer numbers.
- Decide which social media platforms will work for you and start with the platform that will bring committed clients. Boost your business's visibility that reflects your philosophy, values, and beliefs.
- Create a reliable income stream that aligns with your expertise, values, and resources.
- Engage in a caring, respectful manner with all potential clients as you enroll them.
- Develop a clear, customized business plan for startup, maintenance, and growing your business.

Actualize Your Plan: Be prepared to work long hours, especially at first, but also ensure that you balance your work life, even as a nurse entrepreneur.

- Engage with potential clients in a caring, respectful manner as you engage and enroll them in your practice.
- Utilize help from your network, support group, business coach, and experts in practices like yours.

Be Confident: Everything is energy. Embrace and adhere to your spiritual, universal, and energetic values and beliefs.

- Believe in yourself and your skills as an entrepreneur.
- If you do not believe in yourself in your success, it will be the energy you send out to others.
- Do what you can to ensure your success.

Cultivate and Grow: Constantly assess, evaluate, and expand your goals.

- Develop a team that delivers high value care for clients that promotes growth and caring/healing for all who receive your services.
- Constantly appraise your personal and economic goals for the business.
- Grow your support network to assist you in evaluating and expanding business goals.

Starting independent practice can be an exciting prospect, yet it requires a great deal of work and patience. Wearing two hats, that of a businessperson and that of a provider, requires effort and a focus on patient satisfaction/outcomes as well as financial outcomes. Even small practices that start in a home or shared space are businesses that require ongoing care. Whether you are billing insurance companies or getting paid at the time of the patient's visit, it is important to implement a business model so that your practice will survive and thrive. You will be required to work long hours; however, owning your own business allows you to design your practice and practice goals, work flexible hours, and practice in a way that will attract patients and create a practice that is well reimbursed.

As you take these first steps toward becoming a nurse entrepreneur, it may be necessary to access many different community partners. Beginning a business can be a daunting task, but if you have the right team, the right support, and the right ideas, you can do it.

Creating a Business Plan

Business plans typically contain three major elements: organizational plan, marketing plan, and financial plan. The organizational segment describes the management team (i.e., partners, management matrix). The marketing section discusses who may use the service and products/services offered by the business. The financial statement contains the numbers that illustrate how the project is expected to operate over the initial start-up period. An executive summary that outlines key points and introduces the business plan is recommended. This section is often what gains further examination of the business plan (Rich et al., 2019). The executive summary must include a clear and concise outline of the services and products. **Box 24-1** outlines the key elements of the executive summary, and **Box 24-2** combines an actual executive summary of a proposed business.

Box 24-1 Executive Summary

The executive summary is a one- to two-page document that summarizes the opportunity and importance of the proposed business and contains the following elements:

- Description of the present situation and summary of existing conditions, also termed a *gap analysis*
- Description of the new program or proposed solution
- Presentation of options
- Market analysis
- Implementation plan
- Timeline
- Evaluation plan
- Financials

Data from Mary Enzman Hines and Jennifer Gaughan.

Box 24-2 Sample Executive Summary

National healthcare reform, a shortage of primary care physicians, and shifting healthcare delivery models are the driving forces behind the establishment of alternative care models to meet the increasing demand for healthcare services. The Institute of Medicine's 2010 *Future of Nursing* report recommendation to improve access to health care includes allowing APRNs to function to the full extent of their education and training, including the establishment of autonomous practice. The establishment of retail-based clinics is but one outgrowth of that trend. In the state of Colorado, APRNs are allowed to set up autonomous practices, including the provision of health care, the evaluation and treatment of minor acute illness, and the monitoring of stable chronic conditions. Recent advances in insurance company and Medicaid reimbursement have made the reality of nurse practitioner–based clinics financially feasible. These factors, as well as a desire to give back to the community we serve, provide the foundation upon which we have created Integrative Pediatric Health Care of Colorado, LLC.

Integrative Pediatric Health Care of Colorado (IPHC) is a nurse practitioner–owned and operated holistic primary care practice serving children and families of all income levels. The holistic NPs at IPHC specialize in the integration of holistic and conventional healthcare approaches in caring for the unique needs of children. IPHC exemplifies the primary care medical [health care] home model with a philosophy of care rooted in holism. Providers engage with each person as a unique and unified being, encompassing mind, body, and spirit and provide cutting-edge caring primary care services, and achieve the key practice goals of:

- providing high-quality, cost-effective, specialized, holistic primary care to children and families in a medical [health care] home model.
- increasing access to integrative pediatric care in a medically underserved area.
- recruiting and maintaining creative, caring, quality staff that exemplifies a philosophy of caring.
- providing a supportive environment for parents to explore complementary approaches to health care for their child.
- participating in research and utilizing evidence-based practice guidelines to support new knowledge and growth in pediatric health care.
- providing clinical preceptor experiences for advanced practice nursing students in collaboration with area universities and colleges.
- developing a loyal customer base where children receive health care from birth to college; and
- including an onsite retail component, making available to our patients at low-cost plant and botanical-based preparations, common prescriptive medications used in pediatrics, and over-the-counter medications and remedies.

(*continues*)

Box 24-2 Sample Executive Summary *(continued)*

The owners of IPHC are two APRNs (Mary Enzman Hines and Jennifer Gaughan) with more than 60 years of combined experience in pediatrics. The mission and vision of IPHC is supported by a caring, conscientious, efficient staff and includes interprofessional relationships with specialty pediatric providers and a network of specialist providers (e.g., occupational therapy, physical therapy, psychotherapy, speech therapy), including those who practice both conventional and complementary modalities.

The purpose of the following business plan portfolio is to highlight the structure and operational approach of IPHC, explore evidence to support a need for such services, review a market analysis, provide financial statements, provide a timeline, discuss legal implications, and introduce owners and staff.

IPHC owners are proposing a small-business loan agreement with your organization in the amount of $XXXXXX. With these funds, IPHC will achieve start-up goals and create a sustainable, profitable, and unique pediatric practice, allowing us to pay back the loan in 5–7 years.

Data from Mary Enzman Hines and Jennifer Gaughan.

Note: The contents of this executive summary are not to be copied without the expressed permission of the authors.

While the components of a business plan are essentially the same in all organizations, the templates may vary. The process of writing a business plan, coupled with knowledge of macro systems of health care, can result in ensuring success in initiating and operating a successful program or business. The ability to innovate as well as develop an entrepreneurial proposal and solid business plan will prepare nurses to have a strong voice in the financial and business world (Smith et al., 2013; Dossey, 2010).

Financing and Sustaining Practice

Holistic APNs are competent healthcare providers who deliver valuable, cost-effective health care. As the public, government, and insurers recognize the benefits of utilizing holistic APNs, the demand for care will increase. Developing business savvy and carefully planning a practice-based business future can bolster confidence and predict success. No healthcare venture ever succeeds without confident, enthusiastic leadership around a mission that will attract patients. But this rosy outlook can become a liability, especially when dealing with financial projections.

Holistic APNs have not had financial preparation and do not always understand the importance of the financial structure required to sustain a practice. Obtaining financial capital to start a business is the first step in any planning. Proper financial projections include money to purchase equipment and hire personnel and enough operating capital to sustain the practice until it becomes profitable. The amount of funding needed before beginning or opening a practice depends on the type of practice and the business plan. Many financial advisors note the importance of determining the predicted need and increasing that amount by 25 to 50 percent. Capitalization can come from family, a bank, or some combination of these. The first step is developing a working budget for the first year of operation within the business plan.

As a general rule, estimate the amount of money needed to open a practice, and then double it to be sure there is enough. Also, estimate the time required for the practice to become profitable, and double that time as a reasonable estimate for repaying loans. Some of the costs and other items to consider include the following:

- **Equipment**: Equipment can include rented office computers, phones, refrigerator, medical equipment, and supplies. Durable equipment companies and medical supply companies supply office furniture and exam room equipment. Second-hand medical equipment can be found through brokers or advertisements in nursing and medical journals.
- **Salaries**: Salaries can include providers (including your own salary), medical assistants, receptionists, billers/insurance coders, and

office managers. Coders and office managers can make or break a practice financially. If the APN takes on these responsibilities at first, make sure all of the rules of coding are understood so that over- or under-coding does not pose a problem financially or legally. Remember that coding translates into money. Knowledge of laws and statutes regulating healthcare practice as well as the components of human resource management is essential for independent practice. These laws govern how employees must be treated and paid, and they protect the rights of the employees in the workplace.

- **Treatment costs**: These costs include test kits for the Clinical Laboratory Improvement Amendment—waived tests such as urine analysis and strep tests.
- **Health insurance**: Seek funding for health insurance benefits for practice providers and staff.
- **Other insurance**: This encompasses general business liability insurance and malpractice insurance.
- **Funding**: Apply for grants and foundation funding to enable the practice to have foreign language interpreters. Reaching out to the United Way may be an additional funding source.
- **Key relationships**: Maintain a relationship with key professionals outside of the healthcare field to support private practice. Relationships with bankers, attorneys, and accountants will make financial dealings less complex.

Some of these costs may be reduced, shifted, or avoided by focusing the practice on home visits. In a home visit practice, office rental and many other equipment costs will not be required; however, travel costs such as gas, care expenses, and insurance will need to be included. When thinking about starting a practice, consider creating a niche that will bring in patients to the practice, such as a holistic weight loss clinic, a stress reduction clinic, and an acupuncture/acupressure or a holistic pain reduction clinic. Consider being open during times that are convenient for working people, such as evenings and weekends, to attract patients. Consider having day care services or health navigation services (even if patients must pay for these services) to increase accessibility to patients and families. Offer services within the practice setting, such as massage, yoga, or tai chi, that make the practice a one-stop appointment for patients. Determine what services will cost and whether the practice will be a cash-only practice or if insurance will be accepted.

If the economic plan for the practice includes accepting insurance, make an extremely detailed investigation of which insurance plans or payer plans will be accepted, how much each of these payers pay for services provided, how fast they pay, and whether they accept this practice on their insurance panel. Medicare is the largest U.S. insurer, and many other insurance companies follow Medicare rules. As an APN, you may bill the Medicare program directly for services using a national provider identifier (NPI) or an employer's or contractor's NPI. The NPI is a unique 10-digit identification number issued to U.S. healthcare providers by the Centers for Medicare and Medicaid Services. It is important to know exactly which reimbursement levels will be received for services rendered. There is a set amount for each type of visit, treatment, and follow-up based on diagnosis and therapy. Payment is made only on an assignment basis, which means that payment will be the Medicare-allowed amount as payment in full, and the APRN may not bill or collect from the beneficiary any amount other than unmet co-payments, deductibles, and/or coinsurance. For APNs, services are paid 85 percent of the Medicare Physician Fee Schedule amount. Medicaid reimbursement is similar, and in the pediatric population, reimbursements are similarly differential for the APN billing (85% of the Physician Fee Schedule).

Understanding and, in some cases, pursuing reimbursement for APN services may be key to survival for an independent nurse-run practice. To be prepared to adequately and successfully have an independent practice, holistic APNs must be competent clinicians but also well versed in the business/financial constructs for providing care. Understanding the key concepts of holistic

APN roles and definitions, Medicare/Medicaid billing regulations, private insurance regulations, credentialing for privileges in the healthcare setting, inpatient versus outpatient billing issues, the use of Current Procedural Terminology codes, and other topics as defined by the specific setting in which the APN works is critical for success (Smith et al., 2013; Waxman & Barter, 2013). Billing various third-party payers can be accomplished with a variety of medical management software; however, the challenge is the monitoring of claims submitted, tracking the date and amount of payments received, and resubmitting denied claims.

Getting the advice of professionals before developing a business plan or attempting to raise capital is a safe and reasonable step to ensure the sustainability of an independent practice. Connect with an accountant who is an expert in financial management to determine the required funding and the timeframe for the business to turn a profit. The accountant's ability to assist depends on accurate assessments made in the business plan, the market for provided services, a willingness to work hard, and a tolerance to hang in there until the business becomes profitable. Speaking to others in a successful practice venture who have become independent entrepreneurs would be extremely helpful to avoid financial pitfalls. Johnson & Johnson offers a resource on the nurse entrepreneur (www.discovernursing.com/specialty/nurse-entrepreneur). The National Nurses in Business Association website (https://nnbanow.com/) provides valuable information, and the Nurse Entrepreneur website (www.nursingentrepreneurs.com) shares knowledge about opening a business and connecting nurse entrepreneurs in discussions about critical issues.

Federal, state, and local governments offer a wide range of financing programs and grants to help small businesses start and grow their operations. These programs include low-interest loans, venture capital, and scientific and economic development grants. Banks receive monies from the federal government to loan to small business start-up companies. If the services offered in the practice are sufficiently unique and interesting to the community in which the business will be located, it may be possible to obtain grants and loans from within the community itself. Finally, personal funds and family loans are often used to start a business; however, be sure to have all aspects of the loan, including repayment schedules, in writing to avoid problems later.

Starting an independent nursing practice is not easy, but, for the right individual, it is the opportunity of a lifetime to make a difference and to become successful. It requires a lot of work, strength, and perseverance, as well as help from many others in the community and around the country. Holistic nurses are well positioned to offer independent services in a variety of settings that are unique and desired by many, including complementary therapies such as yoga, meditation, Reiki, Therapeutic Touch, Healing Touch, nutritional therapy, and others. Starting a business as a solo practitioner or with a group of like-minded individuals can be a rewarding and thrilling opportunity if the right steps are taken to ensure sustainability and success.

With the changing landscape of healthcare issues in specific communities and populations, holistic APNs are meeting the gaps in care. The following nursing situation depicts the differences that emerge from a holistic approach to providing primary care for children.

This encounter underscores the importance of holistic care, caring-within-practice (Enzman Hines & Gaughan, 2017) integrating person-centered strategies to support children and families. Given the changing landscape of advanced holistic nursing practice, continuous exploration and implementation of holistic approaches necessary to enhance health outcomes for our youngest community members. Comforting nursing interactions impact the pain, anxiety, fear, and distress of families (Bice & Wyatt, 2017).

Caring for diverse, marginalized, underserved families offers many opportunities and challenges. The essence of advanced practice holistic nursing in primary care revolves around a thorough and person-centered approach with the aim of ensuring the overall well-being of children and their families. Family-centered care incorporates health and well-being/becoming that highlights the importance of working together with families to make decisions that promote responsibility and

Nursing Situation

Deon, an African American, 5-day-old newborn, presents to the practice with his mother and grandmother for a newborn visit and follow-up from caesarean section (C/S) delivery. The delivery room record sent electronically by the hospital was reviewed prior to the visit. Angela, Deon's mother, is 25 years old, and this is Angela's second pregnancy and first live birth; her first pregnancy resulted in a stillbirth (G2 P1001). The record revealed that Angela underwent a C/S for tight nuchal cord resulting in "late decels." Once delivered, Deon seemed to recover quickly and their stay in the hospital seemed uneventful. Information about the hospital stay was very technical (delivery information, birthweight, height, weight, APGAR scores, number of pregnancies, lab work [she was group B strep positive at the time of delivery requiring antibiotics], hearing test, and critical congenital heart disease [CCHD] testing).

Upon entering the room, I observed a tearful mother who was trying to smile as I greeted her. Her mother was seated next to her. I pulled my seat up in front of Angela and asked her how she was doing? She shyly replied, "I am okay, just struggling with things." I asked if she felt comfortable, and could she share more about her struggles. She expressed that she was a bit overwhelmed with things. I ask her how she felt the delivery went and she said, "I don't know they said they had to do an emergency C/S." "This is your second child?" I asked. "Well sort of, my first baby was a still birth." Sadness poured over me. She went on to inform me that, "Deon's dad, who was so looking forward to the birth of his son, died a month ago from a seizure." I moved closer and ask her if I could hug her and she nodded her head. The grandmother, whom she is living with, replied, "She is really a strong woman but has been through a lot including having to have a caesarean section for the delivery. They say he had the umbilical cord around his neck."

I paused for a moment to take in the information and the sadness being expressed. During that moment, I reflected, how is Angela dealing with all this loss and joy at the same time? Is she experiencing postpartum depression combined with ongoing grief from the loss of her first child and Deon's father at the same time? What part does sleep deprivation play in this sadness? Who is she as an American woman of African descent, who is a single mom, living with her mother? Is she there for her? How do I approach this woman and not overwhelm her? Angela's mother seemed very supportive but expressed "she is a strong woman, she will just get through it." What does she want me to know about her daughter?

I asked Angela, "How can I help you?" I think to myself, where do I go from here? Angela informs me that she wants me to tell her that Deon will be okay. What does she need to think about over the next few weeks? Can I see Deon, I ask. I open a soft blanket from around Deon and comment, "Oh he is such a good-looking boy! You must be so proud!" Both the grandmother and mother smile, "Yes he is, looks just like his daddy!" My follow-up comments relate to how he is nursing, his sleep cycles, what other things does she notice about him? Angela shares with me that he is breastfeeding well, seems to smile when his eyes are closed but that is probably gas, and he sleeps a lot but when he is awake seems to look around. I comment on his physical features as I complete the physical exam. I ask her what other questions she has and she replies, "Is he going to be okay?"

As the exam and the questions about newborn information unfolded, a transpersonal caring occasion was experienced. I intended to be authentically present, and listen deeply to this woman as she expressed her needs. Realizing how this baby could be a source of joy and challenge for her, how could I convey that I was there to listen and guide her through her journey as a new mother and hoping that I was conveying caring-within-practice (Enzman Hines & Gaughan, 2017).

By the end of the visit, Angela identified that a therapist would be helpful as well as the ability to contact with other single moms. She felt that she could meet Deon's immediate needs with her mother's support. A mutual plan was developed including the name of a therapist who specializes in grief and loss, breastfeeding information and lactation consultants (with background information about each), information about single-parent mommy's groups, resources about raising a child as a single parent, and informational material about her newborn and subsequent visit information. I reassured her this was a lot of information, but she could read and access the information over the next few weeks as time allowed. I also offered the grandmother resources for her ongoing role as a grandparent. We discussed parenting challenges as a single parent and moving through grief. The encounter came to a natural close and Angela shared, "Thank you for taking the time to see me as a mother and woman and listening to my story." Angela and I hugged again and told her I looked forward to hearing more about her story in subsequent visits.

As the encounter came to a close, I was left with many questions, including what she was experiencing as a "single mom" who was an American woman of African descent and the challenges that may be in her future. I have had subsequent visits with Deon and Angela, and Deon is a happy, thriving baby. Angela established care with a therapist and a mommy's group. Angela shared during a visit for Deon that she had gotten through the anniversary of Deon's father's death and focused on the gifts she had received in her life and working on positive affirmations during hard times. She has returned to work as a human resource representative and is learning to balance work, parenting, and self-care as a single parent. We are learning more about each other with each of Deon's visits.

personalized care approaches. Health promotion efforts empower families with healthcare knowledge and fosters a culture of well-being. Cultural competence ensures that holistic advanced practice in pediatrics can navigate through individual patient sociocultural backgrounds to provide individualized care (Enzman Hines & Gaughan, 2017; Saif et al., 2023). Developmental considerations involve assessments and early interventions that support growth and development. Emotional support and counselling help address the complexities related to a child's health issues, ultimately improving well-being/wellbecoming. Additionally, the integration of technology and educational materials aids in enhancing communication, making linkages with consultations, and offering health resources.[23] Providing holistic care for children and families, holistic PNPs integrate multiple patterns of knowing to address the needs of the child and family (Lee et al., 2017).

Implications

This chapter presents how holistic APN entrepreneurs have the potential to create models of care to address the gaps in care for individuals, communities, and global populations. Holistic APNs have the knowledge and skills to address the healthcare needs of at-risk, underserved, and marginalized populations. Holistic APNs now more than ever are in the position to advance a caring, healing covenant with patients as holistic nurse entrepreneurs to create new models of health care. From a holistic perspective, holistic APNs address the whole of human experience while incorporating complexity, systems thinking, and multiple patterns of knowing in nursing. They also engage in interprofessional collaboration to achieve desired outcomes for diverse patient populations. As entrepreneurs, their journey in creation of innovative healthcare models has the potential for having great impact on individuals and communities. Advanced practice entrepreneurs have the potential to impact economic growth and make meaningful contributions to health care, society, and policy (Alexander & Shirey, 2021).

Clinical Practice

Current changes in the healthcare arena require the development of clinical skills that are patient-centered, holistic/integrative, and focused on health, well-being, and wellbecoming. Emerging from the COVID-19 pandemic, holistic health care is now realized as an essential approach for nursing. Holistic APNs have a keen understanding of the care needs and gaps evident in the current healthcare systems. They are in a unique position as nurse leaders to provide holistic, patient-centered care, address the gaps in care for vulnerable and underserved populations, and create new models for providing health care. The scope of entrepreneurial practice depends on the economic infrastructures (e.g., reimbursement, billing, collection) and legal/regulatory standards of the discipline. The scholarship, creativity, and practice of holistic APNs will ensure a sustained impact not only on individual practices, but also to the global world of interdisciplinary healthcare delivery and population health policy (Thorne, 2014). This creative work must always be done within the context of the principles and philosophies of holistic nursing.

Education

Holistic APN entrepreneurs are the change agents who bring new ways of thinking, reasoning, and performing within a holistic approach and leadership. Essential coursework is missing in much of graduate nursing education to prepare holistic APNs for roles as entrepreneurs in independent practice. Preparation in business essentials (e.g., finance, accounting, business law, strategic planning, operations management) and entrepreneurial opportunities can equip holistic APNs in fulfilling their leadership roles within independent practice. With an ability to develop new ideas and creative strategies combined with specialists' skills and knowledge, holistic nurses will create new and exciting products and services that improve the health of patients. Entrepreneurial skills provide the holistic APN with opportunities for developing meaningful and satisfying approaches to practice.

Research

Holistic APNs are introduced to multiple sources of data, information, and outcomes within evidence-informed practice. There are many questions/ideas that emerge for holistic APN entrepreneurs, including:

- What are the gaps within vulnerable, marginalized, and underserved populations that will require innovations in health care?
- What are the models and theories that inform holistic entrepreneurial nursing practice?
- What are sustainable models for entrepreneurial practice?
- How to use multiple patterns of knowing to research questions that will inform holistic nursing practice.
- Developing patient satisfaction strategies focused on evaluating the care provided by holistic APN entrepreneurs.
- What skills and knowledge will guide the creation of new models of holistic health care, resulting from researching specific contributions holistic APNs make in an ever-changing healthcare milieu?

Policy

The Affordable Care Act (Mach & Kinzer, 2018) challenges healthcare providers to develop new systems and structures for promoting the health of individuals and populations in the United States. Promoting systems focused on health and well-being is a growing reality to address the chronic conditions plaguing and increasing the cost of the healthcare system in the United States. Cost-effective holistic health care puts patients in charge of their own health, allowing the patient and provider/team to be active partners in care. Creating a healthcare system focused on holistic approaches to person-centered care values will empower each patient to make decisions based on health beliefs and a sense of wholeness and will move our entire healthcare system away from a disease-oriented model to a wellness, wellbecoming model. Individual challenges for Advanced Holistic Nurse–Board Certified (AHN-BCs)/Advanced Practice Holistic Nurse–Board Certified (APHN-BCs) will include examining and overcoming barriers present in current state and national legislation, patient reimbursement processes, and funding sources for creating innovative holistic practices addressing the evolving healthcare needs of individuals and local, national, and global populations.

Conclusion

The increasing globalization of health care, changing demographics, expanding diversity of populations, and rapid technological changes mandate that nurses possess a breadth of skills and competencies to provide holistic, culturally sensitive health care (Morgan & Yoder, 2012).

Other influencers of health care include the rising cost of health care, the lasting effects of the COVID-19 pandemic on global health, an expanding aging population, rising mental health needs, the role of advanced technology in healthcare documentation and monitoring, and the rising numbers of uninsured Americans (Morgan & Yoder, 2012; DeNisco & Stewart, 2024).

Advanced APNs who are entrepreneurs have the specialty knowledge, skills, and experience to design and implement healthcare systems that will address underserved, diverse, and marginalized populations in various communities (e.g., rural and urban). One of the greatest challenges for the future roles of holistic APN entrepreneurs is focusing on healing within a healthcare system that predominantly embraces a reductionistic view of health care.

In December 2014, the National Center for Complementary Medicine changed its name to the National Center for Complementary and Integrative Health. This provides a clear and strong message that holistic health care with the patient at the center of decision making is the way of the future. The focus on holistic health care provides an impetus for holistic nurses to become increasingly active as healthcare providers using holistic therapies and care principles. Preparing nurses to become entrepreneurs can only strengthen the profession and allow holistic APNs who have the desire to move into more independent practices and become substantive members of the healthcare team.

References

Alexander, S., & Shirey, M. (2021). Advanced nursing practice: Pathway to entrepreneurship. In J. Fulton, A. Goudreau, & L. Swartzell (Eds.), *Foundations of clinical nurse specialist practice* (3rd ed.). Spring Publishing.

American Association of Nurse Practitioners (AANP). (2025). *State practice environment*. https://www.aanp.org/advocacy/state/state-practice-environment

American College of Nurse-Midwives, Accreditation Commission for Midwifery Education, and American Midwifery Certification Board. (2014). *Midwifery in the United States and the consensus model for APRN regulation*. www.midwife.org/ACNM/files/ccLibraryFiles/Filename/000000001458/LACE_White_Paper_2011.pdf

American Nurses Association & American Holistic Nurses Association (ANA & AHNA). (2019). *Holistic nursing: Scope and standards of practice* (3rd ed.). Nursesbooks.org.

Bagheri, A., & Akbair, M. (2018). The impact of entrepreneurial leadership on nurses' innovation behavior. *Journal of Nursing Scholarship, 50*(1), 28–35.

Bice, A. A., & Wyatt, T. H. (2017). Holistic comfort interventions for pediatric nursing procedures: A systematic review. *Journal of Holistic Nursing, 35*(3), 280–295. https://doi.org/10.1177/0898010116660397

Darbyshire, P., (2014). An idea whose time has come: Nursing entrepreneurialism. *Whitieria Nursing and Health Journal, 21*, 9–14.

Darbyshire, P., Downes, M., Collins, C., & Dyer, S. (2005). Moving from institutional dependence to entrepreneurialism. Creating and funding a collaborative research and practice development position. *Journal of Clinical Nursing, 14*(8), 926–934.

DeNisco, S., & Stewart, J. (2024). Historical perspectives: The art and science of nurse practitionering and advanced practice nursing. In S. DeNisco (Ed.). *Advanced practice nursing: Essential knowledge for the profession* (5th ed.) (pp. 21–41). Jones & Bartlett Learning.

Dossey, B. M. (2010). Holistic nursing: From Florence Nightingale's historical legacy to 21st-century global nursing. *Alternative Therapies in Health and Medicine, 16*(5), 14–16.

Enzman Hines M., & Gaughan, J. (2017). Advanced holistic nursing practice narratives: A view of caring praxis. *Journal of Holistic Nursing, 35*(4), 328–341. https://doi.org/10.1177/0898010117715849

Enzman Hines, M. (2009). Reflective practice: How we know what we know. *Beginnings, 29*(2), 3–5.

Gillis, C. (2011). The nurse as social entrepreneur: Revisiting our roots and raising our voices. *Nursing Outlook, 59*(5), 256–257.

Institute of Medicine (US) & Committee on Quality of Health Care in America. (2021). *Crossing the quality chasm: A new health system for the 21st century*. National Academies Press (US).

Institute of Medicine. (2010). *The future of nursing: Leading change, advancing health*. The National Academies Press. https://nap.nationalacademies.org/resource/12956/Future-of-Nursing-2010-Report-Brief.pdf

Lee, H., Kim, A., Meong, A., & Seo, M. (2017). Pediatric nurse practitioners' clinical competencies and knowing patterns in nursing: Focus group interviews. *Contemporary Nurse, 53*(5), 515–523. https://doi.org/10.1080/10376178.2017.1315827

Liu, C., Hebert, P., Douglas, J., Neely, E., Suic, C., Reddy, A., Sales, A., & Wong, E. (2020). Outcomes of primary care delivery by nurse practitioners: Utilization, cost, and quality of care. *Health Services Research, 55*(2), 178–189.

Mach, A. L., & Kinzer, J. (2018, June 27). *Legislative actions to modify the Affordable Care Act in the 111th–115th Congresses*. https://www.congress.gov/crs-product/R45244

McDonald, D. (2011). Nurse to know: An entrepreneurial spirit soars. *Canadian nurse, 107*(1), 30–31.

Morgan, S., & Yoder, L. H. (2011). A concept analysis of person-centered care. *Journal Holistic Nursing, 30*(1), 6–15. https://doi.org/10.1177/0898010111412189

Phillips, J. (2018). Nursing science, nursing theory: Nurse atheists, nurse agnostics, nurse theists. *Nursing Science Quarterly, 31*(2), 105–108.

Rich, C., Vermooij, M., & Wadhwa, S. (2019). *Health entrepreneurship: A practical guide*. Taylor & Francis Group.

Saif, N. A. A., Alharthi, M. S., Alshammari, A. M., Altamimi, A. M., Alanazi, M.A., Hawbani, R. F., Alanazi, N. W., Alromuhi, M. A., Alnashar, A. K., Alzain, S. A., ALZain, A. A., & Aldhim, W. A. (2023). Pediatric nursing in primary care: Strategies for holistic child and family support. *Journal of Survey in Fisheries Sciences, 10*(5), 252–255.

Smith, M. C., Zahourek, R., Enzman Hines, M., Engebretson, J., & Wind Wardell, D. (2013). Holistic nurses' stories of personal healing. *Journal of Holistic Nursing, 31*(3), 173–187.

Thorne, S. (2014). What constitutes core disciplinary knowledge? *Nursing Inquiry, 21*(1), 1–2. https://doi.org/10.1111/nin.12062

Vannucci, M., & Weinstein, S. (2017). The nurse entrepreneur: Empowerment needs, challenges, and self-care practices. *Nursing: Research and Reviews*, 7, 57–66. https://doi.org/10.2147/NRR.S98407

Waxman, K. T., & Barter, M. (2013). Entrepreneurial leadership: Innovation and business acumen. In K. T. Waxman (Ed.), *Financial and business management for the Doctor of Nursing practice* (pp. 241–259). Springer.

World Health Organization (WHO). (2008, May). *Integrated health services: What and why?* (Technical Brief No. 1). https://terrance.who.int/mediacentre/data/sage/SAGE_Docs_Ppt_Apr2014/10_session_child_health_services/Apr2014_session10_integrated_health_services.pdf#:~:text=This%20Technical%20Brief%20is%20intended,of%20a%20rather%20polarized%20debate.

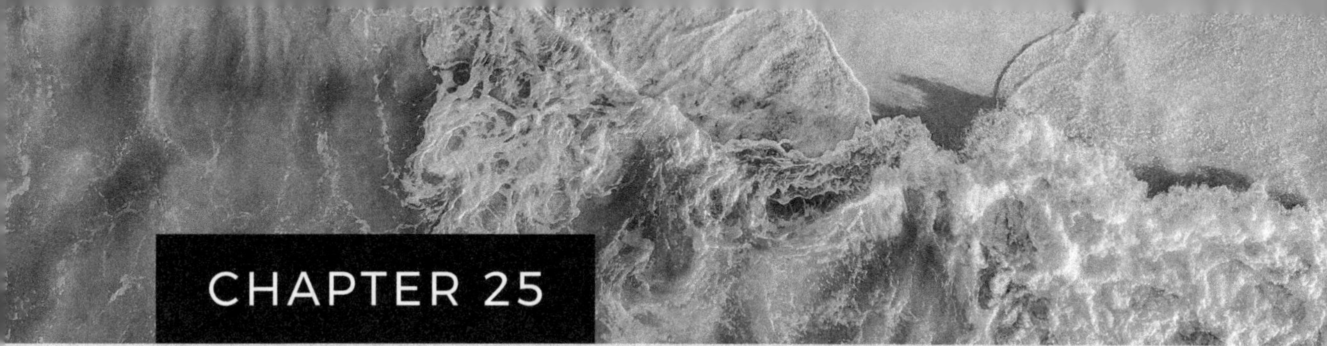

CHAPTER 25

Narrative Reflections of Advanced Holistic Nurses

Karen M. Avino

NURSE HEALER OBJECTIVES

- Articulate potential changes in practice that can result in a new outcome.
- Examine the significance of client stories as related to your holistic practice.
- Create opportunities to enhance your practice with holistic core values and interventions.

The Sharing of Professional Experiences

Narrative reflection is the idea that people are made up of interacting stories and that the situations that they bring to their stories are influenced and shaped by cultural communications in written, verbal, or visual forms. Narrative reflection allows for "restorying" communications that provide an opportunity for reconsidering, reappreciating, and reauthoring the story and relationship (Madigan, 2019). Each person has their own unique story and interpretation of their life's journey. For clients, storytelling may lead to gaining insight into and considering new strategies for moving forward.

For holistic nurses, authentically listening and connecting to the story enables insight into the cause and effect of the entangled variables that affect health and healing. The sharing of experiences of client encounters, self-care activities, various creative nursing interventions, methods of working with clients, and ways of implementing the Holistic Nursing Core Competencies and Core Values is critical to advancing nursing practice. Working in conventional healthcare settings, nurses may not be exposed to interventions that can be implemented through integrating the healing arts with technical competence. Nurses exposed to a holistic nursing community can learn about the many ways of knowing client needs and the numerous methods of creating an environment for the ultimate outcome of holistic healing. Therefore, narrative nursing situations are an essential way to share the story from the nurses' perspective that allows for personal development of new perspectives for client care.

Some of the holistic core values used by nurses daily are obvious, and some are less so. Therefore, nursing situations are a vehicle to document the critical path for envisioning the real-life context of human nature. This chapter, dedicated to narrative reflections, relies on the gracious gifts from fellow nurses who share their lived experiences of distinctive, holistic, and caring moments. Exploring how nurses' actions, interventions, or recommendations can shape an experience and, likewise, how a client can influence the nurse is invaluable. It is through the reader's interpretation and reflection that insight into holistic client care can be understood at a deeper level.

This chapter intends that the following narrative reflections provide a process of sharing a story in its complexity and describe the unique ability of holistic nurses to create an environment for healing. We are grateful to all nurses who value the complex relationships of health, illness, and wellness and weave together both the scientific foundations and the art of nursing in their practice.

Reference

Madigan, S. (2019). Overview. In *Narrative therapy* (2nd ed.). American Psychological Association.

Narrative Reflections of Holistic Nurses

C.H.E.R.I.S.H. Valentine's Day

Connected Hearts Empathetically Restoring Intentional Shared Healing

Focus area: Healing hearts: A day of stress reduction for healthcare professionals (reestablished post-COVID-19 pandemic)

Holistic Nurse: Debra J. DePasqua, MSN, NE-BC, Medical-Surgical Nurse, HNB-BC, HSMI, IAC

Place of Employment: Middlesex Health System, Middletown, CT

Nursing Specialty: Nursing Administrative Supervisor, Co-Chairperson of the Holistic CARE Team (HCT)

Holistic Intervention Specialization: Integrative Aromatherapy

Setting: Healing and nurturing occur from the inside out! The inception of Connected Hearts Empathetically Restoring Intentional Shared Healing (C.H.E.R.I.S.H.) was driven by a local elementary school tragedy in 2012, with the demise of many young children. The distress and pain were felt by the entire state of Connecticut, if not globally. The Holistic CARE Team (HCT), a subcommittee of the health systems nursing department, wanted to support the first responders who were shocked by the catastrophic loss of so many young lives in a meaningful way. Connected Hearts Empathetically Restoring Intentional Shared Healing (C.H.E.R.I.S.H.) was created to raise funds for the cause and support nurses and other healthcare professionals within our community hospital.

It had been an annual event until the emergence of the COVID-19 pandemic in 2020, which prohibited the "connection" that C.H.E.R.I.S.H. espoused and thus disallowed the event. The significantly changed environment that ensued during and beyond COVID-19 has left nurses with moral injuries in need of attention and healing. Nurse HEROs (High Expectation and Risk Occupation) affected by such deeply distressing experiences must realize that self-care is not selfish, but essential to nurturing their well-being (Hossain & Clatty, 2021).

Holistic Core Values and Competencies Identified: Florence Nightingale's wisdom and her philosophy of holism in health care focused on unity, wellness, and the interrelationship of human beings, events, and the environment. The theory emphasizes to *put the person in the best place for nature to act upon to heal.* Moreover, nurses must take care of themselves first before they can effectively care for others.

Self-stewardship is the skill of tending to and nurturing one's well-being (Nightingale, 1969). Self-care strategies aim to combat moral injuries and build resilience (Hossain & Clatty, 2021). The holistic nurse emphasizes the practices of self-care that enhance the parasympathetic nervous system, such as intentionality, presence, mindfulness, and therapeutic use of self and patterning of wellness in others, thereby building moral resilience (American Holistic Nurses Association & American Nurses Association, 2019; Hossain & Clatty, 2021).

Holistic Nursing Methods, Skills, or Interventions and Exploration of Human Experiences: Holistic nursing focuses on promoting health and wellness by supporting healthcare staff to find peace, comfort, harmony, and balance. Living beings radiate electromagnetic fields involved in homeostasis that aim to restore balance and health at the cellular level. When we are stressed, our equilibrium is *dis-eased* or out of balance. When we enter the biofield of another with the intent to heal, we are changed. The biofields cross and interact as energy pathways are exchanged. Aromatherapy, touch, sound healing, and practitioners of energy therapies such as Reiki, reflexology, and massage aim to influence the subtle energy fields surrounding the body of the recipient to enhance physical, mental, emotional, and spiritual health. Moreover, the mere presence of a caring person can be healing (Dossey & Keegan, 2016).

To that end, the HCT reintroduced a Healing Hearts Day on Valentine's Day 2025, C.H.E.R.I.S.H. It is offered in a tranquil, welcoming, healing space that we strive to create in a hospital conference room. The HCT intends to provide a setting for staff to restore balance and health and give themselves permission for self-care, even at work. The goal of the therapies is to ensure that the dimensions of self-physical, mental, emotional, and spiritual are attended to away from the fray of their workspace, even for a short time (American Holistic Nurses Association & American Nurses Association, 2019; Hossain & Clatty, 2021). Integrative medicine practitioners and volunteers offered their healing hands for the event. "It is not uncommon to find like-minded people pulling together to bring intentional thoughts into reality. Tapping into one's senses provides a sense of connection that can be individual yet widespread" (C. Mohrlein, personal communication, March 31, 2025).

Many of the participants offered their impressions of the event. The setting of the "caring, calming, welcoming" (C. Marotta, personal communication, April 6, 2025) healing environment empowers the body's natural healing potential. It offers a safe space, equipped to heal and support self-compassion. Upon entering the space, there is a board of Post-it hearts that invite the participant to write their intention of the planned experience (e.g., peaceful, refresh and renew, quiet time, etc.) and then share their intention with the practitioner, who prepares their environment by being present with a silent pause. Tocco Della Mani: *Touch of the hands* (a Middlesex Health H.C.T. creation to avoid the use of the word *massage*) with lavender (*Lavandula angustifolia*) essential oil in a carrier oil is offered upon arrival to the space.

"In my experience, the healing environment at the C.H.E.R.I.S.H events is welcoming. When you walk into the space, there is a palpable sense of calm, soft lighting, and soothing scents from the aromatherapy" (L. Jansky, personal communication, April 8, 2025). Himalayan salt lamps and strings of white lights enhance the space. Sound healing music plays in the background and sets the tone for unwinding, while relaxation slides are depicted on a projection screen. There is an inviting sitting area arranged with beverages of lemon water and herbal tea, delectable heart-shaped chocolates, a soothing water fountain, a comfortable temperature, and sound healing in a zero-gravity chair with a vibroacoustic pad and headphones.

Additionally, black privacy curtains separate the therapy sections to foster relaxation and mindfulness. "I feel like the C.H.E.R.I.S.H. [team] does a great job working within the limitations of the physical space. Each station for the different healing practices was thoughtfully arranged to create a sense of peace and comfort" (L. Jansky, personal communication, April 8, 2025).

"[An] intentional bowl is a beautiful way to help release what no longer serves us, creating space for what matters most. It becomes a moment of self-care, reflection, and renewal, offering a chance to connect with your well-being. As people came to [my] table, they were invited to place a piece of paper into the bowl of water, watching it soften as the writing dissolved. During that moment, they could witness the act of letting go. The concept behind this simple ritual is to release something painful with love and make room for joy. Though the act is small, it provides a powerful visual reminder of the importance of letting go and creating space for healing and positivity" (S. Peterson, personal communication, April 14, 2025).

> "I had some major losses in my life and struggles that took a toll on me. My brother-in-law passed away at [Middlesex Health] Hospice Service. I struggled with being the family member, not [his]

> hospice nurse. I felt that I cheated him and my sister [because of the role conflict."] Also, "I had a dear loved one who had an accidental overdose on cocaine and alcohol. He is fine now, but it is still a daily struggle [for me] to support this family member. I reached out to EAP [Employee Assistance Program] and my PCP [Primary Care Provider]; they suggested I request intermittent FMLA [Family Medical Leave of Absence] to take mental health days while I struggle with all of this. The EAP counsellor advised me to do something for myself on those days to help my mental health...to help get myself better. That is when I signed up for C.H.E.R.I.S.H. I honestly had never... paid attention to it, as I was always working. I scheduled a massage and a Reiki appointment. Both were so wonderful, relaxing, and rejuvenating for my physical and mental health. It was quiet, peaceful, and I appreciated the workers not talking but allowing me to decompress...I wrote an affirmation on the [heart] board, ...self-care, mental health care, and letting go. I also wrote on the paper that dissolved in water to wash away what was heavy on my mind. I have since taken more time for myself by scheduling a facial in my town. I won a pizza basket in the raffle! I look forward to C.H.E.R.I.S.H. in the future and now appreciate the time I take for myself and my mental health. I found it imperative, especially in my role as a hospice home care nurse. Thank you again for a great day for me" (D. Mathews, personal communication, April 3, 2025).

Pet therapy is offered by hospital volunteers who share their four-legged friends with attendees. Participants were observed sitting on the floor to immerse themselves in the furry friends' heartwarming space. This interaction has therapeutic benefits by reducing stress and prompting healing and well-being.

A member of the HCT, Kathleen Ochowski, RN, introduced the six pillars of lifestyle medicine interventions. She provided educational resources and handouts encompassing whole food, plant-based nutrition, physical activity, stress management, avoidance of risky substances, restorative sleep, and social connection. The activity was designed to be interactive, aiming to teach participants strategies for preventing chronic conditions. Evaluations of the program included positive feedback on the experience.

> "I have remarkable gratitude to you for coordinating this event ...your passion, care, commitment, innovation, preparation, and intentions are so genuine, important, and highly respected. Your attention to detail, safety, quality, evidence-based practice, and a therapeutic healing environment is ideal and excellent. The event was marketed and promoted to share the love of self and others, focusing on employees and volunteers, and that is so appreciated and important." (C. Marotta, personal communication, April 6, 2025).

> "I feel blessed after attending the C.H.E.R.I.S.H. event, where I received a gifted Reiki session. This healing energy experience enhanced my self-acceptance, confidence, and inner strength. I cherish the transformational energy from the experience. The Reiki Master was superb, passionate, experienced, and educated me about [the] ancient therapy as well" (C. Marotta, personal communication, April 6, 2025).

One limitation, as evidenced by feedback when participants were asked to describe their transformation or healing outcome, was "The sessions are not long enough! While the 20-minute chair massage was not long enough for me to experience a deep sense of relaxation, I do feel that it helped me feel more centered, especially after the busy morning I had. Overall, I love this event and appreciate all the hard work that goes into making it happen. Thank you to everyone involved in putting it together" (S. Lee, personal communication, March 31, 2025).

> "The C.H.E.R.I.S.H. event was a heartfelt invitation that reminded me of the healing environment we create as nurses. While our roles are often filled with many tasks, it served as a beautiful reminder that the true heart of our work—compassion and presence—was powerfully embodied that day. As nurses, we frequently find ourselves absorbed in the "doing, but the C.H.E.R.I.S.H. event reminded me that the 'being' is at the essence of our profession. It provided a valuable opportunity to pause and reflect on my role, not just as an individual, but as part of a broader healthcare system. I truly appreciated the focus on self-care and the variety of healing modalities. It was an enriching chance to reconnect with my well-being and reflect on the profound connections we create with those we serve. Thank you" (S. Peterson, personal communication, April 14, 2025).

Every year, I am grateful for this brief but quite consequential reminder about self-care. The fact that the event takes place at our place of work, during our workday, reinforces the power of taking that moment for an honest check-in with ourselves, both in mind and body. That little pause truly does make each day healthier and more productive. I love the reminder that can and should happen every day...and yes, even at work! Oh, and it was nice to see everyone, too!" (E. DePierro, personal communication, April 4, 2025).

Additionally, the team collected 180 pounds of nonperishable food items and held a basket raffle, raising $831, adding both generosity and a touch of fun to the healing day; the proceeds benefit the local food pantry. Supporting our community makes a tangible difference in playing a vital role for so many families in need and brings a little hope to the table. "I was personally touched by the sense of community gratitude, given the significant need for people during these challenging times. It is amazing to see that an act of kindness can build connections and leave one with a greater feeling of empathy, purpose, and overall happiness" (C. Mohrlein, personal communication, March 31, 2025). "I was happy to support such a meaningful cause" (S. Lee, personal communication, March 31, 2025).

Reflections: C.H.E.R.I.S.H. was initially envisioned as a response to a major and significant tragedy. It has developed into an annual event, except for the "pandemic years." It certainly validates the need and provides opportunities for self-care and a time to experience healing therapies, albeit short sessions! The feedback was valuable to me as a holistic nurse; I care for nurses and other healthcare professionals! It truly healed my soul to observe nurses and other healthcare professionals participate and then share their heartfelt feedback with me about their experiences. My involvement as a planner and coordinator, my feelings and passion as a holistic nurse, and the lessons learned were mirrored in the reflections of those who participated! I am wholeheartedly grateful for the support of Middlesex Health as a leading organization that supports the health and well-being of its nurses and all staff.

References

American Holistic Nurses Association & American Nurses Association. (2019). *Holistic nursing: Scope and standards of practice* (3rd ed.). American Nurses Association.

Dossey, B., & Keegan, L. (2016). *Holistic nursing: A handbook for practice* (7th ed.). Jones & Bartlett Learning.

Hossain, F., & Clatty, A. (2021). Self-care strategies in response to nurses' moral injury during COVID-19 pandemic. Nursing Ethics, 28(1), 23–32. https://doi.org/10.1177/0969733020961825

Nightingale, F. (1969). *Notes on nursing: What it is, and what it is not* (Forward by Virginia M. Dunbar). Dover Publications.

The "Problem"–Complex Patient

Focus Area: Imagery and Hypnosis

Holistic Nurse: Rothlyn P. Zahourek, PhD, RN, PMHCNS-BC (ret), AHN-BC (ret), FAAN

Place of Employment: Retired, Vignette was from St Vincent's Hospital Outpatient Alcoholism Treatment Program, NYC; retired from a clinical psych-mental health practice and consulting in Amherst, MA

Nursing Specialty: Psych-Mental Health and Holistic Nursing

Holistic Intervention Specialization: Imagery, clinical hypnosis, energy healing

Setting: A private psychotherapy practice as well as a clinical specialist in Alcoholism Treatment facilities

Nursing Situation: Father Tim, a 55-year-old, unemployed, self-appointed minister in a spiritualist nondenominational church, was referred to the outpatient alcoholism treatment unit. He was "not doing well" and was "slipping" frequently in his attempts to manage his dependence on both alcohol and Valium. He had also missed several outpatient treatment appointments. He was what we might call a "difficult," problematic, and complex patient. He lived alone and described having no friends. Due to childhood cerebral palsy and numerous reparative surgeries to his back and legs, he suffered chronic pain that severely compromised his gait. While it was difficult and painful to walk with his "scissors" gait, he described walking the distance of Manhattan, even though it caused his pain to escalate. He had not engaged in the treatment program (not attending group therapy or Alcoholics Anonymous meetings). He had been assigned to me as his counsellor because it was known that I had previously developed a program for pain management using imagery and hypnosis in another state. I considered the possibility that I might be able to help him engage in the program and subsequently recover.

As holistic nurses, we are accustomed to working with challenging and complex clients, and we are not afraid to try unconventional approaches that might seem unorthodox to some conventional practitioners.

During my assessment, we discussed how the pain was interfering with his life and his capacity for sobriety. He described his gait as a *scissor gate*, which was immediately apparent to anyone observing him. Just observing his walking, it was clear how difficult it was. I informed him about my experiences working with burned patients and using relaxation, imagery, and hypnosis for pain management (an example of storytelling, which itself is a therapeutic intervention). He was captivated by my examples. Did he want to try these methods? He replied with an extremely enthusiastic "yes."

During my assessment, I asked him to describe his pain and what it meant to him. I then offered him blank paper and colored pens, asking him to draw a picture of himself with the pain or just the pain, whatever he chose. He chose a black pen and drew a picture of a head (a plain circle) with dots for the eyes and nose and a grimace for a mouth. He drew the head with a neck but no body. He added scowl lines to his forehead.

Drawing a picture of oneself with an illness or problematic symptom is another technique to engage a person and foster their unconscious attention by shifting from a dominant verbal to the imagery process. This encourages the possibility of a more emotional and unconscious representation of a problem, symptom, situation, or illness. This simple technique opens the door to increased understanding for both the nurse and the client regarding a problematic symptom and/or situation, as well as the possible means for intervention and change. Commonly, when people are asked, they exclaim, "I'M NOT AN ARTIST!" With encouragement and some multicolored felt-tip pens, most people, in my experience, can engage. This simple technique has helped me learn how people view and experience their symptomatic problems that I may not have discovered in months of psychotherapy.

Next in the process of assessment, I asked, "What are your preferred means to rest and relax? What helps promote pain relief and comfort?" He replied that he had not found much other than walking, meditating, and taking Valium and alcohol. I asked what images might help him relax and be comforting for him. He replied that one was the coolness you can feel in an old stone church. It's quiet and meditative. He also loved thinking about a warm tropical beach. His descriptions were part of the assessment that then became the first phase of the introduction to and experience with imagery/hypnosis interventions. He chose to use beach imagery for the first treatment.

I asked him to get as comfortable as possible in the chair and to take a lovely full breath. I instructed him to close his eyes. I asked, "Please tell me more about that place. What colors do you notice? Temperatures? What are you doing? Who's with you? How are you feeling?" During the treatment sessions, he was able to relax and described feeling more comfortable.

This process enhanced my understanding of how he uses his imagination, how he may respond to further imagery treatments, and how he views his life situation. He was enthusiastic and hopeful. I gave him instructions to find a comfortable place to relax at home and use this image of the beautiful beach each day.

We scheduled more sessions for enhancing his imagery experience. We added positive therapeutic suggestions for comfort while encouraging his capacity to decrease drinking and Valium use. I also wove in AA (Alcoholics Anonymous) slogans into the imagery exercises, e.g. "Let go and let God," "One day at a time," and "Take it easy." He was engaged and was doing well with more sober days and better pain management with NSAIDs and the new relaxation/imagery techniques. After a couple of months of regular sessions, he was improving on all fronts. I again asked him to draw a picture of himself and his pain. He chose a brown marker and drew another stick figure, but this time, he drew a whole figure. He was holding his crutches out from his body, his face was smiling; underneath his feet, he wrote wavy lines and the words, "I feel good!"

Holistic Nursing Core Values and Competencies identified: Several Core Values were demonstrated, including the Holistic Caring Process, Holistic Communication, Therapeutic Relationships, Healing Environments, and Cultural Care. Developing a therapeutic alliance with him, accepting his difficulties with sobriety, and "meeting him where he was at" all reflect the above values. Through recognizing his strengths, determination, and willingness to try something different (imagery, positive suggestions of hypnosis) to manage other problematic behaviors (addiction), we became "partners" in his recovery.

Holistic Nursing Methods, Skills, or Interventions: Hypnosis and Imagery were used.

Reflections: First, I engaged him as a whole person. He wasn't just a relapsing alcoholic and addict but an individual with other problems as well as strengths. He had strengths and gifts that I capitalized on, and I engaged him as a partner in a holistic caring process of healing. Second, I utilized his capacity for imagery and accepting therapeutic suggestions.

Holistic Nursing Patient Care

Focus Area: Enhanced Sleep and Decreased Anxiety through the Spiritual Practice of Prayer

Holistic Nurse Name and Credentials: Cheryl A. Passel RN PhD AHN-BC

Place of Employment: University of Wisconsin–Green Bay

Nursing Specialty: Mental Health; Older Adults, and Planetary Health

Holistic Intervention Specialization: Yoga Instructor RYT-200

Setting: Academia/College Professor

Nursing Situation: During the day shift, a new resident had been admitted. I was drawn into her room, where I noticed a 2-foot statue of St. Francis of Assisi on her windowsill. We established a rapport, and she shared the story behind her St. Francis statue. Around 2 a.m., her call light went off, and I entered her room to find her in a panic. She expressed her fear of falling asleep due to a flashback of being resuscitated. I learned that she had suffered a massive heart attack and undergone CPR on her front porch. I stayed with her, encouraging her to take deep breaths. As I glanced around her room, I noticed other religious items in addition to the statue, so I asked if she would like me to pray with her. She responded, "I would like that." I remembered the prayer to St. Francis of Assisi, and as I began to recite the first few lines, and she began to pray with me. I noticed her breathing gradually slow, and her face relaxed. I remained with her until she fell asleep.

The next night I worked, I stopped by the patient's room to check her vital signs. She thanked me for helping her fall asleep the previous night and asked if I could return to her room to recite a prayer with her on the nights I worked; I gladly agreed.

Holistic Nursing Core Values and Competencies Identified: The Holistic Nursing Core Competencies of Holistic Communication, Therapeutic Relationships, and Healing Environments were identified. Before offering the healing modality of prayer, my patient was fearful of her environment and was unable to rest. As I entered the patient's room, I was aware of several religious items and recognized the significance they held in her life. She was fearful, and I demonstrated compassion and empathy by offering her a comforting measure to help her relax.

Holistic Nursing Methods, Skills, or Interventions: I offered to pray for the patient and I gave her my presence; I stayed with her until she fell asleep.

Reflections: This experience I hold near and dear to my heart. As the months passed, I spent many hours with this patient during my free time. I became acquainted with her family, and she introduced me to the Third Order of Secular Franciscans (this is how she received her statue of St. Francis). I eventually became a Third Order Franciscan, and she attended my final profession!

The small gesture of offering my patient a prayer and an extra 15 minutes of my time made all of the difference on the first night of her admission; she was able to get a good night's sleep. I recognize the difference I can make in a person's life each day I walk into a room by being present, listening with intention, and offering my gifts for healing. I am forever grateful to be a holistic nurse.

Chronic Care by the Holistic Nurse Practitioner

Focus Area: Pain and Stress Management During Chronic Illness

Holistic Nurse: Susan Wenzinger, MSN, RN, ANP-BC, AHWC, RYT

Place of Employment: Full Bloom Health and Yoga, Vestal, New York

Nursing Specialty: Chronic Illness Support

Holistic Intervention Specialization: Energy Medicine/Reiki

Setting: Outpatient

Nursing Situation: Throughout my holistic nursing career, there have been many meaningful encounters. One person stands out in my mind, however. It involves P.S., a 63-year-old woman who experienced rheumatoid arthritis (RA). Her RA medication regimen had been advanced from anti-inflammatories to steroids, to disease-modifying agents, and finally to the latest biologic agents. On both clinical and radiologic examinations, her arthritis appeared to be reasonably well-managed with rare flares in her shoulders or right knee. In addition to RA, she was also diagnosed with fibromyalgia syndrome (FMS), for which she had been prescribed muscle relaxants and different antidepressants at varying dosages to help her manage the pain.

Despite the various medication regimens, she experienced daily generalized pain that was non-relenting and debilitating. The pain interfered with her sleep to the point that she was exhausted during the day. She verbalized feelings of frustration because she couldn't get the pain under control. Her chronic pain meant that she could not meet her personal goal of doing many of the things she loved, such as gardening, further adding to her frustration and stress.

She had been followed in the rheumatology practice primarily by the physician; on occasion, she was seen by one of the nurse practitioners. I had known this person for approximately eight years, and each time I noticed her, it seemed she was at the status quo. She would report both generalized muscle and specific joint pain, verbalize frustration, and appear sad and depressed.

On a recent appointment, she became teary, voicing feelings of sadness and increased depression. We reviewed her care plan, and it seemed that every possible combination of medications, along with mental health counseling and physical therapy, had been trialed to no avail. This appointment occurred shortly after completion of my training as a Reiki practitioner, and it occurred to me to offer her Reiki energy, which has been shown in studies to relieve anxiety and pain (Eliopoulos, 2014; Rand, 2005). I briefly discussed the principles behind Reiki energy, then asked her if she would like to sit quietly for a few minutes while I shared healing energy with her. She agreed, and I proceeded to treat her briefly for a few minutes. After the session, she verbalized feeling more relaxed and noted that her pain level had even decreased somewhat. We agreed to continue her current medications without making any changes to be able to assess the effectiveness of the Reiki treatment.

Given the initial positive effects, she readily accepted a one-hour follow-up appointment for a full-body Reiki treatment. What started as one Reiki session soon became monthly sessions continuing for more than a year. At each appointment, she invariably reported some degree of pain, but she also reported improvement in the quality of her sleep, less daytime fatigue, and an ability to be more engaged during the day. Consequently, she began to feel somewhat less frustrated and depressed. Both she and her family were amazed at the improvement in her quality of life. She shared with me at one appointment that she felt so well, she quit taking all of her medications! Unfortunately, not long after that, she had a major flare in her rheumatoid arthritis, at which point she decided that the arthritis medications had been more effective than she realized. She felt, however, that she could get along without the potpourri of other medications, including antidepressants, muscle relaxants, and pain medications. While accepting her limitations, she felt well enough to join her daughter gardening once again, and she was also able to share in the care of her grandchild, both of which had a positive impact on her well-being (Bauer-Wu, 2011).

Holistic Nursing Core Values and Competencies identified: Holistic Theories (Model of Whole-Person Caring); Self-Reflection and Self-Care; Holistic Caring Process; Holistic Communication, Therapeutic Relationships, and Healing Environment.

This is one specific situation in which I applied holistic nursing principles. It was an opportunity for me to experience and share the value of the holistic approach when caring for others, particularly those with pain and chronic illness. It reminded me, as the nurse, to engage in self-care practices so that I did not feel helpless and frustrated like the person for whom I was caring. And it was an opportunity to make a difference by applying holistic nursing theory, concepts, and research in this specific client situation.

Holistic Nursing Methods, Skills or Interventions: Energy Medicine: Reiki

Reflection: As I reflected on this person's life and health, considering the Model of Whole-Person Caring, I was reminded that the spiritual dimension may be viewed as the foundation of one's being (Thornton, 2002). While the rheumatologist cared primarily for her physical being, other aspects of her being were overlooked. It was clear that my role as the holistic nurse was to offer care that extended beyond her physical needs. As we discussed her feelings, it became obvious to her that her negative emotions were associated with much of her pain experience. We identified a circular pattern connecting pain, limitation, frustration, and depression. She felt strongly that if she could manage her pain, she would feel more in control and the other aspects of her being would feel healthier, a concept supported in the literature (Levine, 1991). She did not believe that different medications would be helpful but was open to trying a nonmedical intervention. Once she experienced a Reiki treatment, her awareness of her spiritual dimension grew. She acknowledged a belief in God and felt the support of her family; this, in turn, helped her to feel less isolated. She gradually returned to her practice of reading, meditation, and prayer each morning, practices she had set aside because she didn't feel well enough to engage. I offered to remember her in my daily prayers, and she readily accepted. Studies show that when a person is the object of prayer, whether or not they are aware of it, they tend to have more positive outcomes (Dossey, 1996). As a holistic nurse, this situation was an opportunity to have a long-term impact on another person's care and quality of life and, in turn, be challenged and positively impacted at the same time.

References

Bauer-Wu, S. (2011). *Leaves falling gently: Living fully with serious & life-limiting illness through mindfulness, compassion & connectedness.* New Harbinger Publications, Inc.

Dossey, L. (1996). *Prayer is good medicine.* HarperCollins.

Eliopoulos, C. (2014). *Invitation to holistic health: A guide to living a balanced life.* Jones & Bartlett Learning.

Levine, B. (1991). *Your body believes every word you say.* Aslan Publishing.

Rand, W. (2005). *The Reiki touch booklet.* Sounds True.

Thornton, L. (2002). The art & science of whole-person caring. *International Journal for Human Caring, 6*(2), 38–47.

Empowered Healing: A Nurse Coaching Case of Grief, Metabolic Imbalance, and Lifestyle Change

Focus Area: Holistic and Integrative Health and Wellness Nurse Coaching for Grief, Lifestyle Change, Mindset, and Subconscious Healing

Holistic Nurse: Mary Cohen, MSN-Ed, RN, AHN-BC, HWNC-BC, Certified Consulting Hypnotist, NLP/Time-Line Practitioner, Functional Medicine Nursing

Place of Employment: Joyful Wellness LLC—Private Practice, New York.

Nursing Specialty: Integrative Health and Wellness Transformative Nurse Coach

Holistic Intervention Specialization: Advanced Holistic Integrative Health and Wellness, Nurse Coaching, Hypnosis, Functional Nutrition, Timeline Therapy®, Trauma and Somatic Practice

Setting: Private Coaching Practice (virtual sessions, online and in-person classes and programs)

Nursing Situation: Anthony is a 67-year-old retired man living with type 2 diabetes, fibromyalgia, and a history of depression. He reaches out seeking hypnosis to process the grief of losing his wife three years ago. After selling their home and relocating to a gated community hours away from his stepchildren,

Anthony feels emotionally isolated and unmotivated. Though he lives near his sisters for part of the year; he stays withdrawn from social and community life.

The nurse coach has supported Anthony through weekly virtual sessions over the past three months and currently. Their work evolves from grief support to lifestyle and metabolic health transformation. With deep roots in his Italian heritage—where bread was part of every meal—Anthony carries emotional eating habits shaped by comfort, culture, and early family patterns.

Together, they establish SMART goals and use food-mood journaling to bring awareness to cravings, emotions, and routines. Through hypnosis, Anthony accesses an inner sanctuary—a calm river—and anchors the experience with American flute music. In one pivotal session, he envisions himself in the gazebo, where he proposes to his wife. That image stays with him, allowing grief and love to exist together and becoming a meaningful part of his healing.

Over time, Anthony adjusted his eating schedule, reduced processed carbohydrates, and walked after meals. He slowed his eating, recognizing the stress patterns that once shaped his behavior. His A1C dropped from 6.7 to 6.1, and he lost 10 pounds.

Anthony continues receiving 90-minute weekly sessions integrating hypnosis, mindset and emotional processing, and functional nutrition support. Between sessions, he engages with hypnosis recordings customized to his goals, continues to journal his food and emotions, and walks one hour daily, especially after meals.

Evaluation: Anthony builds consistent habits, lowers his A1C, and begins reconnecting with his purpose and meaning in life. He feels more confident, grounded, and open to re-engaging socially, which marks a shift from his earlier sense of disconnection.

Holistic Nursing Core Values and Competencies Identified

1. Holistic Philosophy, Theories, and Ethics—The nurse coach centers the relationship on whole-person healing, guided by Watson's Transpersonal Caring and Dossey's Integrative Nurse Coaching Theory.
2. Holistic Self-Reflection, Development, and Self-Care—The nurse coach's five-year healing journey equips them with the presence and integrity needed to support clients in profound personal transformation.
3. Holistic Caring Process—The nurse coach follows the six-step nurse coaching process while staying flexible and attuned to the client's emotional and physical readiness. The nurse coach remains grounded, listens deeply and intently, asks open questions, and responds to nonverbal cues with empathy.
4. Holistic Communication and Healing Environment—The nurse coach uses somatic awareness and cultural sensitivity to create a safe, secure, and supportive space for healing.
5. Holistic Education and Research—Instead of directing the client, the nurse coach invites insight and discovery, empowering the client to choose changes that align with his values and goals.

Holistic Nursing Methods, Skills, or Interventions

- Hypnosis and guided imagery for grief and behavior change
- SMART goals and food-mood journaling for structure and insight
- Anchoring techniques using music for emotional regulation
- Mindful eating and post-meal walk to support metabolic health
- Functional nutrition coaching cocreated with client input

Reflections: The nurse coach asks thoughtful, open-ended questions and listens with intention. They pay close attention to Anthony's voice, posture, and energy, noticing subtle changes that signal when something meaningful is stirring beneath the surface. As he talks through memories and moments of loss, his eyes well up. Tears come naturally—not forced—and are met with steady presence and quiet understanding.

Their connection deepens as Anthony begins shifting his habits and opening up emotionally. One session stands out. During hypnosis, Anthony visualizes himself standing in the gazebo where he once proposed to his wife. The memory stops him. His voice catches, and the tears come again—not just from sadness but from love. In that moment, something softens. The image becomes a bridge, letting him hold the grief without being consumed and allowing space for healing to begin.

From Survival to Thriving—A Trauma-Informed Holistic Approach for an Early Career

Hospice Nurse

Focus Area: Trauma Recovery and Nervous System Regulation in Early Career Nurses

Holistic Nurse: Lorre Laws, PhD, RN, NC

Place of Employment: Haelan Academy, a nonprofit organization serving nurses worldwide

Nursing Specialty: Nurse-Specific Traumatization; Hospice and Palliative Care

Holistic Intervention Specialization: Trauma-Informed Nurse Coaching, Polyvagal-Informed Self-Regulation

Setting: Private Practice (Virtual Nurse Coaching)

Nursing Situation: Haley, an early-career hospice nurse, entered practice with only a few months of mentorship before taking on a full caseload, double that of her peers. Lacking basic ergonomic support, she spent hours nightly charting on her phone, often until 2 a.m.

Within six months, she regretted her career choice. The situation worsened when her employer shifted to a salary model, leaving her uncompensated for 20+ hours of weekly overtime. Haley, burdened by student loans, mistakenly believed that she was burned out. She sought my support, feeling trapped and hopeless.

Through our work, it became clear that Haley was not just burned out but experiencing nurse-specific traumatization—a distinct, cumulative stress response common in healthcare settings (Laws, 2024). Recognizing this distinction was pivotal, we shifted our focus from surface-level symptom relief to addressing the roots of her distress.

Holistic Principles Guiding Care: My approach was grounded in holistic nursing's Core Values: Honoring the Whole Person, Therapeutic Partnership, and Self-Reflection (AHNA, 2019). Drawing from the evidence-based framework offered in the *Nursing Our Healer's Heart* book, I helped Haley understand her nervous system's responses as adaptive, not personal failings.

Interventions

Awareness and Attunement: Mindful body scans, breathwork, and daily check-ins to notice shifts in her state.

- **Micro-Regulation:** Short grounding exercises and intentional movement integrated throughout her day.
- **Self-Compassion and Boundaries:** Reframing self-care as professional responsibility; practicing assertive communication and setting boundaries around work hours.
- **Co-Regulation:** Seeking support from trusted colleagues and loved ones to anchor herself during difficult days (Porges, 2022).

Plan

- Set daily self-check-in and micro-regulation goals.
- Develop scripts for boundary-setting with her employer.
- Track changes in physical symptoms, emotional state, and work satisfaction.

Evaluation: Within weeks, Haley reported improved sleep, reduced anxiety, and greater clarity at work. She became more confident advocating for herself and distinguishing her needs from unrealistic workplace demands. Over several months, her "burnout" symptoms resolved—not because her workload lessened, but because her nervous system was no longer trapped in survival mode. Ultimately, Haley changed employers from a place of grounded self-advocacy, finding a role that prioritized nurse well-being and competitive compensation. She now describes herself as thriving.

Holistic Nursing Core Values and Competencies

- Holistic Philosophy, Theories, and Ethics
- Holistic Nurse Self-Reflection, Self-Development, and Self-Care
- Holistic Caring Process

- Holistic Communication and Therapeutic Relationship
- Healing Environments (AHNA, 2019)

Holistic Nursing Methods, Skills, or Interventions

- Trauma-informed nurse coaching
- Polyvagal-informed self-regulation
- Mindfulness and body awareness
- Boundary-setting and assertive communication
- Co-regulation and community support

Reflections: Haley's journey affirmed the necessity of trauma-informed, holistic care for nurses—not as an afterthought, but as a foundation for professional longevity and well-being. Her transformation illustrates that "burnout" is often unrecognized traumatization, requiring interventions that address both body and mind. This experience deepened my conviction that healing begins with understanding the nervous system and cocreating environments where nurses can thrive. As holistic nurses, our role is to guide clients back to safety, agency, and wholeness—one regulated breath at a time.

References

American Nurses Association & American Holistic Nurses Association. (2019). *Holistic nursing: Scope and standards of practice* (3rd ed.). Nursesbooks.org.

Laws, L. (2024). *Nursing our healer's heart: A recovery guide for nurse trauma & burnout.* Collective Ink.

Porges, S. W. (2022). *Polyvagal theory: The transformative power of feeling safe.* W. W. Norton & Company.

Integrative Nurse Coaching

Focus Area: Witnessing the Journey

Holistic Nurse: Karla Rodriguez, DNP, CNE, NC-BC, DipACLM

Place of Employment: New York University, New York, NY

Nursing Specialty: Undergraduate faculty—Medical-surgical adult

Holistic Intervention Specialization: Awareness practices, qigong

Setting: Virtual private practice

Nursing Situation: A 74-year-old female, retired nurse practitioner, has been a client of mine for over three years.

Past medical history: Waldenstrom macroglobulinemia (a type of non-Hodgkin's lymphoma), diagnosed since age 55. Received chemotherapy and radiation and is being followed by Dana-Farber Cancer Institute. Under surveillance now and monitoring for proteins in urine (currently 2+) as well as blood count. She has Meniere's disease with profound hearing loss, left more than right, wears a left cochlear implant, and has peripheral neuropathy. Two hip replacements in the past. She has a central line port on her chest from the chemotherapy treatments she received in the recent past with plans for port removal shortly.

Medications: Melatonin 60 mg daily, multivitamin daily, CBD gummies for rheumatoid arthritis, iron supplement bid, MiraLAX daily, B-complex daily, alpha lipoic acid 600 mg daily, Losartan, Neurontin for peripheral neuropathy, Duloxetine for chronic musculoskeletal pain, and Felodipine for hypertension. AffloVest 30 minutes a day—she had pneumonia last year. Was recently prescribed prednisone, 5 mg daily for weight gain. Her BMI is under 19.

Employment history: Worked full time as a family nurse practitioner at a clinic. Continues to work part time at the doctor's office and also volunteers at a nonprofit providing in-service training to staff.

Social history: Lives alone in a condominium. Divorced. Has friends, especially a male friend, whom she has known for many years, in her circle. Likes plays and musicals.

Background: I have known my client since I began nurse coaching in 2022, and I feel we have developed an appreciation for one another. We have gone through many meaningful events together. I was fortunate that she chose me when it was the first time she underwent chemotherapy and radiation. She expressed considerable concern, particularly because she had different plans in mind, as this was around the time of her retirement. As my client, we have virtual sessions every 2 weeks. I always start by asking how she is feeling, and at the end of our session, we conclude with an awareness practice that includes some qigong exercises while sitting down and working on our head and neck. More details are described below.

Holistic Nursing Core Values and Competencies Identified: For the Holistic Nursing Core Values, I have been incorporating Self-Reflection, Self-Development, and Self-Care. Since beginning our sessions, my client and I have built a meaningful and trusting connection. This connection was fostered by attuning to her preferences, allowing her to guide the conversation based on her needs in each session. I incorporated:

- **Awareness:** Developing mindfulness and insight into one's values, thoughts, behaviors, and reactions.
- **Professional Integration:** Aligning one's values with holistic nursing principles.
- **Lifelong Learning:** Committing to continuous growth in knowledge, emotional intelligence, and spiritual maturity.
- **Transformative Practice:** Using experiences, challenges, and self-inquiry as catalysts for growth.
- **Inner Healing:** Engaging in practices (e.g., journaling, meditation or qigong, supervision) that foster more profound healing and clarity.

The Holistic Nursing Core Values that were demonstrated through our sessions have been Therapeutic Communication and Self-Reflection. I ask her for permission first before asking pertinent questions. What is most important to identify here is that our virtual sessions are closed-captioned, so she is able to read what I am saying. Despite having the cochlear implant, it can still be hard to hear when communicating virtually. As for self-reflection, I refer to questions I learned through my nurse coaching education, which help guide me in establishing aspects of her experience. I always gauge our conversations as a measure in what kind of questions I will ask her, which can open up to other contents of dialogue.

Our goals are set collaboratively, focusing on both emotional well-being and practical tasks. Recently, she identified two goals: completing her tax filing (after an extension) and initiating her divorce paperwork. These goals were self-identified, and my role has been to hold space, offer reflective feedback, and support her in breaking down these tasks into manageable steps.

Health Journey and Therapeutic Insight

My client is a member of Al-Anon, having been deeply affected by the alcoholism of both a former partner and family members. Through our sessions, she has expressed the complex emotions and realizations that have emerged as she navigates her own health challenges. One profound insight she shared is the irony of now being in the patient role—experiencing firsthand how difficult it can be to manage one's health within the healthcare system.

She has become more vocal about the differences she perceives in the quality of care received from her providers, particularly noting the impact of poor bedside manners and inadequate assessments. This has been eye-opening for her, especially as a healthcare professional who always valued *partnering* with patients—engaging with them rather than only instructing them. The transition from caregiver to care receiver has been humbling and, at times, frustrating, but it has also deepened her empathy and understanding of patient vulnerability.

This lived experience has not only affirmed the importance of holistic, patient-centered care but also strengthened her resolve to continue embodying those principles in her own practice.

Integrating Modalities and Life Transitions in Holistic Coaching

Modalities

Throughout our coaching sessions, I have incorporated several holistic modalities—such as awareness practice and guided imagery—tailored to meet my client's needs in the moment. Energy work, particularly qigong, has played a key role in our sessions, emphasizing the integration of body, mind, and spirit. Qigong serves as a bridge between movement, breath, and intentional awareness—supporting both her physical and psychological healing. We've recently incorporated seated qigong exercises focused on the head, neck, hands, and lower back. These practices have been particularly meaningful to her; she not only welcomes them but also shares reflections on how she feels afterward—physically, emotionally, and energetically. Each session begins and ends with the gentle resonance of a chime, creating a grounding and mindful structure. These techniques are not only therapeutic but also sustainable, offering her tools she can use independently outside of our sessions. This supports the holistic goal of fostering self-efficacy and long-term well-being.

Creating a healing environment is also important. Our sessions tend to run early in the morning and she likes to be in natural light with her cup of coffee. Now that she has moved to another location, she no longer sees her friend, a squirrel, who used to visit her outside her window. She was significantly melancholy about that. With this experience, I tried to convey to her that even though things are different now, she can find new ways to feel connected—to her friends, to nature, and to the sense of joy their friendship brought her. This event has inspired me to appreciate those around me. I plan on asking her again if she wants to address this, as she may wish for further healing, and for the comfort of knowing that love doesn't disappear, even when someone or something is no longer near.

Life Transitions

Amidst these practices, my client has undergone significant life changes in 2025. She transitioned from renting to purchasing a condominium, signaling a new phase of independence and stability. She has now formally filed for divorce. While she has no children, these personal milestones represent powerful steps in reclaiming her narrative and creating space for healing and growth.

With our sessions lasting 45 minutes, and the time we have spent together, I hope that the changes she is going through will bring greater alignment with her values, clarity of purpose, and a more empowered way of being. She is seeking many things: improved circumstances, deeper relationships, and personal growth. Ultimately, she wants to feel that her actions and environment are moving toward something more fulfilling, peaceful, and impactful now that she is in a new phase in her life.

We have reviewed characteristics she can work on such as resilience, self-awareness, empathy, creativity, and a strong sense of purpose. Along the way, she has cultivated mindfulness and patience over time. Together, we were able to identify qualities that help her navigate ambiguity, remain centered under pressure, and find meaning even in struggle.

The external resources that were important to my client included supportive relationships, such as her friends, mentors, communities, access to knowledge, financial stability, and professional networks. She has been attending a support system for those who have Waldenstrom macroglobulinemia and also is working with a social worker through Dana-Farber Cancer Institute.

Creating a Safe, Responsive, and Ongoing Holistic Coaching Relationship

Both my client and I ensure a private, distraction-free environment for our sessions. We agreed that our space remains uninterrupted—silencing phones and eliminating external disruptions—to create a container of presence and respect. This intentional space has become an integral part of our work together.

A simple, yet meaningful, moment arose when she mentioned how much she appreciated the meditation chime at the end of our sessions. I hadn't realized she could hear it clearly, but once she expressed its value, I made it a consistent part of our closing practice. This kind of feedback exemplifies the responsive and cocreated nature of our relationship—hallmarks of holistic nursing and coaching.

As we near the third year of working together, I introduced the Integrative Health and Wellness Assessment (IHWA) again to help her reflect on areas of strength, progress, and potential growth. The goal is not to impose change but to invite reflection and shared decision-making on whether she wants to explore new areas or continue deepening work in existing ones. This process honors her autonomy and the evolving nature of our therapeutic journey.

Evaluation: Outcomes were evident both verbally and behaviorally. She frequently expresses that our sessions have helped her process emotional challenges and find clarity. The consistency of our meetings, her continued engagement, and her initiation of concrete action steps (e.g., gathering tax documents and requesting legal information) reflect her growing sense of agency. The reciprocal tone of our interactions and her willingness to share deeply are signs of trust, empowerment, and therapeutic rapport—core indicators of holistic nursing effectiveness.

Since I have known my client, we have developed a deep connection with one another as she has shared many past experiences. This was partly due to discerning the topics she wanted to focus on and then leading our work together from there. She is highly committed as we have been meeting every 2 weeks. The tone of our conversations is reciprocal. She talks first and explains to me the events that occurred over the past 2 weeks. She has expressed numerous times how the sessions have helped her in dealing with situations she is going through and ways to address them. She wants to focus on completing tasks, such as filing her taxes (she has requested an extension) and filing her divorce papers.

Reflections: Working with my client has deepened my understanding of the *art of presence and listening*. This experience shaped me by reinforcing the power of *being with* rather than *doing for*. I've learned to attune to subtle cues—emotional, verbal, and energetic—and respond from a place of compassion rather than urgency to "fix."

Emotionally, this work evoked *humility, empathy, and reverence*. I felt honored to witness my client's vulnerabilities and inner strengths. It affirmed my path as a holistic nurse by reminding me that healing often arises not only from interventions but from *sacred witnessing* and *holding space*.

I've learned that within every client is a reservoir of wisdom and resilience. My role, in this client's case, is to reflect that back—helping her reconnect with her capacity to love, to grieve, and to find meaning. This approach fosters self-efficacy and aligns perfectly with holistic nursing values: empowering the whole person—mind, body, and spirit.

Implications

Clinical Practice

Through authentically listening and connecting to the client's story, valuable insight is gained on the entangled variables that affect health and healing.

Education

Experiential opportunities to listen to the client's story and reflect on what was learned will help nursing students understand the importance of the totality of the human experience.

Research

New research opportunities can be identified through the information received during a narrative reflection.

Policy

Narrative reflections are a powerful tool to highlight the impact of health policies on the human experience.

Conclusion

The narrative reflections of holistic nurses present themselves in various forms. This expression of holistic nursing enables the personal philosophy of practice to emerge, providing each individual nurse with a unique approach in various practice settings. Globally, the message is the same; holistic nurses strive to help others reach their internal resources, to help heal the whole person, and to reach optimal health.

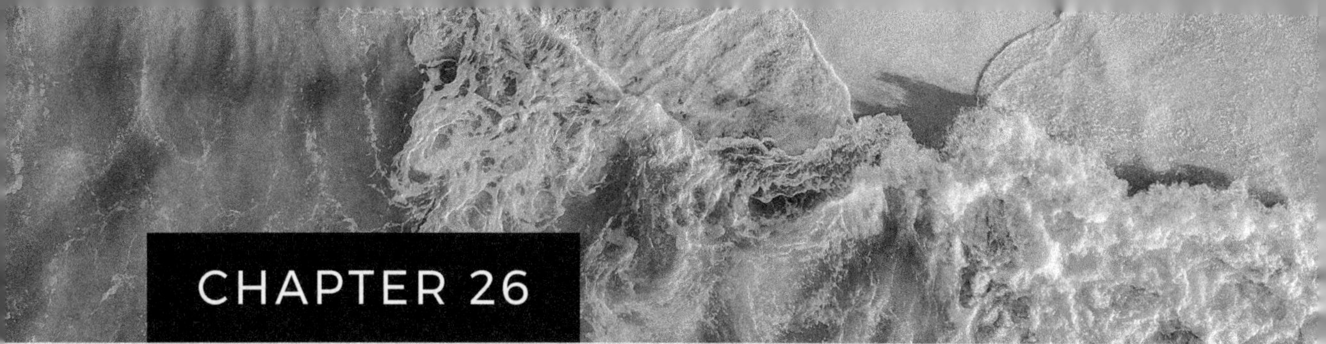

CHAPTER 26

Nurse Coaching

Karen M. Avino and Deborah McElligott

NURSE HEALER OBJECTIVES

- Define the professional nurse coach.
- Compare the nursing process to the nurse coaching process.
- Examine the Theory of Integrative Nurse Coaching©

DEFINITIONS

Professional nurse coach: A board-certified registered nurse (RN) who incorporates a holistic perspective with coaching skills into professional nursing practice. This perspective, as applied to both self and client in a coaching interaction, emerges from an awareness that effective change evolves from within oneself before it can be manifested and maintained externally. The professional nurse coach works with the whole person to utilize principles and modalities that integrate body-mind-emotion-spirit-environment (Southard et al., 2021).

Professional nurse coaching: A skilled, purposeful, results-oriented, and structured relationship-centered interaction with clients provided by registered nurses to promote achievement of client goals (Southard et al., 2021).

Theory of Integrative Nurse Coaching© (TINC): A grand nursing theory with philosophical assumptions of wholeness, the person-environment energy field, alternating rhythms, patterns, change, and healing. TINC's five components are: Nurse Coach Self-Development (self-reflection, self-assessment, self-evaluation, self-care); Integrality, Intentionality, and Change; Integrative Life Pattern, Healing, and Wellbecoming Framework (ILPHW); Awareness and Choice; and Listening to the Story with HEART (Healing, Energy, Awareness, Resonancy, Transformation) (Avino & France, forthcoming).

The Evolution of Nurse Coaching and the Field of Health Coaching

It is well known that coaching has existed for some time in the field of human performance, specifically in athletics and employee development. Recently, nurses have added coaching skills to their professional practice. In 2013, the American Holistic Nurses Credentialing Corporation (AHNCC) began a nationally and internationally recognized Nurse Coach Certification examination (American Holistic Nurses Credentialing Corporation, n.d.). Nursing, recognizing the importance of improving health through lifestyle changes, is leading the shift in health care from disease care to disease prevention, improved health, and enhanced well-being. Nurses constitute the largest group of healthcare providers and are uniquely situated for this role. The caring nature of nurses' relationships with clients allows them to develop a unique partnership to assess, strategize, and plan for healthy lifestyle changes.

Professional nursing practice is rooted in health promotion efforts to assist clients in achieving optimal health and well-being and nurses utilize professional nursing knowledge and skills in their role as coaches.

Professional nurse coaches are emerging as leaders who are informing governments, regulatory agencies, businesses, and organizations about the important part they play in achieving health improvement of the nation and the world at large.

The Art and Science of Nurse Coaching

Coaching is a systematic and skilled process grounded in scholarly, evidence-based professional nursing practice. Nurse coaches incorporate approaches to nursing practice that are integrative and integral and include the work of numerous nurse scholars. At the heart of nurse coaching is support for the client's healing process as it manifests in body-mind-spirit. Nurse coaches recognize that by being open and curious, and by asking powerful questions, they can guide clients through a reflective healing process while also providing them with choices in determining priorities for change.

The quality of human caring is central to the relationship between the nurse coach and the client. The nurse is fully present in the coaching relationship, honoring the client's wholeness. This allows clients a safe environment in which to express their goals, hopes, and dreams, as well as a setting where their vulnerability can be authentically shared. Nurse coaches utilize a full spectrum of coaching strategies and skills to engage the client in meeting desired goals, including a variety of integrative and complementary therapies to create a healing environment. *The Art and Science of Nurse Coaching: A Provider's Guide to Scope and Competencies* (2nd ed.) (Southard, 2021) clarified nursing perspectives concerning the role of nurse coaching in four key ways:

1. It specified the philosophy, beliefs, and values of the nurse coach and the scope of practice.
2. It articulated how *The Art and Science of Nurse Coaching* aligns with the American Nurses Association's *Nursing: Scope and Standards of Practice* (American Nurses Association, 2015).
3. It provided the basis for continued interprofessional conversations among professional health and wellness coaches and lay health and wellness coaches.
4. It provided the foundation for an international certification process in professional nurse coaching.

Nurse coaches are guided in their skill development, critical thinking, and decision making by the following five resources for professional practice:

1. *Nursing: Scope and Standards of* Practice (3rd ed.), outlines the expectations of the professional role of registered nurses within the scope and standards of professional nurse practice and competencies (American Nurses Association, 2015)
2. *Code of Ethics for Nurses with Interpretive Statements* lists the nine provisions that establish the ethical framework for registered nurses across all roles, levels, and settings (American Nurses Association, 2025)
3. *Nursing's Social Policy Statement: The Essence of the Profession* conceptualizes and defines nursing practice and describes the social context of nursing (American Nurses Association, 2010)
4. *The art & science of nurse coaching: the provider's guide to coaching scope & competencies* (2nd ed.), is a resource for professional nurse coach practice for certification and credentialing (Southard, 2021)
5. *Integrative nurse coaching: A guide for praxis* is a comprehensive nurse coach textbook that describes the theoretical foundation, clinical relevance, and practical application of the nurse coaching model (Avino & France, forthcoming).

Professional Nurse Coaching Practice Settings

Nurse coaches work with individuals and groups and are found in all areas of nursing practice, employed as staff nurses, ambulatory care nurses, case managers, advanced practice registered nurses, nurse faculty, nurse researchers, educators, administrators, nurse entrepreneurs, and nurse coaches in private practice. For some, nurse coaching is their primary role. The depth and breadth to which registered nurses engage in the total scope of nurse coach practice depend on their education, experience, role, entrepreneurial skills, goals and the population they serve.

Improved nurse and client satisfaction are just some of the beneficial outcomes for the profession (Dossey, 2015a). A qualitative study found that nurse satisfaction at the Veterans Health Administration Hospitals has improved following nurse coaching education (Dossey, 2015a).

Another survey (Ross et al., 2018) reported that among nurse coaches,

1. 70.7 percent had higher job/career satisfaction;
2. 84.8 percent improved their own health/health behaviors; and
3. 80.3 percent improved interpersonal relationships with friends, family, and coworkers.

These are significant findings to consider. About 194,500 openings for RNs are projected each year, on average, over the decade. Many of those openings are expected to result from the need to replace workers who transfer to different occupations or exit the labor force, such as to retire (Bureau of Labor Statistics, 2025). In fact, it is projected that 1 million experienced RNs will retire by 2030 and that client care will be affected; at the same time, employment of RNs is projected to grow 6 percent from 2023 to 2033, faster than the average for all occupations (Buerhaus et al., 2017). Improving nurse satisfaction through nurse coaching programs to control attrition and maintain experienced nurses in healthcare roles is essential when considering the accelerating rate of RN retirements.

Organizations are recognizing the value of nurse coaching programs as the nurse coach professional practice model of care supports organizations' journey toward Magnet status attainment, meets the criteria of the American Nurses Credentialing Center Magnet Recognition Program, and augments the criteria required for the American Nurses Credentialing Center Practice Transition Accreditation Program as an accredited RN fellowship model for organizations to transition RNs into new practice roles.

Professional Nurse Coaching Scope of Practice

Nurse coaching is grounded in the principles and core values of professional nursing. Effective nurse coaching interactions involve the development of a nurse coach–client coaching partnership, creation of a safe space, and sensitivity to client issues of trust and vulnerability as a basis for further exploration (Dossey, 2015b). The nurse coach must be able to structure a coaching session, explore client readiness for coaching, facilitate achievement of the client's desired goals, and cocreate a means of determining and evaluating desired outcomes and goals (Southard, 2021).

The versatility of nurse coaching practice model enhances many areas of professional nursing work. **Table 26-1** not only highlights career practice area opportunities for nurse coaches but, most importantly, demonstrates how nurse coaching is the overarching umbrella that enhances other nursing practice areas across the care continuum. This is demonstrated in all areas and specialties of nursing practice.

Nurse Coaching Core Values

The following five professional nurse coaching core values are adapted from and congruent with *Holistic Nursing: Scope and Standards of* Practice (3rd ed.) (American Nurses Association, 2019):

- **Core value 1**: Nurse coach philosophy, theories, and ethics
- **Core value 2**: Nurse coach self-development (self-reflection, self-assessment, self-evaluation, and self-care)
- **Core value 3**: Nurse coaching process
- **Core value 4**: Nurse coach communication, coaching environment
- **Core value 5**: Nurse coach education, research, and leadership

Table 26-1 Nurse Coaching Across the Continuum of Care

Stage of Care	Role of the Nurse Coach	Key Activities
Preventive Care & Wellness	**Health Promoter & Educator**	Focus on lifestyle modifications (diet, exercise, stress management, sleep), disease prevention, and risk factor reduction. They lead wellness programs in systems, corporations, or community settings and provide individual care and group workshops.
Acute Care (Hospital)	**Patient Advocate & Navigator**	Help patients and families understand complex medical information and treatment plans. They provide emotional support, facilitate communication and partnership with the interdisciplinary team, and begin planning for discharge and post-acute needs.
Chronic Disease Management	**Guide for Self-Management**	Support patients with chronic conditions in setting and achieving self-management goals. They use specialized coaching strategies to help patients overcome barriers, track progress, and adjust lifestyle habits to manage symptoms, improve outcomes, and reverse disease.
Transitional Care	**Care Coordinator & Continuity Facilitator**	Ensure seamless transitions between care settings. Educate symptom management, coach medication engagement, and encourage follow-up appointments to reduce readmissions and ensure continuity of care.
End-of-Life Care	**Supportive Partner**	Provide emotional and spiritual support to the patient and family, helping them find meaning, cope with grief, and focus on quality of life and personal values, even in illness.

Used with Permission. Integrative Nurse Coach Academy. (2025).

These core values and the nurse coaching competencies define professional practice and are aligned with *Nursing: Scope and Standards of Practice* (3rd ed.) (American Nurses Association, 2015). Professional nurse coaching capabilities are acquired by additional training and practice and enhance foundational professional nursing skills.

Nurse Coaching and Change

Wellness is integrated and congruent functioning aimed at reaching one's highest potential. Nurse coaches work with individuals to help them improve their overall wellness aimed at achieving a greater sense of well-being and balance in their lives. *Human flourishing* is when an individual finds purpose and creates meaning in life, however defined; it includes taking charge of one's own health. Nurse coaching helps clients to flourish by making healthy choices and adopting healthier behaviors. Nurse coaches see clients as whole beings, each with the capacity to connect deeply with their own inner wisdom and truth.

Self-development (self-reflection, self-assessment, self-evaluation, and self-care) promotes the awareness of a deepened personal exploration leading to greater life fulfillment and human potential.

Coaching is an opportunity for self-development through taking small steps for change, promoting and acknowledging success, and then building on that to achieve further success.

In coaching sessions, the client may access vulnerable moments and share pain and suffering. *Pain* is a physical and/or emotional discomfort or experience; *suffering* is the story people create around pain (Dossey, 2015b). Signs of suffering may be physical, mental, emotional, social, behavioral, and/or spiritual. This is why it is so important for nurse coaches to practice self-care and develop a reflective practice to strengthen their own capacity to sit with the pain and the suffering clients express without trying to fix the discomfort. A guiding phrase to remember is "soft front and strong back." This relates to the nurse coach's capacity to bear witness and engage in inner stillness and to be with the suffering fully in the moment, bearing witness without judgment or consuming the client's pain.

Clients seek professional coaching for many reasons, including helping them explore possibilities and new directions in life, celebrating successes and identifying opportunities for personal and professional development, enhancing quality of life, and improving relationships. Clients who turn to coaching for such reasons usually are not focused solely on problems to overcome or issues to manage but are seeking opportunities to enrich a current way of being.

Other clients come with specific problems and health challenges, seeking nurse coaching to improve management of acute or chronic conditions. What separates nurses from other health coaches is their vast knowledge in pathophysiology and disease management. One study looked at nurse coaching interventions in clients with various chronic conditions and found nearly all (11 out of 13) studies reported statistically significant outcomes in improved treatment adherence, reduced hospital readmission rates, and improved disease biomarkers (Vincent & Sanchez-Birkhead, 2013). Other studies on the effects of nurse coaching interventions have shown improvement in dyspnea and quality of life in clients with chronic obstructive pulmonary disease (Rehman et al., 2017) and significantly higher self-efficacy scores in clients diagnosed with diabetes (Young et al., 2014).

Another study looked at the lived experience of adults with chronic disease receiving nurse coaching. The following eight themes emerged regarding participants' new insights:

1. Seeking guidance to navigate life's challenges
2. Entering a safe sacred place
3. Feeling empowered and accountable
4. Developing strategies to access different ways of knowing
5. Finding the answers within
6. Making healthy behavioral changes
7. Forming a new caring relationship with self
8. Transforming to a brand-new approach to life (Delaney & Bark, 2019)

The challenges leading clients to nurse coaching may be related to self-esteem and self-image, fear and self-confidence, and general adaptation to actual or perceived situations that must be addressed before they can focus on health changes. Other clients seek coaching to learn to handle personal and workplace challenges and stressors or to learn new behaviors in relation to improving health through nutrition, exercise, weight management, enhanced sleep, or stress management.

Employee wellness, especially in the health care arena, presents opportunities for nurse coaches to support the work of all health professionals. Another important area for nurse coaching is in working with clients who are facing end-of-life issues, either their own or those of loved ones, as well as those clients who are living with loss and grief.

By using a client-centered, relationship-centered process, the nurse coach accompanies the client through the change and discovery processes. Held within this safe relationship and environment, the coaching journey can arrive at a successful outcome.

Coaching Conversations

A nurse coaching session has a beginning (reasons for seeking coaching, a greeting, quick update), a middle (where the majority of time is spent), and an end (agreeing on the next session date, reviewing action plans and other possibilities, completing the coaching session). After the client determines the topic for the coaching session, the nurse coach uses presence, intention, intuition, and deep listening to determine the most powerful questions to ask the client.

Use of silence, often referred to as "the power of the pause," throughout a coaching conversation allows time for both the client and the nurse coach to reflect on the process of discovery and insight. Further possibilities also emerge in the session, and the nurse coach may rephrase what the client shares, providing an opportunity to delve deeper into the client's story.

As the coach listens to the client's responses, they need to remember that insights and *aha* moments are often examples of the mind grasping something new (Southard et al., 2021). This insight is often transitory and not yet embodied as a lived experience. This is where the coaching agreement and continuing sessions evolve to guide the client toward desired skill-building and committing to action.

Not all coaching leads directly to taking action. Insights can be useful in understanding barriers to change that get in the way of achieving goals. Assisting a client to recognize the need for an adjustment in attitude or challenging a belief may, in and of itself, be the catalyst for change.

The nurse coach is aware that although clients may be expressive and make many internal connections, this does not indicate an embodiment of insights, goals, and actions. For a change to become embodied, a practice must be repeated multiple times. This leads to the creation of new capacities and competencies. Clients who learn to continuously practice self-awareness and self-observation become able to understand and recognize thoughts, actions, behaviors, body sensations, and postures in the moment when they occur and how they relate to the desired changes.

The transtheoretical model of change is important in nurse coaching because determining client readiness is necessary (Prochaska et al., 1995). The challenge of change also includes the client's willingness to sustain new behaviors and ways of being. The five stages of change are (1) precontemplation, (2) contemplation, (3) preparation, (4) action, and (5) maintenance; each stage is predictable and identifiable. Motivational interviewing and appreciative inquiry are essential skills that the nurse coach can use to help clients recognize resistance, ambivalence, and change talk that are important factors in making change happen (Dart, 2011; Southard et al., 2020).

The Nursing Process and the Nurse Coaching Process

The nursing process involves six focal areas: assessment, diagnosis, outcomes, plan, implementation, and evaluation. The nurse coaching process uses the holistic caring process (Southard et al., 2021) with a shift in terminology and meaning to understand and incorporate the client's subjective experience

- from *assessment* to establishing the relationship and identifying readiness for change;
- from *diagnosis* to identifying opportunities, issues, and concerns;
- from *outcomes* to establishing client-centered goals;
- from *planning* to creating the structure of the coaching interaction;
- from *implementation* to empowering clients to reach goals; and
- from *evaluation* to assisting clients to determine the extent to which goals were achieved.

The nurse coach understands that growth and improved health, wholeness, and well-being are the result of an ongoing journey that is ever-expanding and transformative.

Assessment: Establishing Relationship and Identifying Readiness for Change

In a coaching model, assessment is dynamic and ongoing, and the nurse coach begins by becoming fully present with self and client before initiating the coaching interaction. The session proceeds with an assessment, establishing a relationship with the client and listening to the client's subjective experience or story. The foundation for coaching is laid during the assessment phase of the coaching interaction as one establishes the relationship and identifies readiness for change. The nurse coach helps the client assess readiness for change and determines if the client's concerns are appropriate for coaching or if the client would be better served by other services and resources.

Diagnosis: Identifying Opportunities, Issues, and Concerns

The nurse coach and the client together explore assessment data to determine areas for change. There is no attempt or need to assign labels or to establish a diagnosis. Instead, the nurse coaches are open to multiple fluid interpretations of an unfolding interaction in partnership with the client. This process identifies opportunities and issues related to growth, overall health, wholeness, and well-being. Opportunities for celebrating well-being are explored. The nurse coach understands that acknowledgment promotes and reinforces previous successes and serves to enhance further achievements.

Outcomes: Establishing Client-Centered Goals

The nurse coach assists the client in identifying goals that will lead to the desired change. The nurse coach values the evolution and process of change as it unfolds, employing an overall approach to each coaching interaction that facilitates the achievement of client goals.

Creating the Structure of the Coaching Interaction (Plan)

The nurse coach and the client cocreate a coaching plan that identifies strategies to attain goals. The coaching interaction is guided by a coaching agreement that identifies parameters of the coaching relationship, including coach and client responsibilities.

Implementation: Empowering Clients to Reach Goals

The nurse coach supports the client's coaching plan while simultaneously remaining open to emerging goals based on new insights, learning, and achievements. Support for new and expanded goals employs a variety of communication skills to facilitate client learning and growth, such as motivational interviewing, appreciative inquiry, deep listening, and powerful questioning.

In partnership with the client, the nurse coach facilitates learning and achievement by cocreating awareness, designing actions, setting goals, planning progress, and addressing accountability. The nurse coach chooses interventions based on the client's statements and actions, acting with intention and curiosity in a manner that assists the client to achieve their goals. Nursing knowledge and a variety of additional skills appropriate to the coaching relationship are utilized within the coaching milieu.

Evaluation: Assisting Clients to Determine the Extent to Which Goals Were Achieved

The nurse coach partners with the client to evaluate progress toward attainment of goals. The evaluation of coaching (aka the nursing intervention) is done primarily by the client, not the nurse, and is based on the client's perception of success and achievement of client-centered goals.

The Theory of Integrative Nurse Coaching© and the Integrative Nurse Coach® Leadership Model

Health and wellness coaching is a multidimensional concept across the healthcare professions, and it acquires various interpretations

Box 26-1 The Theory of Integrative Nurse Coaching© and the Integrative Nurse Coach® Leadership Model: Five Components

Component 1: Integrative Nurse Coach Self-Development (Self-Reflection, Self-Assessment, Self-Evaluation, Self-Care)
Component 2: Integrality, Intentionality, and Change
Component 3: Integrative Life Pattern, Healing, and Wellbecoming Framework.
Component 4: Awareness and Choice
Component 5: Listening with HEART (Healing, Energy, Awareness, Resiliency, Transformation)

Used with permission. Avino, K., & France, N. (forthcoming). *Integrative nurse coaching: A guide for praxis*. International Nurse Coach Association.

depending on the discipline from which it is viewed. The Theory of Integrative Nurse Coaching© (TINC) contains healing, the metaparadigm in nursing theory, patterns of knowing in nursing, and the five components of Integrative Nurse Coaching (**Box 26-1**), referred to as *theoretical niches* that acquire the TINC meaning and context within the component in which it resides (Dossey, 2015b). Nurse coaches, with their leadership capacities, interactions with clients, and other interprofessional collaborations, are leaders in the evolution of healthy people living in a healthy world. The information on the Integrative Health and Wellness Assessment tool supports the TINC. The five components of TINC are incorporated into the Integrative Nurse Coach Leadership Model.

The Integrative Nurse Coach Leadership Model expands nursing's vision of how to create a culture of health and well-being (Dossey & Luck, 2015). Nurses are challenged to be leaders and the driving force in healthcare reform and in the health and wellness coaching movement. Nurse coaches are uniquely positioned to engage individuals in hospitals, clinics, and communities in the process of behavior change for advancement toward healthier people living on a healthy planet—local to global.

The Nurse Coach Five-Step Process

The nurse coach five-step process actualizes and integrates the TINC. The steps are as follows (Dossey, 2015a):

- **Process 1**: Connecting to the story
- **Process 2**: Deep listening and skillful questioning
- **Process 3**: Inviting opportunities, potentials, and changes
- **Process 4**: Practicing, integrating, and embodying change
- **Process 5**: Guiding and supporting the transforming self

Process 1: Connecting to the Story

Before the coaching session begins, the nurse coach becomes fully present, centered, and grounded. This allows the nurse coach to be completely attentive to the client's topic and the elements of the story. This includes noticing both the affective and energetic state of the client, as well as the content of what the person presents in the initial meeting.

As a starting point, the client may bring a topic, specific intention, or goal to the coaching session. The client provides the subject and direction of the coaching conversation, while the nurse coach conveys curiosity and remains open and attentive. Topics for exploration may be generated by the client's responses and reactions to evaluation tools such as the Integrative Health and Wellness Assessment. If the client cannot identify a topic for the coaching conversation, the nurse coach, through skillful questioning and/or awareness practices, can assist the client in identifying what is being hoped for.

Nurse coaches align their intentions with clients' goals and attend to clients' subjective experiences and internal frames of reference. This builds trust and respect. Belief in the client's capacity to connect with their inner resources, wisdom, and potential supports the client's journey toward desired changes and personal goals. Being authentically present throughout the client's process of self-discovery makes it easier for the nurse coach to step back from the nurse-as-expert role, honoring the wisdom of "less is more" in the coaching conversation.

Process 2: Deep Listening and Skillful Questioning

The nurse coach lets go of trying to "fix" a client through deep listening and skillful questioning. If the client moves into vulnerable moments, bearing witness to the client's narrative is essential. *Bearing witness* to a story means being present with patience and respect for things just as they are. This includes learning to be with the client's joys and successes as well as giving full permission for the client to express pain and suffering. Being curious and open is attending to the present moment, allowing whatever emerges to come forth. By bringing awareness to one's own inner wisdom, wealth of experience, and intuition, the nurse coach draws from inner resources to guide the direction of the questioning. Cultivating a connection with the client that communicates safety and respect creates the opportunity for the client to explore vulnerability, doubts, and challenges as well as strengths, potential, and successes.

Skillful questions move the client toward goals by identifying attitudes, behaviors, and beliefs that have led to past successes and accomplishments. They also help identify blocks and obstacles, both internal and external, that have created limitations. Skillful questioning supports the client in identifying habits of thought and feeling that are self-defeating. Bringing awareness to these patterns provides the client with the possibility of making different choices.

When issues arise in coaching that are outside the scope of the nurse coach's expertise, it is the coach's duty to make that clear to the client and offer to connect them to other services. It is essential that the nurse coach be knowledgeable about the spectrum of community resources and have referral information for professional colleagues who may be more appropriate for the client.

Process 3: Inviting Opportunities, Potentials, and Changes

The nurse coach recognizes and respects the client's subjective experiences, perceptions, learning style, and culture (e.g., beliefs, values, and customs), in addition to upholding the values of honesty, sincerity, personal integrity, and professional ethics. Nurse coaching includes planning and negotiating clear actions by developing SMART goals and agreements as part of the coaching conversation. Reevaluating the effectiveness or appropriateness of the goals and agreements is in keeping with the coaching process, as is altering or creating new action plans when appropriate.

The nurse coach and the client explore which plans have been kept and reexamine those that have not been realized. Periodically reviewing the coaching plan with the client stimulates engagement and helps to identify barriers to change. Holding the person accountable for planned actions, results, and related time frames allows progress to continue as part of the dynamics within a trusting relationship.

A client's new ideas, behaviors, and actions may feel uncomfortable, or even risky, as old patterns and habits are challenged. A client's fear of failure is a commonly experienced variable but may be soothed through the nurse coach's offering of ongoing support. When unrealistic or unmanageable goals are established, the nurse coach suggests that the client apply the "50-percent rule," cutting a goal in half to maximize the potential for initial success.

Process 4: Practicing, Integrating, and Embodying Change

Employing deep listening and powerful questioning, the nurse coach focuses on what the client is communicating. Changing behavior means practicing, integrating, and embodying change and bringing this awareness to day-to-day activities. This awareness opens the opportunity for the client to choose to take new actions and create new ways of thinking and being. This helps in planning ahead, rather than engaging in mindless, habituated behavior. This embodied change brings the possibility of being liberated from self-defeating patterns and thoughts with the spirit of engagement in new health behaviors and choices.

Encouraging and supporting the client in experimenting and applying what has been learned from the coaching interaction leads to new behaviors and sustained change. The nurse coach is an ally in this relationship by being mindful of the power inherent in the coaching relationship. The nurse coach offers encouragement and feedback that is nonjudgmental, respectful, and appropriate, therefore freeing the client to express strong feelings without fear of judgment. Clients who understand their own patterns of resistance gain an opportunity for self-awareness and growth.

When assessing the quality of a client's communication, the nurse coach attends to the person's breath pattern, facial expressions, body language, vocal quality, and energy. When clients acknowledge that change is hard, they can identify their resistance and ambivalence to change.

Process 5: Guiding and Supporting the Transforming Self

The integral perspective is that every individual is always negotiating their lived experience at present on many levels. People are observing their present interaction while at the same time being affected and shaped by past experiences, some remembered and some forgotten. Individuals function in a bio-psycho-social-environmental-spiritual reality. Both challenges and opportunities can present themselves in any of these aspects of being.

Skillfully, the nurse coach assists clients in exploring and navigating the narrative of their life stories. Profound changes can occur in this coaching journey when clients are introduced to the power of their imagination. Introducing clients to meditative and imagery awareness practices may offer them an opportunity to identify metaphors, images, or words that resonate with their story. The intimate, personally meaningful quality of these experiences can help in keeping clients aligned with envisioned hopes and intentions. These images, metaphors, and other creative aspects of the coaching experience become useful resources that may be referred to frequently in coaching sessions. These symbols and stories are not static. They become part of a transformative process that can release or reconcile parts of clients' stories that no longer serve them. This coaching discovery process inspires clients to be open to broader perspectives and new ways of being.

As demonstrated in **Figure 26-1**, the client's current self includes their current reality. As changes are made, the old story remains but also opens into another way of being and transcends into the changing and transforming self. The nurse coach recognizes this new way of being and acknowledges the changed behaviors and new commitments.

This process assists the client in recognizing what was effective in moving forward. Clarity in what works provides the client with a strong

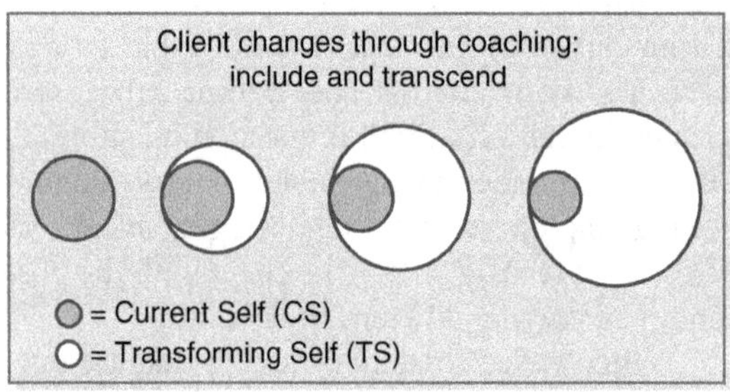

Figure 26-1 Client changes through coaching.

Legend: Clients bring to coaching their current self (CS) and life story. Through coaching, the client's CS opens to new opportunities, potentials, and change. The CS begins to shift, and a transforming self (TS) emerges, with the outer circle going from black (CS) to gray. With the widening of awareness, transformation (TS) occurs, allowing desired goals and changes to be realized.

Nursing Situation

A Walk Toward Change

Maria, the nurse coach, glanced at the clock as she prepared her notes and herself for the next patient. Mr. Johnson was scheduled for a coaching session—his first one since being referred by his primary care provider due to rising blood pressure and early signs of diabetes.

The door opened and in walked Mr. Johnson, a man in his early fifties with kind eyes and a heavy gait. He smiled politely but looked tired—tired in a way that went beyond lack of sleep. "Good to see you again, Mr. Johnson," Maria said warmly, gesturing for him to take a seat in the cozy, private coaching room. "Can I get you some water before we start?"

He declined with a shake of his head and sank into the chair. "I'm here because my doctor keeps pushing this lifestyle change thing," he said without prompting. "Lose weight, exercise more, watch my carbs. It's always something."

Maria nodded, listening intently.

"I've tried a bunch of times," he continued. "I join the gym, eat salad for a week, and then I'm back to old habits. It never sticks."

Maria leaned in slightly, her tone calm and reflective. "It sounds like you've put a lot of effort in before, and it's frustrating when it doesn't lead to lasting change."

He exhaled deeply. "Yeah. Feels like I'm always failing. Maybe I'm just not built for it."

Maria paused, letting his words hang for a moment. Then she said gently, "That's a hard place to be. And yet, here you are. That tells me something—maybe that part of you still wants to try."

Mr. Johnson looked down at his hands, then gave a small nod. "I just don't want to end up like my brother. He's on insulin now, can barely move around. I'm heading in that direction."

"That sounds scary," Maria said, validating his concern. "You want to avoid that path. Can I ask—if things *could* go differently this time, what would you hope for?"

He paused, thinking. "I guess I'd like to feel less tired. Not get so winded going up the stairs. And yeah... stay off more medication."

Maria smiled. "Those are powerful goals. So, there's this part of you that's tired and frustrated—but there's also a part that really wants to feel better, stay independent, and avoid more meds."

"Exactly," he said. "But I don't know where to start anymore."

"Well," Maria said, her voice encouraging, "what's one small thing you think you *could* try? Not a big overhaul—just one small step to get started?"

Mr. Johnson thought for a moment. "You know... I used to take walks after dinner, just around the block. I kind of liked it. Maybe I could do that again. A couple times a week."

Maria's face lit up. "That sounds like a great idea—familiar, manageable, and something you even enjoyed. How would it feel to give that a try this week?"

"I think I could do that," he said, sitting up a little straighter. "Fifteen minutes. Twice a week."

Maria reached for her notepad. "Let's write that down. You're choosing the goal, and it's a meaningful one. How confident on a scale of 1 to 10 are you that you would be able to accomplish walking 15 minutes, twice this week?"

Mr. Johnson replied, "A 9."

"Congratulations," said Maria. "It sounds as though you will be successful in accomplishing your goal. Let's plan a check-in next week to see how it goes."

For the first time in the session, Mr. Johnson smiled.

As he left, his steps seemed just a little lighter.

foundation on which to build when future challenges occur. This recognition also provides more insights and elicits opportunities for new commitments or actions. The client's old worldview and assumptions have been challenged. The transforming self becomes integrated into the broadened sense of self, leading to increased self-efficacy, self-esteem, and confidence.

Implications

Clinical Practice

As the growing body of research demonstrates, integrating nurse coaching into practice will improve client outcomes and client and nurse satisfaction.

Education

Teaching and learning about nurse coaching in basic and advanced nursing curricula is imperative in the movement to transform our healthcare system from a disease orientation to one of health promotion, focusing on both the nurse and the client.

Research

Continued studies on client outcomes and engagement resulting from nurse coaching will provide the data to recognize nurse coaching as a critical nursing specialty.

Policy

The advanced knowledge base of nurses highlights the importance of the nurse coach's role in healthcare. Distinguishing the difference between nonprofessional and professionally educated health and wellness coaches is essential.

Global Health

Worldwide, individuals are becoming increasingly proactive in their approach to health, prioritizing preventive measures such as healthy eating, exercise, and stress management to prevent illness and enhance overall quality of life. Globally, healthcare providers are taking an interest in these health and wellness approaches.

Conclusion

Nurse coaches are uniquely positioned to engage individuals in the process of meaningful and health-promoting behavioral change. With a renewed focus on prevention and wellness in healthcare reform, now is an essential time for the nursing profession to expand its visibility in the emerging coaching paradigm. Professional nurse coaching promotes opportunities for nurses to practice to the full extent of their education and experience, leading to healthy people living in a healthy nation on a healthy planet.

References

American Holistic Nurses Credentialing Corporation. (n.d.). *Holistic nurses certification*. www.ahncc.org/certificationprocess.html

American Nurses Association. (2010). *Nursing's social policy statement: The essence of the profession*. Nursesbooks.org.

American Nurses Association. (2015). *Nursing: Scope and standards of practice* (3rd ed.). Nursesbooks.org.

American Nurses Association. (2019). *Holistic nursing: Scope and standards of practice* (3rd ed.). American Nurses Association, Inc.

American Nurses Association. (2025). *Code of ethics for nurses with interpretive statements*. Nursesbooks.org.

Avino, K., & France, N. (forthcoming). *Integrative nurse coaching: A guide for praxis*. International Nurse Coach Association.

Buerhaus, P., Skinner, L. E., Auerbach, D. I., & Staiger, D. O. (2017). Four challenges facing the nursing workforce in the United States. *Journal of Nursing Regulation*, *8*(2), 40–46.

Bureau of Labor Statistics, U.S. Department of Labor. (2025, June 20). Occupational outlook handbook, *registered nurses*. https://www.bls.gov/ooh/healthcare/registered-nurses.htm

Dart, M. A. (2011). *Motivational interviewing in nursing practice*. Jones & Bartlett Learning.

Delaney, C., & Bark, L. (2019). The experience of holistic nurse coaching for patients with chronic conditions. *Journal of Holistic Nursing*, *37*(3), 225–237. https://journals.sagepub.com/doi/abs/10.1177/0898010119837109

Dossey, B. M. (2015a). Stories, strengths, and the nurse coach 5-step process. In B. M. Dossey, S. Luck, & B. G. Schaub

(Eds.), *Nurse coaching: Integrative approaches for health and wellbeing* (pp. 85–108). International Nurse Coach Association.

Dossey, B. M. (2015b). Theory of integrative nurse coaching. In B. M. Dossey, S. Luck, & B. G. Schaub (Eds.), *Nurse coaching: Integrative approaches for health and wellbeing*. International Nurse Coach Association.

Dossey, B. M., & Luck, S. (2015). Nurse coaching and leadership. In B. M. Dossey, S. Luck, & B. G. Schaub (Eds.), *Nurse coaching: Integrative approaches for health and wellbeing* (pp. 387–402). International Nurse Coach Association.

Prochaska, J., Norcross, J. C., & Di Clemente, C. C. (1995). *Changing for good: A revolutionary six-stage program for overcoming bad habits and moving your life positively forward.* HarperCollins.

Rehman, H., Karpman, C., Douglas, K. V., & Benzo, R. P. (2017). Effect of a motivational interviewing-based health coaching on quality of life in subjects with COPD. *Respiratory Care*, 62, 1043–1048.

Ross, A., Brooks, A. T., Yang, L., Touchton-Leonard, K., Raju, S., & Bevans, M. (2018). Results of a national survey of certified nurse coaches with implications for advanced practice nurses. *Journal of the American Association of Nurse Practitioners, 30*(5), 251–261. https://doi.org/10.1097/JXX.0000000000000041

Southard, M. E., Bark, L., & Hess, D. (2020). Motivational interviewing and appreciative inquiry. In B. M. Dossey & L. Keegan (Eds.), *Holistic nursing: A handbook for practice* (8th ed., pp. 541–555). Jones & Bartlett Learning.

Southard, M. E., Dossey, B. M., Bark, L., & Schaub, B. G. (2021). *The art and science of nurse coaching: The provider's guide to coaching scope and competencies* (2nd ed.). American Nurses Association.

Vincent, A. E., & Sanchez-Birkhead, A. (2013). Evaluation of the effectiveness of nurse coaching in improving health outcomes in chronic conditions. *Holistic Nursing Practice,* 27(3), 148–161.

Young, H., Miyamoto, S., Ward, D., Dharmar, M., Tang-Feldman, Y., & Berglund, L. (2014). Sustained effects of a nurse coaching intervention via telehealth to improve health behavior change in diabetes. *Telemedicine Journal and e-Health*, *20*, 828–834.

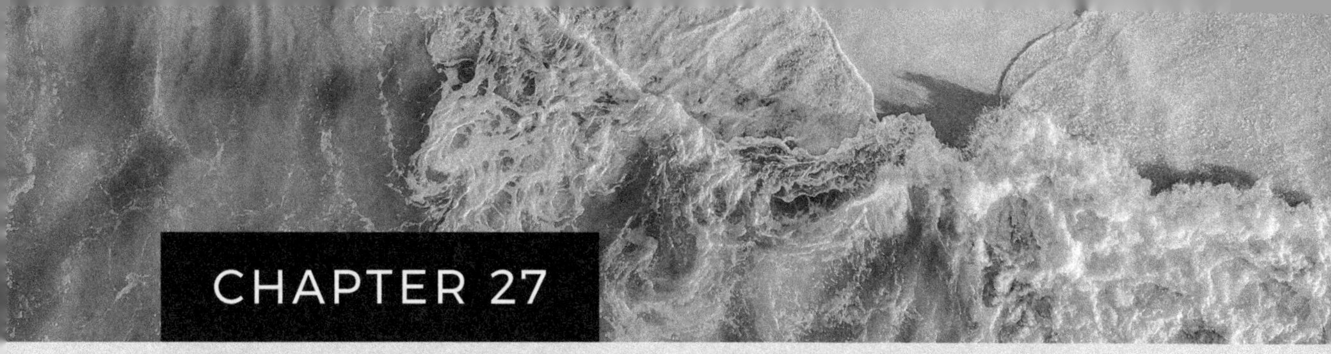

CHAPTER 27

Holistic Mental Health

Bonney Gulino Schaub and Mary Beth White

NURSE HEALER OBJECTIVES

- The reader will experience an expansion of the concept of mental health to include dormant mind–body potentials in every patient.
- The reader will experience a detailed clinical study of how the awakening of mind–body potentials aided a patient experiencing anxiety and depression.
- The reader will get a perspective on the increasing mental health needs of both health professionals and their patients.

DEFINITIONS

Collective unconscious: The culturally influenced self, organized around group and ancestral/genetic ways of thinking and behaving.

Conscious Self: The abiding presence of awareness itself, noticing both our internal and external experiences.

Field of consciousness: All perceptions available to us at any given moment.

Higher unconscious: The spiritual self, oriented around joy, purpose, interconnectedness, and experienced as guiding inner wisdom through words, images, physical sensations, and/or emotions.

Imagery: The method that activates the brain's creative imagination and causes mind–body changes.

Lower unconscious: The survival-based self, oriented around aggression, fear, escape (fight-flight-freeze).

Middle unconscious: The social-conditioned self, organized around seeking approval and avoiding disapproval.

Mind–body: The interaction effect of mental and emotional activity on the physical body; the interaction effect of body processes and changes on the mental and emotional status of the patient.

Transpersonal: Meaning "beyond the personality," it refers to spiritual and creative thoughts and feelings that change our perspective and can lead to breakthrough decisions.

Vulnerability: The awareness of life's unpredictability and of our limited ability to control events in our personal life; the awareness of and sensitivity to change and loss as inevitable facts of life.

Introduction

"Holistic mental health" is a general term referring to the mental–emotional practices that can awaken dormant potentials in our patients and clients. These potentials can be categorized as experiences of peace, inner wisdom, purpose, and oneness to reduce suffering (Schaub & Schaub, 2015).

While other holistic practices may address changes in heart rate, blood pressure, muscle tension, and so on, holistic mental health practices need to be an aspect of care in any health and well-being context. It can bring changes to the individual's capacity to cope, understand, relax, focus, and make healthy choices in the face of physical or mental distress (Schaub & Simon, 2019). The nurse–healer trained in holistic mental health practices can guide and train patients in self-compassion and self-care methods that will remain useful throughout their life, regardless of the onset of a particular illness or crisis. In addition, holistic mental health practices are helpful for clinicians in reducing their stress and enhancing their presence and empathy as an aspect of job performance and satisfaction. Health care is such a demanding field, and nurses and other clinicians often describe feeling overwhelmed by critically ill patients, time constraints, and the pressure to do more with less.

Holistic Mental Health Practice

We begin with a brief history and overview of a holistic mental health perspective. The chapter then provides an extensive account of an advanced practice holistic nurse coach in private practice caring for a woman who is struggling with a medical challenge and anxiety. In the process of this patient's care, other mental health challenges become evident, including depression, PTSD, cognitive decline, grief, pain management, and substance misuse. The treatment included the implementation of meditation, mental imagery, energy awareness, and other mental and emotional caring skills. This case study shows how these methods can become an integral part of nursing education for both holistic patient care and professional self-care.

Guiding a person to experience connection with their profound inner wisdom, their sense of meaning and purpose, and recognition of what they are hoping for will be presented. This includes learning about the implementation of transpersonal clinical skills, such as meditation and mental imagery. As one example, two holistic nurses created a treatment protocol using Clinical Meditation and Imagery (CMI) to ease the pain of patients with spinal cord injuries. They stated that CMI "offers a low-risk, low-cost therapeutic option for people with spinal cord injury to self-manage their pain experience" (Zanca et al., 2022). These practices are presented because they create positive mental, emotional, transpersonal, and physical changes in a wide variety of patient issues. They have risen into the public consciousness through the many studies of mindfulness and its application in hospitals and clinics, including their use for improved attention and stress reduction as self-care for nurses. This need was seen to increase dramatically because of the COVID-19 pandemic, which dramatically increased stress in an already stressed nursing workforce. In one local example, my neighborhood hospital became a total COVID ICU treatment center. In the very beginning of the pandemic, just before the precautionary protocols had been implemented, one of the nurses died from this disease. Nurses also experienced fear of going home and being with their family. Many of them immediately took all their work clothing off, put it in the washing machine, and took a shower before any close contact with loved ones.

This unprecedented traumatic time challenged the well-being and resilience of all the healthcare workers. They were placed on 12-hour shifts from 8 a.m. to 8 p.m. or 8 p.m. to 8 a.m. Every caregiver's workload increased, and many believed there was insufficient personal protective equipment available. They all needed to wear masks and protective garments, which heightened the sense of isolation. I established an online support group that was open to any nurse who was open to connecting with their colleagues with caring and compassion. I also offered meditation and imagery sessions so the nurses could share and connect with their inner peace and wisdom (Munn et al., 2021). They were also caring for dying patients daily. A small group of the overall caregivers had experience in ICU treatment, but now every unit was a COVID ICU. This was quite a challenge for nurses. One nurse commented in the group that all their experience was in labor and delivery and newborn nursery. They had never experienced the death of a patient (Otis et al., 2025). In this study, Otis created a team comprised of two registered nurses (RNs), one patient manager, a chaplain, a nurse researcher, the staff resilience coordinator, and the chief nurse executive to create a Post-Death Care Team Protocol.

For staff working the night shift, restaurants and other food suppliers sent large amounts of prepared food, which was served outside in tents. On weekends, local bands set up outside the food tents and played music to the great pleasure of all. Residents were donating money to support the people providing services to the hospital. This was a moving example of the value of communal support, the nurturance of delicious food, and the joyful creativity of the musicians. Nurses also expressed feeling peaceful looking up at the star-filled sky, and some even spoke of hearing owls singing.

In a study that was conducted to explore the need for connection and kinship during the pandemic, the researchers studied the factors that helped in modifying the stress and despair caregivers were experiencing. For example, Pearson (2022) cited earlier research that "high quality social connections were uniquely important in maintaining mental health during the pandemic." The implication in this study points to carefully assessing the quality of kinship relationships.

Mental health is an aspect of any client/patient/colleague relationship that nurses participate in. I first found this out as a nursing student at Adelphi University in the early 1970s. Adelphi had an excellent nursing faculty, several of whom had received their graduate education at New York University, which was one of the pioneering nursing schools that brought a holistic perspective into nursing practice. One of the faculty, Dolores Krieger, was even creating the practice of Therapeutic Touch and supporting research that proved its effectiveness. This pioneering practice recognized and worked with the power of energy and consciousness in health care. A few of the psychology nursing faculty had studied at Rutgers University, where Hildegard Peplau, in the early 1950s, was a pioneer in creating a nursing model of emotional health and well-being. She spoke of a person's innate capacity for self-healing and growth. She expressed that the interactions that occur between the nurse and patient have a significant effect on patient outcomes. She believed that every person is unique and possesses the capacity to learn, develop, and change. She emphasized the importance of the nurse in collaborating with the patient to support and activate this process. She also stresses the importance of the nurse's self-awareness and self-knowledge so that the nurse can know how to be fully present with the patient, free of their own issues (Peplau, 1952).

Students at Adelphi were fortunate to have a whole semester in psychiatric nursing. We learned about the medical diagnostic categories of psychiatric illnesses, including the associated behaviors and prescribed medications. There was an emphasis on identifying and exploring the behaviors and emotional aspects of the various conditions. Feelings of anxiety, depression, fear, alienation, and other emotional states were not only experienced by individuals with a diagnosis. Our first clinical setting for this course was in a psychiatric hospital. We spent time on a unit, and each of us was assigned to a particular patient. It was a surprise to learn that we were not supposed to look at the patient's chart or know their diagnosis. We spent over an hour with the individual on several visits. We were to get to know them, learn about their life experience, and learn their perception of why they were in the hospital and what they were experiencing.

One patient was a well-educated young woman from an affluent family, but had run away from home to live in New York city where she had previously gone to college. She was found living on the street and struggling to survive. We met several times before she shared her story. She feared that if she told the nurse about her father's abuse, she would not be believed. This patient was considered delusional and paranoid as well as depressed.

When she informed friends about her abuse, and her father found out what they had been told, he threatened them and told them she was lying. She feared he might harm the nurse if he found out what his daughter had shared with her. The patient was reassured that all the information was confidential. Thankfully, today, there is more recognition of child abuse that occurs in families, no matter the socioeconomic status.

In a significant study on the long-term impact of trauma, "dissociation is highly associated with trauma, comprising part of the diagnostic criteria for PTSD and involving both depersonalization and derealization." In this study, the authors describe it as the death of the self. "Trauma can rupture the self and splinter it apart …while part of the self continues to endure, offering in an impoverished form, another part is irredeemably lost" (Dorothy & Hughes, 2023). This is important to know because of the possibility of misdiagnosis and assuming the patient is psychotic. Children who experience abuse of any kind often feel shame, thinking they deserve it or even that this behavior from the parent or other adult is "normal."

There is now greater awareness and concern about the growing number of suicides by preteens aged 8 to 12 years old. The research focused on the period from 2001 to 2022. It was also noted that the incidence has been increasing by 8 percent annually since 2008. The highest increase was in Native American/Alaskan Native, Asian/Pacific Islander, and Hispanic preteen females. Hanging and suffocation were the most common methods, but firearm use is rapidly rising. The highest overall incidence was in Black preteens. The vast array of possible sources of trauma is undoubtedly a significant factor in these statistics (Ruch et al., 2024).

An example is a program created in Alaska that addressed the struggle of suicidal youth. The suicide rate of Alaska Native youth was double the national rate. The highest incidence occurred in Native American and Alaska Native males living in rural areas. The significant health issue of suicidality was attributed to cultural disruptions brought about by colonialism and historical trauma. The plan was to bring youth together to revitalize their culture. This included developing a sense of belongingness by learning about traditional knowledge and skills. Learning about wellness practices, storytelling, and engaging in team sports and exercises were all valuable components, but the most important was to experience a deep connection to the community (Barnett et al., 2020). This sense of not belonging is such a powerful element with so many people we interact with in our communities and our practices. Children may live with out experiencing a sense of belongingness for many reasons, such as body image dysmorphia, ethnicity, and LGBTQ identity. As this distress is noticed, it is important to note any sense of suicidal thinking.

Bonney, in her first nursing job, was working nights on a surgical unit. One night, she was caring for a patient in her mid-30s who was gravely ill, struggling, and unable to sleep. This was a challenging experience, and she received guidance and some support from the night nursing supervisor. When she expressed her difficulty, the supervisor said it would be helpful to ask the patient what she was hoping for. Feeling surprised by this suggestion, she thought, "She doesn't want to die." The nursing supervisor, Cathy Fanslow, helped her understand that everyone has hopes for something, and it is helpful to be able to reflect on it and express it. Cathy went on to become a pioneer in the creation of hospice care and hospice nursing. She also wrote about the importance and power of hope for all of us (Fanslow-Brunjes, 2008).

In returning to the patient and asking what she was hoping for, the surprising response was a smile, and then the patient said, "That's a great question." She expressed that there were some friends she wanted to connect with. She decided she would call them in the morning.

Bonney's next clinical setting was an inpatient private psychiatric unit in a general hospital setting. This was a short-term unit where the psychiatrist admitted patients with whom they were working. The patient's treatment was based on the orders from their private psychiatrist. All the nurses had patients assigned to them as their primary care patients.

Bonney had been interested in meditation and yoga for years before becoming a nurse. She had a strong bond with Jerry, the nurse's aide who was an artist and very much interested in meditation as well. This was long before there was any integration of yoga, meditation, or any other "spiritual" practices in health care. In one example, this interest proved helpful for a teenage patient.

The unit was in the general hospital, and so there were often patients with emotional struggles due to medical challenges. A teenage girl with cystic fibrosis was admitted, struggling with anxiety and difficulty breathing, which is a significant aspect of this condition. She was afraid to fall asleep because she might stop breathing. One of the other patients on the unit was a woman who had been practicing and teaching yoga for many years. She was admitted because she felt compelled to do her practice constantly and could not stop. She was pacing the unit, even at night. When this young woman was admitted, the yoga teacher said, "I can definitely help her."

The nurses told her she couldn't do that without consent from her doctor and her parents. The charge nurse spoke with her psychiatrist, telling him that the yoga teacher was very experienced. The young girl was interested, and we thought it might be comforting for his patient to try the breathing practices. He agreed to this saying, "Obviously I can't write it as an order, but let her try it."

The effect was spectacular. They worked together extensively for a couple of days. The young girl loved that she was able to experience her breath in a positive way. She was able to be discharged because her mood had changed. The yoga teacher became calm and connected to a personal sense of peace and purpose from the help she had given this young patient. The nursing staff sensed that the parents were planning to have their daughter stay connected with the yoga teacher.

Another fascinating patient on the unit was a young woman who was a professional illustrator and a single mom. She was having feelings of disorientation, and concerned friends were worried about her. One of them stayed with her to help care for her child. They were also concerned because her artwork had become drastically different. All of it was now nonrepresentational, with many geometric and swirling images. She was seen by a private psychiatrist who hospitalized her, fearing that she was having a psychotic break. In extended meetings with this patient, Bonney became interested in the fact that the patient had become deeply connected with a local group that was practicing whirling as part of their interest in Sufiism. This emerged as she was feeling the need to whirl in her hospital room. Bonney and Jerry concurred that we thought she wasn't psychotic, but that she was entering into altered mental states from the whirling. They were also aware that Sufi and other Islamic art is not representational. It is full of geometric patterns and symbols.

In speaking with this patient's doctor, who had not yet started her on antipsychotic meds, he was very open and curious about what Bonney and Jerry were saying. He expressed that he had a personal interest in meditation. He said he didn't think she was psychotic, and he wanted to explore this with her. She was discharged and continued to work with this psychiatrist in his private practice.

Since Jerry and I were talking about meditation and spiritual consciousness a lot on the unit, our unit clerk said, "Bonney, you need to talk with my brother-in-law, Pat. He's a psychologist and he's studying a psychology that includes spirituality and consciousness. I think it's something from Italy."

That was how I learned about Psychosynthesis. This was my first connection to the holistic perspective of transpersonal psychology. At the beginning of the 20th century, both Roberto Assagioli, a psychiatrist in Florence, Italy, and Carl Jung, a psychiatrist in Zurich, Switzerland, became involved in the then-revolutionary movement of Sigmund Freud's psychoanalysis as a new way to view psychiatric patients. Jung became Assagioli's clinical supervisor. Assagioli went on to become the first psychoanalyst in Italy.

He left the psychoanalytic movement a year later because of its dismissal of any interest in or respect for spirituality. (Jung left a few years later because of "political" struggles with Freud.) Assagioli began to use the term "psychosynthesis" to indicate the need to integrate the many competing and contradictory impulses in human nature (e.g., survival instinct, social approval, spiritual seeking). He also began to use the term "transpersonal" (simply meaning "beyond the personality") rather than "spiritual" because it was free of religious connotations. His last book was a collection of essays entitled *Transpersonal Development: The Dimension Beyond Psychosynthesis* (Assagioli, 1991).

He combined many techniques in his work, including exploration of the past, rational analysis, meditation, mental imagery, creative expression, and energy practices. Probably his most outstanding contribution was providing both scientific validity and effective techniques for the discovery and awakening of a patient's *higher self*, an innate resource of the higher brain–mind. He was advocating the reality and potentials of interconnectedness and pervading emotional peace and joy of the higher region of the brain 75 years before the current neuroscience interest in studying the benefits of meditation. Assagioli advocated that a key component of all therapy should be the awakening of this brain–mind state.

In 1952, Hildegard Peplau wrote that it was an important aspect of nursing to recognize and mobilize a person's innate capacity for self-healing and growth. This involved the nurse partnering with clients to assist them in realizing that these potentials were within them. She also wanted nurses to have personal self-knowledge and self-awareness of these aspects of self (Peplau, 1952).

Helen Erickson continued and elaborated on the clinical uses of a patient's deeper resources with a particular appreciation for the "inner voice" that provides a source of meaning and guidance. In Helen Erickson's emphasis on the importance of *Self-Knowing* she described the power of this voice:

> Our inner voice is not our conscience; it is not massaged or shaped by society or social norms. It comes directly from our Soul. It draws energy (and therefore, knowledge, or intelligence) from the Universe and imparts energy, created by our holistic being, back to the Universe. *Our inner voice is an aggregate of knowledge drawn from our Soul and knowledge driven from the Universe.* (Erickson, 2006)

Another important figure in holistic and transpersonal mental health, Larry Dossey, MD, described "…a sense of oneness, unity, and unbroken wholeness is a universal, distinguishing characteristic of transpersonal experiences. This is often accompanied by a sense of joy and fulfillment, and the feeling that the world is being sensed the way it really is, an unbroken whole" (Schaub & Schaub, 2015, p. X111).

Since Assagioli lived and had his practice in Florence, he appreciated the power of the massive resources of magnificent art throughout the city. With patients in his private practice, he suggested that they identify the art and places that brought them peace and joy. He was also connected to studying the vast array of meditation practices. He recognized that being present with beautiful art and natural settings could be an effective meditation practice.

In a study conducted at the University of California in Berkeley, there was an exploration of an individual's experiences of awe and the effect it had. They characterized awe as a distinct emotion. It arises in encounters that are vast and expansive. They also cited it as a vast cross-cultural phenomenon that was experienced in positive group encounters that reflected kindness and courage. The awe-inducing pathways they cited were feeling deep immersion with nature, mystical encounters, and spirituality, where there was a sense of connecting to the divine or higher powers, experiences of collective movement that are experienced through music, singing, dancing, or chanting. They noted that music was one of the most common elicitors of awe. They also cited the use of psychedelics. The conclusion was that awe experiences lead to better mental and physical health outcomes consistent with the goals of holistic mental health nursing.

Coming from a similar spirit, a study occurred at an arboretum in California. The researchers found that participants who were brought to places where they could gaze at peaceful water settings, whether it was a pool or a pond or other sources, experienced a lowering of their blood pressure and heart rate (Coss & Keller, 2022).

In Italy, there is a growing recognition of the therapeutic effect of natural settings, which are referred to as "green prescriptions" by health professionals (Droli et al., 2024).

These important insights and perspectives highlight the importance of being able to work with a client/patient by being curious and open to learning what they personally experience as health promoting. The individual's life story and psychological experiences are not typically explored in patient assessment. The focus is on the specific health challenge that is the reason for the admission. It is important to be fully present with patients so they feel they can share personal aspects of what they are experiencing.

Another source of awe is when people have breakthrough creative and spiritual insights. These can be referred to as "transpersonal" (meaning "beyond the personality"). Transpersonal practices, principally the clinical uses of various forms of meditation and mental imagery, are easy to learn and can quickly reduce fear and distress in medical patients whether on the unit or in the office. I first used these practices on the inpatient cancer and cardiac units and substance misuse of a major suburban hospital in the late 1970s.

I subsequently went on to train nurses and other health professionals in the United States, Canada, and Europe. In 2015, nurses working at a local Veterans Administration hospital with the veterans struggling with profound PTSD were able to get a grant to train the staff in these holistic mental health methods.

The training lasted 15 sessions. The staff provided feedback that the practices were both professionally and personally beneficial. The Veterans Administration then sponsored us to create and publish a book on the training: *Transpersonal Development: Cultivating the Human Resources of Peace, Wisdom, Purpose, and Oneness.*

Nursing Situation

In an example from chapter author Mary Beth White's practice, this nursing situation describes the clinical use of holistic mental health practices in addressing anxiety, depression, PTSD, cognitive decline, grief, and substance misuse.

June, a 47-year-old married White female with mild anxiety and PTSD, was referred to the holistic nurse coach by her primary care provider after experiencing side effects (lethargy and insomnia) from a trial of sertraline. She wanted "a more natural approach" rather than a different medication. She was in her second marriage, which she described as "very happy." They are raising an 11-year-old daughter from her prior marriage. Her first husband died during military service when her daughter was 3. June is a stay-at-home mom. June's parents live close by, and her 70-year-old mother was under evaluation for early Alzheimer's.

During the initial assessment, June reported wanting to be able not to get upset about "little things" like worrying about what to cook for dinner, or what color to paint her daughter's room. She also wanted to be more successful at convincing her parents that it is no longer safe for her mom to drive. When June is increasingly bothered by ruminating thoughts, her instinct is to calm them by having a glass of wine. In the past, one glass turned into two, then three glasses, and soon the bottle could be empty. This was her pattern after her first husband died. Over the past 6 years, she has stopped all alcohol use.

Mary Beth guided June in these following three transpersonal holistic mental health practices as a major element of her care.

Hope/Deeper Hope (Schaub & Schaub, 2015)

Steps

1. Make your body comfortable and let the chair hold you...lower or close your eyes...
2. Now follow your breathing...don't do anything to it...just let it be the way it is...you're just noticing it...
3. In a moment, I'm going to ask you to ask yourself two questions. When you ask the first question, try not to think up the answer. Just ask the question and be open to whatever comes to you. If nothing comes to you, that's fine...then we'll go on to the second question...
4. Now, for a moment, go back to your breath...
5. And now ask yourself this question...just be open to what comes to you...Here's the question: "In the way that my life is going now, what am I hoping for?"
6. Pause 30 seconds and then say, "And now let yourself go deeper and ask yourself: 'What is my deeper hope'?"

Wait two minutes and then say, "And now let go of the practice and turn your attention to noticing how you are..."

Wait thirty seconds and then say, "And when you feel ready, at your own pace, begin to come back to the room..."

If you were asked about your hopes and deepest hopes, you would *think* of answers. But when you enter the meditative state and ask the same questions, answers come to you from your guiding inner wisdom. June's response to this experience was feeling the joy and lightness she had soon after her first wedding when she found out she was pregnant. Life seemed open and expansive and full of hope. She now wanted that feeling back. She then shared how she tried to hide from her current husband the fear that could derail her when he went away on work-related trips.

During a *Centering* exercise, June got distracted by the hands-on-belly technique as she disliked her "middle age pouch." Instead, placing her hands on her thighs allowed her to relax better. She also found it easier to focus on her feet on the floor as her mind was "constantly whirring."

Centering (Schaub & Schaub, 2015)

Steps

1. Gently shake your hands for a while...
2. Now place one hand just under your navel and place your other hand on top of the first hand...
3. Now slowly let your awareness go down to your hands and notice the sensations of one hand touching the other...
4. Now begin to notice the rising and falling of your belly underneath your hands...Let yourself become interested in the sensations of the rising and falling...Nothing else to do...Nothing special has to happen...Just noticing the rising and falling...Wait three minutes and then say, "And now let go of the practice and turn your attention to noticing how you are..." Wait thirty seconds and then say, "And when you feel ready, at your own pace, begin to come back to the room..."

Discussion

In a recent experience of teaching clinical meditation at a Veterans Administration hospital, this hands-on-belly technique proved to be the favorite practice. A television news report featured the training, and the veteran selected to demonstrate meditation for the cameras also chose the hands-on-belly practice for its effectiveness and simplicity.

Over time, June's ability to stay in the present during relaxation exercises grew. In between visits, she began a yoga practice at a local YMCA and there she also found a supportive community of friends. Her transpersonal nurse coaching sessions became more sporadic as her anxiety lessened.

One day, she came in to report she had found a growth in her abdomen and the biopsy diagnosed a liposarcoma in need of surgical removal and oncology treatment. She wanted the nurse coach's support as she decided which surgeon to pick. She had gone to two consultants and knew she had to decide ASAP. Although nervous, she was surprised to note how well she was handling the news. She wondered if this meant she was really healthier than she had been in the past when confronted with difficult life situations.

In response to this client's distress about choices she had to make in regard to her treatment and who to work with, her nurse coach guided her into a meditative imagery reflection. She was guided to peacefully connect with her breath. When she was in a peaceful state, the nurse suggested that she connected to the place in her body that she felt needed her attention and care. During an imagery exercise, she experienced herself miniaturized and inside the growth in her belly. She described the interior of the mass as a red-purple blob whose walls were coated with glistening egg-like sacs, "like the roe eggs on sushi." She found herself in her tumor with one of the surgeons, one she had seen earlier that day. He handed her a sledgehammer and they both started smashing the "eggs." They were laughing and steadying themselves to not fall into the slimy mess. When all of the "eggs" were popped, she and the surgeon exited via doors on opposite sides of the mass. As she came out of the experience, she described feeling exhausted yet exhilarated and a belief that "I got this." She chose to use the other surgeon. The mass was removed without complications and without evidence of metastasis. To decrease her chance of recurrence, radiation therapy was advised.

The nurse coach and June continued to work together biweekly while she was undergoing radiation therapy. One day, midway through her radiation treatment schedule, she came in anxious about dying. The nurse coach led her through the *Center of Awareness* exercise (*I have a body, and I am more than my body ...*) June sat quietly for a long time, then emerged with a big smile.

> As I relaxed more and more into your voice, I began to feel weird sensations on either side of my rib cage and I noticed I was actually growing wings. It was bizarre. Then, I heard the voice of my first husband calling my name, and I could see him. He was surrounded by all the dogs that had passed and that I had loved in my life. They were so happy to see me! Then, my uncle, my grandmother, and grandfather showed up. Everyone was smiling and cheering for me saying "We got you, June. No matter what happens, we got you!!" And they do! I have a team. Team June.

Five years later, June is fine and cancer-free. She describes these imagery experiences as seminal, life-changing, and mind-altering events for which she is forever grateful.

Center of Awareness (Schaub & Schaub, 2015)

This practice helps you to identify with the centrality of awareness in your life.

Steps

1. Close your eyes...let the chair hold you...drop your shoulders...
2. Find your breath, either in your nose, your chest, or your belly...begin to tune into your breath...
3. Leaving some of your attention on your breath, bring the rest of your attention into your mind, and in there say to yourself slowly several times, "I have feelings, and I am more than my feelings..." (Pause 30 seconds)
4. And now say to yourself several times, "I have a mind, and I am more than my mind..." (Pause 30 seconds)
5. And now say to yourself several times, "I have a body, and I am more than my body..." (Pause 30 seconds)
6. And now say to yourself several times, "I am a center of awareness..." (Pause 30 seconds)
7. And now, begin to link the phrase "I am a center of awareness" to each in-breath, and then breathe out normally. Try this for a while... Wait one minute and then say, "And now notice how you are..." Wait one minute and then say, "And now, at your own pace, begin to return to the room and open your eyes."

Discussion

Sometimes, clients feel baffled by this meditation. Any of us can become completely identified with our feelings, mind, and body as who we are—and of course they are significantly real. However, equally real is your awareness itself. As we've discussed, you only have the experience of your feelings, mind, and body because you have awareness. Awareness precedes experience. This practice helps you to identify with awareness itself as your own true, continuous nature while everything else in you and around you is changing.

Integration

- **Clinical practice:** Provides a deeper understanding of the diversity and complexity of the psychological components in a patient's medical situation and overall well-being.
- **Education:** Increases training in the psychological and psychosocial aspects of health and illness.
- **Research:** Increase studies of the interaction between psychological states and health and healing status.
- **Policy:** Increased training in psychological health within nursing curricula and also within the clinical environments.
- **Global health:** Expand outlooks on health trends to include psychological pressures and crises.

Conclusion

This chapter's intent was to bring the holistic mental health and psychological aspects of patient care into broader focus. Seeing the patient as fitting into a diagnostic category and ignoring their bio-psycho-social-spiritual context limits the efficacy of treatment. The range of studies and interactions in this chapter seeks to give holistic mental health examples of working with our patients' multidimensionality.

References

Assagioli, R. (1991). *Transpersonal development: The dimension beyond psychosynthesis*. The Aquarian Press.

Barnett, J. D., Schmidt, T. C., Trainor, B., & Wexler, L. (2020). A pilot evaluation of culture camps to increase Alaska Native youth wellness. *Health Promotion Practice, 21*(3), 363–371.

Coss, R. G., & Keller, C. M. (2022). Transient decreases in blood pressure and heart rate with increased subjective level of relaxation while viewing water compared with adjacent ground. *Journal of Environmental Psychology, 81*(101794).

Dorothy, J., & Hughes, E. (2023). The death of the self in posttraumatic experience. *Philosophical Psychology, 38*, 168–188. https//doi.org/10.1080/09515089.2023.2294776

Droli, M., Cargneltti, E., Qualizza, S., Canzonieri, V., Simon, S. D., Costa, C., Droli, E., & Vassallo, F. G., (2024). Enlightening health professionals' predisposition toward green prescriptions in Italy. *Academia Mental Health & Well-Being*. https://doi.org/10.20935/MHealthWellB7367

Erickson, H. L. (Ed.) (2006). *Modeling and role-modeling: A view from the client's world*. Unicorns Unlimited.

Fanslow-Brunjes, C. (2008). *Using the power of hope to cope with dying: The four stages of hope*. Quill Driver Books.

Munn, L., Lui, T., Swick, M., Rose, R., Broyhill, B., New, L., & Gibbs, M. (2021). Well-being and resilience among health care workers during the COVID-19 pandemic: A cross-sectional study. *The American Journal of Nursing, 121*(8), 24–34.

Otis, E., Reid, K. B., Sink, L. K., Scherle, P. A., & Greene-Morris, J. (2025). Supporting nurses when a patient dies. *American Journal of Nursing, 125*(7).

Pearson, G. S. (2022). Kinship influences on adult mental health during a pandemic. *Journal of the American Psychiatric Nurses Association. 28*(6), 431–432.

Peplau, H. E. (1952). *Interpersonal relations in nursing*. G.P. Putnam's Sons.

Ruch, D. A., Horowitz, L. M., Hughes, J. L., Sarkisian, K., Luby, J. L., Fontanella, C. A., & Bridge, J. A. (2024). Suicide in US preteens aged 8 to 12 Years, 2001 to 2022. *JAMA Network Open*, 7(7), e2424664. https://digitalcommons.wustl.edu/oa_4/3959

Schaub, R., & Schaub, B. G. (2015). *Transpersonal development: Cultivating the human resources of peace, wisdom, purpose and oneness*. florencepress.com.

Schaub, R., & Simon, B. (2019). *Easing diabetes distress*. https://www.integrativepractitioner.com/whole-systems-medicine/easing-diabetes-distress

Zanca, J., Gilchrist, C., & Ortiz, C. (2022). Pilot clinical trial of clinical meditation and imagery intervention for chronic pain after spinal cord injury. *Journal of Spinal Cord Medicine, 45*(3), 339–353.

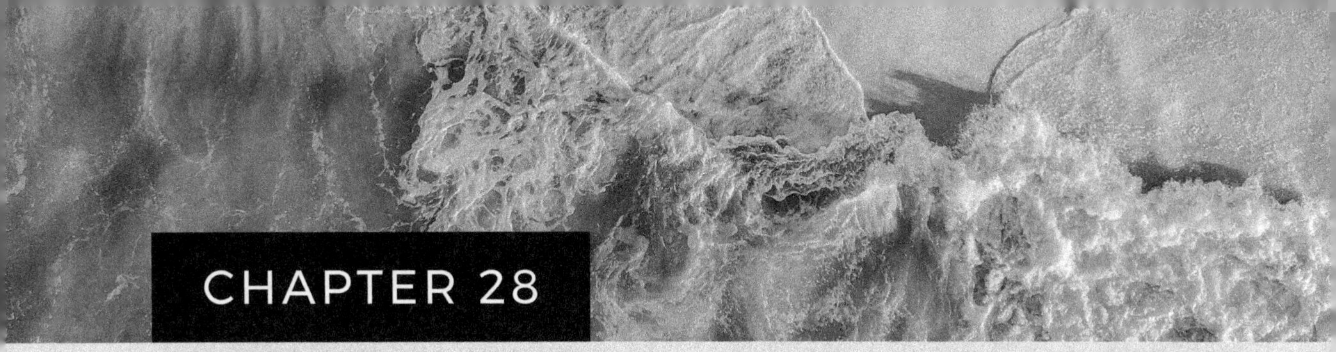

CHAPTER 28

Holistic Nursing's Role in Plant Medicine

Carey S. Cadieux and Stephanie Van Hope

NURSE HEALER OBJECTIVES

- Identify the current and potential future roles of holistic nurses as they advocate for and lead practices that include the use of plant medicines.
- Define the therapeutic benefits of the medicinal use of cannabis.
- Consider the upregulation of the endocannabinoid system (ECS) in relation to maintaining homeostasis.
- Discuss the deep history of sacred entheogen use in traditional cultures.
- Identify indications and outcomes of entheogenic therapy (psilocybin, LSD, MDMA) in current research.

DEFINITIONS

Cannabis: The preferred designation of the flowering herbal plant species *Cannabis sativa* L., belonging to the genus *Cannabis* L., which belongs to the Cannabaceae family (United States Department of Agriculture, n.d.). Commonly known as "marijuana."

Endocannabinoid system: A widespread neuromodulatory system that plays an important role in central nervous system development, synaptic plasticity, and the response to both environmental and endogenous insults. The endocannabinoid system is made up of cannabinoid receptors, endogenous cannabinoids or endocannabinoids, and the enzymes that synthesize and degrade the endocannabinoids (Foster, 2021).

Entheogen[1]: A substance that, when consumed, can engender a spiritual or sacred experience. Psychoactive drugs have profound effects on consciousness. Any substance that is believed to bring about profound revelations. From the Greek *entheos*, divinely inspired (Collins Dictionary, 2024).

Psychedelic[1]: A powerful psychoactive substance that alters perception, mood, and cognitive processes, often through serotonergic pathways; may induce visual phenomenon, ego dissolution, and mystical experiences (Timmermann et al., 2022).

Introduction

A holistic paradigm calls for nurses to consider both pharmacologic and nonpharmacologic approaches to foster well-being while alleviating burdensome symptoms of the disease process. Grounded in a human-centered approach to care and caring, nurses' covenant with society identifies us as agents invested in a return to wholeness

[1] Note that while the terms *entheogen*, *psychedelic*, and *sacred medicine* have subtly different meanings, they are used to describe different aspects or contexts of the same substances within this chapter.

through a deep regard for humanity. In addition, holism invites us to deepen our knowledge of Indigenous cultural practices, transcultural traditions, and sacred medicinal and herbal interventions and to address mental, emotional, spiritual, cultural, and existential health-related factors. The field encourages us to use whatever legal and ethical means are available to best position the patient and family to promote homeostasis and healing. The purpose of this chapter is to spark scholarly dialogue and create new academic and clinical possibilities for holistic nurses regarding the use of plant medicines across practice, research, education, and cultural and policy settings.

Despite over 100 years of federal outlawing in the United States, the legal use of plant medicine—both cannabis and entheogens, such as psilocybin—has been a sensitive and widely debated topic at the national policy level for decades. However, rigorous scientific trials and studies continue to validate their efficacy in myriad domains despite ongoing prohibition concerns. The use of medical cannabis in the United States has boomed so quickly in recent years that ready access to it has been noted as the new healthcare disparity, most negatively impacting the poorest Americans (Cunningham et al., 2022). Psychedelic drugs are now accessible to many Americans through a patchwork of state legislative reforms. This shift requires a consensus on treatment models, healthcare providers' education and guidance, and implementation and regulation planning (Siegel et al., 2023).

These ongoing policy changes and the growing body of evidence related to plant medicines reflect an evolving consciousness among policymakers and the healthcare system regarding the healing applications of these substances. While many cultures have historically used these substances in their sacred rituals and spiritual practices, the science around their effectiveness is beginning to demonstrate their medical necessity. Because of this, holistic nurses must be at the forefront of these significant scientific and scholarly advancements, regardless of personal views or biases.

This chapter provides an in-depth discussion of cannabis, including a description of the endocannabinoid system (ECS), cannabis as the most studied and widely used plant entheogen, and the necessary information about adverse effects, cannabis use disorder, and withdrawal. A brief history of the sacred lineage of entheogens is described, as well as a review of past and current clinical science that supports inspiring outcomes for various populations. Culture is considered, as many sacred plant medicines were originally used and later preserved by Indigenous populations.

Why Cannabis?

In 2018, the National Council of State Boards of Nursing (2018) issued a report that called for all nurses to obtain education on the six essential areas of knowledge necessary for working with medicinal cannabis patients (**Box 28-1**). The rationale for this was that patients were widely using medical cannabis and looking to healthcare providers to effectively support their safe and effective use of cannabis; however, cannabis as medicine was

Box 28-1 Essential Areas for Nurses Working with Medical Cannabis Patients

1. The nurse shall have a working knowledge of the current state of legalization of medical and recreational cannabis use.
2. The nurse shall have a working knowledge of the jurisdiction's Medical Marijuana Program.
3. The nurse shall have an understanding of the endocannabinoid system, cannabinoid receptors, cannabinoids, and the interactions between them.
4. The nurse shall have an understanding of cannabis pharmacology and the research associated with the medical use of cannabis.
5. The nurse shall be able to identify the safety considerations for patient use of cannabis.
6. The nurse shall approach the patient without judgment regarding the patient's choice of treatment or preferences in managing pain and other distressing symptoms.

Reproduced from National Council of State Boards of Nursing (2018). Part I: Current legislation, scientific literature review, and nursing implications. *Journal of Nursing Regulation, 9*(2), S6–S21.

not included in healthcare provider's curricula. While it is beyond the scope of this chapter to thoroughly address each of these essential knowledge areas, the reader should take note of the ethical obligation to educate themselves on these six areas accordingly. The following will support the holistic nurse's beginning knowledge of the human ECS and homeostasis, endocannabinoid deficiency issues, and upregulation of the ECS through holistic modalities. In addition, a brief discussion about the sacred nature of the plant is included, and the spiritual–cultural implications related to cannabis prohibition are considered.

The Endocannabinoid System

Dr. Ralph Mechoulam was a pioneer in discovering the endocannabinoid system (ECS), a body-cellular-based receptor system, in the mid-1990s, when he isolated and cloned the first cannabinoid receptor (Foster, 2021). The ECS is a central regulatory system within our bodies and is known to be the largest receptor system. The ECS and the endocannabinoids it produces are found throughout the body, including the brain, vital organs, connective tissue, glands, and immune cells. The ECS supports our body's ability to maintain homeostasis by controlling central and peripheral nervous system functions, energy uptake processes, immune responses, reproduction, and cellular fate (Foster, 2021).

The two most studied ECS receptors in the human body are CB_1 (found primarily in the nervous system, gonads, organs, and connective tissue) and CB_2 (found primarily in the immune system) (Foster, 2021). These receptors are embedded on the cellular membranes. Our bodies make their own cannabis-like substances that interact with the CB_1 and CB_2 receptors, namely the lipid-based anandamide and 2-arachidonoylglycerol (2-AG); we call these "endocannabinoids." Endocannabinoids are not stored in the body; they must be made on demand by cell membranes to maintain homeostasis, and they are subsequently broken down. Anandamide and 2-AG are lipids made by arachidonic acid derivatives, and they are not stored; rather, they are degraded by the enzymes monoacylglycerol lipase and fatty acid amide hydrolase (FAAH).

The cellular membrane cannabinoid receptors CB_1 and CB_2 send information backward (retrograde transmission) from the postsynaptic to the presynaptic nerve receptors, supporting homeostasis. The endocannabinoids are released from depolarized postsynaptic neurons in a calcium-dependent manner; therefore, they act in a retrograde fashion with the presynaptic cannabinoid receptors to suppress various neurotransmitter releases. Endocannabinoids work on both excitatory and inhibitory presynaptic fibers (Foster, 2021).

For example, when a neuron releases gamma aminobutyric acid (GABA) or glutamate (presynaptic), it aims for a target cell in the postsynaptic area. The endocannabinoids, meanwhile, are synthesized and released from the target postsynaptic cell, traveling backward (retrograde transmission) across the synapse toward the neuron that is releasing the GABA or glutamate and focusing on its CB_1 receptor. The CB_1 receptor that is impacted by the endocannabinoid then inhibits the release of many excitatory and inhibitory neurotransmitters, with the target cell influencing its own synaptic signals through the use of endocannabinoids (Maccarrone et al., 2023).

The ECS is extremely complex, and it needs to be well cared for. An endocannabinoid deficiency occurs when one does not make enough endocannabinoids to maintain homeostasis. This can result in illness or disease. Research has suggested that migraines, irritable bowel syndrome, fibromyalgia, and other chronic conditions may be related to an underlying endocannabinoid system deficiency. Indeed, if the ECS is not functioning properly, exogenous supplementation of phytocannabinoids can help support homeostasis (Maccarrone et al., 2023).

Phytocannabinoids

The Cannabis Plant

There are over 500 compounds in the cannabis plant, many of which interact directly with the ECS to support homeostasis and well-being (Parmelee et al., 2021). Phytocannabinoids can be defined as the plant components that interact with the ECS, and it is believed that using cannabis as a whole plant creates an entourage effect of sorts, where the combination of phytocannabinoids and terpenes best supports ECS functioning in comparison to isolating or synthesizing individual cannabinoids. A good example of this is the synthetic medication Marinol (dronabinol, which contains the cannabinoid delta-9-tetrahydrocannabinol [THC] only) not being as effective as the whole plant cannabis medicine in managing pain and nausea. There are over 100 cannabinoids in the cannabis plant and many terpenes or essential oils, and they all potentially interact with the ECS. The two most studied phytocannabinoids are THC and cannabidiol (CBD) (Parmelee et al., 2021). The following depicts how these cannabinoids interact with the ECS:

- **THC**: This is a psychoactive cannabinoid that interacts primarily with CB_1 receptors, though it may also influence CB_2 receptors, and is commonly used as an anti-emetic, appetite stimulant, anti-inflammatory, and for pain relief.
- **CBD**: This interacts primarily with the immune system and CB_2 receptors, though it also modulates CB_1 receptors. CBD may help to decrease inflammation, and it has neuroprotective and antioxidative impacts.
- **Terpenes**: These are the essential oils that give the cannabis plant its distinctive aroma. Terpenes may also act on both receptors, and they can enhance cannabis's therapeutic potential. There are over 100 terpenes present in cannabis. For example, linalool, which is also found in the lavender plant, has an aroma that may act as an anxiolytic agent.
- **Other therapeutic compounds**: These include esters, ketones, lactones, fatty acids, and steroids (Parmelee et al., 2021).

Other Cannabinoid Plants

Cannabis is not the only plant that interacts with the ECS. Many plants can help support homeostasis. The list includes black peppercorns, rosemary, and copaiba (all contain beta-caryophyllene, which acts as a CB_2 agonist and supports immune system function), black truffles (which create their own anandamide), chocolate (contains substances that inhibit FAAH enzyme, which therefore inhibits the breakdown of anandamide), echinacea (whose components interact with CB_2 receptors to support the immune system and decrease inflammation), kava (for sedation and pain relief; interacts with CB_1), and liverwort (contains perrottetinene, which interacts with the CB_1 receptor with a similar structure to THC). Plants high in flavonoids help to sustain the life of our endocannabinoids, extending the time before they are broken down and increasing the efficiency of the ECS (Clark, 2021).

Cannabis Ingestion Methods

Cannabis can be ingested in many different forms to interact with the ECS, including:

- As a raw plant and juicing (delivers raw cannabinoids: tetrahydrocannabinolic acid [THCA] anti-inflammatory, antiemetic, neuroprotective, anticonvulsant, and cannabidiolic acid CBDA, which is antiemetic and an antianxiety agent).
- Topically (use nano- or ionized particles or omega fats; have variable-onset duration, localized action).
- Orally (20–30% absorption: oils, capsules, tinctures, and edibles).
- Oromucosally (nabiximols spray, tinctures, lozenges).
- Via inhalation (10–60% absorption, very rapid onset, smoking or vaping).
- Via suppositories (may be helpful for specific GI symptoms).
- Via concentrates (shatter, dabs; high THC increases side effects) (Parmelee et al., 2021).

Adverse Effects, Cannabis Use Disorder, and Withdrawal

Cannabis's side effects are believed to be caused primarily by THC and may include euphoria, drowsiness, dizziness, dry mouth, dry eyes, anxiety, nausea, blurred vision, headache, and cognitive impairment. Slightly rarer adverse effects may include orthostatic hypotension, dysphoria, psychosis, paranoia, depression, ataxia, tachycardia, diarrhea, and cannabis hyperemesis (Clark, 2021). Cannabis use disorder risk is greater in young men in their teens–mid-20s and is often associated with other substance use issues and mental health disorders; this diagnosis has an 11-point criteria (American Psychiatric Association, 2021).

Withdrawal from cannabis has often been compared to similar withdrawal symptoms as from caffeine. Symptoms may include anxiety, depression, decreased appetite, headaches, insomnia, irritability, muscle tension, nausea, and nightmares/vivid dreams (Clark, 2021). There are no approved medicinal treatments for cannabis withdrawal, and most people experience only mild symptoms. Even people who use small amounts of cannabis regularly without experiencing clinical cannabis use disorder criteria may experience withdrawal symptoms.

Holistic Modalities

Holistic modalities are known to potentiate the health of the ECS by reducing stress, making it easier for the body to maintain homeostasis, and supporting the production of one's own endocannabinoids (Clark, 2021).

Diet

A diet with balanced omega-3 and omega-6 fatty acids helps to feed the ECS what it needs to manufacture and break down endocannabinoids. Anti-inflammatory diets help to place less strain on the ECS, and flavonoids (the colorful components found in fruits and vegetables, legumes, soy products, and tea) may help modulate CB_2 receptors and delay the breakdown of anandamide (Armeli et al., 2021).

Exercise

The runner's high, long thought to be endorphins, is more closely related to the release of anandamide. Sustained aerobic activity of moderate to high intensity, undertaken freely, may also increase CB_1 density (Matei et al., 2023). Humans are wired to be active and to run, and the release of the bliss molecule may be in some senses addictive. The enhancement of the ECS through exercise is known to uplift mood and decrease feelings of depression and anxiety (Gupta et al., 2024).

Acupuncture, Osteopathy, Massage

Electroacupuncture has been shown to activate CB_2 receptors and reduce inflammation and proinflammatory cytokines while also releasing anandamide and enhancing pain nociception (Ho et al., 2023). Osteopathy, manipulation techniques, and massage also support ECS tone (Buonomini et al., 2024).

Many of nursing's holistic modalities require that we love and cherish the other, that we support patients in learning, and that we offer care with loving-kindness; these acts of loving-kindness may also enhance the tone of the ECS, as patients' stress lowers and homeostasis is more easily attained. In addition to supplementing with exogenous cannabinoids, the holistic nurse supports the medical cannabis patient with coaching around upregulating the ECS and the caring–healing environment (Clark, 2021).

Cannabis: Sacred Nature

The era of global cannabis prohibition is slowly coming to a close as its physiological healing properties are recognized through both scientific endeavors and human experience. As the stigma around cannabis use dissipates and this herbal medicine becomes more widely available, we must ensure that we consider the cultural and historical background of the spiritual and sacred nature of the plant.

Culturally, cannabis has been used in spiritual and religious rituals for thousands of years. The Egyptian Goddess of Wisdom, Sehsat, was depicted as being connected to the cannabis leaf from above her head. Shiva prepared Bhang from the hemp plant and gave it to the people of the

Himalayas. Cannabis has been used in the worship of the Hindu dark goddess of life and death Kali Ma. Freya, the Germanic pagan Norse love goddess, was celebrated as cannabis was harvested through erotic festivals and ingestion of cannabis (Clark, 2023).

Due to prohibition and lack of funding for spiritual research, there is little in the way of scientific evidence around the use of cannabis as a spiritual growth tool. Heide et al. (2021) surveyed 1,087 people and found that 66 percent reported spiritual benefits from cannabis.

Historically, from Rastafarian culture to Sufism and Hinduism, cannabis has been used as a tool for introspection, meditation, connecting to the self, and as a tool to open to the divine (Gray, 2016). Cannabis is a tool that, when used with the proper intentions and practices, may help us to "relax down into direct and intuitive heart perception and the wisdom of the body . . . cannabis can help us enter deeply into the present . . . it can help us awaken from the illusion of separateness" (Gray, p. 6). Part of the future of cannabinoid medicines may include the evidence-based exploration of how cannabis can support spiritual growth and evolution.

While people in legal, adult-use states in the United States can use cannabis to explore spirituality, it is an area that is under-researched. In medical cannabis states, spiritual issues are generally not formally considered during the medical cannabis recommendation process. There is potential in the future to return to the roots of cannabis's spiritual nature.

Cannabis and Social Justice Issues

As holistic nurses, we are charged with addressing social justice issues and inequities. In October of 2022, President Biden issued a blanket pardon of convictions for simple possession. Despite having the same cannabis usage rates, Black people are 3.73 times more likely than White people to be arrested for cannabis possession (Yang et al., 2023). Cannabis businesses in the United States remain predominantly White, with 80 percent being owned by White people. People of color also experience a lack of inclusivity in the cannabis business and research realms. As cannabis is one of the world's most widely researched plant medicines, we must work to follow best practices for ethical research design, support the inclusion of research scientists from underrepresented groups, and advocate for more equitable cannabis policy at the state and federal levels (Martin-Willet et al., 2023). The harms of over 100 years of cannabis plant prohibition lay heavily in the people of color communities, and holistic nurses should be committed to addressing these harms.

As we reflect on the sacred nature of cannabis, we move into an expanded conversation on several other medicines that have been used among different cultures and traditions for healing, health, and spiritual growth.

Sacred Medicine in Traditional Cultures

While psychedelic science has experienced a "renaissance" in the last 20 years, sacred medicines, such as psilocybin mushrooms, peyote, ayahuasca, iboga, *Huachuma*, *Salvia divinorum*, and others have been used for millennia and continue to be used today within cultures around the world. In traditional cultures, these medicines are considered plant teachers held with the highest reverence and embedded within rich and complex traditions. Ayahuasca (called by many names such as *yagé*, *nixi pae*, *caapi*) is held as a sacrament by over 160 distinct cultural groups in South America. Psilocybin mushrooms were known to Aztec people as *Teonanacatl*, meaning "flesh of the gods." The yearly journey to collect peyote medicine for the Huichol people of Mexico is a sacred pilgrimage known as "Wirikuta." Iboga ceremonies within the African Bwiti tradition accompany initiation rites and provide an avenue to contact ancestral spirits (Schultes et al., 1998).

Within these cultures, contact with sacred medicine is a communal and ceremonial experience facilitated by expert guides—known to Westerners as medicine men and women, shamans, curanderos/as, and roadmen. These guides enter into apprenticeships that last years or decades and may require sacrifices such as abstinence from certain foods, substances, and sex. These medicine carriers are knowledgeable of the spiritual realm that the plant allows contact with. Tools of shamanic practice include sound and song healing, purification rituals, and the use of sacred instruments. It is to the lineages of medicine carriers of these intact traditions that the Western psychedelic renaissance owes a debt of gratitude and would be wise to look to for guidance. Indeed, indigenous leaders have provided guidelines on how researchers can respectfully collaborate (Celidwen et al., 2023).

Sacred medicine traditions transform to accommodate the cultures they reside within for a variety of reasons, including the effects of colonialism. While shamans of the Shipibo-Conibo ayahuasca tradition sing *icaros* (sacred songs) in their Shipibo, mestizo (mixed heritage) shamans of the same region also sing in Spanish or in a blend of languages. The Mazatec people of Oaxaca, Mexico, incorporate the mythology of Catholicism into their mushroom and *Salvia divinorum* ceremonies. The *huachuma* cactus, sacred to the people of the Andes mountains, became known as "San Pedro," named for the saint who holds the keys to the kingdom of heaven. When peyote, local to the desert of northern Mexico, migrated northward to the Plains tribes in the mid-1800s, ceremonies began being held in tipis incorporating the song styles of these tribal groups. These ceremonies evolved into the ceremony of the Native American Church, which also honors elements of Christianity. The Church of Santo Daime, which originated in the 1930s in Acre, Brazil, holds ayahuasca as a sacrament and blends indigenous traditions, Catholicism, and the Orisha tradition of the West African diaspora. Today, a variety of approaches to working with psychedelics are evolving in the United States. On one end of the spectrum is a purely medical model with little or no cultural or humanistic support. On the other end is full embedment within community religious and spiritual practice backed by the Religious Freedom Restoration Act, with a variety of approaches in between that incorporate psycho-emotional and spiritual support within a clinical approach.

Clinical and Legal History

Lysergic acid diethylamide (LSD) was first synthesized from ergot alkaloids by Sandoz pharmaceutical scientist Albert Hofmann in 1938 but remained impractical to mass produce until industrial advances in the 1950s. Meanwhile, in 1955, amateur mycologists Gordon and Valentina Wasson traveled to Oaxaca, Mexico, and attended a Mazatec *velada*, a sacred mushroom ceremony, with the healer Maria Sabina. Gordon Wasson published an account of his profound experience in a *Life* magazine cover article in 1957, which sparked a great deal of Western interest in "magic mushrooms," and in 1958, Hofmann synthesized psilocybin from mushroom samples (Schultes et al., 1998). A period of research ensued in the 1950s and early 1960s regarding the potential applications of entheogenic substances for physical, emotional, and spiritual purposes. Despite promising results, ethical and safety concerns arose due in part to indiscriminate behavior by some researchers, to the occasional negative consequences of unsupervised community use, and to changing public opinion in a politically turbulent time. In 1970, the Controlled Substances Act classified psilocybin and LSD as Schedule I substances, defined as having no currently accepted medical use and high potential for substance misuse, halting all human subject research.

MDMA (3,4-methylenedioxymethamphetamine), first synthesized in 1912, was explored in the 1970s as an adjunct to psychotherapy. Some consider MDMA an *entheogen*, while others have called it an *empathogen* for its ability to facilitate connection with oneself and with others. In the 1980s, the drug became popular recreationally, and in 1985, it was made a Schedule I drug despite legal protestations from the therapeutic community. Ketamine was first synthesized in 1962 and is a Schedule III substance, defined as having a moderate-to-low potential for physical and psychological dependence. It is commonly used as an anesthetic, as an analgesic, and off-label as an antidepressant. A variety of depressive disorder treatment approaches continue to evolve using ketamine ranging from a solely medical model to various forms of ketamine-assisted psychotherapy due to its Schedule III status.

In the last few years, multiple states and municipalities have decriminalized psychedelic medicines, making it the lowest priority of law enforcement to prosecute. In addition, Oregon has created a statewide system for adult-supported use of psilocybin that licenses producers, service centers, facilitators, and education programs. Of note is that while nurses have begun to serve as licensed facilitators, they cannot function in their role as nurses while facilitating, and there is a lack of clarity from the Oregon State Board of Nursing if doing so puts their nursing license at risk (Wickenhagen, 2024). Colorado has also passed the Natural Medicine Act, which created a Regulated Natural Medicine Access Program for certified facilitators to practice under (Colorado Department of Regulatory Agencies Division of Professions and Occupations, 2025). At the time of this writing, this framework is being implemented. Other states have bills in the legislature proposing similar legal frameworks. The legal and clinical psychedelic landscape is continuously evolving.

Current Clinical Science

In 1991, researcher Rick Strassman completed the onerous process of obtaining federal permission to conduct clinical safety research with human subjects with a Schedule I psychedelic, N,N-Dimethyltryptamine (N,N-DMT), opening the door for further entheogens research. Research is currently being conducted in the United States with a variety of psychedelics such as LSD, N,N-DMT, 5-methoxy-N,N-dimethyltryptamine (5-MeO-DMT), ibogaine, and most notably with psilocybin and MDMA that are now in phase 3 clinical trials. At the time of this writing, approval for the therapeutic use of MDMA has been denied by the Food and Drug Administration (FDA).

Treatment Paradigms

The use of psychedelics in the clinical context differs from the use of these medicines in traditional cultures, as well as from psychotropic medication treatment paradigms in conventional medicine. In studies of psychedelics, patients receive long-term benefits from only one or two dose administrations. Furthermore, it seems from patient reports that the psychedelic experience itself provides therapeutic benefits in addition to any biochemical processes that occur.

In psychedelic treatment paradigms, the therapeutic context in which the entheogen is administered is of great importance. In most psilocybin and LSD studies, participants prepare for the two 8-hour-long dosing sessions of either an entheogen or a non-psychoactive placebo by engaging in multiple therapy sessions with two study therapists, as well as multiple post-dose therapy sessions to explore, understand, and integrate the experience. During the dosing sessions, participants are generally invited to lie down on a comfortable couch in a thoughtfully decorated room, to put on eye shades and headphones playing instrumental music, and to pay attention to their inward experience.

MDMA studies use a modified approach called "MDMA-assisted psychotherapy," in which manualized, patient-centered therapy is provided during dosing sessions.

Outcomes

Psilocybin

In 2006, Roland Griffiths led a pioneering double-blind, placebo-controlled, randomized trial of the effects of psilocybin administered to healthy participants in supportive settings. In this study, psilocybin occasioned complete mystical-type experiences in 22 of the 36 total participants as compared to 4 participants in the placebo group. Notably, 67 percent of the participants rated the experience with psilocybin to be either the single most meaningful experience of their life or among the top five, similar to the birth of a first child or death of a parent, for example (Griffiths et al., 2006, pp. 276–277).

A study of psilocybin for the treatment of cancer-related anxiety and depression reported immediate and large reductions of anxiety and depressive symptoms and increases in quality of life in the psilocybin group as compared to an active placebo group before crossover

(Ross et al., 2021). Clinically significant reductions in depressive disorder symptoms in 60–80 percent of participants remained durable at the 4.5-year follow-up (Agin-Liebes et al., 2020). In a phenomenological analysis of interviews with patients in the previous trial, Belser et al. reported that typical themes reported by patients included "exalted feelings of joy, bliss, and love; embodiment; ineffability; alterations to identity; a movement from feelings of separateness to interconnectedness" (2017, p. 354). Phase III trials of psilocybin for disease-related existential anxiety are currently underway.

Studies have also shown promise for psilocybin as a treatment for major depressive disorder (MDD) and treatment-resistant depression (TRD). In a phase 2 randomized controlled trial of 59 participants with MDD, participants who were administered two separate doses of 25 mg of psilocybin 3 weeks apart had the same levels of reductions in depressive disorder symptoms as participants receiving 6 weeks of daily oral antidepressant medication (Carhart-Harris et al., 2021). On secondary measures of functioning, psychological connectedness and meaning in life, the psilocybin group showed significantly superior responses. A 6-month follow-up study similarly yielded no significant between-group differences in primary measures, with more favorable secondary measures for the psilocybin group (Erritzoe et al., 2024). In a separate phase 2 study of a novel psilocybin analog for MDD, patients experienced robust and sustained improvement in their MDD symptoms at 4 months with 75 percent of participants who received two doses, each at 16 mg, achieving remission and no longer showing signs of depression, for which the FDA granted Breakthrough Therapy Designation (Cybin, 2023). In a phase 2 randomized controlled trial involving 233 participants with TRD who had tapered off all SSRI medications, psilocybin (with psychological support) at a single dose of 25 mg reduced depression scores significantly more than a 1-mg dose over a period of 3 weeks (Goodwin, et al., 2022).

Other studies of psilocybin, such as for the treatment of addiction and anxiety disorder, have also shown positive results. For a comprehensive summary of current clinical research, please refer to the report *Psychedelic Medicine: A Review of Clinical Research for a Class of Rapidly-Emerging Behavioral Health Interventions* (Brainfutures, 2022).

MDMA

Multiple phase 3 studies of MDMA in conjunction with therapy for the treatment of posttraumatic stress disorder (PTSD) have demonstrated superior benefits versus current treatment models. In a randomized controlled trial with 90 participants, three doses of MDMA given in conjunction with manualized therapy over 18 weeks resulted in a significant and robust attenuation of PTSD symptoms and functional impairment (Mitchell et al., 2021). In a similarly designed study with 104 participants over 18 weeks, MDMA with therapy significantly improved PTSD symptoms and functional impairment, compared to placebo with therapy. Of the participants treated with MDMA, 86.5 percent achieved a clinically meaningful benefit and 71.2 percent of participants no longer met the criteria for PTSD by the study's end (Mitchell et al., 2023).

Though FDA regulation of a drug–psychotherapy treatment paradigm is unprecedented, in light of these robust results, it came as a surprise to the psychedelic field that in August 2024, the FDA rejected an application from Lykos Therapeutics to approve MDMA-assisted therapy for PTSD (Lykos Therapeutics, 2024). Concerns cited by the FDA included insufficient evidence of the durability of effect, expectancy bias in participants who had used MDMA prior, and lack of clarity about the contribution of psychotherapy. The FDA recommended the completion of an additional phase 3 trial for reconsideration.

Ketamine

Ketamine, which has been a Schedule III substance since 1970, is used in a variety of settings, modes of administration, and dosages. It is approved as an anesthetic but is used off-label to treat MDD, TRD, acute suicidality, PTSD, and other disorders. It is not considered a classical psychedelic but rather a dissociative, producing feelings of detachment from the environment and/or self. Ketamine is sometimes used within a purely medical model lacking any therapeutic support. It is sometimes combined with therapy during the session at psycholytic doses or before and after the session. With such a wide range of treatment approaches, and without the need to conduct phase 3 trials for FDA approval, ketamine-related research is heterogeneous. At baseline, there is consistent evidence to demonstrate that ketamine is an effective though transient antidepressant and antisuicidal treatment (remission of symptoms usually lasts between 2–4 weeks) as concluded by a systematic review surveying 83 published reports (Walsh et al., 2021). The durability of the effect is thought to be able to be extended by incorporating psychotherapy in a ketamine-assisted therapy model and repeating doses at regular intervals, though further research on optimal protocols is needed. Ketamine treatment is the area within psychedelics with the most robust participation of nurses currently. Registered nurses (RNs) frequently administer ketamine and monitor ketamine participants in clinical settings. Nurses practicing psychotherapy or health coaching can also provide ketamine-assisted therapy and coaching.

Role of Holistic Nurses

Nurses were largely the professionals providing continuous caring presence at the bedside in the psychedelic trials of the 1950s and 1960s and therefore have played a pioneering role in the psychedelic movement (Penn, Dorsen, et al., 2021). Nurses, and holistic nurses in particular, embody many of the competencies of psychedelic therapists: "empathetic abiding presence, trust enhancement, spiritual intelligence, knowledge of the physical and psychological effects of psychedelics, therapist self-awareness and ethical integrity, and proficiency in complementary techniques" (Penn, Phelps, et al., 2021, p. 5). Nurses, as the consistently rated most trusted professionals, are skilled in enhancing trust and maintaining ethical integrity. Holistic nurses, in particular, demonstrate skills of presence, self-awareness, spiritual intelligence, and complementary techniques. Core Value 3 of the *Holistic Nursing: Scope and Standards of Practice* articulates:

> Holistic nurses provide care that recognizes the totality of the human being (the interconnectedness of body, mind, emotion, spirit, social/cultural, relationships, context, environment, and energy) . . . A holistic nurse may also incorporate a number of complementary and integrative approaches (e.g., cognitive restructuring, stress management, visualization and imagery, hypnotherapy, aromatherapy, Therapeutic Touch, Healing Touch) along with conventional nursing interventions. Holistic nurses focus on integrative care interventions that promote healing, peace, comfort, and a subjective sense of well-being for the person. (ANA & AHNA, 2019, p. 27)

Holistic nurses are specialists in creating sacred spaces for healing through presence, intention, and relationship. This expertise can be utilized and expanded upon in the development of healing paradigms for the clinical use of entheogens. Holistic nursing theories, such as Jean Watson's Human Caring and her concept of presence, are well adapted to support the nursing role in psychedelic care (Penn, Phelps, et al., 2021). In addition, holistic nurses are particularly adept at integrating traditional healing practices within modern healthcare paradigms, a crucial skill in honoring and learning from the deep wisdom of indigenous sacred medicine traditions in developing the clinical practice of entheogenic therapy.

Risk Reduction

While psychedelic therapy shows great promise for benefit, psychedelic use in any setting is not risk-free. Serious adverse events have been reported in clinical trials of MDMA, such as increased suicidality, though this is not an unexpected finding in populations with MDD and TRD. Substances such as psilocybin have a favorable toxicity profile (lethal overdose is nearly impossible), but psychological harms remain. In a mixed methods survey of 608 participants who had reported extended difficulties after psychedelic experiences, including in community and recreational settings, participants described feelings of anxiety and fear, existential struggle, social disconnection, depersonalization, and derealization that for a small portion lasted for years. Some of these difficulties were mitigated by having the experience in a facilitated setting (Evans et al., 2023), though facilitation also comes with risks. Similar to any therapeutic setting, a power imbalance between practitioner and client can lead to inappropriate behaviors, particularly sexual misconduct. These risks are potentially heightened with the inhibition of boundaries inherent to psychedelic effects. The psychedelic field is maturing to detect and protect against these risks through facilitator certification, peer supervision, ethics councils, and public education.

Implications

Clinical Practice

Holistic nursing practice must be guided by the legal auspices of state boards of nursing and our scope and standards of practice. Very often, institutional guidelines determine the prescribing and administering of medical cannabis. Currently, nurses can work legally with ketamine; within clinical trials with psilocybin, LSD, and MDMA; and under specific state-regulated service guidelines for psilocybin in Oregon and other natural medicines in Colorado.

Education

It is vital to continue to inform holistic nurses of the evolving science related to plant medicines. Holistic nurses must be educated regarding the evidence and potential current and future uses. Education should include potential benefits, as well as side effects, use disorders, and holistic considerations. Nurses are also ideal professionals to educate the public about the benefits and risks of psychedelic care and ways to reduce harm.

Research

This is a particularly rich time for research related to all plant medicines. Holistic nurses should be encouraged to participate in related research endeavors. As noted previously, many other disciplines are publishing findings related to this science; the dialogue within holistic nursing and nursing in general is expanding but still leaves room for growth.

Policy

As additional medicinal options to treat illness-related symptoms become decriminalized, holistic nurses have a social justice obligation to ensure equitable access for all. Advocacy for access to medicines that may alleviate the mental, emotional, and spiritual–existential symptoms of advanced illness is essential.

Conclusion

The science shows there is a place for sacred and plant medicines to advance the health and well-being of patients. From physical to mental, emotional, and spiritual–existential outcomes, clinical trial participants are experiencing health improvements due to both physiological and mystical mechanisms. Although the field needs further exploration and substantiation, we must look to the future to guide and nurture the dialogue regarding plant medicines in a manner that best serves our communities. Holistic nurses have long been at the forefront of innovation and creative approaches to health and well-being; this realm is no different. It is likely that indications for plant medicines will soon invite us to new ways of doing and being in the clinical environment. But first, we are asked to consider new ways of thinking and seeing to best meet individual and population health needs with evidence-informed care.

References

Agin-Liebes, G., Malone, T., Yalch, M. M., Mennenga, S. E., Ponté, K. L., Guss, J., Bossis, A., Grigsby, J., Fisher, S., & Ross, S. (2020). Long-term follow-up of psilocybin-assisted psychotherapy for psychiatric and existential distress in patients with life-threatening cancer. *Journal of Psychopharmacology, 34*(2), 155–166. https://doi.org/10.1177%2F0269881119897615

American Nurses Association & American Holistic Nurses Association. (2019). *Holistic nursing: Scope and standards of practice* (3rd ed.). American Nurses Association.

American Psychiatric Association. (2021). *Cannabis: Understanding the risks.* https://www.psychiatry.org/news-room/apa-blogs/cannabis-understanding-the-risks

Armeli, F., Bonucci, A., Maggi, E., Pinto, A., & Businaro, R. (2021). Mediterranean diet and neurodegenerative diseases: The neglected role of nutrition in the modulation of the endocannabinoid system. *Biomolecules, 11*(6), 790. https://doi.org/10.3390/biom11060790

Belser, A. B., Agin-Liebes, G., Swift, T. C., Terrana, S., Devenot, N., Friedman, H. L., Guss, J., Bossis, A., & Ross, S. (2017). Patient experiences of psilocybin-assisted psychotherapy: An interpretive phenomenological analysis. *Journal of Humanistic Psychology*, *57*, 354–388. https://doi.org/10.1177/0022167817706884

Brainfutures. (2022). *Psychedelic medicine: A review of clinical research for a class of rapidly-emerging behavioral health interventions.* https://www.brainfutures.org/wp-content/uploads/2022/05/BrainFutures-Psychedelic-Medicine-Report.pdf

Buonomini, C., Bonetti, O., & Novelli, E., Sr. (2024). Osteopathic approach in the stimulation of the endocannabinoid system: A case report. *Cureus*, *16*(2), e54848. https://doi.org/10.7759/cureus.54848

Carhart-Harris, R., Giribaldi, B., Watts, R., BakerJones, M., Murphy-Beiner, A., Murphy, R., Martell, J., Blemings, A., Erritzoe, D., & Nutt, D. J. (2021). Trial of psilocybin versus escitalopram for depression. *The New England Journal of Medicine, 384*, 1402–1411. https://doi.org/10.1056/NEJMoa2032994

Celidwen, Y., Redvers, N., Githaiga, C., Calambás, J., Añaños, K., Chindoy, M. E., Vitale, R., Rojas, J. N., Mondragón, D., Rosalío & Y. V., & Sacbajá, A. (2023). Ethical principles of traditional Indigenous medicine to guide western psychedelic research and practice. *Lancet Regional Health - Americas (Online), 18*, 100410. https://doi.org/10.1016/j.lana.2022.100410

Clark, C. S. (2021). The nurse's role: Providing cannabis care. In C. S. Clark (Ed.), *Cannabis: A handbook for nurses.* Wolters Kluwer.

Clark, C. S. (2023). *The call of the sacred green mother: Spirituality, philosophy, can cannabis care nursing.* American Cannabis Nurses Association Conference, Denver, Colorado.

Collins Dictionary. (2024). *Enthoegen.* https://www.collinsdictionary.com/us/dictionary/english/entheogen

Colorado Department of Regulatory Agencies Division of Professions and Occupations. (2025). *Natural medicine program.* https://dpo.colorado.gov/NaturalMedicine

Cunningham, C. O., Zhang, C., Hollins, M., Wang, M., Singh-Tan, S., & Joudrey, P. J. (2022). Availability of medical cannabis services by racial, social, and geographic characteristics of neighborhoods in New York: A cross-sectional study. *BMC Public Health*, *22*(1), 671. https://doi.org/10.1186/s12889-022-13076-1

Cybin. (2023, November 30). *Cybin reports positive topline data from phase 2 study of CYB003 in major depressive disorder with 79% of patients in remission after two 12mg Doses.* https://ir.cybin.com/investors/news/news-details/2023/Cybin-Reports-Positive-Topline-Data-from-Phase-2-Study-of-CYB003-in-Major-Depressive-Disorder-with-79-of-Patients-in-Remission-after-Two-12mg-Doses/default.aspx

Erritzoe, D., Barba, T., Greenway, K. T., Murphy, R., Martell, J., Giribaldi, B., Timmermann, C., Murphy-Beiner, A., Jones, M. B., Nutt, D., Weiss, B., & Carhart-Harris, R. (2024). Effect of psilocybin versus escitalopram on depression symptom severity in patients with moderate-to-severe major depressive disorder: observational 6-month follow-up of a phase 2, double-blind, randomised, controlled trial. *EClinicalMedicine*, 102799. https://doi.org/10.1016/j.eclinm.2024.102799

Evans, J., Robinson, O. C., Argyri, E. K., Suseelan, S., Murphy-Beiner, A., McAlpine, R., Luke, D., Michelle, K., & Prideaux, E. (2023). Extended difficulties following the use of psychedelic drugs: A mixed methods study. *PLoS One*, *18*(10), e0293349. https://doi.org/10.1371/journal.pone.0293349

Foster, D. (2021). The endocannabinoid system. In C. S. Clark (Ed.), *Cannabis: A handbook for nurses*. Wolters Kluwer.

Goodwin, G. M., Aaronson, S. T., Alvarez, O., Arden, P. C., Baker, A., Bennett, J. C., Bird, C., Blom, R. E., Brennan, C., Brusch, D., Burke, L., Campbell-Coker, K., Carhart-Harris, R., Cattell, J., Daniel, A., DeBattista, C., Dunlop, B. W., Eisen, K., Feifel, D., Forbes, M., … Malievskaia, E. (2022). Single-dose psilocybin for a treatment-resistant episode of major depression. *The New England Journal of Medicine, 387*(18), 1637–1648. https://doi.org/10.1056/NEJMoa2206443

Gray, S. (2016). *Cannabis and spirituality: An explorer's guide to an ancient plant ally*. Parker Street Press.

Griffiths, R. R., Richards, W. A., McCann, U., & Jesse, R. (2006). Psilocybin can occasion mystical-type experiences having substantial and sustained personal meaning and spiritual significance. *Psychopharmacology, 187*(3), 268–283.

Gupta, S., Bharatha, A., Cohall, D., Rahman, S., Haque, M., & Azim Majumder, M. A. (2024). Aerobic exercise and endocannabinoids: A narrative review of stress regulation and brain reward systems. *Cureus*, *16*(3), e55468. https://doi.org/10.7759/cureus.55468

Heide, F. J., Chang, T., Porter, N., Edelson, E., & Walloch, J. C. (2021). Spiritual benefit from cannabis. *Journal of Psychoactive Drugs*, *54*(2), 149–157. https://doi.org/10.1080/02791072.2021.1941443

Ho, T. J., Lin, C. F., Chen, J. K., Kung, Y. L., Wu, L. K., Chang Chien, C. Y., & Huang, C. P. (2023). Electroacupuncture attenuates inflammatory pain via peripheral cannabinoid receptor type 1 signaling pathway in mice. *PLoS One*, *18*(12), e0295432. https://doi.org/10.1371/journal.pone.0295432

Lykos Therapeutics. (2024, August 9). *Lykos Therapeutics announces complete response letter for Midomafetamine capsules for PTSD*. https://news.lykospbc.com/2024-08-09-Lykos-Therapeutics-Announces-Complete-Response-Letter-for-Midomafetamine-Capsules-for-PTSD

Maccarrone, M., Di Marzo, V., Gertsch, J., Grether, U., Howlett, A. C., Hua, T., Makriyannis, A., Piomelli, D., Ueda, N., & van der Stelt, M. (2023). Goods and cads of the endocannabinoid system as a therapeutic target: Lessons learned after 30 years. *Pharmacological Reviews*, *75*(5), 885–958. https://doi.org/10.1124/pharmrev.122.000600

Martin-Willett, R., Stanger, M., James, W., Bryan, A. D., & Bidwell, L. C. (2023). Effects of historical inequity and institutional power on cannabis research: Moving toward equity and inclusion. *PNAS Nexus*, 2(12), 1–7. https://doi.org/10.1093/pnasnexus/pgad383

Matei, D., Trofin, D., Iordan, D. A., Onu, I., Condurache, I., Ionite, C., & Buculei, I. (2023). The endocannabinoid system and physical exercise. *International Journal of Molecular Sciences*, *24*(3), 1989. https://doi.org/10.3390/ijms24031989

Mitchell, J. M., Bogenschutz, M., Lilienstein, A., Harrison, C., Kleiman, S., Parker-Guilbert, K., Ot'alora G., M., Garas, W., Paleos, C., Gorman, I., Nicholas, C., Mithoefer, M., Carlin, S., Poulter, B., Mithoefer, A., Quevedo, S., Wells, G., Klaire, S. S., van der Kolk, B., Tzarfaty, K., … Doblin, R. (2021). MDMA-assisted therapy for severe PTSD: A randomized, double-blind, placebo-controlled phase 3 study. *Nature Medicine*, *27*(6), 1025–1033. https://doi.org/10.1038/s41591-021-01336-3

Mitchell, J. M., Bogenschutz, M., Lilienstein, A., Harrison, C., Kleiman, S., Parker-Guilbert, K., Ot'alora G, M., Garas, W., Paleos, C., Gorman, I., Nicholas, C., Mithoefer, M., Carlin, S., Poulter, B., Mithoefer, A., Quevedo, S., Wells, G., Klaire, S. S., van der Kolk, B., Tzarfaty, K., … Doblin, R. (2023). MDMA-assisted therapy for severe PTSD: A randomized, double-blind, placebo-controlled phase 3 study. *Focus*, *21*(3), 315–328. https://doi.org/10.1176/appi.focus.23021011

National Council of State Boards of Nursing. (2018). Part I: Current legislation, scientific literature review, and nursing implications. *Journal of Nursing Regulation*, *9*(2), S6–S21.

Parmelee, R., Clark, & Sommers, D. (2021). Cannabis pharmacology: From whole plant to pharmaceutical applications. In C. S. Clark (Ed.), *Cannabis: A handbook for nurses*. Wolters Kluwer.

Penn, A., Dorsen, C., Hope, S., & Rosa, W. (2021). CE: Psychedelic-assisted therapy. *The American Journal of Nursing*, *121*(6), 34–40. https://doi.org/10.1097/01.NAJ.0000753464.35523.29

Penn, A. D., Phelps, J., Rosa, W. E., & Watson, J. (2021). Psychedelic-assisted psychotherapy practices and Human Caring Science: Toward a care-informed model of treatment. *The Journal of Humanistic Psychology*, *64*(4), 592–617. https://doi.org/10.1177/00221678211011013

Ross, S., Agin-Liebes, G., Lo, S., Zeifman, R. J., Ghazal, L., Benville, J., Corso, S. F., Real, C. B., Guss, J., Bossis, A., & Mennenga, S. E. (2021). Acute and sustained reductions in loss of meaning and suicidal ideation following psilocybin-assisted psychotherapy for psychiatric and existential distress in life-threatening cancer. *American Chemical Society*, *4*(2), 553–562. https://doi.org/10.1021/acsptsci.1c00020

Schultes, R. E., Hofmann, A., & Ratsch, C. (1998). *Plants of the Gods: Their sacred, healing, and hallucinogenic powers*. Healing Arts.

Siegel, J. S., Daily, J. E., Perry, D. A., & Nicol, G. E. (2023). Psychedelic drug legislative reform and legalization in the US. *JAMA Psychiatry*, *80*(1), 77–83. https://doi.org/10.1001/jamapsychiatry.2022.4101

Timmermann, C., Watts, R., & Dupuis, D. (2022). Towards psychedelic apprenticeship: Developing a gentle touch for the mediation and validation of psychedelic-induced insights and revelations. *Transcultural Psychiatry*, *59*(5), 691–704. https://doi.org/10.1177/13634615221082796

United States Department of Agriculture. (n.d.). Plant profile for *Cannabis sativa* L. https://plants.usda.gov/core/profile?symbol=casa3

Walsh, Z., Mollaahmetoglu, O. M., Rootman, J., Golsof, S., Keeler, J., Marsh, B., Nutt, D. J., & Morgan, C. J. A. (2021). Ketamine for the treatment of mental health and substance use disorders: comprehensive systematic review. *BJPsych Open*, *8*(1), e19. https://doi.org/10.1192/bjo.2021.1061

Wickenhagen, S. (2024). Advice for the nurse considering Oregon's psilocybin services program. *Oregon Board of Nursing Sentinel*, *43*(2), 18.

Yang, Y. T., Berg, C. J., & Burris, S. (2023). Cannabis equity initiatives: Progress, problems, and potentials. *American Journal of Public Health*, *113*(5), 487–489. https://doi.org/10.2105/AJPH.2023.307255

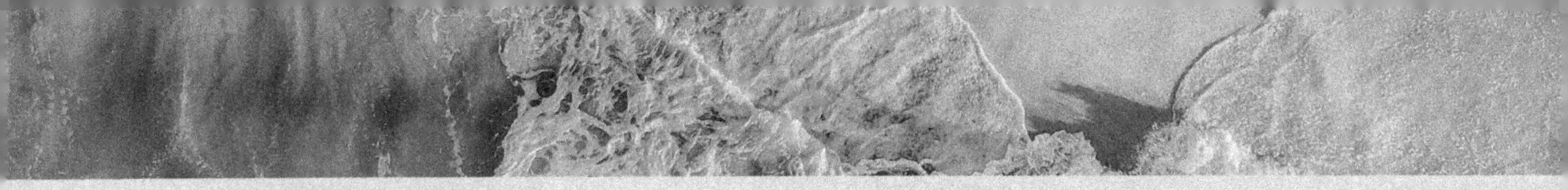

Index

Note: Page numbers followed by *b*, *f*, or *t* indicate materials in boxes, figures, or tables respectively.

D

E

F

I

J

K

L

M

N

Q

R

S

T